LICIT
and
ILLICIT
DRUGS

The Consumers Union Report on Narcotics,
Stimulants, Depressants, Inhalants,
Hallucinogens, and Marijuana —
including Caffeine, Nicotine, and Alcohol

by EDWARD M. BRECHER
and the Editors of CONSUMER REPORTS

LITTLE, BROWN AND COMPANY — BOSTON — TORONTO

COPYRIGHT © 1972 BY CONSUMERS UNION OF UNITED STATES, INC.
ALL RIGHTS RESERVED. NO PART OF THIS BOOK MAY BE REPRODUCED
IN ANY FORM OR BY ANY ELECTRONIC OR MECHANICAL MEANS IN-
CLUDING INFORMATION STORAGE AND RETRIEVAL SYSTEMS WITHOUT
PERMISSION IN WRITING FROM THE PUBLISHER, EXCEPT BY A REVIEWER
WHO MAY QUOTE BRIEF PASSAGES IN A REVIEW.

F

THIS EDITION HAS BEEN PUBLISHED BY LITTLE, BROWN AND COMPANY
FOR DISTRIBUTION TO THE BOOK TRADE.

ACKNOWLEDGMENTS FOR PERMISSION TO REPRINT PREVIOUSLY COPY-
RIGHTED MATERIAL ARE GIVEN ON PAGES 583–593.

Published simultaneously in Canada
by Little, Brown & Company (Canada) Limited

PRINTED IN THE UNITED STATES OF AMERICA

LICIT
and
ILLICIT
DRUGS

4/280   4⁹⁵

362.29
B829l
c. 2

Acknowledgments

Thanks are due to many people for many kinds of help in drafting this Consumers Union Report.

My first and greatest debt is to the late Dr. Charles E. Terry and his associate, Mildred Pellens. In 1969, shortly after starting work on this Report, I stumbled on their 1,042-page classic, *The Opium Problem* (1928)—and I felt as the young poet Keats felt when he first stumbled upon the *Iliad* and *Odyssey*. Terry and Pellens demonstrated that sense can be made of the drug scene only in a historical setting. We cannot approach today's heroin problem with insight so long as we blind ourselves to the altogether different nature of the opiate problem in the nineteenth century. Some knowledge of the bohemian scene of the 1890s and the Greenwich Village scene of the 1920s is almost a prerequisite for understanding the Haight-Ashbury scene of the 1960s. The historical perspective of this Report, no doubt its salient characteristic, is owed to Terry and Pellens.

As the preliminary draft of this book was nearing completion in April 1970, I enjoyed a second similar insight. My task at the moment was to make the youth drug scene, and the value system of the scene's participants, understandable and believable to older readers. As I wrestled with that task, the Canadian Government's Commission of Inquiry into the Non-Medical Use of Drugs, popularly known as the Le Dain Commission, issued its 1970 *Interim Report*. My immediate problem and several others were thereby resolved; and I was heartened to learn that a number of the conclusions I had been reaching independently closely paralleled those of the *Interim Report*. Readers of Parts VIII and IX of this book will find my indebtedness to the commission apparent and acknowledged on many pages.

At various stages, preliminary drafts of chapters of this book were circulated to authorities directly concerned with each chapter—in most cases the men and women whose work was reviewed in that chapter. Their comments, corrections, and suggestions proved most helpful in preparing the final draft. While none of them is responsible for any of the views here expressed, to them belongs the credit for the deletion of many doubtful passages. For helping me to avoid numerous errors, and in many cases for wise counsel as well, let me thank the following:

[v]

Virginia Apgar, M.D.

Robert A. Maslansky, M.D.

Mitchell B. Balter, Ph.D.

Charles Medawar

Herbert Benson, M.D.

Glen D. Mellinger, Ph.D.

Thomas H. Bewley, M.D.

Helen H. Nowlis, Ph.D.

Judge Andrew Bucaro

Vincent Nowlis, Ph.D.

Charles E. Cherubin, M.D.

Marie E. Nyswander, M.D.

Emmett P. Davis, M.D.

John A. O'Donnell, Ph.D.

Vincent P. Dole, M.D.

Hugh J. Parry, Ph.D.

Joel Fort, M.D.

Edward A. Preble, Ph.D.

Daniel X. Freedman, M.D.

Ingemar Rexed, Esq.

Frances R. Gearing, M.D.

Richard Evans Schultes, Ph.D.

Avram Goldstein, M.D.

Roger C. Smith, Ph.D.

Samuel Irwin, Ph.D.

Ralph M. Susman, Ph.D.

Harris Isbell, M.D.

Silvan S. Tomkins, Ph.D.

Jerome H. Jaffe, M.D.

Henry L. Verhulst

Lissy F. Jarvik, M.D.

Stephen Waldron, Ph.D.

Murray Jarvik, M.D.

Robert C. Wallach, M.D.

Rufus King, Esq.

Irene Waskow, Ph.D.

John C. Kramer, M.D.

Andrew T. Weil, M.D.

Alfred R. Lindesmith, Ph.D.

H. R. Williams, M.D.

James R. Gamage and Edmund L. Zerkin of STASH—the Student Association for the Study of Hallucinogens, Beloit, Wisconsin—greatly facilitated my marijuana research, and the research of countless others, through their *Comprehensive Guide to the English-Language Literature on Cannabis* and through their courtesy in supplying the texts of rare materials abstracted in the *Comprehensive Guide*. The chapters on methadone in this Report have been enriched by the proceedings of three National Conferences on Methadone Treatment sponsored by NAPAN— the National Association for the Prevention of Addiction to Narcotics.

Jonathan Leff, Director of Special Publications at Consumers Union, was a bulwark of strength throughout the years of work on this Report; and was a collaborator as well as editor during the final months.

Sharon Hammer Sigman prepared and verified the references and brought order out of chaos.

Irene Dee patiently typed and retyped the manuscript, time after time, month after month, year after year.

The rich resources of the Yale University Library, Yale Medical Library, and Yale Medical Historical Library, and the competence and helpfulness of their staffs, made this project feasible.

The staff of the Consumers Union Library proved adept and cooperative in promptly securing materials unavailable even at the Yale Libraries.

Other Consumers Union staff members were also very generous with their help.

Edward M. Brecher

Yelping Hill
West Cornwall, Connecticut

Introduction

This Report originated five years ago in a growing conviction on our part, and on the part of others associated with Consumers Union, that the illicit drug scene in the United States was rapidly becoming intolerable:

- Heroin, marijuana, LSD, cocaine, the amphetamines, the barbiturates, and many other mind-affecting drugs had become readily and increasingly available on the illicit market in many parts of the country.
- The use of illicit drugs, especially by young people, appeared to be increasing year by year.
- The United States had focused its efforts to curb illicit drug use primarily on penalties—arrest, imprisonment, discharge from jobs, expulsion from schools and colleges, social contempt, and exclusion. But those penalties were damaging our society in many ways, most significantly in the criminalization and alienation of large numbers of young people.
- Programs designed to warn children and young people away from drugs had failed to accomplish their purpose; some programs, indeed, were perhaps even contributing to the rising tide of drug use.

An earlier CU publication, *The Consumers Union Report on Smoking and the Public Interest* (1963), had been well received and had had a significant impact on public attitudes toward cigarette smoking. That report had also proved helpful to the Surgeon General's Advisory Committee on Smoking and Health in the drafting of its 1964 report. A similar CU report on drugs seemed urgently needed. In 1967, accordingly, CU's Director of Special Publications was authorized to launch a search for a writer capable of drafting a sound report on illicit drugs, and a start was made toward assembling source materials for such a report.

One of the drafters of CU's 1963 smoking report, Edward M. Brecher, was our choice for the new assignment, and he agreed both to conduct the necessary research and to draft the new report. He set to work early in 1969.*

---

* Mr. Brecher has written for *Consumer Reports* from time to time since 1938. He and his late wife, Ruth E. Brecher, who also participated in the drafting of CU's 1963 smoking report, were recipients of the Albert Lasker Medical Journalism Award for 1963, and of the American Psychiatric Association's Robert T. Morse Writers Award

The present Report was initially planned as a modest handbook on illicit drugs—a slim volume that would describe the pharmacological effects of each drug on the mind and body, and recommend measures for curbing drug misuse. As Mr. Brecher's review of the medical, pharmacological, sociological, psychiatric, and psychological literature proceeded, however, it became clear that such a limited handbook would serve no useful purpose. It might even further muddy the already confused debate on drugs then raging. That debate, it increasingly became apparent, was overemphasizing the supposed pharmacological effects of drugs while paying curiously little attention to the effects of drug laws, drug policies, and drug attitudes. Accordingly, the project as first conceived was expanded in several directions.

First, the major *licit* drugs—caffeine, nicotine, and alcohol—are considered here along with the illicit drugs. Any book about drugs that ignores such socially approved and legally marketed substances, we are convinced, sacrifices its credibility among young readers—and seriously distorts the perspective of older readers. Considering the licit and illicit drugs together makes both groups more readily understandable.

Second, each drug is presented in its historical setting.

Third, the history of drug laws, policies, and attitudes is presented along with the history of the drugs themselves. A historical perspective helps distinguish the direct effects of a drug on mind and body—relatively stable decade after decade—from the effects of laws, policies, and attitudes, which may vary from decade to decade. The practical advantages of that distinction can hardly be overemphasized. For while little can be done to alter the direct impact of a drug on mind or body, a great deal can be done to alter the impact of laws, policies, and attitudes. Out of an integrated review of pharmacological effects, legal effects, and social effects, there emerges at the end of this Report a set of recommendations designed to minimize both adverse pharmacological effects and adverse legal and social effects of drug use.

Our recommendations, it is true, do not constitute a panacea—"six easy ways to eliminate the drug menace." But they do point the way to both short-term and long-term improvements in the present critical situation.

We hope this Report and the historical perspective it provides will prove useful in several ways. At the very least it can warn against further reliance on "solutions" that have repeatedly failed in the past. It can

---

for 1971, "in recognition and appreciation of their distinguished contributions to the public understanding of psychiatry." They were associate editors of *Consumer Reports* in the 1940s, and joint authors of several books, including *The Rays: A History of Radiology in the United States and Canada* (Williams & Wilkins, 1969). Mr. Brecher is the author of *The Sex Researchers* (Little, Brown, 1969).

provide concerned citizens with the historical background needed to evaluate proposals for change. We hope it will help them to contribute wisely to the search for sound fresh solutions.

We also believe that this Report, and especially the recommendations concerning drug attitudes, will help parents and community leaders faced with drug problems in their own families and neighborhoods. Educators responsible for tailoring more effective educational programs will, we hope, find useful information in many chapters. Finally, young people will find here information they can trust about licit and illicit drugs.

Part I of this Report, the longest part, is concerned with the narcotics —primarily opium, morphine, and heroin. Detailed attention is paid to those drugs because their history in the United States has a lesson to teach. The relentless campaign to suppress heroin, since the Harrison Narcotic Act of 1914, has been more prolonged and more intensive than the campaign waged against any other drug. That campaign has failed. Until society recognizes and accepts the reasons for that failure, it can hardly formulate sound laws and policies with respect to any drug. Further, attitudes toward heroin, the most hated and most dreaded drug of all, subtly tinge popular attitudes toward other illicit drugs. Many people tend to transfer to all illicit drugs, even marijuana, the hate and dread aroused by the mere mention of heroin. Hence, a clear understanding of heroin and a rational attitude toward it are prerequisites for a rational approach to other drugs and for formulating effective policies toward drugs in general.

Throughout this book, many descriptions of drug effects will be found. The reader should bear in mind that the effects described will be in the context of who is taking the drug, in what dosage, by what route of administration, and under what circumstances. Thus, a cocktail which makes one drinker sociable and garrulous makes another silent and morose. A man happily drunk on three highballs may find himself suicidally drunk on four. A woman buoyed up by a few drinks on Saturday night may find herself depressed by the same dose the next Saturday night. An alcoholic on a quart of brandy a day may display fewer signs of drunkenness than he did on a couple of beers a few years earlier.

Much the same is true of the other psychoactive drugs reviewed in this Report. Readers who traditionally think in terms of *the* effect of a drug will learn here that even the simplest drugs have a wide range of effects—depending not only on their chemistry but on the ways in which they are used, the laws that govern their use, the user's attitudes and expectations, society's attitudes and expectations, and countless other factors.

The findings of this Report are firmly rooted—as the text and reference notes will demonstrate—in the published scientific literature. Other lines of inquiry, however, have enriched and buttressed the published data. Mr. Brecher visited leading drug research and drug treatment centers from Boston to San Francisco, as well as in Canada, England, Sweden, Denmark, and the Netherlands. He interviewed authorities in many disciplines, and a number of them generously made available unpublished material. He attended major conferences on drug problems. Well-known drug-use centers from Paradiso in Amsterdam and the West End in London to the Haight-Ashbury in San Francisco and Fourth Avenue in Vancouver were included in his research itinerary, and he talked with many drug users—ranging from marijuana smokers to heroin addicts and alcoholics.

This Report was further enriched by Mr. Brecher's participation in two other undertakings. The first was the work of the Ad Hoc Committee on the Treatment and Prevention of Drug Addiction and Drug Abuse, a committee assembled in November 1970 by Dr. Jerome H. Jaffe, associate professor of psychiatry at the University of Chicago–Pritzker School of Medicine, and director of drug abuse programs for the State of Illinois.* This ad hoc committee met in New York, Washington, and San Francisco; the typed transcript of its proceedings ran to more than 1,500 pages. Mr. Brecher also served in 1970–1971 as a member of an advisory panel on evaluation of drug treatment programs, assembled by the Cambridge consulting firm Arthur D. Little, Inc., under a federal contract. Mr. Brecher's participation in these groups significantly broadened his perspectives and thus enriched this Report. The conclusions reached here, of course, are wholly independent of conclusions reached by the Jaffe ad hoc committee and the Arthur D. Little, Inc., advisory panel.

A major problem in publishing a book in any field in which the news media report almost daily developments and discoveries is when to call a halt. For this Report a halt was called on January 1, 1972. Thus developments after that date, and the impact of those developments on what preceded them, are not reflected here. Consumers Union, however, will continue to monitor the field and will report major developments in the pages of *Consumer Reports*. Meanwhile, to Edward M. Brecher goes this special word of appreciation for his extraordinary contribution to a better understanding of licit and illicit drugs and of laws and attitudes concerning them.

THE EDITORS OF CONSUMER REPORTS

Consumers Union
Mount Vernon, New York

* Dr. Jaffe was subsequently, in 1971, appointed director of President Nixon's Special Action Office for Drug Abuse Prevention.

Contents

Contents

Part I

The Narcotics:
Opium, Morphine, Heroin, Methadone, and Others

The most important opiates are opium, morphine, heroin, and
codeine. These drugs belong to the class called *narcotics,* but there are
also nonopiate, synthetic narcotics.*

Opium is a raw natural product—the dried juice of the unripe capsule
of the opium poppy *(Papaver somniferum). Morphine* is the chief
active ingredient in opium; each grain of opium contains about one-tenth
of a grain of morphine. *Heroin* (diacetylmorphine) is produced by
heating morphine in the presence of acetic acid (that found in vinegar).
The heroin is promptly converted back into morphine in the body.
Codeine is also found in small quantity in opium, and there are
numerous other opiates. *Synthetic narcotics* generally resemble morphine
and heroin in their effects but are not derived from opium; examples
are methadone (Dolophine) and meperidine (Demerol).

Opium is usually taken orally or "smoked"—that is, it is heated and its
vapors inhaled. Morphine and heroin can also be sniffed, or injected
under the skin or into a muscle. For maximum effect, it is injected directly
into a vein ("mainlined"). Codeine ordinarily is taken orally; like most
of the lesser opiates and synthetics, it is rarely the drug of choice
among addicts.

Narcotic effects are quite different in medicinal use and in addiction.
Thus, one grain of heroin administered therapeutically to a nonaddict has
approximately the effect of two or three grains of morphine. Among
addicts, however, that ratio may not hold; indeed, it is difficult to distinguish
an addict who takes a grain of heroin a day from one who takes a
grain of morphine a day, or two grains of heroin or morphine a day.

Effects in medicinal use. Narcotics act primarily on the central nervous
system, but through it affect many other organs and systems. Relief
of pain, tranquilization, sedation, sleep, and relief of coughing and diarrhea

---

* This and similar introductory material in Parts II through VIII are designed to
give readers a rapid orientation to the drugs discussed. The introductory data are
not exhaustive; they are subject to numerous detailed qualifications, which appear
in the text following, and are based on current scientific views, which may undergo
change as research advances.

are effects for which these drugs are commonly prescribed; a few patients experience euphoria (a general feeling of well-being or even bliss). Constipation and constriction of the eye pupils are the most common side effects; some patients also experience dysphoria (anxiety, restlessness, fear), nausea, vomiting, dizziness, and shortness of breath. Excessive doses can lead to coma and eventually death, usually from respiratory failure. An effective antidote, nalorphine (Nalline), is available.

Effects in addiction. All narcotics are addicting—the likelihood of addiction varying, it is believed, with the drug, the dose, the route of administration, and especially with the frequency and duration of use. Addicts who take a narcotic regularly develop *tolerance* to most of the effects listed above; that is, the drug has little effect when taken regularly in a uniform dose—but *lack* of the drug produces in addicts a *withdrawal syndrome* that can be severe or even (in extreme cases) fatal.

A person addicted to a narcotic can forestall withdrawal effects by taking any other narcotic—a phenomenon known as *cross-tolerance.*

1.

Nineteenth-century America — a "dope fiend's paradise"

The United States of America during the nineteenth century could quite properly be described as a "dope fiend's paradise."

Opium was on legal sale conveniently and at low prices throughout the century; morphine came into common use during and after the Civil War; and heroin was marketed toward the end of the century. These opiates and countless pharmaceutical preparations containing them "were as freely accessible as aspirin is today." [1] They flowed mostly through five broad channels of distribution, all of them quite legal:

(1) Physicians dispensed opiates directly to patients, or wrote prescriptions for them.

(2) Drugstores sold opiates over the counter to customers without a prescription.

(3) Grocery and general stores as well as pharmacies stocked and sold opiates. An 1883–1885 survey of the state of Iowa, which then had a population of less than 2,000,000, found 3,000 stores in the state where opiates were on sale—and this did not include the physicians who dispensed opiates directly. [2]

(4) For users unable or unwilling to patronize a nearby store, opiates could be ordered by mail.

(5) Finally, there were countless patent medicines on the market containing opium or morphine. They were sold under such names as Ayer's Cherry Pectoral, Mrs. Winslow's Soothing Syrup, Darby's Carminative, Godfrey's Cordial, McMunn's Elixir of Opium, Dover's Powder, [3] and so on. Some were teething syrups for young children, some were "soothing syrups," some were recommended for diarrhea and dysentery or for "women's trouble." They were widely advertised in newspapers and magazines and on billboards as "pain-killers," "cough mixtures," "women's friends," "consumption cures," and so on. [4] One wholesale drug house, it is said, distributed more than 600 proprietary medicines and other products containing opiates. [5]

Most of the opium consumed in the United States during the nineteenth century was legally imported. Morphine was legally manufactured here from the imported opium. [6] But opium poppies were also legally grown within the United States. One early reference—perhaps the earliest —was in a letter from a Philadelphia physician, Dr. Thomas Bond, who wrote to a Pennsylvania farmer on August 24, 1781: "The opium you sent is pure and of good quality. I hope you will take care of the seed." [7] During the War of 1812, opium was scarce, but "some parties produced it in New Hampshire and sold the product at from $10 to $12 per pound." [8]

In 1871 a Massachusetts official reported:

> There are so many channels through which the drug may be brought into the State, that I suppose it would be almost impossible to determine how much foreign opium is used here; but it may easily be shown that the home production increases every year. Opium has been recently made from white poppies, cultivated for the purpose, in Vermont, New Hampshire, and Connecticut, the annual production being estimated by hundreds of pounds, and this has generally been absorbed in the communities where it is made. It has also been brought here from Florida and Louisiana, while comparatively large quantities are regularly sent east from California and Arizona, where its cultivation is becoming an important branch of industry, ten acres of poppies being said to yield, in Arizona, twelve hundred pounds of opium.[9]

Opium was also produced in the Confederate states (Virginia, Tennessee, South Carolina, Georgia) [10] during the Civil War—and perhaps thereafter. Though some states outlawed it earlier, Congress did not ban the cultivation of opium poppies nationally until 1942.[11]

The nineteenth-century distribution system reached into towns, villages, and hamlets as well as the large cities. A New England physician-druggist wrote about 1870:

> In this town I began business twenty years since. The population then at 10,000 has increased only inconsiderably, but my sales have advanced from 50 pounds of opium the first year to 300 pounds now; and of laudanum [opium in alcohol] four times upon what was formerly required. About 50 regular purchasers come to my shop, and as many more, perhaps, are divided among the other three apothecaries in the place. Some country dealers also have their quota of dependents.[12]

A correspondent for the Portland (Maine) *Press* had this to say about opium users in 1868: "In the little village of Auburn . . . at least fifty such (as counted up by a resident apothecary) regularly purchase their supplies hereabouts; and the country grocers too, not a few of them, find occasion for keeping themselves supplied with a stock." [13]

A survey of 10,000 prescriptions filled by thirty-five Boston drugstores in 1888 revealed that 1,481 of them contained opiates. Among prescriptions refilled three or more times, 78 percent contained opiates.[14]

One Massachusetts druggist, asked to review his opiate sales, added a picturesque detail. He had only one steady customer, he reported—"and that a noted temperance lecturer." [15]

Nor was the Middle West different from New England. The *Annual Report* of the Michigan State Board of Health for 1878 reported three opium eaters in the village of Huron (population 437), four opium eaters and one morphine eater in the village of Otisville (population 1,365), 18 opium eaters and 20 morphine eaters in the town of Hillsdale (population 4,189), and so on around the state.[16] Some children were included in the statistics.

Though called "opium eaters" in the medical literature, most nineteenth-century opium users (including Thomas De Quincey, author of *Confessions of an English Opium-Eater*) were in fact opium drinkers; they drank laudanum or other opiate liquids. Similarly "morphine eaters" included many who took morphine by injection or in other ways. In a number of the quotations which follow, "opium eaters" refers generally to morphine as well as opium users. Opium *smokers*, however, were considered to be in a separate category (see Chapter 6).

The nineteenth-century use of opiates was more or less the same in Britain. A classic report on the English industrial system, *The Factory System Illustrated* (1842), by W. Dodd, noted that factory workers of the time used opiates—notably laudanum—to quiet crying babies.[17]

In the official *Report of the Medical Officer of the Privy Council* for 1864 it was observed: "To push the sale of opiate . . . is the great aim of some enterprising wholesale merchants. By druggists it is considered the leading article." [18] The report also noted the giving of opiates to infants; [19] Karl Marx, citing this report in *Capital* (1867), spoke of the English working-class custom of "dosing children with opiates." [20]

In 1873 an English physician reported:

. . . Amongst the three millions and three-quarters [people in London] there are to be found some persons here and there who take [opium] as a luxury, though by far the greater number of those who take it in anything like quantity do so for some old neuralgia or rheumatic malady, and began under medical advice. Neither is it to be found over the agricultural or manufacturing districts, save in the most scattered and casual way. The genuine opium-eating districts are the ague and fen districts of Norfolk and Lincolnshire. There it is not casual, accidental, or rare, but popular, habitual, and common. Anyone who visits such a town as Louth or Wisbeach, and strolls about the streets on a Saturday evening, watching the country people as they do their marketing, may soon satisfy himself that the crowds in the chemists' shops come for opium; and they have a peculiar way of getting it. They go in, lay down their money, and receive the opium pills in exchange without saying a word. For instance, I was at Wisbeach one evening in August 1871; went into a chemist's shop; laid a penny on the counter. The chemist said—"The best?" I nodded. He gave me a pill-box and

[5]

took up the penny; and so the purchase was completed without my having uttered a syllable. You offer money, and get opium as a matter of course. This may show how familiar the custom is. . . .

In these districts it is taken by people of all classes, but especially by the poor and miserable, and by those who in other districts would seek comfort from gin or beer.[21]

Godfrey's Cordial—a mixture of opium, molasses for sweetening, and sassafras for flavoring—was especially popular in England. Dr. C. Fraser Brockington reports that in mid-nineteenth-century Coventry, ten gallons of Godfrey's Cordial—enough for 12,000 doses—was sold weekly, and was administered to 3,000 infants under two years of age.

Even greater quantities of opium mixtures were said to be sold in Nottingham. . . . Every surgeon in Marshland testified to the fact that "there was not a labourer's house in which the bottle of opium was not to be seen, and not a child, but who got it in some form." . . . Wholesale druggists reported the sale of immense quantities of opium; a retail druggist dispensed up to 200 pounds a year—in pills and penny sticks or as Godfrey's Cordial. . . . To some extent this was a practice which had been taken on during the years when malaria was indigenous in the Fens and when, a century before, the poppy had been cultivated for the London market.[22]

The nonmedicinal use of opiates, while legal in both the United States and England, was not considered respectable. Indeed, as an anonymous but perceptive and well-informed American writer noted in the *Catholic World* for September 1881, it was as disreputable as drinking alcoholic beverages—and much harder to detect:

The gentleman who would not be seen in a bar-room, however respectable, or who would not purchase liquor and use it at home, lest the odor might be detected upon his person, procures his supply of morphia and has it in his pocket ready for instantaneous use. It is odorless and occupies but little space. . . . He zealously guards his secret from his nearest friend—for popular wisdom has branded as a disgrace that which he regards as a misfortune. . . .[23]

Opiate use was also frowned upon in some circles as *immoral*—a vice akin to dancing, smoking, theater-going, gambling, or sexual promiscuity. But while deemed immoral, it is important to note that opiate use in the nineteenth century was not subject to the moral sanctions current today. Employees were not fired for addiction. Wives did not divorce their addicted husbands, or husbands their addicted wives. Children were not taken from their homes and lodged in foster homes or institutions because one or both parents were addicted. Addicts continued to participate fully in the life of the community. Addicted children and young people con-

[6]

tinued to go to school, Sunday School, and college. Thus, the nineteenth century avoided one of the most disastrous effects of current narcotics laws and attitudes—the rise of a deviant addict subculture, cut off from respectable society and without a "road back" to respectability.

Our nineteenth-century forbears correctly perceived the major objection to the opiates. *They are addicting.* Though the word "addiction" was seldom used during the nineteenth century, the phenomenon was well understood. The true nature of the narcotic evil becomes visible, the *Catholic World* article pointed out, when someone who has been using an opiate for some time

attempts to give up its use. Suddenly his eyes are opened to his folly and he realizes the startling fact that he is in the toils of a serpent as merciless as the boa-constrictor and as relentless as fate. With a firm determination to free himself he discontinues its use. Now his sufferings begin and steadily increase until they become unbearable. The tortures of Dives are his; but unlike that miser, he has only to stretch forth his hand to find oceans with which to satisfy his thirst. That human nature is not often equal to so extraordinary a self-denial affords little cause for astonishment. . . . Again and again he essays release from a bondage so humiliating, but meets with failure only, and at last submits to his fate—a confirmed opium-eater.[24]

The terms "addicting" and "addiction" will be further discussed later.

Our nineteenth-century forbears also perceived opiate use as a "will-weakening" vice—for surely, they insisted, a man or woman of strong will could stop if he tried hard enough. The fact was generally known that addicts deprived of their opiates (when hospitalized for some illness unrelated to their addiction, for example) would lie or even steal to get their drug, and addicts "cured" of their addiction repeatedly relapsed. Hence there was much talk of the *moral degeneration* caused by the opiates.

Nevertheless, there was very little popular support for a law banning these substances. "Powerful organizations for the suppression . . . of alcoholic stimulants exist throughout the land," [25] the 1881 article in the *Catholic World* noted, but there were no similar anti-opiate organizations.

The reason for this lack of demand for opiate prohibition was quite simple: the drugs were not viewed as a menace to society and, as we shall demonstrate in subsequent chapters, they were not in fact a menace.

2.

Opiates for pain relief, for tranquilization, and for pleasure

Physicians in the nineteenth century as now prescribed opiates for pain. They were also widely prescribed, however, for cough, diarrhea, dysentery, and a host of other illnesses. Physicians often referred to opium or morphine as "G.O.M."—"God's own medicine." Dr. H. H. Kane's 1880 textbook, entitled *The Hypodermic Injection of Morphia. Its History, Advantages, and Dangers. Based on Experience of 360 Physicians*, listed 54 diseases which benefited from morphine injections. They ranged from anemia and angina pectoris through diabetes, insanity, nymphomania, and ovarian neuralgia, to tetanus, vaginismus, and vomiting of pregnancy.[1]

To modern readers, this list may appear to be evidence of the incompetence of nineteenth-century physicians. Yet, for the great majority of these conditions, morphine really was of help—especially in the absence of more specific modern remedies (such as insulin for diabetes). For morphine, as we shall show, can be highly effective in calming—tranquilizing. The nineteenth-century physician used morphine for a wide range of disorders much as the physician today uses meprobamate (Miltown, Equanil), chlordiazepoxide (Librium), and other tranquilizers and sedatives now in style. The effects are quite different in several respects—but the calming or tranquilizing effect is achieved by both groups of drugs.

Yet another nineteenth-century use of opiates was as a substitute for alcohol. As Dr. J. R. Black explained in a paper entitled "Advantages of Substituting the Morphia Habit for the Incurably Alcoholic," published in the *Cincinnati Lancet-Clinic* in 1889, morphine "is less inimical to healthy life than alcohol." It "calms in place of exciting the baser passions, and hence is less productive of acts of violence and crime; in short . . . the use of morphine in place of alcohol is but a choice of evils, and by far the lesser." [2] Then he continued:

> On the score of economy the morphine habit is by far the better. The regular whiskey drinker can be made content in his craving for stimulation, at least for quite a long time, on two or three grains of morphine a day, divided into appropriate portions, and given at regular intervals. If purchased by the drachm at fifty cents this will last him twenty days. Now it is safe to say that a like amount of spirits for the steady drinker cannot be purchased for two and one-half cents a day,* and that the majority of them spend five and ten times that sum a day as a regular thing.

* Comparisons with contemporary doses and prices are difficult, since today's illicit heroin market does not publish statistics. The estimates below are based on a review

On the score, then, of . . . a lessened liability to fearful diseases and the lessened propagation of pathologically inclined blood, I would urge the substitution of morphine instead of alcohol for all to whom such a craving is an incurable propensity. In this way I have been able to bring peacefulness and quiet to many disturbed and distracted homes. . . . Is it not the duty of a physician when he cannot cure an ill, when there is no reasonable ground for hope that it will ever be done, to do the next best thing—advise a course of treatment that will diminish to an immense extent great evils otherwise irremediable? . . .

The mayors and police courts would almost languish for lack of business; the criminal dockets, with their attendant legal functionaries, would have much less to do than they now have—to the profit and well-being of the community. I might, had I time and space, enlarge by statistics to prove the law-abiding qualities of opium-eating peoples, but of this anyone can perceive somewhat for himself, if he carefully watches and reflects on the quiet, introspective gaze of the morphine habitué and compares it with the riotous devil-may-care leer of the drunkard.[4]*

Many physicians did in fact convert alcoholics to morphine. In Kentucky this practice did not die out among older physicians until the late 1930s or early 1940s. The details are reported in a major contribution to the history of opiate addiction, *Narcotics Addicts in Kentucky,* by Dr. John A. O'Donnell, published in 1969 by the National Institute of Mental Health, an arm of the United States Department of Health, Education, and Welfare.

Dr. O'Donnell, then chief of the research branch of the NIMH's Clinical Research Center in Lexington, Kentucky, reported on 266 addicts living in Kentucky who were admitted to the Lexington hospital for drug addiction between 1935 and 1959. Of these 266, at least 152 had a record of alcohol excesses *prior* to becoming addicted to opiates. Among the men in the sample, this relationship was particularly close. "Over one-third of the men [75 out of 212] began their addiction through treatment

---

of the recent literature; they are substantially the same as estimates presented by the Select Committee on Crime of the United States House of Representatives in its January 2, 1971, report: [3]

Although there is wide variation from time to time, from city to city, and even from bag to bag, a typical heroin "bag" today contains 10 milligrams (1/6 grain) of heroin mixed with 90 milligrams of adulterants, and costs five dollars.

Hence, the nineteenth-century morphinist paying 2½ cents a day for 2 or 3 grains of morphine (as in the example above) can be contrasted with today's New York City heroin addict who would have to pay thirty dollars to sixty dollars a day for the equivalent—one or two grains (60 to 120 milligrams or six to twelve bags) of heroin.

* An English physician similarly noted in 1873 that while opium users in Britain might be dirty, slovenly, lazy, lying, and sanctimonious, "they are not uproarious, and don't swear. There are none of the deeds of brutal violence that are inspired by beer, and none of the foul language." [5]

of alcoholism; they were given a narcotic to help in the sobering-up periods . . . , preferred the narcotic to alcohol, and shifted to its use. . . ." [6] In 50 of these 75 cases, it was a physician who gave the alcoholic his first injection of morphine as an alcohol substitute. [7]

One Kentucky physician described a typical case, Dr. O'Donnell reports, in a letter to the Public Health Service Hospital in Lexington at the time of an addict's admission there:

. . . I decided that these symptoms [acute gastritis, jaundice, liver trouble, and possibly heart disease] were due to overuse of alcoholic drinks, and that an alcoholic cirrhosis was developing. The subject would not drink whiskey when he had morphine, and as he already had a habit for morphine I decided that by prescribing morphine for him he would get along better. This has been true, and the patient has had only a few attacks in the past four years of acute pain in the epigastrium and these occurred when the subject was short of morphine. [8]

Dr. O'Donnell takes a guarded but on the whole favorable view of this kind of conversion: ". . . the addict whose drugs came from a stable medical source was no great problem to his community. . . . He became a serious problem only if he engaged in illegal activities to obtain narcotics. The alcoholic was more visible, and his arrests more frequent, though each individual offense was a relatively minor one. But the community attitude was generally more accepting of the alcoholic." [9]

In a community where alcohol and the opiates are equally available and equally approved (or disapproved), Dr. O'Donnell adds, "there are reasons, in the physical effects of addiction and alcoholic intoxication, to believe that . . . narcotic addiction would be less disruptive than alcoholism." [10]

The advantages of converting alcoholics to opiates were also pointed out in 1928 by Dr. Lawrence Kolb, Assistant Surgeon General of the United States Public Health Service, a psychiatrist specializing in problems of drug addiction. "More than any other unstable group," Dr. Kolb wrote, "drunkards are likely to be benefited in their social relations by becoming addicts. When they give up alcohol and start using opium [i.e., morphine or other opiates], they are able to secure the effect for which they are striving without becoming drunk or violent."

Among 33 heavy drinkers who converted to morphine, Dr. Kolb added, only one "continued to drink after he became addicted to morphine, and his drinking was then moderate." [11]

An evaluation of the comparative physiological effects of the opiates versus alcohol is also found in *A Community Mental Health Approach to Drug Addiction,* by Drs. Richard Brotman and Alfred M. Freedman, published in 1968 by the United States Department of Health, Education, and Welfare: " . . . Opiates are far less physically damaging than barbiturates, or amphetamines—or alcohol. . . . The drug-dependent person who abstains from opiates only to turn to other drugs, specifically alcohol, barbiturates, or amphetamines, cannot be said to be making progress." [12]

Dr. Black's 1889 view that an opiate "calms in place of exciting the baser passions" was very widely agreed upon, and was the basis for the widespread use of opiates as tranquilizers. The first recorded use of the word "tranquilizer" in the English language, according to the Oxford English Dictionary, was by Thomas De Quincey, in his *Confessions of an English Opium-Eater* in 1822. Dr. Horatio Day described the tranquilizing role of the opiates in *The Opium Habit* (1868), three years after the close of the Civil War: "Maimed and shattered survivors from a hundred battlefields, diseased and disabled soldiers released from hostile prisons, anguished and hopeless wives and mothers, made so by the slaughter of those who were dearest to them, have found, many of them, temporary relief from their sufferings in opium." [13]

The same tranquilization theme echoed down through the decades. In 1886, Dr. William Pepper, in his *System of Practical Medicine,* pointed out that the range of opium's effects extended from assuaging the oppression of the working class to allaying the ennui of upper-class women.[14] *The American Textbook of Applied Therapeutics* (1896) spoke of patients using narcotics "to soothe their shattered nervous systems." [15] T. C. Allbutt's *System of Medicine* (1905) spoke of morphine as bringing "tranquility and well-being." [16] L. L. Stanley, writing in the *Journal of the American Institute of Criminal Law and Criminology* in 1915, spoke of society women who "indulge in opium to calm their shattered nerves." [17]

During the last half century, the function of the opiates as tranquilizers has been lost from sight. Old truths, however, tend to be rediscovered. An official 1963 publication setting forth the United States Public Health Service's views made the point clearly: "Last century the pain that led to addiction was often physical; today it is mainly psychic. Most of today's addicted persons have discovered, in other words, that opiates relieve their anxieties, tensions, feelings of inadequacy, and other emotional conditions they cannot bring themselves to cope with in a normal way."* [18]

The tranquilizing effects of narcotics were also clearly revealed during a remarkable 1956 study of many hundreds of addicts in Vancouver, British Columbia. This research was reported in a 658-page document[19] (plus a hundred pages of appendices), "Drug Addiction in British Colum-

---

* The Public Health Service report did not, however, define the "normal way" for untrained and unemployed black or Puerto Rican adolescents living in urban slums to cope with "their anxieties, tensions, feelings of inadequacy and other emotional conditions."

bia—A Research Survey," one of the broadest and most insightful ever written on heroin addiction; unfortunately it has never been published. Prepared under the direction of a psychiatrist, Dr. George H. Stevenson, in collaboration with a psychologist, Lewis R. A. Lingley, a social worker, George E. Trasov, and an internist, Dr. Hugh Stansfield, it exists only as a typed manuscript in the Library of the University of British Columbia. A few photocopies have been made, but even large medical libraries lack copies. To make the findings available to a wider audience, as well as for their intrinsic worth, quotations from this report will be frequently used in the chapters that follow.

Among the many inquiries undertaken in the British Columbia study, one sought to determine what mood effects addicts reported experiencing while on heroin. One group of addicts was given a list of seventeen terms descriptive of moods; some of the terms indicated a tranquilizing effect, others a mood-elevating effect. The addicts were asked to check which of the terms described the way they felt.[20]

The 71 addicts made a total of 449 check marks. Only 8 addicts considered the heroin experience "thrilling" and only 11 considered it "joyful" or "jolly"—as contrasted with 65 who said it "relaxed" them and 53 who thought it "relieved worry."

Twentieth-century research, moreover, suggests that even the beneficial effect of the opiates on *physical* pain is in considerable part a tranquilizing effect. One standard method of testing a drug's effects on pain is to apply warmth to a spot on the skin of a laboratory subject, and then gradually raise the temperature until the subject signals that it has become painful. A subject who has received the usual pain-relieving dose of morphine readily recognizes the sensation of pain when so tested—and it takes only a slightly hotter stimulus to produce the sensation. Another common test is to ask a subject to compare two levels of pain, and to place them on a scale ranging from one "dol" (barely painful) to nine "dols" (intolerable).[21] Subjects rate a given stimulus only slightly lower on the dol scale while they are on morphine. If this direct effect on pain *sensations* were the only effect of the opiates, they would be relatively poor pain relievers. Their enormous usefulness in medicine results from the fact that they also alleviate a patient's *fear* of pain, his *anxiety* about the pain, and both his physical and his emotional *reactions* to the pain. In a word, they tranquilize him. (In some other respects, of course, the effects of the opiates are very different from the effects of modern tranquilizers.)

The relation of the opiates to *pleasure* as distinct from tranquility is complex and controversial. There is frequent reference in the medical literature (and in the mass media) to the "kick," "bang," or "rush" that the addict is said to feel immediately after mainlining morphine or heroin.

This rush has even been likened to "an abdominal orgasm"; and the view has been expressed that addicts shoot morphine or heroin *for the purpose* of experiencing this ecstatically pleasurable rush.

There can be no doubt that the injection directly into a vein of a substantial dose of morphine or heroin produces a readily identifiable sensation. Nonaddicts often describe it as a sudden flush of warmth, and some localize it as warmth in the pit of the stomach. Few nonaddicts perceive the rush as particularly pleasurable, however.[22]

Addicts who take opiates by mouth, or who smoke them, or sniff them, or inject them under the skin or into a muscle, do *not* experience a rush— yet they may become as firmly "hooked" as addicts who mainline their drug. Hence, a desire for the rush is *not* the basis for addiction.

In general, the rush appears to be subject to tolerance; that is, the addict who injects the same dose several times a day, day after day, no longer experiences a rush. Doubt surrounds this point, however. Most American black-market heroin is adulterated with quinine—and quinine also produces a rush when mainlined. Moreover, street addicts are not often able to take uniform doses at regular intervals day after day. If an addict waits an hour or two too long for his next "fix," or if his previous fix was of less than the usual potency, he may suffer incipient withdrawal discomfort—and the next fix may produce an inextricably interwoven mixture of relief from withdrawal distress and the rush sensation. (A fuller discussion of physical dependence, the withdrawal syndrome, tolerance, and other aspects of addiction follows in Chapter 10.)

During the nineteenth century, many highly reputable addicts—whose addiction arose during the medicinal use of opiates—insisted that they had never in their lives experienced a moment's pleasure from opiates; they took their drug solely to forestall withdrawal distress and the unpleasant "post-addiction syndrome," to be described below. Today's addicts almost all concede that they get a highly enjoyable bang or rush from their heroin injections. They may, however, be mistaken. For them as for nonaddicts, the rush may be merely an abdominal sensation of warmth. For the addicts, however, the sensation may have a highly charged meaning—since it will generally signal imminent relief from withdrawal distress. It is exceedingly difficult to distinguish a positive feeling of pleasure from the pleasantness that follows the relief of distress or pain. Perhaps there is no difference. Some theorists have even suggested that addicts shoot heroin *in order to achieve withdrawal distress*—a distress that can then be pleasurably relieved by the next fix.

Most addicts who mainline heroin, when asked what happens when they "kick the habit," describe the classic withdrawal syndrome—nausea, vomiting, aches and pains, yawning, sneezing, and so on. When asked what happens after withdrawal, they describe an equally specific "postaddiction syndrome"—a wavering, unstable composite of anxiety, depression, and craving for the drug. The craving is not *continuous* but seems to come and go in waves of varying intensity, for months, even years, after withdrawal. It is particularly likely to return in moments of emotional stress. Following an intense wave of craving, drug-seeking behavior is likely to set in, and the ex-addict relapses. When asked how he feels following a return to heroin, he is likely to reply, "It makes me feel normal again"—that is, it relieves the ex-addict's chronic triad of anxiety, depression, and craving.

It is this view—that an addict takes heroin in order to "feel normal"*— that is hardest for a nonaddict to understand and to believe. Yet it is consonant with everything else that is known about narcotics addiction— and there is not a scrap of scientific evidence to impugn the addict's own view. The ex-addict who returns to heroin, if this view is accepted, is not a pleasure-craving hedonist but an anxious, depressed patient who desperately craves a return to a *normal* mood and state of mind.

The term "craving," used here and later in this Report, is not in good repute among many psychologists today. For craving is a subjective feeling; and like other subjective feelings, subjects may or may not report accurately on its presence or absence. It cannot be objectively measured. In the case of the craving for narcotics, however, we need not rely solely on addicts' subjective reports. We may reliably infer that an ex-addict still suffers from a heroin craving if he goes wandering the streets in search of heroin. If he engages in drug-seeking behavior despite the fact that his whole future, including his future freedom from imprisonment, depends on his remaining abstinent, we may infer that the craving is quite strong—or nagging and persistent, difficult to resist. If he engages in such behavior especially in times of emotional stress, we may infer that the craving recurs or is intensified when stress is experienced. If he again engages in such behavior after years of abstinence from narcotics, we may infer that the craving is long-lived. As we shall see below, both the craving and tendency to drug-seeking behavior are indeed difficult to resist, stress-associated, and long-lasting.

This discussion of the pleasure factor and craving factor in addiction is certainly not definitive. It takes no account, for example, of individual differences—and they are very great. But regardless of details, three central points seem reasonably well established: the addict does not main-line heroin solely or primarily for pleasure; the addicting nature of narcotics is quite distinct from whatever pleasure the drugs may on occasion provide some addicts; relapse results, not from a striving for

* Dr. J. Yerbury Dent, editor of the *British Journal of Addiction*, stated (1952): "An addict is one who cannot be normal without a drug." [23]

pleasure, but from the need for release from the postaddiction syndrome —anxiety, depression, and craving. Thus, the postaddiction syndrome might also be called the "pre-relapse syndrome."

It is commonly stated that anyone who takes heroin daily for a few weeks or longer is in imminent danger of addiction. This is probably true, but it is almost beside the point. The important question is: if someone takes heroin occasionally, what is the likelihood that he will graduate to using it daily for a few weeks or longer—and thus very probably become addicted?

Unfortunately, there are no statistics on which to base an answer to that question. We can only indicate a spectrum of possible outcomes.

At one extreme are the few addicts who report that they "fell in love" with heroin on their first fix. Thereafter they continued uninterruptedly on the drug. They are a small minority—perhaps 2 or 3 percent. At the other extreme are the unaddicted opiate users who maintain that they have used heroin or morphine occasionally—on Saturday nights, for instance—for prolonged periods, perhaps even for years, without becoming addicted. These long-term "weekend users," or "chippers," are also believed to be rare—how rare, nobody knows.

The great majority of addicts fall between these extremes. They report, no doubt truthfully, that they started off as occasional users. They did not intend to become addicted; indeed, they were confident that they would escape addiction by using the drug only on occasion. Then the kinds of occasions on which they used heroin became more numerous, and the intervals shorter. After weeks or months of increasing use, daily use began —and soon thereafter the casual user became an addict.

The likelihood of addiction is said to be affected by the drug used; heroin, for example, is believed to be more likely to lead to addiction than codeine. It is commonly stated that route of use affects the outcome; thus, heroin sniffed or smoked is alleged to be less addicting than heroin injected. Whether this is literally true, or simply due to the fact that a given dose has a greater effect when injected, remains in doubt. The most that can be said is this: there is a great likelihood that anyone who uses a narcotic once will use it again, and then occasionally, and then daily— and will become addicted. No one can tell in advance whether he will be one of the few who reportedly are able to go on using occasionally.

Some young people today, rightly contemptuous of the myth that a single shot of heroin produces addiction, may point out that they have friends who have been weekend users for months, perhaps many months. This may well be true—but there is unfortunately no assurance that their friends, even after months as "chippers," will not soon become daily users—and thereafter addicts.

[15]

As for the possibility of addiction stemming from medically administered narcotics, the medical literature generally cautions physicians to exercise great prudence in prescribing narcotics for the treatment of pain or physical illness, to minimize the likelihood of a patient's developing "dependence." The results of this policy would seem to be something of a mystery. In the nineteenth century, medical treatment was the commonest source of addiction. But today, Dr. Jerome H. Jaffe writes in the 1970 edition of *The Pharmacological Basis of Therapeutics*, edited by Drs. Louis S. Goodman and Alfred Gilman, "Considering the frequency with which opiate analgesics are used in clinical medicine, addiction as a complication of medical treatment is quite uncommon." [24]

No recent study has been reported of just what does happen to patients who receive narcotics medicinally for several days or weeks. Many of them, of course, are terminal patients whose medical treatment ends in death. Some patients, particularly some who have undergone surgery, complain that physicians are *too* prudent—that they do not prescribe enough narcotics, or enough narcotics often enough, to relieve pain; are such complaints valid?

When nonaddicted patients receive medicinal narcotics regularly for an extended period, do they suffer a kind of postaddiction depression, anxiety, and craving when they stop taking the drug? Do they turn for relief to other drugs—for example, to increased consumption of alcohol? (Studies to be reviewed below indicate that a substantial proportion of morphine and heroin addicts who "kick the habit" become skid-row alcoholics.)

The answers to these and related questions are not known. For now, as in the case of other prescription drugs to be discussed in this Report, it is unclear whether physicians are prescribing narcotics prudently, excessively—or overcautiously.

3.

What kinds of people used opiates?

Several characteristics of opiate use under nineteenth-century conditions of low cost and ready legal availability will strike contemporary readers as strange.

First, most users of narcotics in those days were women. An 1878 survey of 1,313 opiate users in Michigan, for example, found that 803 of them (61.2 percent) were females.[1] An 1880 Chicago study similarly reported: "Among the 235 habitual opium eaters, 169 were found to be females, a proportion of about 3 to 1."[2] An Iowa survey in 1885 showed 63.8 percent females.[3]

The use of opiates by prostitutes did not fully account for this excess of women in the user population. Thus the Chicago report noted: "Of the 169 females, about one-third belong to that class known as prostitutes. Deducting these, we still have among those taking the different kinds of opiates, 2 females to 1 male."[4]

The widespread medical custom of prescribing opiates for menstrual and menopausal discomforts, and the many proprietary opiates advertised for "female troubles," no doubt contributed to this excess of female opiate users. A 1914 Tennessee survey, which found that two-thirds of the users were women, noted also that two-thirds of the women were between twenty-five and fifty-five.[5] "The first twenty years of this period," the survey report commented, "is about the age when the stresses of life begin to make themselves felt with women, and includes the beginning of the menopause period. [Nineteenth-century women, on the average, reached menopause somewhat earlier than twentieth-century women do.] It appears reasonable, therefore, to ascribe to this part of female life, no small portion of the addiction among women."[6]

The extent to which alcohol-drinking by women was frowned upon may also have contributed to the excess of women among opiate users. Husbands drank alcohol in the saloon; wives took opium at home.

After passage of the Harrison Narcotic Act in 1914, the sex ratio in addiction altered drastically. By 1918 a "Special Committee on Investigation" appointed by the Secretary of the Treasury could report that "drug addiction is about equally prevalent in both sexes."[7] Thereafter the sex ratio continued to change. Estimates during the 1960s indicated that males outnumbered females among known addicts by five to one or more.[8]

A second remarkable fact about the nineteenth-century use of opiates in the United States was the age of the users. The 1880 Chicago survey showed an average age for males of 41.4 years and for females of 39.4 years.[9] In the small towns of Iowa in 1885, the average age of 235 users was 46.5 years.[10] The 1914 Tennessee survey showed an average age of 50.[11] Today, in contrast, nearly half of all addicts known to the Federal Bureau of Narcotics and Dangerous Drugs are 30 or younger, and only 13.6 percent are over 40.[12] The age at which they *started* taking narcotics is, of course, much earlier—usually in the teens or early twenties. Thus one aftermath of the twentieth-century narcotic laws has been a shift in the brunt of the addiction problem from menopausal females to adolescent males.

A third interesting fact was the socioeconomic status of nineteenth-century narcotics users. The Massachusetts State Board of Health reported in 1889[13] on 612 answers to the question: "What classes of people use opium in your community?" (Here, as in much of the nineteenth-century literature, "opium" included morphine and other opiates.) Replies from 446 druggists and 166 physicians are shown in Table 1.

The 1881 *Catholic World* article, cited above, said much the same thing more eloquently:

> Opium-eating, unlike the use of alcoholic stimulants, is an aristocratic vice and prevails more extensively among the wealthy and educated classes than among those of inferior social position; but no class is exempt from its blighting influence. The merchant, lawyer, and physician are to be found among the host who sacrifice the choicest treasures of life at the shrine of Opium. The slaves of Alcohol may be clothed in rags, but vassals of the monarch who sits enthroned on the poppy are generally found dressed in purple and fine linen.[14]

The 1885 Iowa survey similarly noted that the majority of opiate users "are to be found among the educated and most honored and useful members of society." [15]

Finally, there is no evidence of any disproportionate use of opiates among black people during the nineteenth century; indeed, there are few references to their use of opiates at all. Surveys made in 1913 in Jacksonville, Florida, and throughout the state of Tennessee in 1914, turned up a much *lower* proportion of opiate users among blacks than among whites.[16] The high proportion of black people among known opiate addicts during the 1950s and 1960s is a quite recent development,* visible chiefly

---

* Among 68,864 opiate addicts known to the Bureau of Narcotics and Dangerous Drugs as of December 31, 1970, 48.4 percent were said to be black.[17] The great majority of addicts, however, were not known to the bureau. The high proportion of black people among *known* addicts may result at least in part from the greater likeli-

A. ACCORDING TO 446 DRUGGISTS

Socioeconomic Class of User	Percentage of Total Replies
All classes	22
Middle class	22
Upper class	7
Lower class	7
Miscellaneous	20
Don't know	22

B. ACCORDING TO 166 PHYSICIANS

Type or Socioeconomic Class of Patient	Percentage of Total Replies
All classes	30
Upper class	22
Middle and upper classes	12
Middle class	3
Lower class	6
Nervous women	14
Don't know	8

Table 1. Classes of Opium Users, 1889.

since World War II. It appears to be closely related to a shift in the channels of heroin distribution (see below) and not to any predilection of black people for opiates. Since the late 1960s heroin use has increased again among youthful middle-class whites; this increase will be discussed in Chapter 20.

The enormous shift in the characteristics of narcotic addicts after 1914, the further shift in the late 1960s, and evidence of similar changes from time to time and from place to place in the kinds of people who use other drugs, to be reviewed in subsequent chapters, should warn against placing excessive reliance on studies equating particular personality characteristics with a tendency to use a particular drug. There is an enormous literature of such studies—purporting to show, for example, that opiate addicts are excessively close to their mothers, or display masochistic tendencies, or that marijuana smokers are psychopathic or introverted. The most such

hood that a black addict will get arrested or otherwise come to the attention of the bureau.

a study can prove, however, is that at a particular time, in a particular place, under a particular set of laws and popular attitudes, morphine or heroin or some other drug tends to attract users of a particular stripe. By the time such a study is completed, the typology of drug use may well have shifted.

4.

Effects of opium, morphine, and heroin on addicts

The popular view of the effects of narcotics on addicts was eloquently expressed in a 1962 decision of the Supreme Court of the United States:

To be a confirmed drug addict is to be one of the walking dead. . . . The teeth have rotted out, the appetite is lost, and the stomach and intestines don't function properly. The gall bladder becomes inflamed; eyes and skin turn a bilious yellow; in some cases membranes of the nose turn a flaming red; the partition separating the nostrils is eaten away—breathing is difficult. Oxygen in the blood decreases; bronchitis and tuberculosis develop. Good traits of character disappear and bad ones emerge. Sex organs become affected. Veins collapse and livid purplish scars remain. Boils and abscesses plague the skin; gnawing pain racks the body. Nerves snap; vicious twitching develops. Imaginary and fantastic fears blight the mind and sometimes complete insanity results. Often times, too, death comes—much too early in life. . . . Such is the torment of being a drug addict; such is the plague of being one of the walking dead.[1]

The scientific basis for this opinion, however, is not easy to find. In 1956, when Dr. George H. Stevenson and his British Columbia associates made their inquiry into narcotics addiction, they exhaustively reviewed the medical literature on the subject.

"When we began this project," they explained,

. . . it was immediately apparent to us that the actual deleterious effects of addiction on the addict, and on society, should be clearly understood. . . . To our surprise we have not been able to locate even one scientific study on the proved harmful effects of addiction. Earlier investigators had apparently assumed that the ill effects were so obvious as not to need scientific verification. . . . We have assembled over 500 documents on various phases of addiction . . ., but not one of them offers a clear-cut, scientifically valid statement on this problem.[2]

A likely place to seek such a statement, the Stevenson group assumed, was in *The Traffic in Narcotics* (1953), by United States Commissioner of Narcotics Harry J. Anslinger, in collaboration with United States Attorney William F. Tompkins. Yet Anslinger and Tompkins had "only a single reference to the harmful effects of narcotic drugs, in which they quote another authority to the effect that the use of narcotic drugs leads to 'a decrease in the potential social productivity of the addict.' " Even this statement, the Stevenson group added, "is not supported in the book by any scientific evidence." [3]

The British Columbia report continued:

We finally wrote to some of the most eminent research workers in the field of drug addiction, explaining our problem and requesting scientific data on the deleterious effects of narcotic drugs. They indicated, in their reply, that there was no real evidence of brain damage or other serious organic disease resulting from the continued use of narcotics (morphine and related substances), but that there was undoubted psychological and social damage. However, they made no differentiation between such damage as might be caused by narcotics and that which might have been present before addiction, or might have been caused, at least in part, by other factors. Moreover, they were unable to direct us to any actual studies on the alleged harmful effects of narcotic drugs.

At a later date we also consulted officials of the United Nations Commission on Narcotic Drugs, and they, too, were unable to direct us to any scientific studies on the actual damaging effects of morphine or heroin addiction. . . .

The Narcotic Control Division of the Canadian Government's Department of Health and Welfare was likewise unable to direct us to scientific studies on this subject.[4]

A review of the literature since the 1956 British Columbia study, undertaken in preparation of this Consumers Union Report, has been only slightly more rewarding. Almost all of the deleterious effects ordinarily attributed to the opiates, indeed, appear to be the effects of the narcotics laws instead.

By far the most serious deleterious effects of being a narcotics addict in the United States today are the risks of arrest and imprisonment, infectious disease,* and impoverishment—all traceable to the narcotics laws, to vigorous enforcement of those laws, and to the resulting excessive black-market prices for narcotics. Here, however, we are concerned with the effects of opiate use on addicts under conditions of low cost and legal availability—in other words, the effects of the drugs themselves as distinct from the effects of economic, social, and legal factors.

The classical clinical study of the effects of prolonged opiate use on the human body was performed in the narcotics wards of the Philadelphia

---

* When opiates are cheap, addicts generally eat them, sniff them, or smoke them (as an estimated 90 to 95 percent of American heroin users in Vietnam did in 1971; [5] see Chapter 20). When the drug cost is high, the same effects are achieved by injecting smaller amounts subcutaneously ("skin-popping") or intravenously ("mainlining"). Such injections, often carried out with crude and unsterile implements, contribute to the risk of infectious disease among addicts. The likelihood of infection is further increased by United States laws making it a crime to possess or sell needles, syringes, or other paraphernalia without a prescription; addicts minimize the risk of arrest by sharing their injection equipment—thus inviting cross-infection.

General Hospital during the 1920s, under the impeccable auspices of the Committee on Drug Addictions of the Bureau of Social Hygiene—a Rockefeller-financed agency—and of the Philadelphia Committee for the Clinical Study of Opium Addiction. In charge were two physicians, Drs. Arthur B. Light and Edward G. Torrance, assisted by a biochemist, Dr. Walter G. Karr, and by Edith G. Fry and William A. Wolff. The results were published by the American Medical Association in the *A.M.A. Archives of Internal Medicine* (1929), and in a book, *Opium Addiction.*[6] The findings of this study are still cited as authoritative in medical textbooks.

In all, 861 male addicts—80 percent of them addicted to heroin and the others to morphine or other opiates—participated in various phases of this study. Most of them were between twenty and forty years of age. They came to the hospital more or less voluntarily (in some cases, no doubt, to escape arrest) for the stated purpose of being "cured." Most of them were criminals and most of them were poor; then as now, affluent addicts did not go to a city hospital for treatment. Here is the broad general conclusion which Dr. Light and his associates reached:

The study shows that morphine addiction is not characterized by physical deterioration or impairment of physical fitness aside from the addiction per se. There is no evidence of change in the circulatory, hepatic, renal or endocrine functions. When it is considered that these subjects had been addicted for at least five years, some of them for as long as twenty years, these negative observations are highly significant.[7]

Details of the study were equally striking. For example, the narcotics addict is popularly portrayed as lean, gaunt, emaciated. A subgroup of about 100 addicts out of the 861 in the Philadelphia study was maintained on adequate doses of morphine and intensively examined and tested while thus maintained. Only four of the 100 were grossly underweight— emaciated. Six of the 100 were grossly overweight—obese. The group as a whole weighed within two-tenths of one percent of the norm for their height and age, as determined by Metropolitan Life Insurance Company standards. Yet these addicts before hospitalization had been taking on the average 21 grains of morphine or heroin per day[8]—more than 30 times the usual dose of the New York City street addict in 1971.

The explanation for the weight findings, which could hardly be more normal, is quite simple. The addicts in the Philadelphia study had ready access to both hospital food and hospital morphine. Under these conditions, they ate well and thrived. The emaciated addict usually described in other studies is one who starves himself to save money for black-market drugs—an ordeal he is able to bear more easily because of the tranquilizing effect of the drugs. The Philadelphia study established that addicts eat like anyone else when both food and drugs are readily available.

The addict is also customarily portrayed as sallow-complexioned. But, Dr. Light and his associates noted, "this change in color was practically always present in patients who lived a rather unhygienic, sedentary life. On the other hand, the skin of those who followed healthy outdoor occupations had the color of excellent health." [9]

The Philadelphia group did notice "a slight degree of anemia" in some of their addicts on admission. This may be present, they added, "when the addict is forced to live in poor hygienic surroundings [and] when all his funds are required to purchase the drug at the expense of sufficient nourishing foods." [10]

Dr. Light and his associates confirmed that 60 percent of the Philadelphia addict group "exhibited a particularly high degree of pyorrhea and dental caries"—but "one must bear in mind that these people are notorious in their lack of care of the teeth and failure to consult a dentist." [11] Malnutrition may also have been a factor. Whatever the cause, there is no evidence that narcotics "rot the teeth." The 1956 British Columbia study also noted a high degree of tooth decay among imprisoned addicts —but found comparable decay in a comparison group of prisoners who were *not* addicted.[12] Perhaps the chief effect of narcotics on the teeth is to enable an addict to bear toothaches uncomplainingly.

Many of the Philadelphia addicts showed chronically inflamed throats and an atypical blood-pressure change when they stood up after lying down. Both of these signs, the Philadelphia researchers noted, are to be expected in excessive cigarette smokers—and all of their narcotics addicts also smoked cigarettes excessively.[13]

A similar study made at Bellevue Hospital in New York City yielded similar findings. Dr. George B. Wallace summed up both studies: "It was shown that continued taking of opium or any of its derivatives resulted in no measurable organic damage. The addict when not deprived of his opium showed no abnormal behavior which distinguished him from a non-addict." [14]

"Since these studies appeared," Dr. Harris Isbell, director of the Public Health Service's Addiction Research Center in Lexington, pointed out in 1958, "it has not been possible to maintain that addiction to morphine causes marked physical deterioration *per se*." [15]

Through the years, this has been the view of authorities familiar with addiction. Thus Dr. Walter G. Karr, the University of Pennsylvania biochemist who participated in the Light-Torrance Study, reported in 1932: "The addict under his normal tolerance of morphine is medically a well man." [16]

In 1940 Dr. Nathan B. Eddy, after reviewing the world literature on morphine to that date, concluded similarly: "Given an addict who is receiving [adequate] morphine . . . the deviations from normal physiological behavior are minor [and] for the most part within the range of normal variations." [17]

Three other authorities who had long worked with heroin addicts from New York City's slums—Drs. Richard Brotman, Alan S. Meyer, and Alfred M. Freedman—had this to add in 1965: "Medical knowledge has long since laid to rest the myth that opiates inevitably and observably harm the body." [18]

Further confirmation of this point was reported in 1967 by a specialist in human metabolism, Dr. Vincent P. Dole of the Rockefeller University, and his wife, Dr. Marie Nyswander, a psychiatrist with broad experience among addicts (see Chapter 14). After examining and testing addicts who had long been addicted to heroin,* Dr. Dole made a significant comparison: "Cigarette smoking is unquestionably more damaging to the human body than heroin." [20]

There is a similar disparity between the popular and the scientific views of the effects of the opiates on the human mind. In 1938, Dr. Lawrence Kolb, Assistant Surgeon General of the United States Public Health Service, and first superintendent of the service's hospital for addicts in Lexington, Kentucky, and Dr. W. F. Ossenfort reported that of more than 3,000 addicts admitted to the hospital at Lexington, not one suffered from a psychosis caused by opiates.[21]

In 1946, Drs. A. Z. Pfeffer and D. C. Ruble compared 600 male addict prisoners at the Lexington hospital with male nonaddict prisoners serving sentences of the same length. Psychoses were no more common among the addicts than among the nonaddicts. Controlled tests showed that there had been no intellectual deterioration due to morphine. Drs. Pfeffer and Ruble concluded: "The data of this study indicate that the habitual use of morphine does not cause a chronic psychosis or an organic type of deterioration." [22]

In 1956 Dr. Marie Nyswander noted similarly: "The incidence of insanity among addicts is the same as in the general population." [23]

Also in 1956, Dr. George H. Stevenson and his British Columbia associates gave complete neurological and psychiatric examinations to imprisoned addicts, and questioned them and their relatives in an attempt

---

* Drs. Dole and Nyswander found a somewhat higher level of white blood cells in the blood of some addicts prior to treatment—an effect others had noted earlier. White blood cells, of course, protect the body from infections; but an excess of them is worrisome because it may be a sign of bone-marrow pathology or of infection somewhere in the body. The bone marrow of these addicts, however, was normal, and no other infection was detected.[19]

to find mental deterioration. They reported: "As to possible damage to the brain, the result of lengthy use of heroin, we can only say that neurologic and psychiatric examinations have not revealed evidence of brain damage. . . . This is in marked contrast to the prolonged and heavy use of alcohol, which in combination with other factors can cause pathologic changes in brains, and reflects such damage in intellectual and emotional deterioration, as well as convulsions, neuritis, and even psychosis." [24]

The British Columbia report continued:

Our psychological studies do not support the common assertion that long continued heroin use produces appreciable psychological deterioration. So far as we can determine, the personality characteristics commonly seen in addicts are assumed to have been largely present before their addiction, and the same characteristics are commonly seen in most recidivist [relapsing] delinquents who do not use narcotic drugs.

Moreover, it is not evident that these personality weaknesses are aggravated or made worse *by addiction as such.* Years of crime, years of prison, years of unemployment, years of anti-social hostility (and society's anti-addict hostility), years of immorality—these can hardly be expected to strengthen a personality and eradicate its weaknesses. If "years of addiction" is added to these other unfavorable behavioral and environmental factors, why should the personality deterioration (if measurable) be attributed to drug addiction as if it were the only responsible factor? [25]

Drs. Harris Isbell and H. F. Fraser of the Public Health Service addiction center in Lexington, Kentucky, reported in 1950: "Morphine does not cause any permanent reduction in intelligence." [26]

The British Columbia group in 1956 went to considerable pains to check this finding. They dug up old child guidance clinic records and other childhood test records that could be compared with tests run on the same subjects following years of addiction to heroin. If a promising child with a high I.Q. turned into a dull adult opiate addict with a low I.Q., opiates might be suspected as the cause of the deterioration. The cases studied, however, pointed in the opposite direction. In a number of cases, addicts who had normal or superior I.Q.'s while addicted were found to have had subnormal I.Q.'s as children. The British Columbia researchers accordingly abandoned this line of investigation, on the ground that "the comparative psychological results were undependable." [27] The British Columbia report also noted: "We found most of the addicts very likeable people. On the whole, they were friendly, cooperative, interested and eager to talk freely and frankly about themselves. Many of them have sensitive minds, are interested in their own psychological reactions and in philosophical problems generally. They were, on the whole, not self-conscious, were self-possessed, courteous and helpful." [28]

In 1962 Dr. Kolb added that "Chronic psychoses as a result of the excessive use of opiates are virtually non-existent." [29]

In 1963, Deputy Commissioner Henry Brill of the New York State Department of Mental Hygiene, chairman of the American Medical Association's narcotics committee, after a survey of 35,000 mental hospital patients, summarized the data in these terms: "In spite of a very long tradition to the contrary, clinical experience and statistical studies clearly prove that psychosis is not one of 'the pains of addiction.' Organic deterioration is regularly produced by alcohol in sufficient amount but is unknown with opiates, and the functional psychoses which are occasionally encountered after withdrawal are clearly coincidental, being manifestations of a latent demonstrable pre-existing condition." [30]

Such views had long been commonly accepted among physicians. "That individuals may take morphine or some other opiate for twenty years or more without showing intellectual or moral deterioration," Dr. Kolb wrote in 1925,

is a common experience of every physician who has studied the subject. . . .

The criterion for lack of deterioration in individuals originally useful and in good standing in the community has been continued employment in useful occupations, the respect of associates, living in conformity with accepted social customs, avoidance of legal prosecution except those brought about by violations of narcotic laws, undiminished mental activity, and unchanged personality, or, when this could not be determined, the possession of a personality that would be considered by psychiatrists to be within the range presented by nervously normal individuals or mild psychoneurotics.

We think it must be accepted that a man is morally and mentally normal who graduates in medicine, marries and raises a family of useful children, practices medicine for thirty or forty years, never becomes involved in questionable transactions, takes a part in the affairs of the community, and is looked upon as one of its leading citizens. The same applies to a lawyer who worked himself up from a poor boy to one of the leading attorneys in his county, who became addicted to morphine following a severe abdominal disease with recurrence and two operations, and who continued to practice his profession with undiminished vigor in spite of his physical malady and the addiction.

Such cases as are cited above, and they are not uncommon, have taken as much as 15 grains [900 milligrams] of morphine daily for years without losing one day's work because of the morphine.[31]

There is thus general agreement throughout the medical and psychiatric literature that the overall effects of opium, morphine, and heroin on the addict's mind and body under conditions of low price and ready availability are on the whole amazingly bland. When we turn from overall effects to detailed effects, however, there is somewhat less unanimity of expert opinion.

Effect on sexual potency and libido.   It is impossible to supply a succinct and authoritative account of the specific effects of opiates—or other drugs—on sexual behavior and response, for two reasons. First, as noted in the Introduction, no psychoactive drug has uniform effects. The effects vary from person to person and from time to time in a specific person. They vary with dose, with the expectations and desires of the user, and with the circumstances surrounding use. Thus one user may report that a drug is a sexual stimulant; another may report that the same drug is a sexual depressant.

Second, nobody has studied the sexual effects of drugs under controlled laboratory conditions. For most drugs, we can hardly even offer an informed guess—except to suggest that the sexual effects (whether favorable or unfavorable) are probably less specific and less impressive than is usually alleged.

With respect to heroin and the other opiates, there is some anecdotal and some survey information. Both male and female addicts generally report that the opiates reduce sexual desire. This is no doubt an unwelcome side effect for many people—though it has also been suggested that some people turn to opiates *because* these drugs shield them from distressing sexual desires.

Many addicts report that the opiates have an effect on male sexual performance which they find desirable; ejaculation is delayed or even blocked altogether, so that coitus can be greatly prolonged or even continued indefinitely. It is said that in India during the nineteenth century this was a major reason for taking opium.

Male sexual potency is retained, at least in part, except when very large doses are taken.*

The addicts studied in the 1956 British Columbia study were highly active sexually—starting at an early age and continuing with many partners—*before* they became addicted. Almost all sexual activity, both before and after addiction, was heterosexual.

"In the heterosexual aspects," the British Columbia group reported, "it is well known that opium and its derivatives exert a mild aphrodisiac action for a time, but after heavy drug use has developed, the heterosexual

---

* Dr. Lawrence Kolb reported (1925): ". . . It was learned from addicts in this series [of 230 cases studied] that [male sexual] potency is not completely abolished until the daily dose of heroin or morphine is 15–30 grains [900 to 1,800 milligrams— $450 to $900 worth per day at 1971 New York City black-market prices]. Desire is reduced by much smaller doses, but considerable potency remains. One thirty-five-year addict raised ten children. Others addicted for years had families of average size, and men beyond sixty who had been addicted twenty years or more reported sexual competency." [32]

urges are less strong and potency is commonly reduced." [33] Forty-nine of
fifty men in the British Columbia study said that narcotics decreased their
libido; [34] the decrease, however, was from a remarkably high pre-addic-
tion level. Among the women, 13 out of 21 reported decreased libido when
on heroin. One, however, reported increased libido, and 7 reported no
change.[35]

A 1970 study revealed that many Philadelphia addicts thought their
sexual functioning was adversely affected while they were on heroin.
The study did not differentiate, however, between the effects of the heroin
itself and the other depressing aspects of the street addict's way of life.[36]

Perhaps the best evidence for a depressant effect of heroin on both
potency and libido is the fact that addicts who complain of reduced libido
and impaired sexual performance while on heroin report prompt improvement when they "kick the habit." In a group of 13 ex-addicts intensively
studied at St. Luke's Hospital in New York City, for example, all "claimed
their sexual problems disappeared during detoxification, whether in hospitals, detention, jails, etc." [37] There are even reports of spontaneous
orgasm in males during withdrawal from opiates. All of the evidence
suggests that heroin temporarily depresses rather than permanently
damages sexual function.

Effect on menstruation. Some women addicts stop menstruating while
on heroin; others report delayed menstruation and other menstrual irregularities. Most observers consider this a direct effect of the heroin—
though Drs. George Blinick, Robert C. Wallach, and Eulogio Jerez, on the
basis of experience with hundreds of young women addicts at the Beth
Israel Medical Center in New York, believe that menstrual irregularities
may result in part at least from the generally stressful life which addicts
lead on the streets of New York. [38]

Effect on likelihood of pregnancy. Women addicts can become pregnant while on heroin, but the likelihood of pregnancy is reduced. How
much of the reduction is due to the heroin itself and how much is traceable to other aspects of being a heroin addict in the United States today
(malnutrition, infection, and so on) is not known.

Effect on childbirth. It is often stated that pregnant addicts suffer "a
high incidence of maternal complications such as toxemia, abruptio
placentae, retained placenta, postpartum hemorrhage, prematurity by
weight, breech delivery, and high neonatal morbidity and mortality." [39]
This may be true. Such complications of pregnancy, however, are also associated with poverty, malnutrition, infection, and lack of prenatal care.
No controlled studies have been made of the relative incidence of complications of pregnancy among addicted and nonaddicted women from
the same neighborhood and socioeconomic status.

The findings of Drs. Blinick, Wallach, and Jerez cast some doubt on the conventional view. They studied 100 consecutive births to addicts at Beth Israel. Many of the mothers suffered from malnutrition, and 18 had positive blood tests for syphilis. Many earned their living by prostitution. Individual mothers also suffered from such conditions unfavorable to a healthy pregnancy as cancer (carcinoma *in situ* of the cervix), rheumatic fever, anemia, hepatitis and other forms of liver disease, epilepsy, and Class A diabetes. One addict had had ten babies; another was over forty years old; many had a history of using other drugs in addition to heroin. Almost all were heavy cigarette smokers. Two had had prior cesarean sections. Despite this concentration of unfavorable antecedent conditions, 88 of the 100 mothers gave uneventful birth to healthy babies.* The chief divergence from normal noted was low birth weight—a condition known to be associated with poverty and with cigarette smoking. Breech deliveries were also frequent; these were probably associated with low birth weight and thus with cigarette smoking and poverty. "In this series, contrary to reports and expectations," the Beth Israel team summed up, "there have been few serious complications." [41]

In a series of 230 babies born at Beth Israel to addicted mothers, only two had congenital defects [42]—a rate which would be considered low in a group of nonaddicted mothers.

Effect on babies born to addicted mothers. Morphine and heroin, like alcohol and nicotine, are believed to pass through the placenta and reach the unborn baby. They are also believed to enter the mother's milk, so that a breast-fed baby is maintained on the drug and is weaned from the drug as it is weaned from the breast. There are numerous reports of withdrawal symptoms in babies who are not breast-fed; and at some hospitals opiates or other drugs are administered if a baby born to an addicted mother exhibits what appear to be opiate withdrawal symptoms.

There is not full agreement, however, on the conventional views summarized above. Thus Drs. Blinick, Wallach, and Jerez have some doubts concerning the passage of opiates to the fetus. "Placental transfer of narcotics prior to and during labor is poorly understood and the conclusions of experimentation are open to doubt," they report.[43]

"The minute amounts of morphine that pass the placenta barrier," Dr. Blinick reported sometime later, "cannot be detected by ordinary biochemical methods." [44] In the Beth Israel series of 100 consecutive births to heroin addicts, it proved unnecessary to administer opiates to the babies. The many reports that such babies require opiates are all based on clinical judgment; no one has divided babies into two groups at random

* The standard test for the condition of a baby at birth, the "one-minute Apgar test," rates such factors as breathing, crying, color, etc. The scale runs from 0 to 10. Eighty-nine of the 100 babies born to heroin addicts had high (8, 9, or 10) Apgar scores.[40]

to see whether babies who receive opiates do better than babies who merely receive good care.

Dr. Saul Blatman, the pediatrician at Beth Israel in charge of the care of the babies in the Blinick-Wallach-Jerez sample, points out that many infants born to heroin addicts, like many born to other ill or poverty-stricken mothers, suffer from low birth weight and other signs of immaturity. The symptoms commonly attributed to heroin "withdrawal" may thus in fact be due to immaturity of the nervous system. Indeed, "when we talk about symptomatology in the baby, we should not label these babies as addicted, because there is no indication that they are." Dr. Blatman similarly urges that the term "withdrawal symptoms" as applied to the babies of addicts "is an unsatisfactory term, which we should eliminate."

Dr. Blatman warns particularly against "standing orders" to administer opiates or other drugs to these babies; where standing orders are in effect, "many of these babies are often 'snowed under' by depressant medication starting soon after birth." While hyperirritable babies born to addicted mothers (like those born to nonaddicted mothers) may need medication—phenobarbital, chlorpromazine, or in some instances paregoric (an opiate)—the treatment should be individualized and matched to each baby's need.[45]

In sum, many babies born to addicted mothers are born in excellent health; others suffer a handicap. How much of this handicap is traceable to the heroin and how much to malnutrition, infection, and other adverse factors has not been determined.

We shall return to these subjects—sexual libido and potency, menstrual functions, pregnancy, and childbirth—in Chapter 16.

Effect on diagnosis of illness. An addict on morphine or heroin can feel and recognize pain. By making him more tolerant of pain, however, an opiate may lead him to postpone seeing a doctor or dentist when pain arises; thus treatment may in some cases be delayed and cure made more difficult or impossible. Poverty, of course, may also delay medical and dental treatment.

Effect on pupils of the eyes. Opiates produce in most users a constriction of the pupils of the eyes, which can decrease ability to see well in the dark. This effect usually persists, even with prolonged use of opiates.

Effect on digestion. The opiates are constipating. Indeed, codeine and opium itself (as tincture of opium or paregoric) are commonly used as a treatment for diarrhea. Some addicts must compensate for this constipating effect by taking a laxative or other aid to elimination; others have no long-term problem. "Street" heroin is sometimes adulterated with mannite, a mild laxative, to counteract the constipating effect.

Effect on stability of mood. A very serious shortcoming of the opiates in common use, morphine and heroin, is their brief period of action. An addict must take his drug two, three, or even four times a day to forestall withdrawal symptoms. Addicts whose supply is uncertain may thus tend to "bounce" from a satisfied to an incipient withdrawal state several times a day.

Effect on sweat glands. Some addicts report profuse perspiration, even after long periods on heroin or other opiates.

Other side effects. Any survey of heroin users turns up a wide variety of other complaints; headaches, joint pains, hiccups, diarrhea, nervousness, running nose, difficulty urinating, and unhappiness were among the side effects reported in a recent Stanford University survey.[46] These reports no doubt result at least in part from the natural human tendency of addicts and nonaddicts alike to attribute whatever happens to whatever drug one currently happens to be taking.

These, then, are the deleterious physiological effects on addicts traceable to the opiates themselves. Those traceable to the narcotics laws, and to the heroin black market flourishing under those laws—including the so-called heroin overdose deaths—will be discussed in Chapter 12.

5.

Some eminent narcotics addicts

The United States Supreme Court's 1962 characterization of the drug addict as "one of the walking dead" can no doubt be illustrated many times over among addicts living under twentieth-century conditions of high opiate prices, vigorous law enforcement, repeated imprisonment, social ignominy, and periodic unavailability of opiates. The court's major error was to attribute the effects it so vividly described to the drugs themselves rather than to the narcotics laws and to the social conditions under which addicts live today. To illustrate, let us consider the effects of opiate addiction on a few distinguished addicts who throughout their lives had adequate access to continuing supplies.

Perhaps the most remarkable case was that of Dr. William Stewart Halsted (1852-1922), one of the greatest of American surgeons. Halsted, the scion of a distinguished New York family, and captain of the Yale football team, entered the practice of medicine in New York in the 1870s and soon became one of the promising young surgeons of the city. Interested in research as well as in performing operations, he was among the first to experiment with cocaine—a stimulant drug similar to our modern amphetamines (see Part V). With a small group of associates, Halsted discovered that cocaine injected near a nerve produces *local anesthesia* in the area served by that nerve. This was the first local anesthetic, and its discovery was a major contribution to surgery.

Unfortunately, Halsted had also injected cocaine into himself numerous times. "Cocaine hunger fastened its dreadful hold on him," Sir Wilder Penfield, another famed surgeon, later noted. "He tried to carry on. But a confused and unworthy period of medical practice ensued. Finally he vanished from the world he had known. Months later he returned to New York but, somehow, the brilliant and gay extrovert seemed brilliant and gay no longer." [1]

What had happened to Halsted during the period of his disappearance? A part of the secret was revealed in 1930, eight years after his death. Then Halsted's closest friend, Dr. William Henry Welch, one of the four distinguished founders of the Johns Hopkins Medical School, stated that he (Welch) had hired a schooner and, with three trusted sailors, had slowly sailed with Halsted to the Windward Islands and back in order to keep Halsted away from cocaine.

The effort was not successful. Halsted relapsed and next went to Butler Hospital in Providence, where he spent several months. Again he relapsed, and again he went to Butler Hospital. Halsted's biographers reported that thereafter he was cured. Through magnificent strength of will, after an epochal struggle, he had cast off his cocaine addiction and gone on to fame and fortune as one of the four distinguished founders of the Hopkins. Or so the story went.

In 1969, however, on the occasion of the eightieth anniversary of the opening of the Johns Hopkins Hospital, a "small black book closed with a lock and key of silver" [2] was opened for the first time. This book contained the "secret history" of the Hopkins written by another of its four eminent founders, Sir William Osler. Sir William revealed that Halsted had cured his cocaine habit by turning to morphine.

Thus Halsted was a morphine addict at the age of thirty-four, when Welch invited him in 1886 to join the distinguished group then laying the foundations for what was soon to become the country's most distinguished medical school. Welch knew, of course, of Halsted's addiction, and therefore gave him only a minor appointment at first. Halsted, however, did so brilliantly that he was soon made chief of surgery and thus joined Osler, Welch, and Billings as one of the Hopkins "Big Four."

"When we recommended him as full surgeon," Osler wrote in his secret history, ". . . I believed, and Welch did too, that he was no longer addicted to morphia. He had worked so well and so energetically that it did not seem possible that he could take the drug and do so much.

About six months after the full position had been given, I saw him in a severe chill [evidently a withdrawal symptom caused by Halsted's seeking to give up morphine once again] and this was the first intimation I had that he was still taking morphia. Subsequently I had many talks about it and gained his full confidence. He had never been able to reduce the amount to less than three grains [180 milligrams] daily; on this he could do his work comfortably and maintain his excellent physical vigor (for he was a very muscular fellow). I do not think that anyone suspected him, not even Welch. [3]

While on morphine Halsted married into a distinguished Southern family; his wife had been head nurse in the operating rooms at the Hopkins. They lived together in "complete mutual devotion" until Halsted's death thirty-two years later.

Halsted's skill and ingenuity as a surgeon during his years of addiction to morphine earned him national and international renown. For Lister's concept of *antisepsis*—measures to kill germs in operation wounds—Halsted substituted *asepsis*: measures to keep germs out of the wound in the first place. In this and other ways, he pioneered techniques for minimizing the damage done to delicate tissues during an operation. Precision became his surgical trademark. A British surgeon, Lord Moynihan, admiringly described the Halsted technique at the operating table as one of "frequently light, swift, sparing movements with the sharpest of knives, instead of free, heavy-handed deep cutting; of no hemorrhage or the minimum of hemorrhage instead of the severance of many vessels, each bleeding freely until clipped." [4] For pioneering improvements such as these, Halsted became widely known as "the father of modern surgery."

In 1898, at the age of forty-six, Osler's secret history notes, Halsted reduced his daily morphine to a grain and a half (90 milligrams) a day. Thereafter the surviving record is silent—though Osler in 1912 expressed a hope that Halsted had "possibly" given up morphine.[5] Halsted died in 1922, at the age of seventy and at the pinnacle of his exacting profession, following a surgical operation. He remained in good health, active, esteemed, and in all probability addicted, until the end.

Unfortunately, we have no physical or psychological test data on Halsted following his decades of addiction to morphine. We do have such data, however, on another addicted physician, known in the medical literature as "Doctor X." A complete case history of Doctor X was published in the *Stanford Medical Bulletin* in 1942 by Dr. Windsor C. Cutting of the Stanford University Medical School.[6] The following account is taken from that report.

Doctor X was born in 1858 and entered medical school in 1878. Two years later he began spitting blood. His illness was diagnosed as tuberculosis, and he was sent home with a bottle of "Scott's Emulsion," to which a quarter of a grain of morphine per dose had been added. Six months later he was well enough to return to medical school—"but found that, when he did not take his prescription, he had a 'craving.'"

To be without the drug for 24 hours made him nervous, sleepless, nauseated, and subject to hot flashes. On the other hand, when he took morphine, he experienced no excitement, but a "delightful sensation of strength—bodily and mentally," and could "concentrate upon [his] work to a remarkable degree." He therefore took morphine by mouth, usually twice a day.

Doctor X graduated from medical school among the top ten members of his class, interned in a large city hospital, and entered practice—first in an Eastern industrial town, later in the Far West. ". . . His addiction caused him little inconvenience," except that he was, like most addicts, constipated. He weighed only 114 pounds at his heaviest—but he was short, and had had tuberculosis. Sometimes he went for a few days, or even weeks, without the drug, but then "suddenly the overpowering desire would come," and he would start taking morphine again.

Doctor X married twice, and had three children. On three occasions he took cures—"but each time returned to the drug after periods of as long as a year. Thus the habit continued over many years."

In 1925, the forty-fifth year of his addiction, Doctor X got into trouble with the authorities for the first time. "His addiction came to the attention of the state board of medical examiners." This meant, of course, that he might lose his license to practice medicine. He therefore took the cure a fourth time—and this time remained abstinent for six years. "Then, during the course of a severe infection, he was given morphine, and has continued taking it until the present [eleven years later]. The average daily dose at present is 2½ grains (150 mg.) taken hypodermically." This is several times the daily dose of a typical New York City addict of the 1970s.

Doctor X continued to practice medicine until he retired at the age of eighty-one, in 1939. Three years later, at the age of eighty-four, he was subjected to a thorough physical examination. Departures from the normal were few for a man of eighty-four in the sixty-second year of his addiction. "The evidence of damage is surprisingly slight," Dr. Cutting summed up, "as regards both physical and mental functions." The only serious disease from which Doctor X suffered was pulmonary emphysema—a disease associated with his cigarette smoking rather than with narcotics addiction.

Psychological tests were administered to the eighty-four-year-old physician by Miss Vee Jane Holt of Stanford. "The evidence is very clear," she wrote,

that Doctor X has been, and is yet, a person of very superior mental ability, even when compared with persons much younger than himself. Scores on the information and comprehension tests . . . are significantly above mean score of persons *in their twenties*—the age level at which intellectual function is generally regarded as maximal—and therefore almost certainly far above those of the average person at his own age level. On the solution of arithmetic problems . . . he did as well as the average person of 45 to 49 years of age.

He did well on several other tests as well. Indeed, he failed only one test. When given a series of five random numbers—such as 5–3–8–2–6—he was able to repeat them forward but not backward. (The reader might try this test on himself.) "This is a typically hard operation for old persons," the psychologist explained.

Another noteworthy case of a distinguished addict was reported in 1962 by Commissioner Harry J. Anslinger of the Federal Bureau of Narcotics. "This addict," Commissioner Anslinger stated, "was one of the most influential members of the United States Congress. He headed one of the powerful committees of Congress. His decisions and statements helped to shape and direct the destiny of the United States and the free world." Commissioner Anslinger heard of this man's addiction, recognized the political damage that might follow exposure, and therefore arranged a continuing supply of drugs for the elderly Congressman from a pharmacy on the outskirts of Washington. When a nationally syndicated columnist got a tip on the story from the pharmacist, Commissioner Anslinger staved off exposure by warning the journalist that "the Harrison Narcotic Act provided a two-year jail term for anyone revealing the narcotic records of a drug store."[7] The Congressman died in office, still legislating, still addicted, and still unexposed.[*]

That many addicts live lives as respectable as those of Dr. Halsted, Dr. X, and Commissioner Anslinger's friend in Congress is well established. In 1950 Dr. Eugene J. Morhous of the Clifton Springs Sanitarium and Clinic in Clifton Springs, New York, reviewed the records of 142 narcotics addicts treated for their addiction at that expensive private institution. The average age of these mid-twentieth-century addicts, as in the nineteenth century, was forty-nine years; the oldest was eighty-one. A substantial proportion of the patients (46.1 percent) were women. The occupations represented are shown below.

Occupation	Number of Patients
Housewife	45
Physician	40
Businessman	13
Physician's wife	6
Nurse	5
Salesman	5
Clerical worker	4
Broker	3
Teacher	3
Druggist	2
Clergyman	2
Mechanic	2
Chemist	1
Actor	1
Composer	1
Dentist	1
Banker	1
Lawyer	1
Undertaker	1
Optician	1
Student	1
Reporter	1
No Occupation	2[9]

---

[*] Commissioner Anslinger also told the story of a Naval Academy graduate who, despite his addiction to narcotics, "held the rank of commander and was co-author of 32 books, some of them best-sellers."[8]

There is little doubt that many addicts today are like those Dr. Morhous described in 1950. The Ad Hoc Panel on Narcotic and Drug Abuse of President Kennedy's 1962 White House Conference on Narcotic and Drug Abuse indicated that "a significant number of persons in the higher socioeconomic classes regularly receive narcotic drugs without detection or apprehension by enforcement agencies." Among its grounds for this belief the Ad Hoc Panel cited "individual reports from public figures, chance findings among hospitalized patients, and comments by practicing physicians." [10]

Incredible as it may seem, even a few poverty-stricken American addicts today make a reasonably successful adjustment to their addiction. "It doesn't happen often," Dr. Marie Nyswander concedes, "but once in a while, one of the so-called vilest addicts in East Harlem finds a doctor who gives him drugs or he gets an easy source from a friend. Under these conditions, he is likely to keep a job, maintain his family intact, and cut out his criminal activity. We see more of this kind of adjustment among middle-class and wealthy addicts who either have a medical disease which gives them a legal excuse for acquiring a regular supply, or who discover a brave doctor. With these people you see no social deterioration. I've yet to see a well-to-do addict arrested." [11]

Referring to today's addicts, Dr. Jerome H. Jaffe—now Director of President Nixon's Special Action Office for Drug Abuse Prevention—has this to say in Goodman and Gilman's textbook (1970):

> The addict who is able to obtain an adequate supply of drugs through legitimate channels and has adequate funds usually dresses properly, maintains his nutrition, and is able to discharge his social and occupational obligations with reasonable efficiency. He usually remains in good health, suffers little inconvenience, and is, in general, difficult to distinguish from other persons.[12]

Dr. Morhous's 1950 study points in the same direction. "A great majority of these persons," Dr. Morhous noted, "were actively engaged in their chosen livelihoods, and some had even made definite upward gains since they had become addicted to narcotic drugs." [13]

The Federal Bureau of Narcotics has through the years insisted that all or substantially all narcotics addicts are criminals who support themselves by preying on society. During testimony before a Senate Committee in 1964, for example, when Federal Narcotics Commissioner Henry Giordano was asked whether addicts can hold jobs and lead useful lives, he replied: "I would say absolutely no. I have never seen any that have been able to efficiently operate while under drugs. This doesn't mean that they can't do some jobs. But the efficiency is impaired and generally they are unable to hold a job. In many cases they are unskilled and it makes it even more difficult." [14]

There is reason to believe, however, that the files of the Federal Bureau of Narcotics itself contain evidence to the contrary. The only occasion, so far as is known, when those files were opened to outsiders was during the 1960s, when a Boston consulting firm, Arthur D. Little, Inc., was employed to make one study of addiction problems for the President's Commission on Crime and another for the National Institute of Mental Health.

In July 1969, Dr. Stephen Waldron of Arthur D. Little, Inc., presented some of the findings of these two studies in testimony before the House Select Committee on Crime. The Federal Bureau of Narcotics files and the Lexington data, he reported, independently led to the same conclusion, that "roughly 30 percent of all the drug abusers actually are legitimate people, in the sense that they have a job which they keep—whether because of, or in spite of, using drugs, it is hard to tell.

They tend to be professional people, doctors and lawyers, quite a number of housewives, some musicians but not too many, people who appear to the outside world to be fairly normal, and people who do not seem to get in trouble with the law, except after long periods of use, when they may get picked up through a contact, or in some cases where they turn themselves in for treatment in the Public Health Service Hospital.[15]

Further confirmation comes from Vietnam, where only slightly adulterated heroin became readily available to members of the United States armed forces during 1970 and 1971. Tens of thousands of young Americans tried it, and thousands became addicted. Despite daily use of doses of heroin far larger than those commonly available in the United States, these men continued to perform their military duties without detection, and in some cases with distinction. Indeed, military personnel addicted to heroin were indistinguishable to their superior officers from their unaddicted comrades-in-arms—so indistinguishable that military authorities found it necessary to introduce urine tests to identify heroin users. Addicted military personnel whose terms of duty expired before the urine tests were introduced sometimes re-enlisted—either while in Vietnam or after sampling civilian life and civilian heroin in the United States—in order to be close to the supply of low-cost, high-quality Vietnam heroin; these addicts were welcomed back into service with open arms, for their addiction was clinically undetectable.[16] (For a further discussion of heroin addiction in Vietnam, see Chapter 20).

But what of the "street addicts," those who earn their living by theft, mugging, prostitution, and petty graft or rackets? For them, heroin has been described as an escape from "psychological problems and from the responsibilities of social and personal relationships—in short, an escape from life." [17] These addicts have been characterized as "passive, anxious, inadequate," [18] and as "retreatists and double failures who cannot qualify for either legitimate or illegitimate careers." [19]

Even with respect to such street addicts, however, there are differences of opinion. The 1956 British Columbia report, for example, observes that the typical street addict finds in heroin

a purpose in an otherwise purposeless life. The activities of the drug addict become a full-time job. Formerly living with no real objective, with indolence and unemployment perhaps intimately related, the addict now finds he has to hustle. If he is going to use drugs steadily he must find each day, by illegal means, the funds for the purchase of his drugs. This usually involves daily thieving, the sale to a "fence" or to beer parlor habitués . . . of the goods he has stolen, the locating of a drug pedlar, negotiating for his supply, then the actual securing of the drugs at a designated time and place, followed by the locating of a presumably secure place where he can inject his drugs and rest and relax for several hours after the injection. He may take his last injection of the day at midnight, having in reserve a supply for his first "fix" the following morning on awakening. A program such as this keeps the addict busy all day. He has no time for boredom. He has barely time enough after each injection to enjoy the effects before he may have to start another phase of this cycle. In other words, the addict now has a job, a full-time job . . . not governed by regular hours as is most legal employment. [20]

A remarkably similar profile of the addict's life on the streets of New York City today, entitled "Taking Care of Business," was presented in the March 1969 issue of the *International Journal of the Addictions* by an anthropologist, Professor Edward A. Preble of the Manhattan State Hospital Drug Addiction Unit, and an economist, John J. Casey, Jr., of Georgetown University. Preble and Casey studied hard-core urban addicts from the heart of New York City's slums—mostly black or Puerto Rican, but with Irish, Italian, and Jewish addicts among them.

Addicts in New York City, Preble and Casey report, are

actively engaged in meaningful activities and relationships seven days a week. The brief moments of euphoria after each administration of a small amount of heroin constitute a small fraction of their daily lives. The rest of the time they are aggressively pursuing a career that is exacting, challenging, adventurous, and rewarding. They are always on the move and must be alert, flexible, and resourceful. The surest way to identify heroin users in a slum neighborhood is to observe the way people walk. The heroin user walks with a fast, purposeful stride, as if he is late for an important appointment—indeed, he is. He is hustling (robbing or stealing), trying to sell stolen goods, avoiding the police, looking for a heroin dealer with a good bag (the street retail unit of heroin), coming back from copping (buying heroin), looking for a safe place to take the drug, or looking for someone who beat (cheated) him—among other things. He is, in short, *taking care of business,* a phrase which is so common with heroin users that they use it in response to words of greeting, such as "how you doing?" and "what's happening?" *Taking care of biz* is the common abbreviation. *Ripping and running* is an older phrase which also refers to their busy lives. For them, if not for their middle and upper class counterparts (a small minority of opiate addicts), the quest for heroin is the quest for a meaningful life, not an escape from life. And the meaning does not lie, primarily, in the effects of the drug on their minds and bodies; it lies in the gratification of accomplishing a series of challenging, exciting tasks, every day of the week.[21]

Typical of the New York street addict, Preble and Casey add, was one who told them: "When I'm on the way home with the bag safely in my pocket, and I haven't been caught stealing all day, and I didn't get beat and the cops didn't get me—I feel like a working man coming home; he's worked hard, but he knows he's done something. . . ." The *feeling* of hard work rewarded by accomplishment, this addict continued, was strong "even though I know it's not true."

"If anyone can be called passive in the slums," Preble and Casey conclude, "it is not the heroin user, but the one who submits to and accepts [slum] conditions."[22]

6.

Opium smoking is outlawed

To summarize the data reviewed so far, opiates taken daily in large doses by addicts were not a social menace under nineteenth-century conditions, and were not perceived as a menace. Opium, morphine, and heroin could be legally purchased without a prescription, and there was little demand for opiate prohibition. But there was one exception to this general tolerance of the opiates. In 1875, the City of San Francisco adopted an ordinance prohibiting the smoking of opium in smoking-houses or "dens." [1]

The roots of this ordinance were racist rather than health-oriented, and were concerned with what today is known as "life-style." Opium smoking was introduced into the United States by tens of thousands of Chinese men and boys imported during the 1850s and 1860s to build the great Western railroads.* The Chinese laborers then drifted into San Francisco and other cities, and accepted employment of various kinds at low wages —giving rise to waves of anti-Chinese hostility. Soon white men and even women were smoking opium side by side with the Chinese, a life-style which was widely disapproved. The San Francisco authorities, we are told, learned upon investigation that "many women and young girls, as well as young men of respectable family, were being induced to visit the [Chinese opium-smoking] dens, where they were ruined morally and

---

* Professor Jonathan Spence of the Department of History, Yale University, presented a fascinating account of opium smoking in nineteenth-century China at the Conference on Local Control and Social Protest during the Ch'ing Period, held at Honolulu, Hawaii, from June 27 to July 2, 1971. He reported, for example, that "opium was highly regarded in China, both as a medicinal drug (that checked diarrhea and served as a febrifuge), and as an aphrodisiac. Therefore people might become addicted either because they took opium intensively during an illness—for instance in the great cholera epidemic of 1821—or because they had vigor, leisure and money and wanted to make the best of it.

"Those who ate regularly and well did not suffer physiologically from their addiction, but for the poor, addiction was a serious health hazard (even though, ironically, it was often first taken for health reasons), since scarce cash resources were put to opium rather than food purchases. The rewards for the poor were a blurring of the pains of prolonged labor, and an increase in work capacity over short periods of time. Thus there was heavy addiction among coolies and chair-bearers, and among such groups as boatmen who had to work their boats upstream, and stone-cutters working out-of-doors in cold weather. The last Chinese to become addicted seem to have been the peasants, though as they grew more opium crops the incidence of heavy opium smoking rose, and by 1902 one could find entire rural communities that were in desperate straits because addiction had become almost total. By the late Ch'ing, it seems that no major occupational group was without its addicts." [2]

otherwise."* [4] The 1875 ordinance followed, "forbidding the practice under penalty of a heavy fine or imprisonment or both. Many arrests were made, and the punishment was prompt and thorough." [5]

This first law, however, like so many subsequent antinarcotics laws, failed to work despite the promptness and thoroughness of the punishment. When opium dens became illegal, "the vice was indulged in much less openly, but none the less extensively, for although the larger smoking-houses were closed, the small dens in Chinatown were well patronized, and the vice grew surely and steadily." [6] Indeed, the new law "seemed to add zest to their enjoyment." [7]

A similar ordinance was passed in Virginia City, Nevada, the following year. [8] This also failed to accomplish its purpose; hence the State of

---

* One white girl of good family and education began opium smoking at sixteen in San Francisco in 1880, later became a prostitute, moved to Victoria, British Columbia, and was found in an opium den in 1884 by a Royal Commission. The transcript of her answers to questions reads, in part:

Q. Why did you commence to smoke opium?
A. Why do people commence to drink? Trouble, I suppose led me to smoke. I think it is better than drink. People who smoke opium do not kick up rows; they injure no one but themselves, and I do not think they injure themselves very much.
Q. . . . Why do you smoke [now]?
A. Because I must; I could not live without it. I smoke partly because of the quiet enjoyment it gives, but mainly to escape from the horrors which would ensue did I not smoke. To be twenty-four hours without smoking is to suffer worse tortures than the lost.
Q. But does not the smoking make you wretched, just as drinking would?
A. No; I require about twelve pipes, then I fall into a state of somnolence and complete rest. When I awake I feel all right, and can attend to fixing-up the house. I am brisk, and can work as well as anybody else. I do not feel sick or nervous, neither have I the inclination to smoke more opium.
Q. Then why do you return to the use of the drug?
A. Ah! that's it; there is a time when my hands fail me; tears fall from my eyes; I am ready to sink; then I come here and for a few bits have a smoke which sets me right. There is too much nonsense talked about opium-smoking. Life without it would be unendurable, I am in excellent health; but, I suppose, every one has their own troubles, and I have mine.
Q. I do not want to be offensive, but are you what is called a fast woman?
A. I am. But you would be greatly mistaken if you imagined that all the women who come here to smoke are of that character. In San Francisco I have known some of the first people visit opium houses, and many respectable people do the same here.
Q. Are women of your class generally addicted to opium-smoking?
A. No; they are more addicted to drink, and drink does them far more harm. Drink excites passions, whereas this allays it; and when a fast woman drinks she goes to ruin pretty quick. . . .
Q. Have you anything else to add . . . ?
A. No; I will say this, though: that if opium houses were licensed as drinking saloons are one need not have to come into such holes as this to smoke. There would be nice rooms with nice couches, and the degradation would be mitigated. At all events I think the government that will not license an opium saloon should shut up public houses and hotels where they sell vitriol for whiskey and brandy, and where men kill themselves with a certainty and a rapidity beyond the power of opium.[3]

Nevada passed a more stringent act a year or two later.[9] Other states and cities voted similar statutes soon after.

When these laws failed as well, Congress took a hand. Before opium can be smoked, it must be specially prepared; and weak opium containing less than the usual amount of morphine is used in its preparation. In 1883, Congress raised the tariff on opium prepared for smoking from $6 to $10 a pound; [10] and in 1887 it prohibited altogether the importation of the kind of weak opium—that containing less than 9 percent morphine—used for preparing smoking opium. The 1887 law also prohibited the importation of opium by Chinese, and a law three years later limited the manufacture of smoking opium to American citizens.[11]

The results of these steps were set forth in a letter dated January 12, 1888, from the Secretary of the Treasury of the United States to the Speaker of the House of Representatives. The effect, he wrote, had been "to stimulate smuggling, extensively practiced by systematic organizations [presumably the Chinese "tongs" or mutual benefit societies] on the Pacific coast. Recently completed facilities for transcontinental transportation have enabled the opium smugglers to extend their illicit traffic to our Northern border. Although all possible efforts have been made by this Department to suppress the traffic, it is found practically impossible to do so." [12]

The law was not changed, however; indeed, the tariff on smoking opium was further increased, from $10 to $12 per pound in 1890. Then, in 1897, it was reduced to $6 a pound—"experience having at last taught that it could not bear a higher rate without begetting an extensive surreptitious manufacture or serious smuggling operations." Following the reduction in the tariff, "the amount that passed through the customs houses . . . progressively increased." [13]

Throughout this period, states and cities continued to pass laws against opium smoking; by 1914 there were twenty-seven such laws in effect.* Yet the amount of smoking opium legally imported continued to rise steadily, as shown in Table 2.[14]

There was a lesson implicit in these import figures. During more than thirty years of city, state, and federal efforts to suppress opium smoking, the amount smoked per year increased sevenfold—without taking account of smuggled supplies.

In 1909, the importation of smoking opium was prohibited altogether.[15] This law was successful in the sense that smoking opium imported through the customhouses fell to zero, but it did not solve the opium-smoking problem. Congress in January 1914 found it necessary to amend the 1909

* Several of these laws also made it a crime to possess a pipe for the smoking of opium—a precedent for later laws prohibiting the possession of hypodermic needles and syringes without a prescription.

Decade	Pounds of Smoking Opium Imported	Number of Smokers Who Could Be Supplied [a]
1860–69	21,176	8,470
1870–79	48,049	19,219
1880–89	85,988	34.395
1890–99	92,462	36,985
1900–09	148,168	59,267

[a] At 2½ pounds per year.

Table 2. Rise in Legal Importation of Opium, 1860–1909.

law [16] and to pass an additional statute imposing a prohibitive tax ($300 per pound) on opium prepared for smoking within the United States.[17] In December 1914 Congress passed the Harrison Narcotic Act, with far broader provisions [18] (see Chapter 8). Yet as late as 1930, according to Federal Narcotics Commissioner Harry J. Anslinger and United States Attorney William F. Tompkins, "opium dens could be found in almost any American city." [19]

One reason for the failure of these anti-opium-smoking laws, and of subsequent antinarcotics laws, appears obvious. They were aimed at private transactions between willing sellers and willing, usually eager, buyers. Thus there were no *complainants*. Other such laws include the Volstead Act, since repealed, which prohibited the sale of alcoholic beverages; the laws against fornication, homosexual acts, and other sexual acts between consenting individuals in private; the laws against gambling; and the drug laws generally. The phrase "crimes without victims" has been applied to such acts; they can more accurately be called "crimes without complainants." It is hard to cite a law aimed at crimes of this class which has had much effect in curbing the behavior aimed at.*

The mere fact that a law fails to achieve its goal fully is of course not a sufficient reason for repealing it; witness the laws against murder. The basic argument against laws creating crimes without complainants must rest on evidence that they not only fail but also, in the process of failing, do more harm than good. Such evidence exists with respect to the laws

---

* "All laws which can be violated without doing any one an injury are laughed at. Nay, so far are they from doing anything to control the desires and passions of men that, on the contrary, they direct and incite men's thoughts the more toward those very objects; for we always strive toward what is forbidden and desire the things we are not allowed to have. And men of leisure are never deficient in the ingenuity needed to enable them to outwit laws framed to regulate things which cannot be entirely forbidden. . . . He who tries to determine everything by law will foment crime rather than lessen it."—Baruch Spinoza (1632–1677).[20]

against opium smoking. For one effect of these laws was to convert opium smokers to more hazardous forms of opiate use.

"Opium smoking is vastly less vicious than morphine-taking," wrote an American authority on opiates, Dr. Charles B. Towns, in 1912.[21]

Dr. Marie Nyswander also commented on opium smoking, in 1956:

There is a pattern of self-limitation or restraint in opium smoking as practiced in countries where it is socially acceptable. It is common for natives of these countries to indulge in opium smoking one night a week, much as Americans may indulge in alcoholic beverages at a Saturday night party. . . . families who accept opium smoking as part of their culture are mindful of its dangers much as we are mindful of the dangers of overindulgence in alcohol.[22]

The reasons for the lesser harmfulness of opium smoking in moderation are not hard to find. The opium used, as noted above, is of a specially weak type containing less than 9 percent morphine. Only about 10 percent of the morphine in this weak opium enters the vapor, and only a portion of the morphine in the vapor enters the human bloodstream when inhaled. Since the opium is heated rather than burned, only smoke-free vapor is inhaled; there are no "tars" or other carcinogens to cause cancer. The so-called "opium smoker" is actually a vapor inhaler. At a very rough estimate, a smoker would have to smoke 300 or 400 grains of opium to get a dose equivalent to the intravenous injection ("mainlining") of one grain of heroin. Even heavy opium smokers actually smoke less than this daily.* And the opium-smoking dose is necessarily spread over a considerable span of time rather than being absorbed into the bloodstream almost instantaneously, as in mainlining. Surely the nineteenth-century enemies of opium smoking did not and could not foresee that the new laws were starting this country down the dismal road from that relatively innocent "vice" to the intravenous injection of heroin—the dominant form of illegal opiate use today; yet that was in fact the sequel.†

* Dr. Charles B. Towns wrote (1912): "The average opium-smoker consuming twenty-five pills a day gets only the equivalent of about a quarter grain [15 milligrams] of morphine taken hypodermically or of a half grain taken by the mouth. A beginner could not smoke a quarter of that quantity. . . ."[23]

† Dr. Lawrence Kolb wrote (1925): "Case 35, now thirty-eight years of age, started smoking opium twenty years ago [in 1905]. After the importation of smoking opium was prevented by law, he used morphine, and when this could no longer be secured, he changed to heroin." [24] This was the common pattern.

7.

The Pure Food and Drug Act of 1906

A major step forward in the control of opiate addiction was taken in 1906, when Congress passed the first Pure Food and Drug Act despite opposition from the patent-medicine interests. The pressures to pass the act were intense—generated by Dr. Harvey W. Wiley and his crusading journalistic followers, notably Samuel Hopkins Adams,[1] who were known as "muckrakers."

The 1906 act required that medicines containing opiates and certain other drugs must say so on their labels.[2] Later amendments to the act also required that the quantity of each drug be truly stated on the label, and that the drugs meet official standards of identity and purity. Thus, for a time the act actually served to safeguard addicts.

The efforts leading to the 1906 act, the act itself and subsequent amendments, and educational campaigns urging families not to use patent medicines containing opiates, no doubt helped curb the making of new addicts. Indeed, there is evidence of a modest decline in opiate addiction from the peak in the 1890s until 1914.[3]

For those already addicted, however, the protection afforded by the 1906 act and by subsequent amendments was short-lived, for in 1914 Congress passed the Harrison Narcotic Act, which cut off altogether the supply of legal opiates to addicts. As a result, the door was opened wide to adulterated, contaminated, and misbranded black-market narcotics of all kinds. The heroin available on the street in the United States today, for example, is a highly dangerous mixture of small amounts of heroin with large and varying amounts of adulterants. The black market similarly distributes today large quantities of adulterated, contaminated, and misbranded LSD and other drugs. The withdrawal of the protection of the food-and-drug laws from the users of illicit drugs, as we shall show, has been one of the significant factors in reducing addicts to their present miserable status, and in making drug use so damaging today.

8.

The Harrison Narcotic Act (1914)

Through most of the nineteenth and early twentieth centuries, the anti-alcohol forces in the United States were gaining ground. The anti-opiate forces, in contrast, remained weak and poorly organized. Why, then, did opiate prohibition precede alcohol prohibition by five years?

After the Spanish-American War, when the United States War Department took over the chore of governing the Philippine Islands, it inherited a whole system for licensing narcotics addicts and supplying them with opium legally—a system established under Spanish rule. A War Department Commission of Inquiry was appointed under the Right Reverend Charles H. Brent, Episcopal Bishop of the Philippine Islands, to study alternatives to the Spanish system. After taking evidence on programs of narcotics control throughout the Far East, the Brent Commission recommended that narcotics should be subject to international rather than merely national control.[1]

This proposal struck a responsive chord in the United States State Department. For many years, Britain had been criticized for shipping opium grown in India into China; indeed, two nineteenth-century "opium wars" between Britain and China had been fought over this issue. Many Chinese saw opium from India as unfair cut-rate competition for their home-grown product. American missionaries in China complained that British opium was ruining the Chinese people; American traders similarly complained that the silver bullion China was trading for British opium could better be traded for other, perhaps American, products.* The agitation against British opium sales to China continued unabated after 1900. Thus the United States State Department saw a way not only to solve the War Department's Philippine opium problem but also to please American missionaries and traders. President Theodore Roosevelt in 1906, at the request of Bishop Brent, called for an international opium conference, which was held in Shanghai in 1909. A second conference was held at The Hague in 1911, and out of it came the first international opium agreement, The Hague Convention of 1912, aimed primarily at solving the opium problems of the Far East, especially China.

It was against this background that the Senate in 1914 considered the Harrison narcotic bill. The chief proponent of the measure was Secretary

* Some American traders also sent opium into China on a small scale.[2] Some of New England's world-renowned "China clippers" were in fact opium clippers.

of State William Jennings Bryan, a man of deep prohibitionist and missionary convictions and sympathies. He urged that the law be promptly passed to fulfill United States obligations under the new international treaty.[3]

The supporters of the Harrison bill said little in the Congressional debates (which lasted several days) about the evils of narcotics addiction in the United States. They talked more about the need to implement The Hague Convention of 1912. Even Senator Mann of Mann Act fame, spokesman for the bill in the Senate, talked about international obligations rather than domestic morality.

On its face, moreover, the Harrison bill did not appear to be a prohibition law at all. Its official title was "An Act to provide for the registration of, with collectors of internal revenue, and to impose a special tax upon all persons who produce, import, manufacture, compound, deal in, dispense, sell, distribute, or give away opium or coca leaves, their salts, derivatives, or preparations, and for other purposes."[4] The law specifically provided that manufacturers, importers, pharmacists, and physicians prescribing narcotics should be licensed to do so, at a moderate fee. The patent-medicine manufacturers were exempted even from the licensing and tax provisions, provided that they limited themselves to "preparations and remedies which do not contain more than two grains of opium, or more than one-fourth of a grain of morphine, or more than one-eighth of a grain of heroin . . . in one avoirdupois ounce."[5] Far from appearing to be a prohibition law, the Harrison Narcotic Act on its face was merely a law for the orderly marketing of opium, morphine, heroin, and other drugs—in small quantities over the counter, and in larger quantities on a physician's prescription. Indeed, the right of a physician to prescribe was spelled out in apparently unambiguous terms: "Nothing contained in this section shall apply . . . to the dispensing or distribution of any of the aforesaid drugs to a patient by a physician, dentist, or veterinary surgeon registered under this Act in the course of his professional practice only."[6] Registered physicians were required only to keep records of drugs dispensed or prescribed. It is unlikely that a single legislator realized in 1914 that the law Congress was passing would later be deemed a prohibition law.

The provision protecting physicians, however, contained a joker— hidden in the phrase, "in the course of his professional practice only."[7] After passage of the law, this clause was interpreted by law-enforcement officers to mean that a doctor could not prescribe opiates to an addict to maintain his addiction. Since addiction was not a disease, the argument went, an addict was not a patient, and opiates dispensed to or prescribed for him by a physician were therefore not being supplied "in the course of his professional practice." Thus a law apparently intended to ensure the orderly marketing of narcotics was converted into a law prohibiting the supplying of narcotics to addicts, *even on a physician's prescription.*

Many physicians were arrested under this interpretation, and some were convicted and imprisoned. Even those who escaped conviction had their careers ruined by the publicity. The medical profession quickly learned that to supply opiates to addicts was to court disaster.

The effects of this policy were almost immediately visible. On May 15, 1915, just six weeks after the effective date of the Harrison Act, an editorial in the *New York Medical Journal* declared:

As was expected . . . the immediate effects of the Harrison antinarcotic law were seen in the flocking of drug habitués to hospitals and sanitoriums. Sporadic crimes of violence were reported too, due usually to desperate efforts by addicts to obtain drugs, but occasionally to a delirious state induced by sudden withdrawal. . . .

The really serious results of this legislation, however, will only appear gradually and will not always be recognized as such. These will be the failures of promising careers, the disrupting of happy families, the commission of crimes which will never be traced to their real cause, and the influx into hospitals for the mentally disordered of many who would otherwise live socially competent lives.[8]

Six months later an editorial in *American Medicine* reported:

Narcotic drug addiction is one of the gravest and most important questions confronting the medical profession today. Instead of improving conditions the laws recently passed have made the problem more complex. Honest medical men have found such handicaps and dangers to themselves and their reputations in these laws . . . that they have simply decided to have as little to do as possible with drug addicts or their needs. . . . The druggists are in the same position and for similar reasons many of them have discontinued entirely the sale of narcotic drugs. [The addict] is denied the medical care he urgently needs, open, above-board sources from which he formerly obtained his drug supply are closed to him, and he is driven to the underworld where he can get his drug, but of course, surreptitiously and in violation of the law. . . .

Abuses in the sale of narcotic drugs are increasing. . . . A particular sinister sequence . . . is the character of the places to which [addicts] are forced to go to get their drugs and the type of people with whom they are obliged to mix. The most depraved criminals are often the dispensers of these habit-forming drugs. The moral dangers, as well as the effect on the self-respect of the addict, call for no comment. One has only to think of the stress under which the addict lives, and to recall his lack of funds, to realize the extent to which these . . . afflicted individuals are under the control of the worst elements of society. In respect to female habitués the conditions are worse, if possible. Houses of ill fame are usually their sources of supply, and one has only to think of what repeated visitations to such places mean to countless good women and girls— unblemished in most instances except for an unfortunate addiction to some narcotic drug—to appreciate the terrible menace.[9]

In 1918, after three years of the Harrison Act and its devastating effects, the secretary of the treasury appointed a committee to look into the problem. The chairman of the committee was Congressman Homer T. Rainey; members included a professor of pharmacology from Harvard, a former deputy commissioner of internal revenue responsible for law enforcement, and Dr. A. G. Du Mez, Secretary of the United States Public Health Service. This was the first of a long line of such committees appointed through the years. Among its findings [10] were the following:

- Opium and other narcotic drugs (including cocaine, which Congress had erroneously labeled as a narcotic in 1914) were being used by about a million people.*
- The "underground" traffic in narcotic drugs was about equal to the legitimate medical traffic.
- The "dope peddlers" appeared to have established a national organization, smuggling the drugs in through seaports or across the Canadian or Mexican borders—especially the Canadian border.
- The wrongful use of narcotic drugs had increased since passage of the Harrison Act. Twenty cities, including New York and San Francisco, had reported such increases. (The increase no doubt resulted from the migration of addicts into cities where black markets flourished.)

To stem this apparently rising tide, the 1918 committee, like countless committees since, called for sterner law enforcement. It also recommended more state laws patterned after the Harrison Act.[11]

Congress responded by tightening up the Harrison Act. In 1924, for example, a law was enacted prohibiting the importation of heroin altogether, even for medicinal use. This legislation grew out of the widespread misapprehension that, because of the deteriorating health, behavior, and status of addicts following passage of the Harrison Act and the subsequent conversion of addicts from morphine to heroin, heroin must be a much more damaging drug than opium or morphine. In 1925, Dr. Lawrence Kolb reported on a study of both morphine and heroin addiction: "If there is any difference in the deteriorating effects of morphine and heroin on addicts, it is too slight to be determined clinically."[12] President Johnson's Committee on Law Enforcement and Administration of Justice came to the same conclusion in 1967: "While it is . . . somewhat

* This was almost certainly an overestimate; see Chapter 9.

more rapid in its action, heroin does not differ in any significant pharmacological effect from morphine." [13]

The 1924 ban on heroin did not deter the conversion of morphine addicts to heroin. On the contrary, heroin ousted morphine almost completely from the black market *after* the law was passed.

An editorial in the *Illinois Medical Journal* for June 1926, after eleven years of federal law enforcement, concluded:

The Harrison Narcotic law should never have been placed upon the Statute books of the United States. It is to be granted that the well-meaning blunderers who put it there had in mind only the idea of making it impossible for addicts to secure their supply of "dope" and to prevent unprincipled people from making fortunes, and fattening upon the infirmities of their fellow men.

As is the case with most prohibitive laws, however, this one fell far short of the mark. So far, in fact, that instead of stopping the traffic, those who deal in dope now make double their money from the poor unfortunates upon whom they prey. . . .

The doctor who needs narcotics used in reason to cure and allay human misery finds himself in a pit of trouble. The lawbreaker is in clover. . . . It is costing the United States more to support bootleggers of both narcotics and alcoholics than there is good coming from the farcical laws now on the statute books.

As to the Harrison Narcotic law, it is as with prohibition [of alcohol] legislation. People are beginning to ask, "Who did that, anyway?" [14]

By 1936, twenty-two years after passage of the Harrison Act, an outstanding police authority had reached the same conclusion. He was August Vollmer, former chief of police in Berkeley, California, former professor of police administration at the Universities of Chicago and California, author of a leading textbook on police science, and past president of the International Association of Chiefs of Police. Chief Vollmer wrote:

Stringent laws, spectacular police drives, vigorous prosecution, and imprisonment of addicts and peddlers have proved not only useless and enormously expensive as means of correcting this evil, but they are also unjustifiably and unbelievably cruel in their application to the unfortunate drug victims. Repression has driven this vice underground and produced the narcotic smugglers and supply agents, who have grown wealthy out of this evil practice and who, by devious methods, have stimulated traffic in drugs. Finally, and not the least of the evils associated with repression, the helpless addict has been forced to resort to crime in order to get money for the drug which is absolutely indispensable for his comfortable existence. . . .

Drug addiction, like prostitution and like liquor, is not a police problem; it never has been and never can be solved by policemen. It is first and last a medical problem, and if there is a solution it will be discovered not by police-men, but by scientific and competently trained medical experts whose sole objective will be the reduction and possible eradication of this devastating appetite. There should be intelligent treatment of the incurables in outpatient clinics, hospitalization of those not too far gone to respond to therapeutic measures, and application of the prophylactic principles which medicine applies to all scourges of mankind.[15]

Perhaps the most eloquent and most persistent critic of our narcotics laws, Professor Alfred R. Lindesmith, Indiana University sociologist, had this to say in 1940:

Solemn discussions are carried on about lengthening the addict's already long sentence and as to whether or not he is a good parole risk. The basic question as to why he should be sent to prison at all is scarcely mentioned. Eventually, it is to be hoped that we shall come to see, as most of the civilized countries of the world have seen, that the punishment and imprisonment of addicts is as cruel and pointless as similar treatment for persons infected with syphilis would be. . . .

The treatment of addicts in the United States today is on no higher plane than the persecution of witches of other ages, and like the latter it is to be hoped that it will soon become merely another dark chapter of history.[16]

In 1953, Rufus King, Esq., chairman of the American Bar Association's committee on narcotics,* summed up his personal views in the *Yale Law Journal:*

The true addict, by universally accepted definitions, is totally enslaved to his habit. He will do anything to fend off the illness, marked by physical and emotional agony, that results from abstinence. So long as society will not traffic with him on any terms, he must remain the abject servitor of his vicious nemesis, the peddler. The addict *will* commit crimes—mostly petty offenses like shop-lifting and prostitution—to get the price the peddler asks. He *will* peddle dope and make new addicts if those are his master's terms. Drugs are a commodity of trifling intrinsic value. All the billions our society has spent enforcing criminal measures against the addict have had the sole practical result of protecting the peddler's market, artificially inflating his prices, and keeping his profits fantas-tically high. No other nation hounds its addicts as we do, and no other nation faces anything remotely resembling our problem.[17]

In 1957, Dr. Karl M. Bowman, one of this country's foremost psychi-atrists and authorities on narcotics, concluded similarly:

For the past 40 years we have been trying the mainly punitive approach; we have increased penalties, we have hounded the drug addict, and we have

* And author, in 1972, of *The Drug Hang-up: America's Fifty-Year Folly* (Norton).

brought out the idea that any person who takes drugs is a most dangerous criminal and a menace to society. We have perpetuated the myth that addiction to opiates is the great cause of crimes of violence and of sex crimes. In spite of the statements of the most eminent medical authorities in this country and elsewhere, this type of propaganda still continues, coming to a large extent from the enforcement bureaus of federal and state governments. Our whole dealing with the problem of drug addiction for the past 40 years has been a sorry mess.[18]

Also in 1957, Dr. Robert S. de Ropp, biochemist and writer on mind-affecting drugs, added this comment:

Just why the alcoholic is tolerated as a sick man while the opiate addict is persecuted as a criminal is hard to understand. There is, in the present attitude of society in the United States toward opiate addicts, much the same hysteria, superstition, and plain cruelty as characterized the attitude of our forefathers toward witches. Legislation reflects this cruelty and superstition. Prison sentences up to 40 years are now being imposed and the death sentence has been introduced. Perhaps one should feel thankful that the legislators have not yet reached the point of burning addicts alive. If one insists on relying on terrorism to cope with a problem which is essentially medical one may as well be logical and "go the whole hog." [19]

In 1958, a study of the narcotics problem published by the Joint Committee on Narcotic Drugs of the American Bar Association and American Medical Association declared:

Stringent law enforcement has its place in any system of controlling narcotic drugs. However, it is by no means the complete answer to American problems of drug addiction. In the first place it is doubtful whether drug addicts can be deterred from using drugs by threats of jail or prison sentences. The belief that fear of punishment is a vital factor in deterring an addict from using drugs rests upon a superficial view of the drug addiction process and the nature of drug addiction. . . . The very severity of law enforcement tends to increase the price of drugs on the illicit market and the profits to be made therefrom. The lure of profits and the risks of the traffic simply challenge the ingenuity of the underworld peddlers to find new channels of distribution and new customers, so that profits can be maintained. . . .[20]

Dr. Jerome H. Jaffe remarked in the 1965 edition of Goodman and Gilman's textbook:

. . . Much of the ill health, crime, degeneracy, and low standard of living are the result not of drug effects, but of the social structure that makes it a criminal act to obtain or to use opiates for their subjective effects. . . . It seems reasonable to wonder if providing addicts with a legitimate source of drugs might not be worthwhile, even if it did not make them our most productive citizens and did not completely eliminate the illicit market but resulted merely in a marked reduction in crime, disease, social degradation, and human misery.[21]

9.

"Tightening up" the Harrison Act

Very few countries followed the United States policy of relying on prohibition laws to curb the narcotics menace. But Canada did, and so did the forty-eight states and the Canadian provinces. The failure of those prohibition laws did not lead to a change in policy. Instead, newer and stricter laws were enacted. By 1970, Congress had passed 55* federal drug laws to supplement the 1914 Harrison Act.[1] A list of the antinarcotics laws voted by the fifty state legislatures would run far into the hundreds. Canada's Parliament and provincial legislatures similarly amended old laws and passed new ones over the years.[2]

Many of the United States federal and state laws, and the Canadian laws, were passed to stiffen the penalties for narcotics offenses. The maximum penalty specified in the three 1909 federal laws was two years' imprisonment. The 1914 Harrison Act increased this maximum to five years. In 1922 a maximum federal penalty of ten years' imprisonment was enacted.† Subsequently state laws were stiffened to provide twenty-year, forty-year, and even ninety-nine-year maximum sentences. Life imprisonment and the death sentence were added to both federal and some state antinarcotics laws during the 1950s.

Increased maximums, however, did not curb the narcotics black market. The chief effect of such penalties appeared to be as a kind of tranquilizer or opiate on public opinion, persuading the public that severe measures were at last being taken against addiction.

When high maximum sentences failed, "softhearted" judges, unwilling to invoke the maximum penalties, were blamed. In fact, few offenders actually drew maximum sentences. Hence federal laws, many state laws, and the Canadian laws were amended to provide high mandatory *minimum* sentences. Under these laws, a judge could not levy a lesser sentence after a defendant pleaded guilty or was convicted. Neither probation nor a suspended sentence was allowed.‡

---

* This number, moreover, is incomplete in a significant respect. It excludes the Volstead (Alcohol Prohibition) Act of 1919—and the many subsequent laws designed to stamp out the drinking of alcohol between 1920 and 1933, when alcohol was also an illicit drug.

† In 1922, Canada added whippjng and deportation to its penalties.[3]

‡ The extreme mandatory punishment provision was enacted in Connecticut in 1955; it decreed that a judge *must* impose life imprisonment for a third offense—even if all three offenses were merely for possession of a narcotic (or marijuana).[4] Referring to similar Canadian proposals, the 1956 British Columbia report noted: "One is im-

Dr. Stanley Yolles, then director of the National Institute of Mental Health, testified against mandatory minimum sentences before the House Select Committee on Crime in the fall of 1969:

This type of law has no place in a system devised to control an illness. It has no place being used for individuals who are addicted to drugs.

This type of law angers us as doctors, because it should not apply to people who are sick. It destroys hope on the part of the person sentenced—hope of help, hope for starting a fresh life. It's totally contradictory to the whole concept of medicine. A prison experience is often psychologically shattering. The young person is exposed to sexual assault. He may for the first time in his life learn criminal ways. Such mandatory sentences *destroy* the prospects of rehabilitation.

. . . I feel that judges have to be free to deal with violators of drug laws as individuals, not as a class of criminals. In my field, treatment is always tailored to the individual's needs. I feel the same should be true in dealing, under the law, with addicts and drug abusers. Why on earth must we class the street addict, who sells to support his habit, with the big operator who pushes the narcotics wholesale? The former is a sick person who needs medical help and rehabilitation. The latter is a criminal who is living off the misery of the addicts. Many laws on the books don't allow for this distinction.

As a result, what we have in our prisons and Federal hospitals, like Lexington, are many young people serving *irrationally* long sentences, some up to 20 years. In no other field has there been such a punitive approach. And let's not forget this is an illness mainly of young people—the very age group with the highest potential for rehabilitation, yes, and cure.

These laws came about by sometimes well-intentioned people who placed too much confidence in the principle of deterrents. But if mandatory penalties were that effective, what is the rationale for limiting them only to drug abuse offenders? Why not extend them to thieves, burglars, murderers? Even murderers with life sentences can come up for parole after about seven years.[6]

Soon after this testimony, the acting chairman of the House subcommittee before which Dr. Yolles had testified—Congressman Albert Watson of South Carolina—stated on the floor of the House:

"Dr. Yolles's views are an affront to every decent, law-abiding citizen in America. At a time when we are on the verge of a narcotics crisis, a supposedly responsible Federal official comes along with the incredibly ridiculous idea of dropping mandatory jail sentences for those who push dope, even for those adults selling hard drugs to minors."[7]

In a subsequent interview, Congressman Watson added: "I have called for [Dr. Yolles's] resignation because of the simple belief that it's too much to ask the American taxpayer to pay the salary of any individual

---

pressed with the fact that imprisonment, even for life, is recommended for certain people because they prefer heroin to alcohol!"[5]

who publicly espouses a position which we consider so detrimental in our fight to control the drug abuse problem. . . ." [8]

When mandatory minimum sentences failed to close down the black markets, "softhearted" parole boards were blamed. Congress and a number of state legislatures accordingly passed laws depriving narcotics law violators of eligibility for parole * or time off for good behavior. An addict sentenced to life imprisonment under these no-mitigation-of-sentence laws would actually have to spend the rest of his life in prison.

The first addict sentenced to life imprisonment under the federal no-mitigation law was twenty-one years old, born in Mexico, epileptic, with an I.Q. of 69. He had recently been released after fourteen months in a California state mental hospital. His offense was selling small amounts of heroin to another addict—a seventeen-year-old employed as a stool pigeon by the Federal Bureau of Narcotics.[9] It was the defendant's first federal offense, and his first narcotics offense. Fortunately, the Constitution gives the President the power—which Congress cannot take away—"to grant reprieves and pardons." President John F. Kennedy reduced this and a number of similar sentences.

What have been the accomplishments during the past half-century of the legal provisions described here and in the next few pages? The fact is that the use of such methods has not made heroin unavailable or even difficult to secure. The main accomplishment of law enforcement has been to raise black-market prices.

At times, law-enforcement officials have pointed with pride to this achievement. Thus Federal Narcotics Commissioner Harry J. Anslinger and United States Attorney William F. Tompkins noted in 1952 that heroin, which had been available in the United States during the early 1920s at $25 to $50 an ounce, and which was still available in Turkey at $100 an ounce, was currently selling in the United States at $3,000 an ounce.[10] More recently, however, even law-enforcement officials have come to realize that this price escalation is at best a mixed blessing. As one New York City police precinct commander told a New York *Times* reporter in September 1969, when prices increase, addicts simply steal more.[11]

Another common explanation of the failure of the most Draconian laws to close down or even seriously to curtail the black market concerned the difficulties of securing a conviction in court. Hence various laws have been passed and legal principles developed to make conviction of narcotics offenders surer and easier. A typical example is the way in which the verb "to sell" and the noun "sale" have been legally redefined.

One state court, for example, has held that "The 'sale' of narcotics

*Depriving addicts of parole eligibility meant that at the end of their terms they were simply turned loose on the streets without even nominal parole supervision.

prohibited by criminal statutes is much broader in scope than the concept of a sale which obtains in other branches of the law. It may include a transfer by gift as well as one for consideration in money." [12]

Another opinion holds that "a mere gift" or even "an offer to sell" constitutes a sale if the product in question is narcotics, "notwithstanding the fact that no consideration is paid or that the sale is not fully completed by payment of the agreed price." * [13]

Another device to make conviction easier is embodied in a series of state and federal laws designed to shift the burden of proof in narcotics cases from the prosecution to the defense. A 1922 federal law and some similar state laws, for example, provide that the prosecution need not prove that the defendant is in illegal possession of narcotics; the burden is on the defendant to prove that his possession is legal.† Similarly, various "presumptions of law" have been built into the narcotics statutes. In a trial for possession of heroin, for example, it is a "presumption of law" (which the defendant must rebut if he can) that the heroin was smuggled into the country, and that the smuggling occurred after passage of the law prohibiting the importation of heroin.

Under some state laws, an *intent to provide narcotics* to a minor is punishable by imprisonment—even though no narcotics are in fact provided. And New York State has made it a crime to "loiter for the purpose of using narcotics," even though no narcotics are used, and even though the actual use of narcotics is not a crime.[16]

Conviction is also made easier by a wide range of laws making narcotic offenses out of ancillary matters—such as selling, or buying, or even possessing without a prescription a hypodermic syringe, or needle, or other equipment for the administration of narcotics. Hundreds of persons each year in New York City alone are convicted of such "narcotic offenses."

When these and other efforts to make narcotics convictions easier failed to curb the black market, various "status laws" were enacted. These laws made it a crime merely to *be* an addict; it was not even necessary to possess a drug or a syringe in order to be sentenced to imprisonment. At this point, however, the Supreme Court called a halt; it ruled in 1962 that imprisonment merely for being an addict was cruel and unusual punishment prohibited by the Bill of Rights to the Constitution.‡ [17]

---

* A 1927 Canadian law included under "sale" the sale of substances represented to be narcotics—even if they were innocent substances.[14]

† "Whenever on trial for a violation of this subsection the defendant is shown to have or to have had possession of the narcotic drug, such possession shall be deemed sufficient evidence to authorize conviction unless the defendant explains the possession to the satisfaction of the jury." [15]

‡ The 1962 decision did not, however, remove the taint of criminality from addiction. Both *purchase* and *possession* of narcotics can still be punished, in part on the

New York, California, and the federal government have since gotten around this decision by imprisoning ("confining") defendants in closed institutions called "rehabilitation centers." The imprisonment procedure is called "civil commitment," thus avoiding constitutional restraints.

The laws making *conviction* of narcotics offenders easier have been accompanied by laws making the *arrest* of narcotics suspects easier. If a policeman suspects a man, for example, of having committed a narcotics offense, he can arrest him without a warrant. Ordinarily search warrants may be served only by day; a special provision of some narcotics laws makes it legal to serve a narcotics search warrant at any hour of the night as well. The Nixon administration's 1970 "no-knock law," permitting narcotics agents under certain circumstances to enter private premises without knocking, was merely the most recent of these many futile efforts to curb narcotics addiction by facilitating arrests.

All of the above approaches are based on a simple premise: that arresting, convicting, and imprisoning a narcotics addict will deter him and others from using narcotics. The 1956 British Columbia study provides cogent evidence against this premise.

On the basis of many kinds of data, Dr. Stevenson and his associates demonstrated that about 900 addicts were subject to criminal sanctions in British Columbia in 1955.[18] (Doctors, nurses, and other health professionals, whose addiction was associated with easy access to narcotics, as well as those addicted through medical treatment, were excluded from the total, since they were less harshly punished in Canada at that time.) Of the 900 arrestable addicts, 516 were sentenced to prison between September 1, 1954, and April 15, 1956—a period of 19½ months. Quite a few, indeed, were sentenced two or even three times during that brief period —so that the total number of prison sentences imposed came to 755. And quite a few of the 900 addicts were immune from arrest and conviction during the 19½ months of the study because they spent the entire period in prison.

Of 100 consecutive addicts admitted to prison during the last three months of the study, 56 had been imprisoned at least once before during the previous 16½ months. Indeed, among these 100 convicted addicts, only *three* were serving their first term, "many of the remainder having had from five to twenty previous convictions."[19]

On an average day, the British Columbia report continued, 550 of the province's 900 addicts were in prison. Thirty-two narcotics officers were

---

theory that anyone possessing narcotics is *in a position* to sell them. It is, of course, impossible to take a narcotic without first possessing it. At most, the 1962 Supreme Court decision changes the kind of evidence which the police must assemble to secure the criminal conviction of an addict.

employed full time in suppressing the narcotics traffic—an average of one full-time narcotics officer for every eleven addicts at large. Yet the number of addicts did not decrease. Not a few addicts, the report noted, were "again sentenced to prison only a few weeks after completing penitentiary sentences of two to five years." [20] Imprisonment, in short—even on so intensive a scale as this—is not a cure for addiction, or even an effective deterrent. Nor is a ratio of one full-time narcotics officer for every eleven addicts sufficient to curb a black market.

Statistics for cities in the United States are rarely so complete or so reliable, but they point in the same direction. A recent example is New York City, where the police department markedly stepped up its anti-narcotic activities during the first ten months of 1969. The number of men assigned to the narcotics division was increased from 340 to 500; all other members of the force were instructed to be on the alert for narcotics offenses; and other new measures were introduced. The results were superficially impressive: narcotics arrests rose from 18,764 during the first ten months of 1968 to 27,868 during the first ten months of 1969—a rise of almost 50 percent.

When David Burnham of the New York *Times* interviewed police officials concerned with the narcotics drive, however, he found little optimism. The officials told Burnham they found "no evidence that the increased police effort was having much of an impact on the availability of drugs."

"The only way you would know the increased arrests were really making a dent is if there was a drug panic on the street—which there isn't," Burnham quoted one police official as explaining. "The use of illegal drugs is almost completely a medical problem, which the police are unable to handle. But until the public comes to understand this fact, we'll continue to go through the motions." [21]

Another police official added: "You could have 100,000 cops and not stop the drugs."

In 1971, another antinarcotics drive was launched in New York City; but by September of that year its failure was generally admitted. Nine hundred pounds of heroin—nearly 40 million 10-milligram doses—had been seized in New York between May and September, United States Attorney Whitney North Seymour, Jr., announced. This was nearly three times the total amount of heroin seized by the United States Bureau of Customs at all borders during the entire year ending June 30, 1970. But the heightened law-enforcement efforts and the vast increase in heroin seizures had not made "the slightest ripple" in the heroin supply of the metropolitan area. Prices had not gone up. "The suppliers are able to meet the demand regardless of what we do on the law-enforcement part," Mr. Seymour was quoted as saying.[22]

The same has been true with only temporary exceptions ever since 1914. Indeed, after more than a half-century of intensive law-enforcement efforts, this "success" can be claimed: while the population has doubled, the number of addicts has apparently increased only moderately.

During the ten years following passage of the Harrison Act, estimates of the number of opiate addicts in the United States at the time it was passed ranged from 100,000 to 1,000,000. Opponents of the Harrison Act argued that there were only 100,000 addicts or so before 1914 and that addiction was on the increase; proponents of the law alleged that there had been a million addicts before 1914 and that the number was declining. Neither group offered evidence to support its figures.

In 1924 the United States Public Health Service published the estimate of Drs. Lawrence Kolb and A. G. Du Mez. In contrast to others, Kolb and Du Mez collected and studied reliable data from citywide and statewide surveys, from duties paid on opiate imports, from examination of military recruits, and from other sources. They were able to demonstrate that the number of opiate addicts in the United States prior to the Harrison Act was certainly less than 246,000, and probably in the vicinity of 215,000.[23]

With respect to the number of opiate addicts in the United States in 1971, most estimates start with the number of "active" addicts "known to the Bureau of Narcotics and Dangerous Drugs." This number stood at 68,864 on December 31, 1970, up from 68,088 a year earlier. This, of course, is a woeful understatement; in some cities more addicts have applied for methadone maintenance treatment of their addiction (see Chapter 14) than are found on the bureau list for those cities. The question is by what factor the bureau list must be multiplied to achieve a realistic estimate.

Using what it calls a "capture-recapture method," the Federal Bureau of Narcotics and Dangerous Drugs concluded in 1971: ". . . It is virtually certain that the number of addicts in 1969 falls somewhere between 285,000 and 345,000. The best estimate of the number of addicts for that year is 315,000." [24] The estimate of the National Institute of Mental Health in 1971, based on a wide range of data, was 250,000 addicts.[25] In this Report, we use both the bureau and NIMH estimates in placing the number of addicts at between 250,000 and 315,000 in 1971.

The only conclusion possible from either the bureau estimate or the NIMH estimate is that the decades of enforcement of the Harrison Act and of countless other state and federal laws designed to stamp out opiate addiction have been a losing battle. There were almost certainly more opiate addicts in the United States from 1969 to 1971 than in 1914. And their status, of course, was far worse.

The *per capita* addiction rate, it is true, has declined since 1914—that is, addiction has not increased as rapidly as the population—but at a disastrous cost in human suffering and in social disorder.

Three basic conclusions can be drawn from this brief review of United States narcotics legislation and law enforcement:

• There is little likelihood that further tinkering with the laws—additional legal devices of the kinds here reviewed, or of novel kinds—will prove more successful than the hundreds of such laws already on the books. Legislators who trust in such measures are failing to face the facts. Narcotic addiction remains endemic despite the most ingenious laws and vigorous law enforcement.
• The time has come to end our dependence on repressive legislation and law enforcement as a cure for the narcotics evil, and to explore more rational alternatives.
• The history of the narcotics laws—and of alcohol prohibition (see Part IV)—should warn us against going further in the 1970s down a similar legislative blind alley with respect to marijuana, LSD, the amphetamines, the barbiturates, and other drugs of current concern.

We shall consider alternative approaches later in this Report.

10.

Why our narcotics laws have failed: (1) Heroin is an addicting drug

In 1970 a ruling of the United States Food and Drug Administration was sufficient to limit severely the use of a group of chemicals known as the cyclamates, many tons of which had been marketed annually in the country's favorite soft drinks and in many other food products. No cyclamates were smuggled into the United States following the new regulation; no black market in cyclamates was established; no midnight raids on clandestine cyclamate pushers were organized—indeed, cyclamates were curtailed without (so far as is known) a single sentence of imprisonment being invoked.

Why could not the opiates be calmly and sensibly removed from the market as effortlessly as the cyclamates were? The glib answer, of course, is that the opiates are *addicting*. But "addicting" is a slippery word, often misused. Let us examine a few of its multitudinous meanings.

In Roman law, to be addicted meant to be bound over or delivered over to someone by a judicial sentence; thus a prisoner of war might be addicted to some nobleman or large landowner. In sixteenth-century England, the word had the same meaning; thus a serf might be addicted to a master. But Shakespeare and others of his era perceived the marked similarity between this legal form of addiction and a man's bondage to alcoholic beverages; they therefore spoke of being addicted to alcohol. Poets also spoke of men "addicted to vice," and of young women "addicted to virginity." Dr. Johnson wrote of "addiction to tobacco" and John Stuart Mill of "addiction to bad habits." The concepts of addiction to opium, morphine, and heroin followed quite naturally.

Following the passage of the Harrison Narcotic Act in 1914, however, the meaning of the word "addicting" underwent a subtle change. The original meaning—a drug to which one becomes enslaved—was lost sight of. Many people assumed that any addict could stop taking an addicting drug if he wanted to and if he tried hard enough. The imprisonment of addicts was based on this confusion; addicts were expected to stop taking heroin for fear of imprisonment, or of repeated reimprisonment. We have shown in the previous chapter how that view fell victim to the facts.

Along with these popular views of addiction, various *medical* theories of addiction have arisen. Physicians noted centuries ago that when alcoholics were abruptly deprived of alcohol, they often developed a very serious, indeed life-threatening, condition known as *delirium tremens*. When opium, morphine, and heroin addicts were deprived of their drug, they similarly developed a *withdrawal syndrome* that could be devastating, even fatal.

Dr. Jerome H. Jaffe describes the withdrawal syndrome in Goodman and Gilman's textbook:

The character and the severity of the withdrawal symptoms . . . depend upon many factors, including the particular drug, the total daily dose used, the interval between doses, the duration of use, and the health and personality of the addict. . . . In the case of morphine or heroin . . . lacrimation [excessive tearing], rhinorrhea [running nose], yawning, and perspiration appear . . . the addict may fall into a tossing, restless sleep known as the "yen," which may last several hours but from which he awakens more restless and more miserable than before . . . additional signs and symptoms appear . . . dilated pupils, anorexia [loss of appetite], gooseflesh, restlessness, irritability, and tremor . . . symptoms reach their peak at 48 to 72 hours . . . increasing irritability, insomnia, marked anorexia, violent yawning, severe sneezing, lacrimation, and coryza [cold-like nasal symptoms]. Weakness and depression . . . nausea and vomiting . . . intestinal spasm and diarrhea. Heart rate and blood pressure are elevated. Marked chilliness, alternating with flushing and excessive sweating . . . waves of gooseflesh . . . the skin resembles that of a plucked turkey . . . the basis of the expression "cold turkey" to signify abrupt withdrawal without treatment. Abdominal cramps and pains in the bones and muscles of the back and extremities are also characteristic, as are the muscle spasms and kicking movements that may be the basis for the expression "kicking the habit." Other signs . . . include ejaculations in men and orgasm in women. . . . The failure to take foods and fluids, combined with vomiting, sweating, and diarrhea, results in marked weight loss, dehydration. . . . Occasionally there is cardiovascular collapse. At any point in the course of withdrawal, the administration of a suitable narcotic will completely and dramatically suppress the symptoms of withdrawal.[1]

Physicians thus concluded that drugs such as alcohol and heroin produce a phenomenon known as *physical dependence*. An addicting drug came to mean a drug that produces physical dependence—that is, withdrawal symptoms—when the drug is abruptly discontinued.

Drugs that produce withdrawal symptoms usually also produce, as noted earlier, a phenomenon known as *tolerance*. This means that if the same dose is taken day after day, the effects gradually disappear. Thus a new definition was evolved: an addicting drug is one that produces both withdrawal symptoms and tolerance.

The association of addiction with withdrawal symptoms led naturally to the earliest theory of how addiction could be cured: all that was necessary was to help an addict through his withdrawal crisis. Once withdrawn from the drug, it was widely believed, he could live happily ever after as an ex-addict. This theory goes back at least to 1856, when an

American pharmacologist, Dr. George B. Wood, wrote in his *Treatise on Therapeutics and Pharmacology*:

It is satisfactory to know that this evil habit may be corrected, without great difficulty, if the patient is in earnest; and as the disorders induced by it are mainly functional, that a good degree of health may be restored. . . . The proper method of correcting the evil is by gradually reducing the cause; a diminution of the dose being made every day, so small as to be quite imperceptible in its effects. Supposing, for example, that a fluid ounce of laudanum [opium in alcohol] is taken daily, the abstraction of a minim [one drop] every day would lead to a cure in somewhat more than a year; and the process might be much more rapid than this.[2]

In practice, however, the gradual withdrawal method had difficulties. Few addicts stayed with the withdrawal to the end; for while the first portion of the dose-lowering process was quite easy, suffering eventually set in—and it was thereafter prolonged rather than eased by the inadequate daily doses. As early as 1867, accordingly, a writer in the *British Medical Journal* expressed a contrary view: "Absolute and immediate suspension [of all opiates] is for efficacy the far more reliable plan, being less tedious, less exhausting, less the occasion of hard sufferings."[3]

The debate between these two points of view—abrupt versus gradual withdrawal—continued for decades. But both sides agreed that for either type of treatment to succeed, an addict had to be "in earnest" and "strongly motivated," and to have "will power"; moral weaklings failed.

The major problem with these early "cures" was that patients—whether abruptly or gradually withdrawn from their opiate—promptly relapsed and became addicted again. Nineteenth-century physicians, however, were not discouraged by this tendency to relapse: the patients, they complained, didn't *really* want to give up opiates. Or alternatively, they were weaklings lacking in will power. The fault was not in the treatment but in the patient. This is still a widely held view.

The next step forward in the "cure" of drug addiction was *prolonged* treatment. Patients might be kept in a sanitarium for a month, or six months, or even a year. After enforced abstinence for that long a period, it was universally agreed, opiate addiction must of necessity be entirely cured. After the Harrison Narcotic Act of 1914, this theory was pushed to even further extremes. Addicts were imprisoned for two years, five years, or even longer. When they thereafter promptly returned to their drugs, the same explanations were offered—lack of a *desire* to give up opiates, and lack of *will power*.

At the turn of the century the cure of opiate addiction was attempted on a scale that dwarfs even today's efforts. In 1908, for example, Hugh C. Weir reported in *Putnam's Magazine*: "There are forty institutions in this country advertising a cure for the drug habit, and all of them are largely patronized. One such institution at Atlanta, Georgia, has the names of over 100,000 patients whom it has treated, and there are several others that can show 50,000." [4]

There is no evidence, however, that any addicts were ever actually cured at these "sanitariums." Indeed, the enormous success of the sanitariums depended on the fact that they were "revolving-door institutions." Some addicts came back to the same sanitarium again and again; others drifted from one sanitarium to another. Cases of men and women still addicted after ten or twenty "cures" were matters of common knowledge.

With the rise of the behavioral sciences in the twentieth century— especially psychology, psychiatry, and sociology—the old theories of "poor motivation" and "weak will power" to explain addiction and relapse were not abandoned but simply rephrased. The newer theories fell into three main categories.

Psychological theories. Theories in this group are in general the heirs to the old "weakness of will" approach. Some of them hold that there exists an "addictive personality." The unfortunate possessors of this personality pattern are prone to become addicted, and are also prone to become readdicted after they have been "cured." A restructuring of the personality is therefore needed. There are many variations on this theme —including Freudian views which trace addiction-proneness to factors in early childhood, existential views which associate addiction-proneness with psychological pressures and conflicts in adult life, and so on. What the views have in common is the belief that the secret of addiction lies in the psyche of the addict.

Sociological views. These views hold in general that society creates addicts and causes ex-addicts to relapse into addiction again. The sense of hopelessness and defeat among dwellers in our city slums, the sense, among young people today, of impotence to affect change, the needs of young people to belong to a group and their consequent drift into groups of heroin users—countless sociological factors such as these are cited to explain both addiction and relapse following "cure." An addict relapses, according to some sociological theories, because he returns to the same neighborhood where he became addicted and associates with addicts once more. What these theories have in common is the belief that the secret of addiction lies in the social context.

There are also, of course, combinations of psychological and sociological theories. The best-known of these is the theory underlying Synanon, Daytop, Odyssey House, Phoenix House, and numerous other "therapeutic communities." In such communities, the addict spends months or even years in a milieu designed to restructure his psyche from immature and addiction-prone into strong, self-reliant, no longer in need of a drug

[67]

"crutch." Simultaneously, the therapeutic-community milieu provides the ex-addict with a drug-free social setting in which all the social pressures are directed toward abstinence rather than relapse. The degree of success achieved by these communities, combining the best in both the psychological and the sociological tradition, will be reviewed below.

Biochemical theories. These theories are of recent origin, and are held by only a few experts. They have arisen largely as a result of disenchantment with the practical failure of the psychological and sociological theories. These theories begin with the unchallengeable fact—on which all schools of thought are agreed—that the acute withdrawal symptoms suffered after an addict is deprived of his drug are genuinely biochemical in origin. The cause of these immediate withdrawal symptoms is in the structure of the chemical molecule and its effect on cells of the nervous system. Exposed regularly to opiate molecules the human nervous system adjusts to their presence—that is, becomes dependent upon them. If they are withdrawn, the nervous system becomes very seriously disturbed. The nervous system can readjust only gradually to the *absence* of an opiate in the way in which it initially adjusted to the *presence* of the opiate.

The controversial additional point urged by proponents of the biochemical theory is their conviction that the *long-term* outcome of opium, morphine, or heroin addiction—the craving and the tendency of addicts to resume drug-seeking behavior and to become readdicted months or even years after withdrawal has been successfully achieved—is also a direct effect of the opiate molecule on the nervous system.

Holders of the biochemical view are not absolutists. They concede, for example, that some people are more likely to become addicted and readdicted than others (though they tend to explain these differences in terms of differences in the nervous system as well as childhood upbringing or current psychic stresses). They also concede that some ex-addicts can go without drugs, and that psychological and social factors can increase or decrease the likelihood (or the promptness) of relapse and readdiction. But they focus primary attention on the drug itself, and on its effects on the cells of the nervous system. The secret of addiction, they stress, lies primarily in the chemical molecule.

The vast bulk of the evidence to date, it must be pointed out, favors the psychological and sociological theories. But this may be because the vast bulk of scientific studies throughout the past century has been devoted to a search for psychological and sociological factors. The search for biochemical factors has barely begun (see below). We are hopeful that it will prove rewarding.

Fortunately, one need not here decide among these theories. Perhaps all three are true in part—or perhaps there is a fourth explanation of addiction as yet undiscovered. What can and must be done here, however, is to consider the *consequences* of these theories in the real, nontheoretical world. This can be done by reviewing the success (or failure) of the various treatment programs based on each theory.

The first official United States government theory following passage of the Harrison Narcotic Act of 1914 was a compromise: addicts must be deterred from using drugs by incarceration in an institution *and* helped to give up drugs by receiving therapy while incarcerated. Hence as early as 1919, the Narcotics Unit of the United States Treasury urged Congress to set up a chain of federal "narcotics farms" where addicts could be incarcerated and treated for their addiction. The request was often renewed; but such institutions cost money. Until 1929, Congress preferred to pass punitive rather than therapeutic legislation. Not until 1935 did the first United States Public Health Service hospital for narcotics addicts actually open its doors, in Lexington, Kentucky. It had 1,000 beds and 500 employees. Tens of thousands of addicts have been treated there, some many times over. A second hospital, at Fort Worth, followed a few years later.

Federal Narcotics Commissioner Harry J. Anslinger and United States Attorney William F. Tompkins, in *The Traffic in Narcotics* (1953), reported on the success of the Lexington hospital:

The bright side . . . is the Lexington story. From 1935 to 1952, 18,000 addicts were admitted for treatment. Of these 64 percent never returned for treatment, 21 percent returned a second time, 6 percent a third time, and 9 percent four or more times. These figures should give everyone confidence that the U.S. Public Health Service Hospitals can secure good results in one of medicine's most tremendously difficult tasks.[5]

The flaw in Commissioner Anslinger's figures, obviously, is that they refer only to patients who *returned to Lexington* up to 1952. Addicts released from Lexington who returned to other hospitals, or went to prisons, or who merely continued their addiction at home, or who were to return to Lexington after 1952, were included among the 64 percent who "never returned for treatment."

When we turn from official claims to actual follow-up studies, the figures are very different. One study traced 1,912 Lexington alumni for periods of from one to four and a half years. Only 6.6 percent remained abstinent throughout the follow-up period.[6]

A second study checked on 453 Lexington alumni six months, two years, and five years after release. Only 12 of the 453 (less than 3 percent) were abstinent on all three follow-ups. The failure rate was thus in excess of 97 percent.[7]

The most recent follow-up of Lexington alumni was published in 1965 by Dr. George E. Vaillant, staff psychiatrist at Lexington and later on the Harvard Medical School faculty. Dr. Vaillant reviewed the records of 100 Lexington alumni—fifty white and fifty black—who had been released from the hospital between August 1, 1952, and January 31, 1953. (The outcomes for blacks and whites did not differ significantly.) The follow-up continued for nearly twelve years, through the end of 1964. Unlike most Lexington alumni, moreover, these ex-addicts were provided with aftercare. "For several years after discharge," Dr. Vaillant explained, "virtually all the patients or their families were regularly contacted by a social agency about once every three months. . . .

In spite of these relatively favorable conditions, within two years all but ten of the 100 patients again became addicted—at least temporarily. Of the ten who did not, three died in less than four years after discharge, two turned to alcohol, three had never used narcotics more than once a day and one used drugs intermittently after discharge. In other words, virtually all patients who had been physically addicted and did not die, relapsed.[8]

Two of the three patients who were *not* addicted when they entered Lexington became addicted after discharge. "Subsequent to Lexington the 100 patients served over 350 prison terms and underwent over 200 known voluntary hospitalizations for addiction."[9] Only 11 of the more than 200 voluntary hospitalizations were followed by apparent abstinence from narcotics for periods of one year or longer.

Despite these woeful facts, which are here quoted directly from Dr. Vaillant's own report, the Vaillant study has been cited as evidence that narcotics addiction is readily curable. This curious conclusion arose out of the fact that Dr. Vaillant also published a chart showing only 20 of his 100 addicts still addicted in 1964, twelve years after discharge from Lexington.

What happened to the other 80? Some were dead, some were now addicted to alcohol instead of heroin, some were in prisons, some were in hospitals, some had simply disappeared, and the current status of others remained in doubt.

Twenty-three were classified in the Vaillant chart as doing well in 1964—stably employed and not at the moment addicted, so far as could be determined. In this as in other studies, however, the figures at any given moment of time are misleading. For just as some of the 23 "successes" had become readdicted after leaving Lexington, so some could be expected to become readdicted yet again after completion of the follow-up. The evidence for absence of addiction, moreover, depended on "statements from potentially fallible patients, relatives and parole officers," [10] as Dr. Vaillant himself modestly noted; perhaps at least a few of those classified as ex-addicts were still taking heroin after all.

Citing the Vaillant report as evidence that narcotics addiction is readily curable is an example of how far some people will go to delude themselves and others. A fair summary of the findings, both positive and negative, would go something like this.

At any given time after being "cured" at Lexington, from 10 to 25 percent of graduates may appear to be abstinent, nonalcoholic, employed, and law-abiding. But only a handful at most can maintain this level of functioning throughout the ten-year period after "cure." Almost all become readdicted and reimprisoned early in the decade, and for most the process is repeated over and over again.

The above figures are not to the discredit of Lexington; satisfactory research of several kinds has been done there since 1935. But no cure for narcotics addiction, and no effective deterrent, was found there—or anywhere else.

The high rate of relapse even after prolonged incarceration and treatment can readily be explained in terms of the postwithdrawal syndrome —anxiety, depression, and craving—described in Chapter 2. Prolonged incarceration may postpone the drug-seeking behavior but it does not alleviate that underlying syndrome. Release from prison and from treatment may thereafter trigger an intense new wave of anxiety, depression, and craving—followed by drug-seeking behavior and relapse.

In 1961, California launched its large-scale civil commitment program for narcotics addicts. This program permits addicts to be locked up without first being convicted of a crime. Instead of being called "prisoners" or "prison inmates," the addicts are called "residents"—not of prisons but of "rehabilitation centers." Instead of being under the jurisdiction of prison authorities, the "residents" are held by the California Rehabilitation Center (CRC), to which they are committed for periods of up to seven years. Part of the time is spent "in residence," that is, locked up, and the rest on "outpatient status," that is, on parole. Release is supposed to follow three years of successful parole. (The constitutionality of this program of incarceration without criminal trial and conviction—and of similar New York State and federal "civil commitment" programs—has been repeatedly challenged in the courts. The challenges are from time to time successful in individual cases, but the system as a whole has to date remained impervious to constitutional attacks.)

Between September 1961 and the spring of 1968, Dr. John C. Kramer and Richard A. Bass reported in the *Journal of the American Medical Association*, more than 8,000 addicts or alleged addicts were committed under the CRC program. Of these, 5,200 were still in the program in the spring of 1968. Up to that point, 3,300 had departed. Only 300, however, had been released because of successful completion of three years on parole. The remaining 3,000 who left had gone from the program to prison, or had disappeared, or died, or gotten out on writs of *habeas corpus* or in other ways.[11]

The CRC program, moreover, locked up persons "in imminent danger of becoming addicted" as well as actual addicts. The Kramer-Bass study cited data indicating that a remarkably high proportion of the 300 alleged "successes" were not in fact heroin addicts and never had been. In a sample of the 300 "successes" selected at random for intensive study, more than 40 percent were "atypical." Some denied ever having used opiates. Some were primarily users of nonopiate drugs. Some had used heroin only occasionally, or only briefly, and so on.[12] The Kramer-Bass study also cited reasons for anticipating that the relatively small proportion of "successes" emerging from the program—300 out of 3,300 departures— was unlikely to improve as the program matured. Instead, more and more "residents" were likely to pile up inside the CRC as the years rolled by. Indeed, the 2,600 "residents" locked up in the institution in the spring of 1968 were already overcrowding it, and it became necessary soon thereafter to reduce the residence period in order to make room for more addicts. Meanwhile, narcotics addiction in California continues to be a major problem.*

The figures above, moreover, should not be taken to mean that the California system "cured" 300 out of 3,300 addicts. The 300 were merely *released from parole;* whether or not any of them would live free of heroin after release remained problematic. Many of the 300 have in fact been returned to CRC or imprisoned.

New York City and New York State have the most intense narcotics problem in the United States; it has been estimated that more than half of all American addicts reside there. For this and other reasons, which will become apparent below, several New York efforts to rehabilitate addicts deserve detailed attention.

One widely publicized New York program was launched in 1952 at Riverside Hospital on North Brother Island in the East River. Riverside's 140 beds, it was announced, were to be "devoted exclusively to the treatment, aftercare, and rehabilitation of adolescent narcotics addicts." It was to be very generously staffed—"14 full-time and 9 part-time physicians, 6 psychologists, 9 social workers, and 13 rehabilitation and educational personnel"[14]—a total of 51 professionals plus guards and other

* Dr. John C. Kramer wrote (1969): "Though the [California] program has been useful for a small proportion of those committed, for the majority it has proved to be merely an alternative to prison. The majority have entered a revolving system of admission-release-admission-release, and spend a majority of their commitment incarcerated in an institution which resembles a prison more than it does a hospital." [13]

employees for 141 addicts. It was realized, of course, that all the addicts in New York could not be as lavishly provided with care, including rehabilitation services and aftercare following release; but it was hoped that techniques could be devised at Riverside which might prove generally applicable. Some patients were admitted voluntarily; others were committed to Riverside by the courts. New York State put up a million dollars a year to fund the program.

After five years of Riverside, however, the New York City adolescent narcotics problem remained as acute as ever. Accordingly, in 1957, New York State Health Commissioner Herman Hilleboe, wishing to determine whether the state funds for Riverside were being wisely spent, asked Dr. Ray E. Trussell—then director of the Columbia University School of Public Health—to conduct an evaluation, in which all of the 247 adolescent addicts admitted to Riverside during the calendar year 1955 would be traced and their status determined.

Tracing addicts in the world's largest city proved remarkably easy. "It turned out," Dr. Trussell explained, "that the best way to find these people was to keep an eye on hospital admissions and the admissions to penal institutions." [15] Eighty-six percent of the 247 addicts admitted to Riverside in 1955 were found again in prisons or hospitals—including Riverside Hospital—in 1958.

Dr. Trussell described the end results of the evaluation as "discouraging." Eleven of the 247 addicts were dead—a high death rate for an adolescent population. An additional 228 had been reimprisoned, or rehospitalized, or both, one or more times, following release from Riverside. Of the 247 addicts admitted in 1955, only eight remained alive, unaddicted, unimprisoned, and unhospitalized three years later.

Nor was that the worst of it. New York law, like California law and the law of several other states, provides for the incarceration not only of addicts but of *persons in imminent danger of becoming addicted.* What was most startling, Dr. Trussell reported, was the fact that all eight of the Riverside alumni who remained drug-free in 1958 "to a man swore that they had never been addicted; they had been caught in possession, they had been committed, they had put in their time and gone home, and that was the end of that episode so far as they were concerned." [16] Riverside Hospital records confirmed their nonaddict status in seven of the eight cases. For patients actually addicted, the "success rate [was] zero." [17]

In other words, heroin really is an addicting drug.

Having established with precision that the Riverside Hospital program had failed to rehabilitate even one out of 239 addicts, Dr. Trussell and his associates "had a behind-the-scenes meeting with city and state officials and various public leaders interested in the problem of addiction." [18] Those present agreed that "Riverside Hospital should be closed as an absolute failure." But now a phenomenon common in drug-addiction treatment programs appeared. Just as Lexington continued to go through the motions of rehabilitating addicts for three decades despite mounting evidence that the failure rate exceeded 90 percent, so Riverside went right on functioning with a 100 percent failure rate. Eminent political figures who had taken credit for establishing Riverside, Dr. Trussell learned, were unwilling to face public responsibility for its collapse. Abandonment proved politically impossible. Riverside thus became, like a number of other rehabilitation programs, a kind of false front—assuaging public demand that "something be done about drug addicts" without actually accomplishing anything.

In 1961, Dr. Trussell became New York City's commissioner of hospitals, with direct responsibility for Riverside. "By this time," he later recalled, "the personnel were smuggling drugs in to the patients or the patients were going home on passes and bringing drugs back. We had some unwanted, unplanned pregnancies; the guards were taking advantage of the patients and it was a situation which was certainly highly undesirable from the patients' point of view and as a public investment of tax funds." [19] Such deterioration in morale is not uncommon in closed institutions devoted to the treatment of drug addicts—especially when it is known that the treatment is accomplishing nothing. Competent staff evaporates from such institutions. Following public airing of the scandalous conditions, Dr. Trussell was able to close Riverside Hospital—which was, he said, "one of the most pleasant things I have ever undertaken as an administrator." [20]

What was to take its place? A survey of all known programs, here and in other countries, turned up nothing that really made sense. The most immediate need was, quite simply, for a low-cost "detoxification unit," where addicts could voluntarily go for a few days or weeks to "kick the habit." Most patients who go through a detoxification unit promptly relapse, of course; but at least they experience a few drug-free weeks or months, and after they do relapse, the daily cost of their drugs is lower for a time. In the course of detoxification their numerous other health needs can be met, including the special needs of pregnant addicts. To Dr. Trussell's amazement, he discovered that New York City, despite chronic demands that something be done about the horrors of drug addiction, had failed to set up a single center where addicts could voluntarily go for detoxification. (Most other cities also lacked such centers.)

To provide a detoxification service for women addicts who were pregnant and who wanted to be detoxified, "I got together all the administrators and directors of medicine in my 15 municipal hospitals," Dr. Trussell recalled, "and I said, 'You know, gentlemen, you've got 16,000 beds between you and let's find twenty-five beds for pregnant addicts.' And to my utter amazement I was flatly told where I could go by people who were on my payroll! Further, they formed a committee and sent me a letter saying [in effect], 'Drug addiction is not a medical problem, it's a social and criminal problem, and keep it away from us.' " Thus Dr. Trussell "became aware of the really entrenched negative attitude on the part of the medical leadership in this city toward drug addiction." [21] It was an attitude common in other cities as well—an attitude deeply entrenched ever since federal narcotics officials had begun arresting physicians under the Harrison Narcotic Act of 1914, half a century earlier.

Eventually Dr. Trussell was able to find, on Eighteenth Street in Manhattan, a private proprietary hospital, then known as Manhattan General, which was in financial difficulties and therefore willing to contract with the city to supply detoxification services at the city's expenses. Patients "went in a side door which was used for the delivery of supplies," Dr. Trussell recalled. "They were carefully sequestered from other patients in the hospital and they were treated in a very secretive way." [22] For several years, this remained New York City's only detoxification service.

Two more New York State programs require consideration. In 1956, the New York State Parole Division announced a new plan of intensive follow-up service and parole supervision for selected addicts released from the state's prisons. The publicized central feature of this program was "intensive supervision, using the casework approach in an authoritative setting." [23] The parole officers assigned to the project were specially selected and trained for the job. They were assigned only 30 parolees each instead of the customary 85 or more. In other ways, too, the parolees assigned to this program received more intensive care than is customary.

The head of the project, Meyer H. Diskind, considered the abstinence rates attained by this program "rather favorable"—better, for example, than the rates obtained after hospitalization. A study he published in 1960 reported that of the 344 parolees assigned to the program between November 1, 1956, and October 31, 1959, "119 offenders, or 35 percent, had never been declared delinquent for any reason whatsoever, drugs or otherwise." Another 36 parolees had violated parole—but had not, so far as was known, returned to narcotics. "If we were to add these 36 delinquents to the 119 who made a fully satisfactory adjustment," Mr. Diskind and an associate, George Klonsky, announced, "then 45 percent abstained from drugs while under supervision." [24]

Alas, there were several things wrong with that claim. To cite one example, some of the 119 "successes" had only been out of prison a month or two when their status was determined and their success pronounced. To cite another example, use of narcotics was determined primarily by an "arm check"—examining the addict's arms periodically for needle marks. Addicts on the program knew, of course, that their arms would be checked. How many injected narcotics into their legs, or other portions of their anatomy, or took drugs without injecting them, is not known.

In 1964, Diskind and Klonsky published a further report on the same 344 addicts. It was based in part on the project's own records, and in part on a social-work thesis by Robert F. Hallinan and his associates at the Fordham University School of Social Service. Diskind and Klonsky reported that of 66 successful parolees followed up by Hallinan, "36, or 55 percent, had completely abstained from drug usage since their discharge from parole." Seven others had abstained for periods ranging from three to thirty-six months. "If we were to add the 7 who terminated the habit to the 36 complete abstainers, then 43, or 65 percent, were in an abstention status at the time of the study." [25] Statements such as these, enthusiastically reported in the press decade after decade, have given the public a firm belief that heroin addiction is curable.

A closer look at the figures, however, leads to less optimistic conclusions.

Of the 344 addicts admitted to the program prior to October 31, 1959, only 83 were still in good standing on December 31, 1962. Of these 83, moreover, 17 were either still on parole or had been released from parole after less than seven months of supervision. Thus only 66 parolees (19 percent) were believed (on the basis of arm checks) to have remained free of parole violations or narcotics and to have completed seven months or more of parole.[26]

The 65 percent and 55 percent success figures cited by Diskind and Klonsky in the quotations above applied only to these 66 parolees! When the Fordham University group followed up the 66 "successes" who had been released after seven months or more of parole, they found only 30 still living apparently drug-free and without known legal offenses.[27] Thus, the true success rate for the original 344 addicts was 30 out of 344, or less than 9 percent.

Doubts can be raised, of course, concerning even these 30 alleged "successes." How many of them, for example, had in fact been narcotics addicts? The original sample of 344 consisted of a selected group of addicts with sufficiently modest criminal records to persuade a parole board to release them. It is not unlikely that in this program, as in the Vaillant study, the California Rehabilitation Center program, and the Riverside Hospital program described above, a significant proportion of the 30 "successes" had never in fact been addicted to heroin.

By 1966, the federal program at Lexington, the California Rehabilitation Center program, the Riverside Hospital program, and the New York State "Special Narcotic Project Program" had firmly demonstrated that neither incarceration alone nor incarceration plus treatment nor incarceration followed by intensive parole supervision accomplishes much of value for more than a handful of addicts, and that costs per addict are very high. Despite these demonstrations, New York State in 1966 announced a mammoth new program—the largest and costliest in history—based on precisely the principles that had so often proved a failure before. A total of 4,500 addicts and alleged addicts were to be immured in twenty-six new institutions. These institutions, as in California, were called rehabilitation centers rather than hospitals or prisons. Aftercare was also provided for, and the official in charge of New York State's "Special Narcotic Project Program," described above, was placed in charge of this aspect of the new program. The cost for the first three years was pegged at $200,000,000—most of it for the purchase of old buildings and the construction of new ones in which addicts could be locked up.[28]

At the beginning of 1971, the gargantuan New York State program was still spending money at the rate of $150,000,000 a year.[29] It had failed to publish any statistics from which its success rate could be calculated. Two outside reports on results did become available, however, in February 1971. One was a staff report to New York City Mayor John Lindsay; the other was a report by New York District Attorney Frank S. Hogan.

The state's Narcotic Addiction Control Commission, it was learned, had 5,800 addicts under treatment, out of an estimated 100,000 addicts in the state.[30] To provide similar treatment for the other 94,000 would raise the cost from $150,000,000 a year into the billions.

The Lindsay report further noted that 526 persons had left the program between April and September 1970. But only 97 of these, or 18.4 percent "had completed the aftercare phase of the program without relapsing or absconding." [31]

This did not mean, of course, that 18.4 percent were cured. It meant only that 18.4 percent were now on the street without supervision. The other 81.6 percent had already relapsed or absconded.

Meanwhile, addicts convicted of narcotics law violations were piling up in New York City jails, under intolerable conditions, and prisoners were rioting in protest at the overcrowding. The New York State "civil commitment program" played a curious role in this overcrowding. Addicts, the Hogan report indicated, much preferred a short sentence in prison to three years in a state "rehabilitation" institution.[32] Hence prosecutors were able to persuade them to plead guilty in criminal court, and overcrowd the jails still further, under threat that if they did not plead guilty, they would be committed without a trial to a state "treatment center."

By 1970 even New York Governor Nelson A. Rockefeller, who had launched this mammoth program amid high hopes in 1966, was ready to concede that it had failed. "It is a god-damn serious situation," he told a meeting of clergymen. "I cannot say that we have achieved success. We have not found answers that go to the heart of the problem." [33] Yet the state continued to pour money into the program.*

In 1966, the federal government also established an incarceration-plus-aftercare program patterned on the California model. Preliminary evaluation studies of this National Addiction Rehabilitation Administration (NARA) program, made public in 1971, indicated that the NARA program was approximately as successful as the California and New York State programs described above.[34]

What about Synanon, Daytop, Phoenix House, Odyssey House, and other widely publicized private and semiprivate agencies for the rehabilitation of heroin addicts in a "therapeutic community" setting?

In 1958 Charles E. Dederich established Synanon in California as a treatment center for drug addicts. The center combined the best features of the psychological and sociological theories of addiction. Addicts entering Synanon went through a rigorous psychic restructuring process designed to change their personalities from addiction-prone to stalwart and self-reliant. Simultaneously the Synanon community was structured so as to encourage total abstinence and discourage drug use. Many could not "take it" and withdrew. Others remained in the Synanon community for years—until the rehabilitation process was presumably complete and the likelihood of relapse negligible.

By the mid-1960s, however, even Synanon itself conceded that its program had with few exceptions failed to turn out abstinent alumni. Members apparently cured beyond any possibility of relapse promptly relapsed when they left the sheltering confines of Synanon or of other therapeutic communities to which they had transferred. Dederich himself estimated in 1971 that the relapse rate among Synanon graduates was in the neighborhood of 90 percent.

"We once had the idea of 'graduates,' " he told a reporter. "This was a sop to social workers and professionals who wanted me to say that we were producing 'graduates.' I always wanted to say to them, 'A person with this fatal disease will have to live here all his life.'

"I know damn well if they go out of Synanon they are dead. A few, but very few, have gone out and made it. When they ask me, 'If an addict goes to Synanon, how long will it take?' my answer is, 'If he's lucky, it will take forever.'

"We have had 10,000 to 12,000 persons go through Synanon. Only a small handful who left became ex-drug addicts. Roughly one in ten has stayed clean outside for as much as two years." [35]

Even this one-in-ten success rate, moreover, must be viewed with cau-

* Late in June 1971, an economy-minded state legislature reduced the appropriation for the Rockefeller program, and its gradual dismantling began in July.

tion. For Synanon accepted in the first place only highly motivated addicts who were willing to go through the rigorous Synanon procedures, including "cold turkey" withdrawal. Many "split" within a few days or weeks after entering Synanon—*before* they were formally enrolled or included in the statistics. Synanon procedures applied to an unselected cross section of addicts rather than to this very select group would no doubt yield a far lower success rate.

Despite this record of failure, Synanon was widely hailed throughout the 1960s as evidence that heroin addiction is curable; and many other similar centers were modeled more or less closely on Synanon principles. Reasonably precise figures are available for one such project—Liberty Park Village in New Jersey—for the period prior to 1971. It was founded by a Daytop alumnus, with federal and state financing; its budget totaled $1,670,800 for the year beginning August 1, 1970.[36]

The area served by Liberty Park Village contained an estimated 4,000 heroin addicts. The program ran six "outreach centers," and an estimated one thousand addicts made contact with these centers during the first twenty-two months. Not all of them, however, were accepted for admission to the Village therapeutic community. During the period from January 1969 through October 1970 only 272 of the more promising applicants were selected.

A basic principle of the therapeutic community is its voluntary nature. Addicts are free to leave at any time. Most Liberty Park Village addicts took advantage of this freedom. By the end of 1970, only 22 had "graduated" and only 67 were left in the program. The others had all "split" (absconded), some of them more than once.

Again, this did not mean that Liberty Park Village had "cured" 22 addicts on its $1,670,800-a-year budget. It only meant that 22 had completed the program and returned to the streets, where they might or might not relapse. At the beginning of 1971, it was known that 4 of the 22 "alumni" were back on heroin or in jail. Nothing was known about the other 18—and no effort was being made to find out. Despite the $1,670,800-per-year budget, and despite an additional federal grant for the specific purpose of "evaluating" the program, no funds were available to find out how many of the 18 were back on heroin or in jail.

Yet the most astonishing part of the Liberty Park Village story remains to be told. The New Jersey state officials responsible for supervision of the program, and many ordinary citizens as well, were firmly convinced for a time that it was a success.

Here an explanation is necessary. Despite its woeful overall failure to solve the problems of the 4,000 heroin addicts in its area, Liberty Park Village on any given day has (like other therapeutic communities) a cadre of twenty or thirty bright, alert "ex-addicts" in residence who are doing very well at the moment. Visitors to the project met this core group and were impressed with its progress. So were state officials. "Ex-addict" members of the core group lectured local civic organizations on the good work Liberty Park Village was doing. They also spoke at high schools and other educational institutions. And the message they carried was a very simple one: *heroin addiction is curable.* Indeed, one need only look at them to see that a young man or woman with enough will power could convert himself from a heroin addict to an upright, healthy, personable ex-addict in a year or so. (Late in 1971, the Liberty Park Village program, philosophy, and leadership were altered and a new program was instituted. It is still too early to evaluate this new program.)

Each of the other "therapeutic communities" differs from Synanon and Liberty Park Village in one respect or another. One difference is that even the rudimentary statistics available for Liberty Park Village are not available for many of the others.* Dr. Vincent P. Dole's comment is, "Agencies seldom conceal success." [38]

In general, the outline of all the therapeutic communities follows substantially the following pattern.

Out of the estimated 250,000 to 315,000 heroin addicts in the United States, each therapeutic community selects a handful—perhaps 100 or 200 per year—who are the most highly motivated for cure and who seem to be the "best bets." During their first few months on the program, these most promising recruits are made to work very hard and are sub-

* An unpublished report by George Nash, a sociologist (and currently consultant for program planning and evaluation to the Division of Narcotic and Drug Abuse Control, New Jersey Department of Health), and three associates provides data on Phoenix House programs.[37] Of 157 residents in two Phoenix House units in August and September 1968, the Nash group reported:
40 were still affiliated with the Phoenix House program two years later, of whom
    17 were employees, living on the outside,
    12 were in treatment,
    10 were "elders,"
     1 was the wife of a program director;
117 had left the program, of whom
100 had "split" (absconded without graduating) and
  17 had graduated, of whom
    7 were employed in other narcotics programs, and
    2 were known to have returned to heroin within a year after graduation. This left
    8 graduates who were living on the outside and who, so far as could be determined, were living drug-free.
The 8 graduates believed to be living drug-free on the outside, and not working in the field of narcotics treatment, had been out for less than two years—some of them for much less. It would therefore have been too early to have much confidence in their status as "ex-addicts."
Moreover, at least 19 of the original 157 Phoenix House residents in the study *had never been addicted to heroin:* they had used heroin only occasionally before admission.
Thus, Phoenix House returns only a trickle of ex-addicts to drug-free life on the outside.

jected to severe stresses by those who joined the program earlier. These stresses are an essential part of the program, and are often dubbed "encounter therapy." The purpose is psychological restructuring, combined with sociological adaptation to a drug-free environment. Most addicts cannot take it, and promptly walk out. Their departure is an essential part of the program; for if some do not leave, there is no room for newcomers.

The many who drop out early, however, are not counted as "failures." Indeed, they are not counted at all. The count does not begin until an addict has survived the difficult first few months. Only then is he "admitted" to the therapeutic community—and to the success-failure statistics.

Like Liberty Park Village, the other therapeutic communities have in residence on any given day a cadre of impressive "ex-addicts" who have survived these preliminary months and who arouse the admiration and awe of visitors. What happens to them, however, *after* they graduate?

Significant proportions of them stay on in the therapeutic community as staff members, or leave to found or help found other therapeutic communities. In either case, they remain in a sort of *vise* which enables them to stay abstinent. Day and night they are surrounded by the community; their motivation is high, their opportunities for relapsing few. They continue to "make it" (though many of them report they still crave heroin on occasion).

The success claims made by therapeutic communities refer almost entirely to these continuing community members. Those who apply but are not accepted are forgotten, along with those who do not even apply. Those who drop out during the first months are similarly forgotten. Thus a therapeutic community can (and often does) claim a success rate of 50 percent, or 60 percent, or even higher, despite the fact that only a handful of addicts ever "graduate."

Nor is that the whole of the story. In the entire history of therapeutic communities, no study has ever been published of what happens to alumni who complete the treatment program and *leave* the therapeutic community setting. *Their* success rate remains unknown. The only statistic we have is Charles Dederich's statement (see above) that about 90 percent of the few who successfully graduate from Synanon return to heroin within two years.

One advantage of therapeutic communities sometimes cited is that they accept young addicts who otherwise would have to serve time in prison, with all of the psychological and social deterioration that the prison experience entails. This is no doubt true in many cases—but not in all. A therapeutic community housed in Fairfield Hills Hospital (a state mental institution) in Newtown, Connecticut, accepts addicts who choose hospitalization in lieu of imprisonment. These patients cannot leave except to go to prison. Yet some of them "decide, after they enter the treatment program, that they can 'do easier time' in jail and thus choose to return there. It is estimated that about sixty percent of such patients stay in the program while about forty percent decide they would rather be in jail." [39]

The temporary success of therapeutic communities while addicts remain in residence, followed by a high failure rate when they return to the open community, focuses attention once more on the postaddiction syndrome described earlier. Therapeutic communities have developed quite effective techniques for assuaging these mood disturbances—anxiety, depression, craving—and preventing them from triggering drug-seeking behavior and relapse; but they do not *cure* the syndrome. Thus, leaving a therapeutic community, like leaving prison or a "treatment center," may be followed by a recurrence of anxiety, depression, and drug craving—and, all too often, by relapse to heroin.

None of these comments should be taken as a criticism of the dedicated men and women who are devoting their lives to Synanon, Daytop, Phoenix House, and some other therapeutic communities. They represent a high flowering of the human spirit. So does the minuscule cadre of ex-addicts who continue to live drug-free in the open community after graduation. The failure of the programs is not due to the shortcomings of the staffs or members of therapeutic communities. It results from the fact that *heroin is an addicting drug.*

Synanon, to its credit, now recognizes its inability to graduate "cured" heroin addicts. It no longer presents itself as solely or even primarily a treatment center for heroin addicts, and it no longer claims that it can graduate successful ex-addicts. Rather, it presents itself as a way of life, admits nonaddicts, and states that the goal is to remain in Synanon forever. Other therapeutic communities, too, are increasingly presenting themselves as a way of life rather than a cure for heroin addiction.

Viewed as a way of life, the therapeutic community may have a role to play in American society. It may also have some merit for drug users who use drugs that are *not* addicting. Its merits in that context, however, fall outside the scope of this discussion.

From the narrow point of view of *heroin* addiction, the therapeutic communities, without a single known exception, represent a major disaster, for they have helped persuade the public that heroin addiction is curable, without curing more than a trivial number of addicts.

The message brought to the nation's schools by the therapeutic community "ex-addicts" is also subject to grave question. Their message is that heroin addiction is curable. ("So why be afraid of heroin?" is the natural and obvious corollary.)

The ex-addicts who speak in schools and at civic meetings, it is true, do not portray the cure as easy. They describe it as requiring a heroic effort of will and the ability to endure grave hardships—like climbing a mountain, or like crossing a desert. Young people, of course, are attracted to precisely such challenges.

Let us summarize. No effective cure for heroin addiction has been found—neither rapid withdrawal nor gradual withdrawal, neither the drug sanitariums of the 1900s, nor long terms of imprisonment since 1914, nor Lexington since 1935, nor the California program since 1962, nor the New York State program launched in 1966, nor the National Addiction Rehabilitation Administration program, nor Synanon since 1958, nor the other therapeutic communities. Nor should this uninterrupted series of failures surprise us. *For heroin really is an addicting drug.*

Against the background of this tragic century-long record of failure to cure heroin addiction, let us return briefly to the issue with which this chapter began—the dispute among proponents of psychological, sociological, and biochemical theories of heroin addiction.

The failure of the psychological and sociological approaches, reviewed above at such length, certainly does not *disprove* the psychological and sociological theories of addiction. Perhaps an effective psychological or sociological cure for addiction will be discovered next year. (Certainly some new "cures" will be *announced*.) But the failure to date of the psychological and social approaches helps to explain why a still small yet growing segment of those concerned with addiction problems in the United States is beginning to take more seriously the biochemical theory.*

A study at the Addiction Research Center in Lexington, Kentucky,

---

* Many centers are currently at work on biochemical research designed to establish the precise ways in which the heroin molecule achieves its remarkable effects. While all of them are not directly concerned with the "postaddiction syndrome," their findings are likely to prove relevant to an understanding of that syndrome. Workers concerned with the biochemistry of addiction include Dr. Dole at the Rockefeller University, Dr. Avram Goldstein at the Stanford Medical School, Dr. Peter Lomax at the University of California at Los Angeles, researchers at the Addiction Research Center in Lexington, Kentucky, Dr. E. Leong Way at the University of California–San Francisco Medical Center, Dr. Naim Khazan at the Mt. Sinai School of Medicine in New York City, Dr. Doris H. Clouet of the Narcotic Addiction Control Commission's Testing and Research Laboratory in Brooklyn, New York, Dr. Thomas R. Castles of the Midwest Research Institute in Kansas City, Missouri, Dr. Louis Shuster at Tufts University School of Medicine in Boston, Drs. Conan Kornetsky and Joseph Cochin at Boston University, Dr. Martin W. Adler at Temple University School of Medicine in Philadelphia, Dr. Philip L. Gildenberg at the Cleveland Clinic Foundation, Drs. Frederick W. L. Kerr and Jose Pozuelo of the Mayo Clinic, and no doubt others. To summarize the complex body of data already assembled would exceed the capacity of the authors of this Report and tax the patience of readers. The most that can be said with confidence is that the next few years—perhaps even the coming year—should see the publication of a substantial volume of experimental data throwing additional light on the biochemistry of addiction.

by Dr. William R. Martin and his associates (Drs. Eades, Sloan, Jasinski, Jones, and Wikler) is concerned with long-lasting *physiological* effects of opiate addiction. "We have shown," Dr. Martin reports, "that following withdrawal of patients dependent on morphine and methadone, there is a long-lasting syndrome of physiological abnormalities which has been called protracted abstinence, which appears to be characterized by hyper-responsivity to stressful stimuli and which is associated with relapse to the drug of dependence." [40] The Lexington group's "protracted abstinence syndrome" is no doubt the physiological substrate of the anxiety-depression-craving phenomenon, which we have here called the "post-addiction syndrome."

In other countries, too, the biochemical theory is winning new support. In England, for example, Dr. M. A. Hamilton Russell of the Addiction Research Unit, Institute of Psychiatry, London, has recently urged acceptance of the heart of the biochemical approach: the doctrine that the cravings that ex-addicts experience months or even years after their last "fix," and that lead to drug-seeking behavior and to relapse, are as physiological in nature as the early withdrawal symptoms. "Psychological processes are mediated by physiological events. Intense subjective craving, so long regarded by the unsympathetic as 'merely psychological,' may well be governed by physiological adaptive mechanisms in the hypothalamic reward system which are no less 'physical' than the similar mechanisms . . . responsible for the classical phenomena of opiate withdrawal." [41]

The uninterrupted failure of narcotic addiction "cures" from 1856 to date suggests an altogether new definition of an addicting drug—an operational definition. Let us here formulate such a fresh definition, at least roughly.

An *addicting drug* is one that most users continue to take even though they want to stop, decide to stop, try to stop, and actually succeed in stopping for days, weeks, months, or even years. It is a drug for which men and women will prostitute themselves. It is a drug to which most users return after treatment at Lexington, at the California Rehabilitation Center, at the New York State and City centers, and at Synanon, Daytop, Phoenix House, or Liberty Park Village. It is a drug which most users continue to use despite the threat of long-term imprisonment for its use—and to which they promptly return after experiencing long-term imprisonment.

The *reasons* why opiates produce this curious behavior need not be specified; they may be psychological, sociological, or biochemical. *But this is the kind of behavior these drugs evoke.*

One major virtue of our operational definition is that it specifies precisely what young people should be concerned about, and what parents and public officials should be concerned about. The major reason for not taking opiates is that they are addicting—enslaving—in the ways specified in the definition. If society belittles this enslavement by falsely stressing the curability of heroin addiction, as it was doing throughout the 1960s and as it continues to do, then it should not be surprised that more and more young people turn to heroin. It is society, after all, that has told them that addiction is only temporary.

Readers of this Consumers Union Report need not accept our operational definition of addiction. Nothing that follows depends upon it. But readers are urged to keep the operational definition in mind when reading about "new approaches to drug addiction" or new "cures" or new "rehabilitation programs." The question is not whether a new program is theoretically sound, or honestly motivated, or competently staffed, or adequately financed. The question is whether it can in fact turn out ex-addicts who do not, promptly or after a modest delay, become narcotics addicts again.

But what of the tiny minority of addicts who do succeed in "kicking the habit" permanently? Even if there are only a handful of them, and even if it costs a million dollars apiece to cure them of their addiction, is not the effort worthwhile? Unfortunately, studies of ex-heroin addicts indicate that a substantial proportion of them are at least as badly off following cure as they were during their addiction.

In their 1956 study of heroin addiction in British Columbia, Dr. Stevenson and his associates sought the names and whereabouts of former addicts currently living there drug-free. There turned out to be very few of them. With great diligence, the Stevenson group managed to interview 14 ex-addicts at length, and made full psychological studies of 7—three men and four women. In addition, they talked with a number of others, and secured anecdotal descriptions of a number whom they did not actually meet.

The most striking finding in this study concerned the very close relationship between alcoholism and abstinence from narcotics. In about half of the cases studied, the ex-addicts "merely changed their status from that of drug addicts to alcohol addicts. Many of these were alcoholic before they began the use of narcotics, and have merely returned to their first love." * [42]

The reports on these alcoholic ex-addicts make sorry reading indeed:

* Nineteenth-century physicians were well aware of the tendency of ex-opiate addicts to become alcoholics. Dr. J. B. Mattison, medical director of the Brooklyn Home for Narcotic Inebriants, wrote in 1902, after thirty years of experience with addiction treatment: ". . . Unless care be taken, a drunkard results. The shore of the post-poppy land is strewn with wrecks of those who, after escape from narcotic peril, have taken to rum." [43]

Male, 46: "Has become an end-stage alcoholic, substituting alcohol for heroin."

Male, 30: "Although [he] has discontinued the use of narcotics he has become heavily alcoholic, which endangers his other home and work adjustments and increases the likelihood of subsequent return to the use of narcotics."

Male, 58: "This man has merely exchanged his addiction from narcotic drugs to alcohol, and has made no satisfactory social adjustment. Does no work, repeatedly in gaol for intoxication and petty theft."

Female, 34: "It is obvious that this is not a successful abstention from narcotics, but merely a change in the chemical substance. Has continued in skid road alcoholism, interrupted only by repeated gaol sentences."

Female, 46: "Because of her dependence on alcohol, the child's father left her. . . . Has become a skid road alcoholic and prostitute."

Some of the other British Columbia ex-addicts looked at first glance much more promising. For example:

Male, 52: "Has worked steadily for past twelve years, not using narcotics and rarely using alcohol to excess. Has a good job which provides adequately for wife and himself."

Male, 53: "Since joining A.A. has lived a useful and relatively happy life, and is an asset to the community, working steadily and being helpful to others."

Male, 27: "Has worked steadily, is proud of his home and ownership of its contents, and lives contentedly with his wife and child."

Female, 24: "Has continued to abstain from drugs, in spite of husband's relapse and return to gaol. Takes good care of children and home."

Female, 23: "Has found a new life with her second husband and realizes she is living happily on an entirely different level. Gave birth to first baby. Is an excellent wife, home-maker and mother." [44]

When we examine these nonalcoholic cases more closely, however, two factors appear which should give us pause. First, those who successfully stopped were in some cases far from being long-term or hard-core addicts. The twenty-four-year-old female ex-addict cited above, for example, first used narcotics at seventeen and stopped at twenty, having served a jail sentence in between. Second, only a handful of nonalcoholic ex-addicts could be found in a province with 900 current addicts. Third, the period of abstinence was in some cases still too short to warrant confidence in its permanence.

This third point is illustrated by another portion of the British Columbia study. Of 100 consecutive addict admissions to a penal institution, Dr. Stevenson and his associates reported, 69 had voluntarily discontinued drug use once or several times. An additional 14 had discontinued use of drugs involuntarily during imprisonment—but had continued to abstain voluntarily following release. Of the total of 83 who abstained,

the majority had relapsed in less than a year. But 19 had remained abstinent for two years or longer—a few for as long as five years. Then they
had relapsed and had been imprisoned again.[45] If studied during the
period of abstinence, of course, these 19 addicts would also have looked
like successes. Other studies have similarly reported a high percentage
of relapse, even after periods of abstinence measured in years. The ex-
addict, in short, is commonly also a pre-addict. A "cure" is rarely more
than temporary.

Turning from opiates to alcohol, as noted above, is almost universally
the fate of those who turned initially from alcohol to opiates. All 33 of
the drunkards who turned to morphine in Dr. Lawrence Kolb's study
"resumed drinking when, by cure of their addiction, they abstained
from narcotics for varying periods." [46]

Dr. John A. O'Donnell's classic 1969 study, *Narcotic Addicts in Kentucky* (see Page 9), not only confirms the British Columbia and the
Kolb addict-alcoholic findings but expands them in significant respects.
Dr. O'Donnell and his associates actually interviewed 47 male addicts residing in Kentucky, all former patients at the federal hospital in Lexington, who appeared to be abstaining from narcotics at the time of the
interview. Of the 47, however, 16 were now alcoholics and 4 were barbiturate addicts.* [47]

Dr. O'Donnell also prepared data on the number of years the 212
male addicts in his study spent on narcotics, on alcohol or barbiturates,
and abstinent following discharge from Lexington. *Of the years spent out
of institutions and free of narcotics, more than half were spent on alcohol
or barbiturates.*[48]

Female addicts showed a considerably better record than male addicts
did of abstinence from narcotics, and much less of a tendency to substitute alcohol or barbiturates for narcotics. Even with women included,
however, the overall figures were hardly optimistic. Ninety percent of
all the addicts in the study, male and female together, spent at least a
part of the time following their discharge from Lexington addicted to
narcotics, to alcohol, or to barbiturates.

Among the 10 percent who remained abstinent, moreover, several could
hardly be defined as "voluntarily" abstinent. Here are three O'Donnell
examples:

Case 035 "had used narcotics from about 1907 to 1949. . . . In 1949 he
began to lose his sight, and by 1950 he could not leave the house without
[his wife]. He could not go to physicians, and she would not get narcotics for him." [49]

---

* The difference between alcoholism and barbiturate addiction is negligible. As we
shall demonstrate in Part IV, alcohol is, in many of its effects, a "liquid barbiturate"
and the barbiturates are very much like "solid alcohol."

Case 177 "was abstinent in the latter years of his life because, due to arthritis, he was bedridden. All medications were controlled by his family, and they could make sure that no narcotics were used."

Case 193 "claimed abstinence for 10 years up to the time of followup, attributing it to an exercise of will power. His wife, however, stated that he still begged for drugs constantly. For the first 5 of these 10 years he had been a traveling salesman, and would visit physicians in the towns he passed through to get [morphine] prescriptions. . . . For the last 5 years, however, he was confined to a wheel chair in his home, and during that time she kept him completely abstinent until the last 6 months, during which the family physician prescribed occasional narcotics for him. This was confirmed in detail by the physician." [50]

An example of an "ex-addict" who successfully refrained from narcotics for twelve years following release from Lexington is Dr. O'Donnell's Case Number 088. "Two physicians in his community described him as a chronic alcoholic, and as having been one for years. His local police record showed four arrests between 1957 and 1959, of which one was for driving while intoxicated. . . . State hospital records showed treatment in 1947, 1957, twice in 1959, and again in 1960, always for alcoholism." [51]

Finally, let us consider the very small minority of ex-addicts who manage to refrain permanently from both narcotics and alcohol. Dr. O'Donnell's Kentucky report suggests that even these few may not be quite so fortunate as we would hope.

One of Dr. O'Donnell's "successes," for example, became a compulsive eater after discontinuing narcotics. Though only 5 feet 7 inches tall, he weighed 260 pounds.[52]

Another "success," Case 002, was insane. He was described as

a man who was floridly psychotic, with many religious delusions, during most of the 5-year sentence imposed in 1938 for sale of narcotics. His complete abstinence for more than 20 years after discharge was one of the best-documented in the study, with almost every informant in his community spontaneously mentioning him as one addict who was certainly cured. Among the facts mentioned was that he had attended church and Sunday School for over 300 consecutive Sundays, with several informants suggesting he had "too much religion," that his interest in it was abnormal. The taped interview with him reads like a disjointed revival sermon, and the interviewer saw the subject as a schizophrenic in not quite complete remission. But, however a psychiatrist might diagnose him, the facts indicate that it was an act of choice, even though psychotic rather than rational, which explains his abstinence.[53]

Yet another "success" was Case 183, a formerly addicted physician who at the age of sixty-five was confined to a wheelchair. "His widow stated that he was abstinent from his discharge [from Lexington] to his death.

His daughter confirmed this story, adding that . . . his last words were a request for morphine." [54]

These case histories, and the other evidence concerning the sorry plight of so many ex-addicts, should serve to remind us once again that the addict seeking to "kick the habit" has far more to contend with than just the short-term withdrawal syndrome. Through the months and years which follow withdrawal, he must also continue to contend with the post-addiction syndrome—the wavering composite of anxiety, depression, and craving that so often leads to drug-seeking behavior and to relapse. When opiates are not available, the syndrome leads to alcoholism or to barbiturate addiction, and when even alcohol is not available, as in the case of closely guarded blind or bedridden patients, the postaddiction syndrome continues to mold their lives, even to their dying words.

Toward the end of the 1960s, heroin use spread increasingly into the middle-class, white drug scene. The youthful new addicts differed from the traditional addicts in many ways—socioeconomic class, educational level, life-style, length of addiction, motivation for the use of heroin, and so on. Hopes therefore rose that the new-style addicts might be more readily curable than their predecessors.

The first controlled study of these new-style addicts, however, gives little cause for hope. Among 62 old-style addicts admitted to the Haight-Ashbury Medical Clinic in San Francisco and detoxified after November 1969, 94.8 percent were using heroin again in 1971. Among 115 new-style addicts, 93.3 percent were back on heroin. The difference was not statistically significant. In addition, 9.4 percent of the old-style addicts and 8.3 percent of the new-style addicts were rated as "markedly improved"; they reported that although they were still using heroin, they were using it only once a week or less.[55] Once again, the difference between old-style and new-style addicts was not significant. (For a further discussion of new-style heroin addiction in the "youth drug scene," see Chapter 20.)

11.

Why our narcotics laws have failed: (2) The economics of the black market

Even readers willing at this point to concede that heroin really is an addicting drug may still favor vigorous enforcement of our antinarcotics laws. After all, addicts go without heroin while in prison.* Why not make narcotics unavailable throughout the country? Why not, in short, enforce the narcotics laws?

The answer lies firmly imbedded in the structure of the American heroin black market. Let us examine this industry as we might examine any other commercial enterprise.

The opium poppy can be cultivated almost anywhere, with adequate yields of opium per acre in many soils and climates. While it is often alleged that poppy growing requires special soil and climate, the successful commercial cultivation of opium poppies in Vermont, New Hampshire, Connecticut, Pennsylvania, Virginia, Tennessee, South Carolina, Georgia, Arizona, and California demonstrates that the concentration of poppy cultivation in China, Greece, India, Iran, Laos, Thailand, Turkey, and Yugoslavia, with lesser amounts grown in Bulgaria, Mexico, North Africa, Pakistan, and the Soviet Union, is a legal and economic phenomenon rather than a botanical necessity. It takes hundreds of hours of labor during a short ten-day season to harvest the opium from one acre of poppies; thus commercial production flourishes primarily in countries where surplus labor can be hired for short periods at low hourly rates.

Most of the heroin that reaches the United States black market has come (at least until recently) from Turkey. Farmers there have for years been required by law to sell their entire opium crop to the Turkish government, which resells it to legitimate pharmaceutical manufacturers. Until 1970 or 1971, the official price paid was $7.25 per kilogram (2.2 pounds). By offering more than that, black-market operators have, despite the law, been able to secure all the Turkish opium they want; whatever portion of the crop they don't buy goes to the government and then to the legitimate pharmaceutical manufacturers.[1]

In 1970, American government representatives stationed in Turkey offered a solution to this problem. They persuaded the Turkish government to raise the official price from $7.25 to $10 or $15 per kilogram. The

---

* This statement is only partially true; heroin is readily smuggled into some prisons.

black-market operators thereupon raised *their* price to $25 per kilogram, and continued to secure all the heroin they wanted.[2]

The increase in price did not seriously affect black-market profitability. With opium at $25 per kilogram, the raw-materials cost of the heroin in a $5 New York City bag is only about a quarter of a cent. An increase in the farm price of opium to $100 per kilogram would still take only a penny of the $5-per-bag retail price.

In June 1971, President Nixon announced that the United States government had successfully persuaded Turkey to pass a law banning production of opium altogether after 1972—even legal opium for conversion to medicinal morphine.[3] Such a law, when and if enforced, will certainly have an effect on the legitimate pharmaceutical companies who supply the world's legal morphine. They will have to go elsewhere for their opium. The net effect of this prohibition, when and if it occurs, will be to give the black-market suppliers a monopoly position as the only buyers to whom Turkish farmers can sell their opium.

But while the new law will, when and if enforced, drive the legitimate pharmaceutical companies out of the Turkish opium market, it is unlikely to curtail the availability of black-market opium. The proposed new measure will be only one more law for the Turkish farmers to break when they sell to the black-market entrepreneurs. Alternatively, if efforts are in fact made to enforce the new law, poppy culture may have to move higher into the Turkish hills. Finally, in the unlikely event that the ban on Turkish poppy growing becomes completely effective, the black-market suppliers will no doubt simply follow the legitimate pharmaceutical firms to Asia, Africa, or Latin America for their supplies. Indeed, there is growing evidence of a recent substantial shift in black-market operations from cheap Turkish opium to even cheaper Southeast Asian opium.*

Even if the cultivation of poppies throughout the world should be completely blocked, moreover, the effect would be minimal. There are numerous synthetic opiates today which do not require opium as a raw material.

* In June 1971, for example, a "Special Study Mission" of the United States House of Representatives reported that opium grown in Southeast Asia "is smuggled to the United States by couriers on commercial or military aircraft. Some is mailed to the United States using both commercial and military postal services." One group centered in Bangkok, Thailand, was alleged to utilize "active duty military personnel to ship heroin to the United States through the Army and Air Force Postal System." In confirmation, the Special Study Mission cited United States Bureau of Customs data: from the beginning of March through April 24, 1971, the bureau made 248 seizures of narcotics passing through army and air force post offices. How many shipments passed through unseized was, of course, not known. One package from Bangkok, Thailand, containing 17 pounds of heroin—about 800,000 "fixes"—was seized at Fort Monmouth on April 5, 1971. Southeast Asian heroin is also said to reach the United States through Okinawa, Hong Kong, and other Asian ports.[4] The suppression of this traffic is likely to prove even more difficult than the suppression of the traffic from Turkey through Italy or France to New York.

The formulas of these synthetics are known, and their synthesis is not beyond the skills of black-market chemists. Indeed, heroin itself can be synthesized in the chemical laboratory without using opium. An effective worldwide policing of all sources of raw opium would no doubt result in a conversion of the natural-heroin black market into a black market for synthetic heroin or for a synthetic heroin substitute. Why have black-market entrepreneurs not already shifted to synthetics? The answer is simple. Even at inflated 1971 prices, the black marketeers (like the legitimate pharmaceutical companies) secure natural opium so cheaply that synthetics cannot compete.

After the poppies are grown and the opium harvested, the morphine must be extracted from the opium and converted to heroin. This processing can be quite readily accomplished with simple, inexpensive,* relatively mobile equipment—much less equipment than is needed for the distillation of alcohol on a comparable scale. When one heroin "factory" is closed down, another is set up. The United States was unable to prevent the illegal distillation of alcoholic beverages from 1920 to 1933 (or even today);† preventing the conversion of opium to morphine and then to heroin is a much more difficult undertaking. The bulk of the morphine is converted to heroin in the south of France, because that is where the trade began. It continues to be centered there, presumably because the converters like to live in the south of France. If law enforcement there becomes too troublesome, they can readily take their skills and modest equipment elsewhere.

Faced with these discouraging facts, United States law-enforcement officials have devoted much of their efforts through the years to preventing the *importation* of heroin into the United States. The problems they face at this level can be suggested by a few figures.

There are an estimated 250,000 to 315,000 addicts in the United States, each paying an estimated $20 a day for an estimated 40 milligrams of heroin.[7]

To supply 250,000 addicts with 40 milligrams apiece per day takes less than 25 pounds of heroin per day—four or five tons a year.

Total United States imports of all goods exceed 100,000,000 tons a year. The task of the Bureau of Customs, accordingly, is to find four or five tons of heroin amid 100,000,000 tons of other imports.

The number of persons entering the United States through Customs each year totals more than 200,000,000—4,000,000 per week. One or two travelers can carry concealed on their persons a day's supply of heroin

* Equipment for a factory capable of converting morphine into heroin in kilogram batches costs about $700.[5]

† For every 14 gallons of legal distilled spirits consumed in the United States in 1969, it is estimated that one gallon of bootleg "moonshine" was produced.[6]

for 250,000 addicts; two or three can carry a week's national supply in their luggage. To spot that handful of smugglers among 4,000,000 border crossers each week is a problem not easily solvable. It has certainly not been solved during the decades since 1914. What antismuggling controls really accomplish is to discourage an *increase* in the supply and thus to help maintain high prices.

Few smugglers are caught by means of random border checks, of course. Arrests generally occur when border officials are tipped off to their coming by national and international surveillance networks. Many seizures are in fact made, and widely publicized. But here three other factors tend to limit police effectiveness.

First, the national and international surveillance networks with their paid informers and voluntary informants are an ideal method of spotting *new* entrants into the narcotics industry. An established smuggler or importer faced with fresh competition—especially competition from a supplier who cuts prices—need only pass the word through informers or informants to the surveillance networks and thus to the United States Bureau of Customs. The law-enforcement agents may be completely honest; * even so, the net effect of their efforts is largely to keep out new competitors and thus to buttress the existing heroin distribution system and its price-fixing effectiveness.

Second, increasing the Bureau of Customs heroin seizures has only a trivial effect on the cost of the heroin in a bag. An estimated 6,600 pounds of heroin was smuggled into the United States in the fiscal year ending June 30, 1970. During that year, the Bureau of Customs seized 311 pounds, or less than 5 percent; this was a better-than-average year for the bureau. [10] It meant that foreign suppliers had to ship 6,911 pounds of heroin in order to land 6,600 pounds safely in the United States. Suppose that by herculean efforts and a vast expansion of its staff, the Bureau of Customs manages to quadruple its seizures next year. The net effect will be that European suppliers will have to ship 7,844 pounds instead of 6,911 pounds in order to land 6,600 pounds safely. The additional 933 pounds of heroin intercepted will represent a loss to heroin importers of about $3,500,000. This will add less than two cents to the materials cost of a $5 bag. (The selling price of the bag may go up by more than two cents,

---

* Honesty remains a problem, however. Agents making $10,000 to $12,000 a year must resist bribes totaling many times that sum. In narcotics work, says the chief of the Federal Bureau of Narcotics and Dangerous Drugs, John E. Ingersoll, are "the most fantastic temptations that I have found in some 18 or 19 years of law enforcement." [8] During a twelve-month period ending in November 1969, 49 Federal Bureau of Narcotics agents (39 of them in New York) resigned under fire following investigation. The agents' misconduct took three forms: actual sale of narcotics, participation in a conspiracy to sell, and illegal possession of drugs. In one case, more than $1 million changed hands. [9]

of course; but if so, the rest of the increase will represent added profits to the traffickers.)

Third, the smuggler actually caught is rarely the owner of the heroin seized; he is instead a very well-paid courier (sometimes a sailor, sometimes a minor diplomat, sometimes a college student, sometimes just a traveler). Even if he is caught and imprisoned for life, there are others eager to take his place for a sufficient fee.

On rare occasions, it is true, the seizure of a very large shipment of heroin does cause a temporary shortage of black-market supplies within the United States. This, however, is hardly an objectionable event for the American distributors; on the contrary, it enables them to raise their prices even higher.* Indeed, the profitability of the entire narcotics black market depends on untiring efforts of the law-enforcement agencies to hold the available supply down to the level of effective demand. Only during World War II, when international channels of trade were disrupted on a mammoth scale, was the shortage of smuggled heroin sufficiently acute to curtail significantly the number of addicts receiving their opiates.† [13]

If the price of tomatoes goes up, many housewives will shift to other vegetables. But, as a 1967 Arthur D. Little, Inc., report points out, the demand for opiates is remarkably inelastic. [14] Even at the inflated black-market prices charged in the 1960s, consumers went right on buying heroin. (Alcohol and cigarettes are two other products that display very little demand elasticity.) Vigorous law enforcement, while it can be enormously effective in inflating heroin prices, has relatively little effect on heroin consumption.

The efficiency of American law-enforcement agencies in keeping the price of heroin high in the United States has proved to be a boon primarily to Great Britain, France, Germany, the Scandinavian countries,

---

* Law enforcement produced a temporary shortage of heroin in New York City, for example, in November 1961. Preble and Casey said (1969): "The panic lasted only a few weeks. During this time the demand for the meager supplies of heroin was so great that those who had supplies were able to double and triple their prices and further adulterate the quality, thus realizing sometimes as much as ten times their usual profit. By the time heroin became available again in good supply, the dealers had learned that inferior heroin at inflated prices could find a ready market. Since that time the cost of heroin on the street has continued to climb. . . . A few minor panics—about two a year—help bolster the market. Today an average heroin habit costs the user about $20 a day, as compared to $2 twenty years ago. This fact is responsible for a major social disorder in [New York City] today." [11]

A minor panic developed in New York City late in November 1971, with heroin hard to get; it was generally attributed to the two-month dock strike, which cut off all ocean freight, rather than to law enforcement. The panic ended when the strike was settled.

† During this shortage of imported heroin, opium poppies were again planted in the United States.[12] Congress responded by passing the Opium Poppy Control Act of 1942. The shortage also led to an expansion of opium production in Mexico.

and other nonopium-producing countries throughout the world. Why bother to smuggle heroin into London or Stockholm when you can sell it at far higher prices in the United States? *

Britain's relative freedom from smuggled opiates through the decades has often been attributed to the policy that permitted British physicians to prescribe morphine and heroin for addicts legally. This, as we shall show in Chapter 13, has been one important factor; but American law-enforcement efforts, by stimulating increased prices and thus attracting the world's smugglers, also deserves much credit for Britain's freedom from smuggled heroin.

It is the economics of smuggling, incidentally, that explains why American addicts converted from opium or morphine to heroin after 1914. The difference to the addict is slight,† for heroin is promptly reconverted into morphine after it enters the human body. Addicts now take heroin because that's what the smugglers smuggle. One pound of pure morphine can be easily and cheaply converted into a little more than one pound of pure heroin (diacetylmorphine) by heating it in the presence of acetic acid, some of which it absorbs. The heroin that emerges is more potent, per ounce or per cubic inch, than the morphine that goes into the process; ‡ it is therefore worth more.

* Detective Sergeant Arthur Howard, senior sergeant of the Scotland Yard Drugs Office, reported at a meeting of the British Medico-Legal Society on February 11, 1965, that the black-market price of heroin of medicinal strength and purity in London was then twenty shillings (about $2.80) per grain.[15] Heroin of medicinal strength and purity was not available on the New York retail black market at any price at that time; adulterated heroin of equivalent opiate activity was retailing at about $30. The London black market was very small and unable to raise its prices because an overcharged addict could get his heroin without charge through the National Health Service.

† "It is widely believed amongst addicts," says Dr. J. H. Willis, consultant psychiatrist in drug addiction to Guy's, King's College, and Bexley Hospitals in London, "that heroin possesses some special euphoriant effect; a collective belief which may be shared by many doctors but in fact it is not the case. Studies carried out on nonaddicts and post-addicts have clearly demonstrated that the subjects completely failed to distinguish between the effects of heroin and morphine. What seems likely is that a 'special effect' of heroin as a euphoriant is a myth propagated by narcotics pedlars in the United States. Thus the myth may have an economic basis, since an illicit dealer can sell more doses. Its 'special' effect is then directly linked to its greater potency weight for weight than morphine rather than to a qualitative difference.

"In the same way the drug has acquired a bad reputation as an addictive substance and a special reputation as an analgesic. Whilst it is an excellent analgesic there is little firm evidence that it is more effective than morphine although it is traditionally favoured in terminal illness. This is not to say that it is a drug which should be removed from the pharmacopoeia but merely to highlight the fact that it is a drug that has acquired a reputation for good or ill probably for no really valid reason." [16]

‡ The ability of one milligram of heroin to accomplish as much in medicinal use as two or three milligrams of morphine is believed to result from the greater ease with which a heroin molecule passes through the barrier separating the bloodstream from the brain. Thus more heroin molecules reach the brain and fewer are wastefully excreted. For the addict, however, the difference is slight; he readily develops tolerance to both morphine and heroin, so that neither produces much effect.

One final point concerning smuggling is made in the 1967 Arthur D. Little report. If United States law-enforcement policies become so efficient as to prevent altogether the smuggling of heroin, the black market can readily convert to narcotic concentrates that are a thousand or even ten thousand times more potent, milligram for milligram.[17] A month's supply of such a concentrate for one addict can be hidden under a postage stamp. A few pounds of these concentrates might supply the entire United States addict market for a year. The formulas for these concentrates are known, the raw materials are available, and only small quantities are needed. The skills required are not beyond those possessed by the clandestine chemists who now extract morphine from opium and convert the morphine to heroin, or of better chemists who might be recruited. If the Bureau of Customs should some day develop methods for seizing so much heroin that smuggling became unprofitable, the foreign suppliers could and no doubt would convert to the uninterceptable concentrates—or the concentrates might be manufactured here in the United States, much as black-market amphetamines and LSD are now clandestinely manufactured here (see Parts V and VII).

After importation, the heroin is adulterated or "cut" with other materials. The morphine that physicians legally prescribe for the treatment of pain is also "cut" with a fluid vehicle; pure morphine and pure heroin are too concentrated to be safely injectable into the human body. The objection to the "cutting" of street heroin is not that it occurs, but that it is not properly done, and that unsafe diluents are used. The adulterated heroin that reaches the street has, on the average, about as much opiate activity (10 percent) as the natural product, opium. The net effect of the whole opium–morphine–heroin–adulterated heroin cycle is thus to put the active opiate into its most concentrated form for the smuggling leg of its trip to market.

The 1967 Arthur D. Little report distinguishes three levels of middlemen between the importer and the addict on the street—and estimates buying and selling prices per kilogram (2.2 pounds) of pure heroin at each level as follows.[18]

Supplier	Buying Price	Selling Price
Importer	$10,000	$18,000
Wholesaler	18,000	32,000
Dealer	32,000	70,000
Pusher	70,000	225,000
Addict	225,000	. . .

A more detailed analysis of the New York City heroin market was published in the *International Journal of the Addictions* for March 1969 by

Professor Edward A. Preble and John J. Casey, Jr. The Preble-Casey analysis follows in part.

Heroin contracted for in Europe at $5,000 per kilo (2.2 pounds) will be sold in $5 bags on the street for about one million dollars, after having passed through at least six levels of distribution. . . . The following account does not include all the many variations, but can be taken as a paradigm.

Opium produced in Turkey, India, and Iran is processed into heroin in Lebanon, France, and Italy and prepared for shipment to the East Coast of the United States. A United States importer, through a courier, can buy a kilogram of 80% heroin in Europe for $5,000. . . . The importer, who usually never sees the heroin, sells down the line to a highly trusted customer through intermediaries. If it is a syndicate operation, he would only sell to high level, coded men, known as *captains*. These men are major distributors, referred to as *kilo connections* and, generally, as *the people*.

The *kilo connection* pays $20,000 for the original kilogram *(kilo, kee)*, and gives it a one and one cut (known as *hitting it*), that is, he makes two kilos out of one by adding the common adulterants of milk sugar, mannite (a product from the ash tree used as a mild laxative) and quinine. . . . After the cut, the kilo connection sells down the line in kilos, half kilos and quarter kilos, depending upon the resources of his customers. He will get approximately $10,000 per half kilo for the now adulterated heroin.

The customer of the kilo connection is known as *the connection* in its original sense, meaning that he knows *the people*, even though he is not one of them. He may also be called an *ounce man*. He is a highly trusted customer. . . . Assuming that the connection buys directly from a kilo connection, he will probably give the heroin a one and one cut (make two units of each one), divide the total aggregate into ounces, and sell down the line at $700 per ounce. In addition to the adulteration, the aggregate weight of the product is reduced. Known as a *short count*, this procedure occurs at every succeeding level of distribution. At this stage, however, it is called a *good ounce*, despite the adulteration and reduced weight.

The next man is known as a *dealer in weight*, and is probably the most important figure in the line of distribution. He stands midway between the top and the bottom, and is the first one coming down the line who takes substantial risk of being apprehended by law enforcement officers. He is also the first one who may be a heroin user himself, but usually he is not. He is commonly referred to as one who is *into something* and is respected as a big dealer who has put himself in jeopardy by, as the sayings go, *carrying a felony with him* and *doing the time;* that is, if he gets caught he can expect a long jail sentence. It is said of him that "he let his name go," or "his name gets kicked around," meaning that his identity is known to people in the street. This man usually specializes in *cut ounces*. He may give a two and one cut (make three units of each one) to the good ounce from the connection and sell the resulting quantity for $500 per ounce. The aggregate weight is again reduced, and now the unit is called a *piece* instead of an ounce. Sometimes it is called a *street ounce* or a *vig ounce (vig* is an abbreviation for *vigorish*, which is the term used to designate the high interest on loans charged by loan sharks). In previous years 25 to 30 level teaspoons were supposed to constitute an ounce; today it is 16 to 20.

The next customer is known as a *street dealer*. He buys the *piece* for $500, gives it a one and one cut and makes *bundles,* which consist of 25 $5 bags each. He can usually get seven bundles from each piece, and he sells each bundle for $80. He may also package the heroin in *half-bundles* (ten $5 bags each), which sell for $40, or he may package in *half-loads* (fifteen $3 bags), which sell for $30 each. This man may or may not be a heroin user.

The next distributor is known as a *juggler* [in popular parlance, *pusher*], who is the seller from whom the average street addict buys. He is always a user. He buys bundles for $80 each and sells the 25 bags at about $5 each, making just enough profit to support his own habit, day by day. He may or may not make a small cut, known as *tapping the bags*. He is referred to as someone who is "always high and always short," that is, he always has enough heroin for his own use and is always looking for a few dollars to get enough capital to cop again. . . . The juggler leads a precarious life, both financially and in the risks he takes of getting robbed by fellow addicts or arrested. Most arrests for heroin sales are of the juggler. Financially he is always struggling to stay in the black. If business is a little slow he may start to get sick or impatient and use some of the heroin he needs to sell in order to re-cop. If he does this he is in the red and temporarily out of business. A juggler is considered to be doing well if he has enough money left over after a transaction for cab fare to where he buys the heroin. One informant defined a juggler as a "non-hustling dope fiend who is always messing the money up." [19]

Figure 1, taken from the Preble and Casey report, summarizes the major features of the distribution transactions.

The purpose of this complex, multilayered distribution system is clear: it makes it possible for each participant in the system to deal with only a few others whom he knows and trusts, and thus to minimize his risk of arrest. The 1967 Arthur D. Little report estimates, for example, that the average importer supplies only eight wholesalers, each wholesaler only six retailers, each retailer only six pushers, and each pusher only fifteen addicts. Yet the supplies from the original importer reach 4,320 addicts. [20]

The middlemen (wholesalers and retailers) are liable to arrest—but arresting a middleman is not likely to close down a channel of distribution. One retired middleman told a New York *Times* reporter in September 1969 that he had been making $4,000 a week before his retirement by distributing a relatively small amount of heroin weekly. [21] At a White House press conference in October 1969, the head of the Federal Bureau of Narcotics and Dangerous Drugs, John E. Ingersoll, similarly reported: "The money is terrific. I have seen traffickers who can make $150,000 to $200,000 a year. These are not the big-time fellows. These are the middle level." [22] When a job like that falls vacant through arrest, retirement, or other cause, there are many applicants eager to fill it. No college degree

Distributor	Type of Cut	Adulteration	Percentage Heroin	Rate of Return on Investment
Importer	–		80%	300%
Kilo Connection	1 & 1		40%	100%
Connection	1 & 1		20%	145%
Weight Dealer	2 & 1		6.7%	114%
Street Dealer	1 & 1		3.3%	124%
Juggler	?	?	?	56%

FIGURE 1. The Heroin Market: Chain of Supply, Adulteration Process, and Profit [23]

is required, nor much technical skill or experience. Since the black market keeps few records, the need to pay income tax on the $4,000 a week is less than for most other sources of income; this acts as a multiplier of incentive. Even $1,000 a week is generous pay if no tax is paid on it. If a middleman is prudent, he can retire quite young. Lack of middlemen, in short—like lack of poppy growers, processors, or importers—is not likely to prove the Achilles' heel in the black-market distribution system.

The middlemen lowest on the ladder, the pushers or "jugglers," are often arrested. Indeed, the 1967 Arthur D. Little report estimates that of every seven pushers, one goes to prison each year. Following such an event, there is keen competition among the arrested man's friends, neighbors, and other customers to determine which one of them will be fortunate enough to inherit his "connection"—for "juggling" is a way of life much preferable to stealing or other alternatives open to street addicts. Thus doubling or trebling the number of jugglers or pushers arrested each year has little effect on the distribution system; it simply opens the door of opportunity for additional replacements.

From time to time, enforcement officials find a weak spot in one of the conduits through which drugs flow from the poppy growers overseas to addicts in the United States. When this occurs, the supply is simply re-routed around the weak spot. Failure to close down the opiate black markets during the past fifty-six years of intensive effort suggests that not too much hope should be pinned on the success of future efforts.

The structure of the black market, incidentally, helps to explain why the black-market retailing of narcotics has tended since World War II to center in black inner-city ghettos. The first black markets after 1914 were largely in brothels and red-light districts—neighborhoods where the risk was minimized that passers-by, if they happened upon drug trans-actions, would summon the police. After 1920, the markets tended to shift to speakeasies in the nation's Boweries and skid rows—also areas where residents and the police were inclined to be alienated from one another. The shift after World War II to the alienated black inner-city ghettos was a natural further development.

Narcotics agents followed the traffickers into the black ghettos. Thus, arrest figures and Federal Bureau of Narcotics figures since 1946 have shown a heavy overrepresentation of black inner-city addicts. The true ratios, past and present, of black to white addicts, of impoverished to middle-class addicts, and of inner-city to suburban addicts are unknown.

The evidence is clear, however, that heroin addiction among white, middle-class young people outside the inner cities increased notably in 1970 and 1971 (see Chapter 20). This was the first major extension of the heroin market since the early 1950s—and it is ironic indeed that it coin-cided with the Nixon administration's vigorous law-enforcement campaign against illicit drugs.

12.

The "heroin overdose" mystery and other hazards of addiction

Chapter 4 of this Report reviewed in detail the effects of heroin and other opiates on addicts, including deleterious physiological effects traceable to the drugs themselves. Narcotics addicts today face other physiological hazards that are traceable to the narcotics laws, to the adulteration, contamination, and exorbitant black-market prices that those laws foster, and to other legal and social (as distinct from pharmacological) factors. Dr. Jerome H. Jaffe has described some of these risks in Goodman and Gilman's textbook (1970): "Undoubtedly, the high cost and impurities of illicit drugs in the United States exact their toll. The high incidence of venereal disease reflects the occupational hazard of the many females who earn their drug money through prostitution. The average annual death rate among young, adult heroin addicts is several times higher than that for nonaddicts of similar age and ethnic backgrounds. . . . The suicide rate among adult addicts is likewise considerably higher than that of the general population." [1]

Because "the preferred route of administration is intravenous," Dr. Jaffe continues, "there is sharing of implements of injection and a failure to employ hygienic technics, with a resultant high incidence of endocarditis, and hepatitis, and other infections." [2]

The exorbitant price of black-market heroin, Dr. Jaffe might have added, is one of the factors that makes intravenous injection "the preferred route of administration," for "mainlining" is the cheapest way to forestall withdrawal symptoms. And the laws restricting possession of injection equipment, under penalty of imprisonment, increase the risk of needle-borne infections by encouraging the sharing of implements.

There remains to be considered yet another risk of heroin addiction, the most publicized hazard of all—death from "heroin overdose." Because these deaths are a source of such widespread concern, and also because they are so widely misunderstood, even by authorities on heroin addiction and by addicts themselves, we shall examine the data in detail. Much of the discussion that follows is focused on New York City, since the deaths attributed to heroin overdose are most numerous there and since the New York City data are published in convenient form.

"Prior to 1943, there were relatively few deaths among addicts from overdosage."[3] By the 1950s, however, nearly half of all deaths among New York City addicts were being attributed to "acute reaction to dosage or overdosage."[4] In 1969, about 70 percent of all New York addict deaths were assigned the "overdose" label[5]—and in 1970, the proportion was about 80 percent.[6] The number of deaths so designated by New York City's Office of the Chief Medical Examiner increased from very few or none at all before 1943 to about 800 in 1969 and 1970.[7]

During this same twenty-eight-year span, addict deaths from all other causes—infections, violence, suicide, and so on—increased very little. The enormous increase in number of deaths among addicts shown in Figure 2 was attributed almost entirely to "overdose" deaths.

The number of deaths throughout the United States attributed to heroin overdose from 1943 to date must total many thousands. In New York City it was reported that narcotics, chiefly heroin, were the leading cause of death in 1969 and 1970 in all males aged fifteen to thirty-five,[8] including nonaddicts. This can properly be characterized as an epidemic; the general alarm over these deaths is thoroughly warranted.

There are two relatively simple ways, however, to prevent deaths from heroin overdose.

First, addicts can be warned to take only their usual dose of heroin rather than risking death by taking too much.

Second, even in cases where an addict takes a vastly excessive dose despite the warning, death usually can be readily prevented, for death from an overdose of opiates is ordinarily a slow process. "In cases of fatal poisoning with morphine, the time of death may vary roughly from one to twelve hours."[9] The first signs are lethargy and stupor, followed by prolonged coma. If, after a period of hours, death does ensue, it is usually from respiratory failure. During the minutes or hours following the injection of a potentially fatal overdose, death can be readily forestalled by administering an effective antidote: a narcotic antagonist known as nalorphine (Nalline).[10] Nalorphine brings a victim of opiate overdose out of his stupor or coma within a few minutes. Since there is plenty of time and since nalorphine is stocked in pharmacies and hospital emergency rooms throughout the country, the death of anyone due to heroin overdose is very rarely excusable.

But alas, the two standard precautions against overdose—warnings against taking too much and administration of an antidote—are in fact wholly ineffective in the current crisis, *for the thousands of deaths attributed to heroin overdose are not in fact due to heroin overdose at all.* The evidence falls under three major rubrics.

(1) The deaths *cannot* be due to overdose.
(2) There has *never been any evidence* that they are due to overdose.
(3) There has long been a plethora of evidence demonstrating that they are *not* due to overdose.

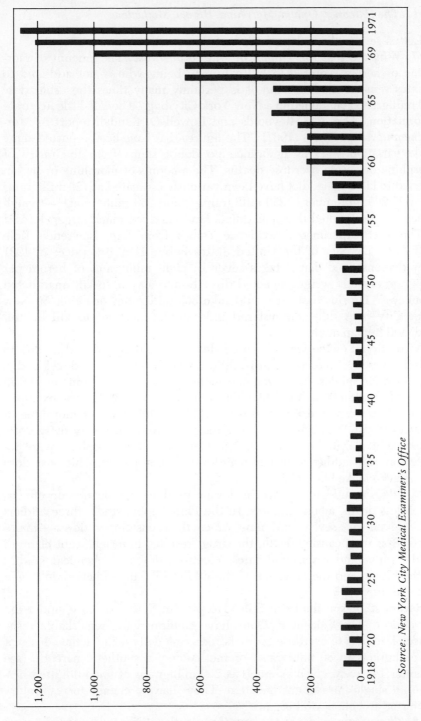

FIGURE 2. Deaths from Narcotics Abuse in New York City, 1918–1971[11]

Source: New York City Medical Examiner's Office

Let us review these three bodies of data in detail.

(1) Why these deaths cannot be due to overdose. The amount of morphine or heroin required to kill a human being who is not addicted to opiates remains in doubt but it is certainly many times the usual dose (10 milligrams) contained in a New York City bag. "There is little accurate information," Drs. A. J. Reynolds and Lowell O. Randall report in *Morphine and Allied Drugs* (1967). "The figures that have been reported show wide variation." [12] This ignorance no doubt stems from the rarity of morphine or heroin overdose deaths. The amounts of morphine or heroin needed to kill a nonaddict have been variously estimated at 120 milligrams (oral),[13] 200 milligrams,[14] 250 milligrams,[15] and 350 milligrams[16]—though it has also been noted that nonaddicts have survived much larger doses.[17]

The best experimental evidence comes from Drs. Lawrence Kolb and A. G. Du Mez of the United States Public Health Service; in 1931 they demonstrated that it takes seven or eight milligrams of heroin per kilogram of body weight, injected directly into a vein, to kill unaddicted monkeys.[18] On this basis, it would take 500 milligrams or more (50 New York City bags full, administered in a single injection) to kill an unaddicted human adult.

Virtually all of the victims whose deaths are falsely labeled as due to heroin overdose, moreover, are addicts who have already developed a tolerance for opiates—and even enormous amounts of morphine or heroin do not kill addicts. In the Philadelphia study of the 1920s, for example, some addicts reported using 28 grains (1,680 milligrams) of morphine or heroin per day.[19] This is forty times the usual New York City daily dose. In one Philadelphia experiment, 1,800 milligrams of morphine were injected into an addict over a two-and-a-half-hour period. This vast dose didn't even make him sick.[20]

Nor does a sudden *increase* in dosage produce significant side effects, much less death, among addicts. In the Philadelphia study, three addicts were given six, seven, and nine times their customary doses—"mainlined." Far from causing death, the drug "resulted in insignificant changes in the pulse and respiration rates, electrocardiogram, chemical studies of the blood, and the behavior of the addict." [21] The addicts didn't even become drowsy.[22]

Recent studies at the Rockefeller Hospital in New York City, under the direction of Dr. Vincent P. Dole, have confirmed the remarkable resistance of addicts to overdose. Addicts receiving daily maintenance doses of 40 milligrams to 80 milligrams of methadone, a synthetic narcotic (see Chapter 14), were given as much as 200 milligrams of unadulterated heroin in a single intravenous injection. They "had no change in respiratory center or any other vital organs." [23]

(2) There is no evidence to show that deaths attributed to overdose are

in fact so caused. Whenever someone takes a drug—whether strychnine, a barbiturate, heroin, or some other substance—and then dies without other apparent cause, the suspicion naturally arises that he *may* have taken too much of the drug and and died of poisoning: an overdose. To confirm or refute this suspicion, an autopsy is performed, following a well-established series of procedures.

If the drug was taken by mouth, for example, the stomach contents and feces are analyzed in order to identify the drug and to determine whether an excessive amount is present. If the drug was injected, the tissues surrounding the injection site are similarly analyzed. The blood, urine, and other body fluids and tissues can also be analyzed and the quantity of drug present determined.

Circumstantial evidence, too, can in some cases establish with reasonable certainty that someone has died of overdose. If a patient fills a prescription for a hundred barbiturate tablets, for example, and is found dead the next morning with only a few tablets left in the bottle, death from barbiturate poisoning is a reasonable hypothesis to be explored. Similarly, if an addict dies after "shooting up," and friends who were present report that he injected many times his usual dose, the possibility of death from heroin overdose deserves serious consideration.

Further, in cases where an addict has died following an injection of heroin, and the syringe he used is found nearby or still sticking in his vein, the contents of the syringe can be examined to determine whether it contained heroin of exceptional strength. And there are other ways of establishing at least a *prima facie* case for an overdose diagnosis.

A conscientious search of the United States medical literature throughout recent decades has failed to turn up a single scientific paper reporting that heroin overdose, as established by these or any other reasonable methods of determining overdose, is in fact a cause of death among American heroin addicts. The evidence that addicts have been dying by the hundreds of heroin overdose is simply nonexistent.

At this point the mystery deepens. If even enormous doses of heroin will not kill an addict, and if there exists no shred of evidence to indicate that addicts or nonaddicts are in fact dying of heroin overdose, why is the overdose myth almost universally accepted? The answer lies in the customs of the United States coroner–medical examiner system.

Whenever anyone dies without a physician in attendance to certify the cause of death, it is the duty of the local coroner or medical examiner to investigate, to have an autopsy performed if indicated, and then formally to determine and record the cause of death. The parents, spouse, or children of the dead person can then ask the coroner for his findings. Newspaper reporters similarly rely on the coroner or medical examiner to explain a newsworthy death. No coroner, of course, wants to be in a position of having to answer "I don't know" to such queries. A coroner is *supposed* to know—and if he doesn't know, he is supposed to find out.

At some point in the history of heroin addiction, probably in the early 1940s, the custom arose among coroners and medical examiners of labeling as "heroin overdose" all deaths among heroin addicts the true cause of which could not be determined. These "overdose" determinations rested on only two findings: (1) that the victim was a heroin addict who "shot up" prior to his death; and (2) that there was no evidence of suicide, violence, infection, or other natural cause.[24] No evidence that the victim had taken a *large* dose was required to warrant a finding of death from overdose. *This curious custom continues today.* Thus, in common coroner and medical examiner parlance, "death from heroin overdose" is synonymous with "death from unknown causes after injecting heroin."

During the 1940s, this custom of convenience did little apparent harm. Most deaths among heroin addicts were due to tetanus, bacterial endocarditis, tuberculosis, and other infections, to violence, or to suicide, and they were properly labeled as such by coroners and medical examiners. It was only an occasional death which baffled the medical examiner, and which was therefore signed out as due to "overdose." But, beginning about 1943, a strange new kind of death began to make its appearance among heroin addicts.[25] The cause of this new kind of death was not known, and remains unknown today—though it is now quite common.

A striking feature of this mysterious new mode of death is its suddenness. Instead of occurring after one or more hours of lethargy, stupor, and coma, as in true overdose cases, death occurs within a few minutes or less—perhaps only a few seconds after the drug is injected. Indeed, "collapse and death are so rapid," one authority reports, "that the syringe was found in the vein of the victim or on the floor after having dropped out of the vein, and the tourniquet was still in place on the arm."[26] This explains in part why nalorphine and other narcotic antagonists, highly effective antidotes in true opiate overdose cases, are useless in the cases falsely labeled overdose.

An even more striking feature of these mysterious deaths is a sudden and massive flooding of the lungs with fluid: pulmonary edema. In many cases it is not even necessary to open the lungs or X-ray them to find the edema; "an abundance of partly dried frothy white edema fluid [is seen] oozing from the nostrils or mouth"[27] when the body is first found. Neither of these features suggests overdose—but since "overdose" has come to be a synonym for "cause unknown," and since the cause of these sudden deaths characterized by lung edema is unknown, they are lumped under the "overdose" rubric.

Not all of the deaths attributed to heroin overdose are necessarily characterized by suddenness and by massive pulmonary edema, but several studies have shown that a high proportion of all "overdose" deaths share these two characteristics.[28]

(3) Evidence demonstrating that these deaths are not due to overdose is plentiful. This evidence has been summarized in a series of scientific papers, beginning in 1966, by New York City's Chief Medical Examiner, Dr. Milton Helpern, and his associate, Deputy Chief Medical Examiner, Dr. Michael M. Baden. At a meeting of the Society for the Study of Addiction held in London in 1966, Dr. Helpern explained that the most conspicuous feature of so-called "overdose" deaths is the massive pulmonary edema. When asked the cause of the edema, he cautiously responded:

> This is a very interesting question. To my knowledge it is not known why the pulmonary edema develops in these cases. . . . This reaction sometimes occurs with the intravenous injections of mixtures, which as far as is known, do not contain any heroin, but possibly some other substance. The reaction does not appear to be specific. It does not seem to be peculiar to one substance, but it is most commonly seen with mixtures in which heroin is the smallest component.[29]

In a paper published in the *New York State Journal of Medicine* for September 15, 1966, Dr. Helpern again cast doubt on the myth that these deaths are due to overdose. "Formerly such acute deaths were attributed to overdose of the heroin contained in the sample injected," Dr. Helpern reported—but he went on to cite several lines of evidence arguing *against* the overdose theory:

> . . . Unexpected acute deaths may occur in some addicts who inject themselves with heroin mixtures even though others who take the same usual . . . dose from the same sample at the same time may suffer no dangerous effect. In some fatal acute cases, the rapidity and type of reaction do not suggest overdose alone but rather an overwhelming shocklike process due to sensitivity to the injected material. The toxicologic examination of the tissues in such fatalities, where the reaction was so rapid that the syringe and needle were still in the vein of the victim when the body was found, demonstrated only the presence of alkaloid, not overdosage. In other acute deaths, in which the circumstances and autopsy findings were positive, the toxicologist could not even find any evidence of alkaloid in the tissues or body fluids. Thus, there does not appear to be any quantitative correlation between the acute fulminating lethal effect and the amount of heroin taken. . . .[30]

Dr. Helpern's associate, Deputy Chief Medical Examiner Baden, went on to further discredit the already implausible overdose theory at a joint meeting of two American Medical Association drug-dependency committees held in Palo Alto, California, in February 1969.

"The majority of deaths," Dr. Baden told the AMA physicians, "are due to an acute reaction to the intravenous injection of the heroin-quinine-sugar mixture. This type of death is often referred to as an 'overdose,' which is a misnomer. Death is not due to a pharmacological overdose in the vast majority of cases." [31]

At the same AMA committee meeting and at a meeting of the Medical Society of the County of New York, Dr. Baden cited six separate lines of evidence overturning the "heroin overdose" theory.

First, when the packets of heroin found near the bodies of dead addicts are examined, they do not differ from ordinary packets. "No qualitative or quantitative differences" are found.[32] This rules out the possibility that some incredibly stupid processor may have filled a bag with pure heroin instead of the usual adulterated mix.

Second, when the syringes used by addicts immediately before dying are examined, the mixture found in them does not contain more heroin than usual.

Third, when the urine of addicts allegedly dead of overdose is analyzed, there is no evidence of overdose.

Fourth, the tissues surrounding the site of the fatal injection show no signs of high heroin concentration.

Fifth, neophytes unaccustomed to heroin rather than addicts tolerant to opiates would be expected to be susceptible to death from overdose. But "almost all of those dying" of alleged overdose, Deputy Chief Medical Examiner Baden reported, "are long-term users."

Sixth, again according to Dr. Baden, "addicts often 'shoot' in a group, all using the same heroin supply, and rarely does more than one addict die at such a time." [33]

These definitive refutations of the heroin overdose theory should, of course, have led to two prompt steps: a warning to addicts that something *other* than overdose is causing these hundreds of addict deaths annually —and an intensive search for the true cause of the deaths. But neither of these steps has been taken. Hence the news media go right on talking about "heroin overdose" deaths. "Death from acute reaction to heroin overdose" and other complicated phrases are also used; these phrases similarly conceal the fact that these deaths are *not* due to overdose.

How can the "heroin overdose" myth not only survive but flourish even after these repeated scientific debunkings? Two stenographic transcripts provide an answer.

The first is the transcript of a press conference held at the Rockefeller University on October 27, 1969, in connection with the Second National Conference on Methadone Treatment. In the course of his remarks to the assembled reporters, Deputy Chief Medical Examiner Baden there discussed at some length a case of what he described as an "addict who died of an overdose of heroin." [34] The reporters present naturally referred thereafter to this death as a "heroin overdose" case.

At the *scientific* meeting held in the same room on the same day, how-ever, Dr. Baden described the same death in quite different terms. To the scientists he stated that the addict in question "died of acute reaction to injection of heroin, a so-called overdose." When even this description was challenged by a fellow physician, who pointed out that addicts don't die following even enormous doses,[35] Dr. Baden went on to explain that "whenever I say 'overdose,' it is in quotation marks." [36]

The reporters, of course, could not see those invisible quotation marks when they listened to Dr. Baden at his press conferences and interviews. They quite naturally took him literally—and continued to inform the public that addicts were dying of overdose.*

Even Chief Medical Examiner Helpern eventually became convinced that the "heroin overdose" publicity emanating from his office was "dangerously wrong." In testimony before the Select Committee on Crime of the United States House of Representatives on June 27, 1970, Dr. Helpern stated:

A difficulty has been that people have considered these fatal reactions the result of overdose. Now, to some people the designation overdose means [taking] more than usual with the implication that if you are careful of how much is taken there is no danger of anything other than the usual effect. This impression which many addicts have is dangerously wrong. [38]

Yet a full year after Dr. Helpern testified, neither he nor Dr. Baden nor anyone else had yet ventured to correct the "dangerously wrong" view that was being foisted on the New York and national news media. Almost everyone who did not read Dr. Helpern's and Dr. Baden's papers in the medical journals still believed that heroin addicts by the hundreds were dying of overdose. Worse yet, nobody had as yet even begun to investigate seriously the crucial question: *If these hundreds of addicts a year aren't dying of overdose, what are they dying of?*

Fortunately, enough is already known to suggest some promising direc-tions for immediate research.

Most deaths from so-called overdose, as noted above, are characterized by suddenness and by pulmonary edema. No other cause of death—such as tetanus, bacterial endocarditis, hepatitis, or a knife or gunshot wound —is found. In approximately 60 percent of autopsies, a 1970 study in-dicates, there is also cerebral edema (accumulation of fluid in the brain) along with widespread fragmentation of the astrocytes (star-shaped cells) in the brain.[39] A death with these characteristics, occurring in a heroin addict, constitutes a dramatic and readily identifiable syndrome which Dr.

---

* Thus in the New York *Times* for December 16, 1969, a reporter was led to state without qualification: "About 800 addicts of all ages died this year from overdoses, according to Dr. Baden." [37]

Helpern has called "acute fatal reaction to the intravenous injection of crude mixtures of heroin and other substances." We shall here apply a less cumbersome label: "Syndrome X."

One clue to the true cause of Syndrome X is its initial appearance about 1943, its relative rarity for the next few years, and its recent rapid increase in frequency. The time sequence obviously suggests that the cause of Syndrome X must be some factor introduced about 1943 and affecting a vastly increased number of addicts during 1969 and 1970. Heroin clearly does not qualify; it was widely used long before 1943. Indeed, a highly significant fact about Syndrome X is that it has become more and more frequent as the amount of heroin in the New York City bag has gone down and down. These deaths are, if anything, associated with "underdose" rather than overdose.

One theory sometimes advanced is that Syndrome X deaths are caused by the *quinine* in the bag. Quinine was introduced as an adulterant of heroin sometime after 1939, when an epidemic of malaria spread by contaminated injection needles hit New York City addicts; [40] thus the time of introduction fits the Syndrome X timetable. Some addicts discovered that the quinine contributed to the sensation known as a "rush" immediately after injection. Heroin traffickers also discovered that the bitter taste of the quinine makes it impossible for addicts to gauge the concentration of heroin in the bag by tasting the mixture. For these and possibly other reasons, quinine has remained a standard adulterant of New York City heroin ever since.

Perhaps the first suggestion that quinine might be causing New York City's Syndrome X deaths came from Dr. F. E. Camps, the United Kingdom Home Office pathologist in charge of investigating opiate deaths in England. At a conference of the Society for the Study of Addiction held in London in September 1966 (which Chief Medical Examiner Helpern attended), Dr. Camps stated: "The only comparable drug to heroin which causes rapid death with pulmonary oedema is quinine. In this case patients start off with discomfort in their chest, and then rapidly die. It is conceivable that this could have some relation to [New York City] heroin deaths." [41]

At the same conference an American pathologist, the late Dr. Rudolph J. Muelling of the University of Kentucky Medical School, added that a type of lung lesion similar to that found in Syndrome X deaths "is found to occur when one studies pure quinine cases. In the United States this kind of lesion has been found in several nurses attempting to induce abortions on themselves. They take the quinine orally and the condition comes on quite rapidly. The patients die of quinine alone." [42]

A second possible cause of Syndrome X deaths can best be illustrated by two examples.

One is the case of "C. G.," a heroin addict long accustomed to main-lining his drug, who one day got drunk, took his "customary injection of heroin and collapsed shortly thereafter." Subsequent X-rays showed lung edema.[43]

Another is the case of a heroin addict whose death was recently reported by Dr. George R. Gay and his associates at the Haight-Ashbury Medical Clinic, San Francisco. This addict first "shot some reds" (that is, barbiturates) and then "fixed" with heroin following the barbiturates. He died of what was diagnosed as "overdose of heroin." [44]

Cases such as these have given rise to the question whether Syndrome X deaths may result from injecting heroin (with or without quinine) into a body already laden with a central-nervous-system depressant such as alcohol or a barbiturate.

Addicts themselves would seem to deserve credit for first suspecting that so-called "heroin overdose" deaths might in fact result from the combined action of alcohol and heroin. Back in 1958, a team headed by Dr. Ray E. Trussell and Mr. Harold Alksne interviewed more than 200 New York City addicts—alumni of the Riverside Hospital addiction treatment program (see Chapter 10). In this as in other pre-1960 studies, few addicts drank alcohol while on heroin, and they did not drink much. When asked why, the addicts commonly gave two reasons.

One was that the effect of alcohol is "offensive" to a man on heroin. "The narcotic alone has an analgesic effect which tends to quiet the individual. Alcohol, on the other hand . . . has the capacity to agitate the individual in his relationships with other people. This generally is offensive to the addict." [45]

The other reason given by addicts in 1958 for not drinking while on heroin is the first extant clue to the possible relationship between alcohol and death from "heroin overdose." Addicts, the Trussell-Alksne team noted, "believe that the use of narcotics and alcohol in combination is dangerous and might possibly lead to the death of an individual." [46] By the 1960s, this awareness of the hazard of shooting heroin while drunk had disappeared from the addict scene. Addicts, like others, were evidently convinced by the official announcements that those deaths were indeed due to heroin overdose.

If the theory is sound that even an ordinary dose of an opiate *injected while drunk* can produce death, then death could occur when an ordinary drunk who is *not* addicted is brought into a hospital emergency room with a painful injury and is given a routine (10 milligram) injection of morphine to ease his pain. Drs. William B. Deichmann and Horace W. Gerarde report in their *Toxicology of Drugs and Chemicals* (1969 edition) that death may in fact occur under such conditions.

"The ordinary safe therapeutic dose of morphine," they warn, in italics,

[111]

in their textbook, *"may be fatal to persons who have been drinking alcoholic beverages.* Morphine in therapeutic doses [similar to the doses commonly injected by addicts] resulted in fatalities in individuals whose blood alcohol levels ranged from 0.22 to 0.27%. Morphine is also synergistic with barbiturates and related drugs." [47] Thus the hazard of death from shooting an opiate while drunk on alcohol or a barbiturate is familiar to some toxicologists even though it has been ignored by authorities on drug addiction—and by coroners and medical examiners—through the years.

If this alcohol-heroin and barbiturate-heroin explanation is correct, the fact is of the utmost practical importance—for hundreds of deaths a year might be prevented by warning addicts not to shoot heroin while drunk on alcohol or barbiturates.

The alcohol-barbiturate hypothesis fits the Syndrome X time schedule. Throughout the nineteenth century and well into the twentieth, opiate addicts were known for their *dislike* of alcohol while on opiates. As noted earlier, they turned to alcohol only when deprived of their opiate supply or when trying to "kick the habit." This remains generally true today; an addict rarely drinks while *on* heroin. He often drinks, however, when his heroin supply runs out and withdrawal symptoms set in. During World War II, many heroin addicts were abruptly deprived of their heroin supply for longer or shorter periods. If some of them turned to alcohol, then connected with a fresh heroin supply and "shot up" while still drunk, the first few identified Syndrome X deaths might have occurred. The recent sharp increase in Syndrome X deaths might similarly be explained by an increased tendency to alternate alcohol or barbiturates with heroin as a result of high heroin prices. As the amount of heroin in the New York City bag went down and down, according to this theory, more and more addicts got drunk—and died of Syndrome X following their next "fix."

Evidence in recent years for the use of alcohol by addicts shortly before their death has been assembled from the New York City files by Drs. Jane McCusker and Charles E. Cherubin. They reviewed 588 city toxicology reports found in the files on addicts who died in 1967. In 549 of these cases, tests for alcohol had been run—and in 43 percent of the cases tested, alcohol was in fact found.[48] (Barbiturates were not reported on.) Their findings led Drs. McCusker and Cherubin to suggest that further research be promptly launched into the possible role of alcohol and the barbiturates in so-called "heroin overdose" cases.

The same suggestion has been tentatively made by Dr. Gay of the Haight-Ashbury Medical Clinic. Thirty-seven percent of the addicts attending the clinic, Dr. Gay states, report using barbiturates "for sedation and sleep" when heroin withdrawal symptoms set in; and 24 percent report using alcohol similarly.[49] Thus the stage is set for shooting heroin while drunk on one or the other—and, perhaps, for sudden death from "overdose."

Two of the most publicized "overdose deaths" of 1970, Dr. Gay informed the National Heroin Conference in June 1971, fit precisely this pattern. These were the deaths of the rock musician Jimi Hendrix and the singer Janis Joplin. Hendrix was known to use both alcohol and barbiturates—and possibly also heroin. Janis Joplin "drank [alcohol] like an F. Scott Fitzgerald legend," Dr. Gay adds—and also used narcotics.[50]

The magazine *Time* reported on October 19, 1970, shortly after Janis Joplin's death:

> The quart bottle of Southern Comfort [whiskey] that she held aloft onstage was at once a symbol of her load and a way of lightening it. As she emptied the bottle, she grew happier, more radiant, and more freaked out. . . .
>
> Last week, on a day that superficially at least seemed to be less lonely than most, Janis Joplin died on the lowest and saddest of notes. Returning to her Hollywood motel room after a late-night recording session and some hard drinking with friends at a nearby bar, she apparently filled a hypodermic needle with heroin and shot it into her left arm. The injection killed her.[51]

Janis Joplin's death, of course, was popularly attributed to "heroin overdose." If the alcohol-barbiturate-heroin theory is correct, her fatal injection of heroin while drunk on alcohol was the prototype of many other deaths similarly mislabeled "overdose."

The British experience with deaths attributed to heroin overdose is consistent with the alcohol-barbiturate hypothesis. Dr. Ramon Gardner of the Bethlem Royal Hospital and Maudsley Hospital in London studied the records of 170 deaths known to have occurred among addicts in Britain during the five-year period 1965 through 1969. Twenty of these deaths were deemed suicides, 24 were traceable to infections, 12 were from natural causes, 11 were drownings, falls, murders, or other accidents, and 6 occurred during treatment (of which two followed abrupt withdrawal of narcotics when the addicts were imprisoned). Eight more were due to overdose of barbiturates or other nonopiate drugs. This left a maximum of 89 mysterious deaths out of 170 which *might* have been caused by accidental opiate overdose—or by something else.[52]

Dr. Gardner then went on to study in more detail 47 of these deaths *possibly* due to heroin overdose. In a number of cases, he found that the addicts had been confined in a hospital, prison, or detention center or had for other reasons been abstinent from opiates for a week or longer, and had thus lost at least a portion of their tolerance for opiates. They had then injected an opiate—some of them on the day of discharge, others within the next day or two. Thus these deaths *might* have been due to overdose—though evidence was lacking that the victims had in fact taken fatally large doses. (Merely doubling or quadrupling the dose, it will be recalled, will not kill even nonaddicts.)

But in at least 21 of the 47 cases, there had been no withdrawal from opiates prior to death, so that tolerance had *not* been lost. And in some cases, the dose preceding death was so small—as little as 20 or 30 milligrams of heroin, for example—as to establish beyond question that overdose was *not* the cause.[53]

These British deaths, accordingly, remain mysterious, like deaths from Syndrome X in the United States. Among several likely explanations, Dr. Gardner himself noted, is the possibility that these addicts may have taken some other drug, perhaps a central-nervous-system depressant, at the same time. Since there is no quinine in British opiates, that drug must be exonerated in the British deaths.

Another British drug authority adds that in Britain as in the United States, "many of those who die, in fact, have taken barbiturates as well [as opiates] at the same time." [54]

It might prove absurdly easy to confirm the alcohol-barbiturate hypothesis. All that might be necessary would be to addict a few monkeys or other primates to heroin, intoxicate them on alcohol or barbiturates, and then inject modest doses of heroin. If the monkeys drop dead of Syndrome X, a warning against shooting heroin while drunk on alcohol or barbiturates might save many hundreds of lives a year throughout the world.

Several other possible explanations of Syndrome X deaths have been offered. No theory has yet been proved. Worse yet, no theory has ever been experimentally tested. The time has surely come to determine the cause (or causes) of Syndrome X and bring to a close this tragic series of deaths. If 800 respectable citizens instead of heroin addicts had dropped dead in New York City of a mysterious syndrome in 1970, a gargantuan research program would no doubt have been promptly launched.

If the Syndrome X deaths are due to quinine or to any other adulterant or contaminant in the bag, the responsibility clearly rests with the American heroin black market for selling unsafe mixes. If the cause of these deaths is the shooting of heroin while drunk on alcohol or barbiturates, the black-market distribution system remains at least indirectly responsible, for it is largely the high cost of black-market heroin that makes heroin users turn to alcohol and barbiturates on occasion—and thus, perhaps, to risk death from Syndrome X.

The two steps which must now be taken are (1) to stop sweeping these mysterious deaths under the carpet by falsely labeling them "overdose" and (2) to launch an intensive clinical and experimental search for what is in fact killing these addicts.

13.

Supplying heroin legally to addicts

The American system of black-market heroin distribution, with its exorbitant prices for contaminated and adulterated heroin, has been described in the previous chapters. It can be contrasted with the American system of *morphine* distribution, which delivers at an amazingly low price some 40,000,000 doses a year of medicinally pure morphine, aseptically packaged and meeting the high standards for injectable products set by the *United States Pharmacopoeia.*

An addict who shifts from black-market heroin to morphine by prescription moves into another world. Suppose, for example, that he has been paying $20 a day for 40 milligrams of heroin mixed with 360 milligrams of hazardous adulterants and contaminants. Armed with a prescription, he can walk into almost any neighborhood pharmacy and secure pure morphine, U.S.P., safely diluted in an appropriate vehicle, and sterilely packaged, at the full retail price of $5 per dram or less. He thus pays about five cents for 40 milligrams of morphine. If heroin were stocked in pharmacies, he could buy 40 milligrams of it, too, on prescription, for about a nickel—as British addicts do.

The question is obvious: Why shouldn't the addict be *encouraged* to secure his opiates legally, on prescription, in pure form, for a nickel a day, rather than be forced by federal and state laws to spend $20 per day in the heroin black market?

Early United States opiate clinics (1912–1924). The suggestion that heroin addicts receive their drug legally is hardly new or revolutionary. Indeed, narcotics-dispensing clinics were established in Florida and Tennessee back in 1912 and 1913. Following passage of the Harrison Narcotic Act in 1914, clinics for supplying addicts with legal heroin at low cost or without charge spread throughout the country; at least 44 of them are known to have been opened by 1920 or 1921.[1]

Some of these clinics actually dispensed morphine or heroin or both. Others gave addicts prescriptions. In either case, the addict received his unadulterated medicinal opiate legally, at low cost or without charge. If enough addicts were thus supplied, it was reasoned, the narcotics black market would wither away; it could hardly support itself by selling opiates solely to nonaddicts. And the task of the police would be greatly simplified. Instead of facing the herculean task of trying to keep narcotics away from addicts, law-enforcement agencies would have the minor task of cleaning out whatever remnants of a black market might continue selling to a few nonaddicted occasional users not registered in the clinics. In short, the clinics would care for the addicts, and the police would maintain an alert against clandestine sales to nonaddicts.

The fascinating history of these narcotics-dispensing clinics is currently being reviewed by Dr. David Musto, a Yale University psychiatrist, and need not here be reported in detail. On the whole, the clinics did a remarkably good job—except for the New York City clinic, which was a woeful failure. Then, as now, the New York City program was a bone of contention between state and city officials, and between Republicans and Democrats at both the state and city levels. The New York City clinic, moreover, was *not* a maintenance clinic. Its function was to give declining doses of opiates to patients until the dose reached zero—gradual withdrawal. Thus, it was a detoxification rather than a maintenance clinic, and its failure cannot be charged against maintenance programs.

In 1920, the Narcotics Unit of the Treasury Department—predecessor of the Federal Bureau of Narcotics—launched a successful campaign to close the dispensing clinics. The case made against them was on its face a plausible one. It was alleged that some addicts secured more morphine or heroin from the clinic than they needed, and sold the balance on the black market. Some addicts supplemented the small amounts of opiate they could get at their local clinic by buying more on the black market. Since the clinics were hurriedly set up, understaffed, and administered by physicians and laymen who knew little about addiction, they no doubt dispensed opiates by mistake to at least a few nonaddicts who then either used the drugs themselves or sold them on the black market. (In some cases, the nonaddict was a chauffeur or other employee sent to stand in line at the clinic on behalf of his addicted employer.) Some criminal addicts, moreover, unquestionably continued to pursue a life of crime while on clinic-supplied opiates. Newspaper readers were particularly shocked by allegations that morphine or heroin was being supplied to prostitutes. Thus a convincing and highly sensational case against the dispensing clinics—especially against the New York City clinic, which received nationwide publicity and condemnation—was easily made in the press.

The questions of the utmost public-health significance, however, were never asked. How extensive was the abuse? Between 1912 and 1924, at least 12,000 addicts received opiates from clinics, and the total was probably much higher.[2] What proportion of the total black-market supply—tens of millions of doses a year—represented diversions from the clinics? If diversions had dropped to zero, would the black-market supply have been reduced by one-half of one percent? One-tenth of one percent? The clinics, unfortunately, were closed down by zealous law-enforcement officials before answers were secured to these and other crucial questions.

Their closing did not curtail the opiate supply; it simply buttressed the monopoly of the black-market suppliers, and returned thousands of addicts to that market.

Another series of questions also went unanswered: How much good did the opiate-dispensing clinics accomplish? How many doctors, lawyers, housewives, and others were enabled to continue their respectable law-abiding lives without being forced to patronize the illicit market? How many women (and men) did the clinics save from being forced to prostitute themselves to pay for black-market heroin? Could an adequate expansion of the maintenance system have prevented the rise of the illicit market in the first place? (This was what happened in Britain; see below.) Could a dispensing clinic drive an existing illicit market out of business?

Dr. Musto's current study of the 1912–1924 dispensing clinics is of great contemporary relevance—for by coincidence, today's methadone-dispensing clinics are similarly under attack, with similar allegations appearing in the news media. Methadone maintenance clinics in 1971 were dispensing more than 9,000,000 doses of methadone annually to an estimated 25,000 addicts. It should hardly have been a cause of surprise (or alarm) that a few doses—perhaps even thousands of doses—were finding their way to the black market, or into the hands of nonaddicts (who could, of course, secure heroin on the black market just as easily). We shall consider this problem in more detail in subsequent chapters.

Later proponents of legal heroin (1936–1965). Despite the closing down of the 1912–1924 clinics by federal law-enforcement officials, the narcotics-dispensing idea never completely died out. In 1936, for example, former Police Chief August Vollmer urged the same basic approach in these terms:

The first step in any plan to alleviate this dreadful affliction should be the establishment of Federal control and dispensation—at cost—of habit-forming drugs. With the profit motive gone . . . the drug peddler would disappear. New addicts would be speedily discovered and through early treatment some of these unfortunate victims might be saved from becoming hopelessly incurable.[3]

In 1952, a Special Committee on Narcotics of the Community Chest and Council of Greater Vancouver, British Columbia, Canada, recommended after thorough study: "The Federal [Canadian] Government should be urged to modify the Opium and Narcotic Drug Act to permit the provinces to establish narcotic clinics where registered narcotic users could receive their minimum required dosages of drug."[4] Such dispensing clinics, the committee predicted, would "protect the life of the addict and support him as a useful member of society." It would also "within a reasonable time eliminate the illegal drug trade. . . . The operation of such clinics would not entail any reduction in the vigilance of law-enforcement agencies,"[5] which would continue to be responsible for keeping narcotics out of reach of nonaddicts.

In 1954, a California citizens' advisory committee to the Attorney General on crime prevention proposed that an addict certified as incurable by a disposition board should legally receive specified doses of narcotics "and thereby remove said addict as a potential market for criminally or illegally secured narcotics."[6]

Also in 1954, Dr. Edward E. Eggston, for the New York state delegation, brought to the annual convention of the American Medical Association a proposal that the AMA go on record as favoring "the establishment of narcotics clinics under the aegis of the Federal Bureau of Narcotics."[7] (The resolution did not pass.)

In 1955, the Medical Society of Richmond County (Staten Island), New York, recommended the "establishment of narcotic clinics in large centers where the problem is acute." It suggested, "Suitable private physicians can care for the occasional addict in isolated areas. . . . The addict will receive his narcotics only at the clinic, hospital, or doctor's office so that he cannot resell them elsewhere."[8]

Also in 1955, the New York Academy of Medicine proposed "taking the profit out of the illicit trade by furnishing drugs to addicts at low cost under federal control."[9] The academy recommended that "clinics be attached to general hospitals, whether federal, municipal, or voluntary, dispensing narcotics to addicts, open 24 hours daily, 7 days a week."[10]

In 1956 the Council on Mental Health of the American Medical Association, while opposing the immediate establishment of substantial numbers of drug-dispensing clinics as urged the previous year by the New York Academy of Medicine, did suggest "the possibility of devising a limited experiment which would test directly the hypothesis that clinics would eliminate the illicit traffic and reduce addiction."[11]

Also in 1956, the American Bar Association and the American Medical Association established a Joint Committee on Narcotic Drugs, which recommended in its 1958 *Interim Report:*

(1) An Outpatient Experimental Clinic for the Treatment of Drug Addicts
   Although it is clear . . . that the so-called clinic approach to drug addiction is the subject of much controversy, the Joint Committee feels that the possibilities of trying some such outpatient facility, on a controlled experimental basis, should be explored, since it can make an invaluable contribution to our knowledge of how to deal with drug addicts in a community, rather than on an institutional basis. It has been suggested that the District of Columbia, being an exclusively federal jurisdiction and immediately accessible to both law-enforcement and public health agencies, might be an advantageous locus for this experiment.[12]

[118]

In 1962, the Ad Hoc Panel on Narcotic Use and Abuse of President Kennedy's White House Conference on Drug Use and Abuse stated that it would "welcome careful, rigorous, and well-monitored research designed to learn if there exist in this country certain addicts who cannot be weaned permanently from drugs, but who can be maintained in a socially acceptable state on an ambulatory basis." [13]

In 1963 the New York Academy of Medicine again recommended that narcotics be prescribed for addicts if deemed necessary in the judgment of a physician.[14]

Also in 1963, President Kennedy's Advisory Commission on Narcotic and Drug Abuse—a commission that grew out of the 1962 White House Conference—endorsed the 1962 suggestion of the Ad Hoc Panel. The advisory commission's *Final Report* urged "that properly designed experiments should be initiated to explore whether ambulatory clinics for the dispensation of maintenance doses to addicts are feasible." [15]

An editorial in the *Wall Street Journal* for April 17, 1963, recommended that Americans "start searching for ways in which the tragic incurables can be put on sustaining doses that will keep them from desperate acts." [16]

In their comprehensive 1964 study of narcotics addiction among New York City adolescents, *The Road to H,* Dr. Isador Chein, professor of psychology at New York University, and his three coauthors concluded that opiates should be dispensed by physicians to addicts:

There is an obvious expedient for reducing the demand [for black-market narcotics]—and that is to make a better quality of narcotics, and far more cheaply, available to addicts on a legal market. There are many advocates, the present writers included, of one variant or another of such a plan; and the numbers seem to be increasing. No one, of course, advocates putting narcotics on the open shelves of supermarkets. The basic idea is to make it completely discretionary with the medical profession whether to prescribe opiate drugs to addicts for reasons having to do only with the patient's addiction. . . .

We think it is high time . . . to call a policy of forcing the addict from degradation to degradation, and all in the name of concern for his welfare, just what it is— vicious, sanctimonious, and hypocritical, and this despite the good intentions and manifest integrity of its sponsors. . . . Every addict is entitled to assessment as an individual and to be offered the best available treatment in the light of his condition, his situation, and his needs. No legislator, no judge, no district attorney, no director of a narcotics bureau, no police inspector, and no narcotics agent is qualified to make such an assessment. If, as a result of such an assessment and continued experience in treating the individual addict, it should be decided that the best available treatment is to continue him on narcotics . . . then he is entitled to this treatment.[17]

An editorial in the New York *Times* for February 27, 1965, stated: "The best hope for smashing the illicit traffic in narcotics lies in the dispensing of drugs under medical controls—particularly at hospitals in the needy sections of the city, where physicians and psychiatrists can initiate well-rounded programs of medicine, counseling, and therapy as a basis for helping addicts overcome their dependence on narcotics." [18]

Also in 1965, the General Board of the National Council of Churches urged that physicians be given full power "to determine the appropriate medical use of drugs in the treatment of addicts." [19]

These were powerful voices demanding a change in the American system of heroin distribution. Yet they were voices crying in the wilderness. Judge Morris Ploscowe explained why, in the *Interim Report* published in 1958 by the Joint ABA-AMA Committee:

> The spearhead of the opposition to legal narcotics clinics has been the present Bureau of Narcotics. For years it has opposed legal clinics and dispensaries for the treatment of drug addicts. Its main weapon against the establishment of present day clinics was the alleged failure of the approximately 44 earlier clinics. . . .[20]

The British experience. Further light on the effects of dispensing morphine and heroin to addicts can be gained from the experience of Britain.

During the nineteenth century, as noted earlier, opiate use in Britain was much like that in the United States. Opiates were on open sale and were dispensed in enormous quantities without a prescription; even babes in arms were given remedies containing opiates. During World War I, it is true, a "Defense of the Realm" regulation forbade the non-prescription sale of opiates to members of the armed forces; but they still could be, and were, sold legally to civilians without a prescription. The United Kingdom, however, was under much the same pressure as the United States to pass a law implementing the 1912 Hague Convention for the international control of narcotics. In 1920, accordingly, Parliament enacted the Dangerous Drugs Act, which, like the Harrison Act in the United States, was designed to hold opiate distribution within medical channels.

In Britain as in the United States, the question naturally arose whether, under the new law, a physician could legally continue to prescribe morphine or heroin to his addicted patients. The British, however, did not leave this crucial question to be decided by law-enforcement officers. Instead, the government appointed a committee of distinguished medical authorities, headed by Sir Humphrey Rolleston, to consider this and other policy matters.

By 1924, when the Rolleston committee met, the disastrous effects of the United States decision to refuse legal opium, morphine, and heroin to addicts were conspicuously visible. Dr. Harry Campbell came to the

United States in 1922 to observe what had been happening during seven years of enforcement of the Harrison Act. What he saw flabbergasted him. Upon his return to England he informed his medical colleagues of the astonishing conditions he had observed:

In the United States of America a drug addict is regarded as a malefactor even though the habit has been acquired through the medicinal use of the drug, as in the case, e.g., of American soldiers who were gassed and otherwise maimed in the Great War [World War I]. The Harrison Narcotic Law was passed in 1914 by the Federal Government of the United States with general popular approval. It places severe restrictions upon the sale of narcotics and upon the medical profession, and necessitated the appointment of a whole army of officials. In consequence of this stringent law a vast clandestine commerce in narcotics has grown up in that country. The small bulk of these drugs renders the evasion of the law comparatively easy, and the country is overrun by an army of peddlers who extort exorbitant prices from their helpless victims. It appears that not only has the Harrison Law failed to diminish the number of drug takers—some contend, indeed, that it has increased their numbers—but, far from bettering the lot of the opiate addict, it has actually worsened it; for without curtailing the supply of the drug it has sent the price up tenfold, and this has had the effect of impoverishing the poorer class of addicts and reducing them to a condition of such abject misery as to render them incapable of gaining an honest livelihood.[21]

Profiting from the American mistake, the Rolleston committee recommended that "with few exceptions addiction to morphine and heroin should be regarded as a manifestation of a morbid state"[22]—that is, an illness that any physician could legally treat by supplying the necessary morphine or heroin.

This recommendation was accepted, and British physicians remained free to prescribe morphine and heroin for addicted patients through the succeeding decades.

One obvious advantage of this system was that it enabled the United Kingdom Home Office to keep tabs on the number of addicts currently receiving morphine or heroin. Some physicians voluntarily notified the Home Office when they added an addict to their roll of patients; other cases were picked up quite easily by periodically checking the special prescription records that physicians and pharmacies were required to keep when they dispensed an opiate.

The results can best be described as magnificent. By 1935, the United Kingdom reported to the League of Nations that there were only 700 addicts left in the entire country.[23] The number of addicts continued gradually to drop after 1935, as old addicts died off and few new ones were recruited, until the official figure of addicts known to the United

Kingdom Home Office reached a low of 301 for the entire country in 1951.[24]

These figures require some minor qualification. Since physicians were not *required* to notify the Home Office directly, the identification of some new addicts was delayed until their names were picked up during the periodic prescription audits. On the other hand, there was a similar delay in striking dead addicts off the list. Thus the figures fairly well represented the number of addicts receiving opiates legally.

Another qualification to the official figures concerns people who might be securing morphine or heroin in other ways than on prescription. There were certainly such uncounted cases. They had several sources of supply. Some British physicians, for example, freely prescribed very large doses of morphine and heroin to their addicted patients. Addicts naturally tended to gravitate to these generous physicians, and a patient receiving more than he really needed might be tempted to share his excess with a friend, or even to sell a part of it.

There was a very firm ceiling on the amount of opiates thus diverted, however. For if the friend or customer became addicted—that is, if he found that he needed a daily supply of the drug in order to keep well and socially functioning—he had only to go to a physician to secure the drug cheaply and legally, with an assurance of medicinal purity and quality. Thereupon he was added to the official count. The addict statistics cited above *include* addicts who secured their initial supplies from a friend or who bought them, and who thereafter turned to a physician when addiction set in.

A major feature of this system, in addition to the way in which it reduced the *number* of addicts to a negligible level, was its effect on law enforcement. There were, of course, violations of the law. Occasionally, for example, a physician or pharmacy failed to keep the required records in sufficient detail. Occasionally someone smuggled in a little heroin—though he could not get American prices for it because very cheap legal heroin was available. Occasionally someone stole morphine or heroin from a chemist's shop or warehouse. Yet law-enforcement officials had a very easy time of it, for their only real concern was to keep narcotics out of the hands of *nonaddicts*. Unlike their opposite numbers in the United States, they were not saddled with the hopeless responsibility of trying to keep narcotics out of the hands of addicts. Nor were the British courts and prisons jammed with narcotics offenders.

During the period from 1924 through the 1950s, Americans visiting Britain were naturally impressed with the British system, and on their return urged that a similar system be tried here. Many of the proposals of committees of the American Medical Association and the American Bar Association, and other similar proposals described above for legal narcotics dispensing in the United States, grew directly out of such visits to Britain.

These proposals were met by condemnation of the British system by United States Commissioner of Narcotics Harry J. Anslinger and the Federal Bureau of Narcotics. Repeated official American statements and speeches alleged, for example, that London, like New York, had a black market in heroin. This was unquestionably true. The market centered around Soho and Piccadilly. What the critics of the British system failed to add was that the market supplied a few dozen "weekend users," perhaps even a hundred or more. To jeopardize the entire system, and the contribution it was making to the nation's health and security, in order to try to stamp out a few peripheral shortcomings was simply not the British way. There was probably also a realization that the publicity accompanying raids on Soho and Piccadilly would attract additional customers and further popularize heroin.

Commissioner Anslinger and others also charged that the British addict count was phony, that Britain had addicts not included in the official reports. This, too, was unquestionably true. What the critics failed to add was that there were dozens of such unreported addicts, perhaps even a few hundred. The American heroin black market, in contrast, supplied tens of thousands of addicts—and made even an approximate count impossible.

Finally, Commissioner Anslinger and others insisted that if the British system worked in Britain, it was because Britain was an island, or because the British were law-abiding citizens, or because of other national differences.* This is a point to which we shall return.

Beginning about 1960, a modest change occurred in the British heroin problem. A group of fifteen Canadians plus a smaller group of Americans migrated to London to take advantage of high-quality, low-cost, legal heroin there—and proceeded to set up a "heroin subculture" on the American and Canadian model. They made a number of friends, and these friends also became addicted.

Only a moderate commercial black market developed, however. For at the very point when a potential black-market customer became addicted, he simply went to a physician and secured high-quality legal heroin without paying the black-market price. The availability of low-cost legal heroin also made it unnecessary for this new crop of British addicts to become thieves or prostitutes.

Nevertheless, the British during the 1960s became understandably

* It has also often been alleged—most recently by Drs. Frederick B. Glaser and John C. Ball in the *Journal of the American Medical Association* [25] in 1971—that the British system worked because it started out half a century ago with only a "negligible" addiction problem. This allegation, as we have shown, does not square with British drug-use history.

Year	British	Canadian	Other	Total
1955	9	0	1	10
1956	10	0	0	10
1957	7	0	0	7
1958	11	0	0	11
1959	10	1	0	11
1960	15	4	4	23
1961	27	24	5	56
1962	49	16	5	70
1963	77	10	3	90
1964	133	15	14	162
Total for decade	348	70	32 [a]	450

[a] Includes: U.S., 13; Jamaican, 8; Indian, 3; Australian, 3; New Zealand, 2; other, 3.

Table 3. New Cases of Heroin Addiction Recorded in the United Kingdom, 1955–1964.[26]

distressed as more and more young people became addicted to heroin. The *numbers* remained exceedingly small by American standards, but the *trend* seemed ominous (see Table 3).

The 162 new heroin addicts reported to the United Kingdom Home Office in 1964 may be contrasted with the 10,012 new addicts reported in that year to the United States Federal Bureau of Narcotics—with the warning that the British count was far more complete than the American count, since the British gave free heroin to those willing to be counted, while Americans who let their addiction become known risked imprisonment. If the British trend continued, of course, that country could expect several thousands of addicts during the 1970s.

In the United States, the Federal Bureau of Narcotics seized on this modest increase with great interest. Before 1960, the official United Kingdom statistics had been dismissed as worthless. Now they were taken as gospel, and word was spread that addiction in Britain had doubled in four years. Before 1960, the bureau had insisted that the British experience was not relevant to American conditions. Now the bureau reversed its field. It pointed to the "failure" of the British system as proof positive that supplying heroin to addicts would fail in the United States as well.

The British, too, reversed their field. Since 1924 they had prided themselves that by avoiding American methods they had avoided the American heroin disaster. Now they began to study American methods, in part because Britain had few experts of its own. With only a few hundred addicts spread through the country a few years before, most British physicians had never treated an addict, had never been concerned with addiction, and had only a hazy understanding of the problem. Since the United States had such an enormous number of addicts, the British naturally concluded that our experts knew better.

The British newspapers and other mass media, moreover, followed American mass-media precedents with alacrity. During the 1960s, they published the same stories with which Americans are so familiar—the annual rise in number of addicts, the arrests of drug pushers, the teen-age boy or girl caught shooting heroin into his arm, a mother's plaintive first-person story of how heroin had ruined her child. Letters to the editor of the *Times* (London) sounded as vindictive as similar American letters in demanding that penalties be escalated. Prison was deemed too good for a heroin addict or pusher. A committee of distinguished physicians, under Lord Brain, recommended fresh measures to curb the heroin menace—which by now was claiming 162 new victims a year.

The 1966 Brain committee recommendations, which are currently in force, significantly improved the basic British system. The committee noted that a few physicians under the old system had been prescribing excessive amounts, that these few overgenerous physicians had naturally attracted many addicts as patients, and that the excess heroin had flowed to the black market. They also noted that many of the new addicts were consulting physicians who had never seen an addict before and who knew nothing about addiction. Accordingly, the prescription of heroin was taken out of the hands of the medical profession as a whole and was concentrated instead in a limited number of clinics staffed by trusted physicians, who would thus be able to gain expertise on drug abuse problems.[27] As Dr. Thomas H. Bewley, the head of one large new London heroin-dispensing clinic, remarked on a visit to the United States, the British had gone back to the old 1912–1924 American system of clinics for dispensing heroin.

The new British restrictions, however, apply *only* to heroin. Any physician can continue to prescribe morphine or methadone—a synthetic opiate that can take the place of heroin. Thus British addicts today are given a choice of drugs and drug sources. They can patronize an ordinary physician and get morphine or methadone, or they can go to one of the new clinics for heroin, morphine, or methadone. Britain never at any time seriously considered following the American policy of keeping opiates away from addicts and thus opening the door to a large-scale heroin black market. The disastrous effects of the American black-market system, and the beneficent effects of their own long-established system, were much too readily visible.

Once again, this British development was seriously misrepresented in the United States. Opponents of opiate dispensing here charged that even the British now conceded that their system was a failure and had abandoned it. American proponents of a better system of opiate distribution were condemned for proposing a plan that even the British had now abandoned. Few readers of this Consumers Union Report, it seems likely, are aware that in Britain today an addict can continue to get high-quality, low-cost heroin, morphine, or methadone legally from clinics—or, if he prefers, morphine or methadone from any medical practitioner.

Through the decades since the Rolleston committee report, British physicians (like their American opposite numbers) hoped to cure heroin addiction and made efforts in that direction. Like the Americans, they rarely succeeded. When the new ripple of addicts hit Britain during the 1960s, treatment facilities were expanded. There is to date no evidence, however, that the new British treatment facilities are having any greater success in achieving "cures" than the United States federal facilities, the California facilities, the New York State facilities, or the therapeutic communities.

Another change in British policy became visible about 1970. By then, a small but significant cadre of medical specialists in addiction problems had been developed within the clinics—men who now knew addicts and their problems at first hand. Excellent research projects were launched at the Addiction Research Unit (ARU) in London and in other centers. These studies were far more reliable than similar American studies, since addicts could speak frankly to the researchers, without fear that they would be imprisoned or that their supplies would be cut off.

Based on this fresh examination of the heroin problem, a growing number of British authorities had by 1970 reached the conclusion that the British "heroin explosion" of the 1960s could be only partly blamed on those few Canadian and American addicts who had migrated to London. Britain's American-style *response* to the modest rise in number of addicts during the first few years of the 1960s had also contributed to the explosion. The Soho and Piccadilly black markets in heroin were by now famous; indeed, they had become tourist attractions. The attention of a whole generation of British young people had been focused on heroin. Warnings against heroin added to the publicity, and each warning became a lure. The whole antiheroin campaign in the mass media was thus one of the factors adding fuel to the heroin explosion. (We shall discuss this process further, as it occurs in the United States, in several subsequent chapters). In short, Britain had begun to adopt American antidrug propaganda methods, and was beginning to reap American-style rewards in terms of a rise in youthful addiction.

A subtle change in British policy resulted from this reassessment. Reassuring statements were issued in 1970 and 1971. The public was informed in headlines that everything was under control—that the number of known addicts was in fact declining. Indeed, the British "heroin explosion" was shown to be in part a mere statistical artifact.

Prior to 1968, as noted above, notification of addicts to the United Kingdom Home Office was voluntary. The result of the 1968 compulsory-notification law, as might have been expected, was a marked rise in the number of addicts reported to the Home Office.[28]

Year	Number Reported
1967	1,729
1968	2,782
1969	2,881

As might also have been expected, however, the compulsory-notification law resulted in duplicate notifications and other statistical "bugs," which swelled the total. To avoid penalties for failure to notify, physicians sent in all doubtful names—including those who received opiates only briefly during the year, those imprisoned, those who died, those who gave up opiates, and so on. To eliminate duplication and other errors, it was necessary to determine the number of addicts receiving opiates *on a given day*—for example, the last day of the year. When overnotification was thus eliminated, the British figures revealed not only a significantly smaller *number* of addicts at the end of 1968 but also a downward trend in 1969 and 1970.[29]

Date	Number Known
December 31, 1968	1,746
December 31, 1969	1,466
December 31, 1970	1,430

These totals, moreover, were not just for *heroin* addicts. As in the United States, efforts were being made to convert heroin addicts to methadone, a synthetic narcotic that has advantages over heroin, to be reviewed in later chapters. The effort had been highly successful. As of December 31, 1970, more than half of all British addicts (732 out of the 1,430) were being maintained on methadone alone. An additional 261 addicts were being maintained without heroin—on morphine (91) or other drugs and drug combinations. Only 140 addicts were being maintained on heroin alone, while 297 were being maintained on combinations of heroin and other drugs.[30] Heroin, in short, was rapidly becoming again a drug of only trivial importance in Britain.

Despite these facts, which could readily have been ascertained from the United Kingdom Home Office or any other informed British source, the *Journal of the American Medical Association* published on May 17, 1971, an article by Drs. F. B. Glaser and J. C. Ball that alleged once again that the British system of opiate maintenance is a myth and that "the British . . . have moved in a direction similar to the United States" with respect to opiates.[31]

The *British Medical Journal* responded on August 7, 1971, with an editorial that was remarkably restrained under the circumstances. It described the *JAMA* article as "an incomplete interpretation of recent developments," and as "one which incidentally invites us to overlook what are still profound differences in emphasis." The British editorial continued:

To suppose that the British prescribing system was discredited by the alarming growth in heroin addiction in the 1960's, and thereafter abandoned, would be a considerable misreading of history. The same essential policy is being maintained as heretofore, with the difference that [heroin] prescribing is limited to specially approved doctors operating from specified clinics and with notification now compulsory. This issue should not be clouded. The British response still permits the prescribing of heroin and still gives central responsibility to the individual physician. And without undue complacency it may be claimed that this policy seems to have some real success in containing what threatened to be an explosive epidemic.[32]

In sum, the British system of supplying morphine, heroin, and other narcotics to addicts is not a failure. It has not been abandoned. Even at its peak in 1968, British heroin addiction was a trivial fraction of the American level, and at least a part of the peak could be attributed to the temporary adoption of American antiheroin propaganda methods.

Morphine, heroin, and other opiates, it is important to note, are not "legal" in Britain in the sense that anyone can buy them. There are strict laws against the unlawful importation, sale, or even possession of these drugs, specifying long prison terms—long by British standards. The police still have a role in ferreting out illegal smuggling, possession, and sales, as in the United States. But the problem is trivial in scale, for few addicts patronize the black market. Physicians and clinics take care of them, while the police protect nonaddicts by maintaining an alert against smugglers and traffickers.

What of other countries?

Visits to Sweden, Denmark, and the Netherlands in the course of preparing this Consumers Union Report confirmed the fact that in none of these countries is a physician threatened with imprisonment for prescribing opiates to addicts. In these countries, as in Britain, physicians take care of the addicts while the police concentrate their efforts on keeping heroin out of the hands of nonaddicts. And in these countries, as in Britain, narcotics addiction, though a worrisome problem, has remained through the decades a small one by American standards.

A review of the literature, moreover, has turned up no other country in the world, except Canada, which tolerates anything approaching the heroin black market in the United States.

Of course, a system which has worked magnificently in Britain for decades (except for a few years in the 1960s), and which also does well in other countries, may not necessarily work equally well in the United States. Accordingly, let us turn next to an examination of how the dispensing of legal opiates to addicts has been working through the decades here at home.

Legal opiates in Kentucky. In his 1969 study, *Narcotics Addicts in Kentucky*, cited earlier, Dr. John A. O'Donnell revealed one of the most closely kept secrets in the history of United States narcotics addiction— the fact that all through the years since the Harrison Act of 1914, a substantial though diminishing number of Kentucky physicians had continued to prescribe legal morphine or other opiates for their addicted patients—and no disaster had resulted.

In the course of his study of Kentucky addicts, Dr. O'Donnell inquired carefully into the question of *where* they had gotten their narcotics. As might be expected, there were many answers. Some obtained the drug from relatives (often a spouse) or friends. Some bought from pushers. A few broke into pharmacies and stole drugs. A few forged prescriptions for narcotics. Seventeen of the 266 addicts in the O'Donnell sample were themselves physicians, pharmacists, or pharmacy employees with direct access to narcotics.[33] But—*in an amazing number of instances, these Kentucky addicts secured their narcotics (usually morphine) quite legally on prescription from their personal physicians.*

Specifically, 67 percent of the men in the sample and 87 percent of the women reported getting their narcotics legally, from a physician or on his prescription, during at least a part of their careers as addicts after 1914.[34] A quarter of the men and more than half of the women reported getting all or the major part of their narcotics legally from a physician *throughout* their careers as addicts.[35]

These latter addicts, Dr. O'Donnell notes, might get their drugs from one physician for a while, then change to another when that physician died or retired. "But these subjects never received narcotics outside of what was, or may have been, a normal physician-patient relationship." [36] Since it is legal for a patient to possess narcotics given him by a physician or secured on prescription, these addicted patients violated no law. Whether or not the physicians broke the law will be considered below.

The likelihood that an addict could secure his drugs legally from a physician depended in considerable part—especially for male addicts—on where in Kentucky he lived. Thirty-eight percent of the male Kentucky addicts residing in villages secured all or most of their drugs legally from a physician, as compared with 19 percent of those living in towns and 11 percent of those living in cities. For women, the comparable percentages were much larger but the differences based on place of residence were smaller: 62 percent in villages, 56 percent in towns, and 46 percent in cities.[37]

Physicians readily confirmed that they were providing opiates for addicts. "For example, the physician who prescribed for 13 subjects in one county confirmed this in all cases but two. In these he did not deny prescribing, but said he did not remember the names, which is credible because both subjects had left town almost twenty years before. In other older cases, he remembered he had prescribed for long periods of time, but could not specify the number of years. In the current and recent cases, however, his description tallied exactly with the accounts given by subjects."[38]

How did physicians justify their prescription of narcotics to addicts after 1914? And how did they get away with it? Dr. O'Donnell's report suggests that no two cases were alike; they ranged from cases in which the medical prescription of narcotics was clearly justified by current illness to cases where it was simply a business transaction, with the addict buying medicinal morphine from a doctor instead of adulterated heroin from a pusher.

It is not illegal for a physician, in Kentucky or anywhere else, to prescribe an opiate for a patient who needs relief for a physical illness, even if he happens also to be an addict. In general, Dr. O'Donnell explains, "elderly addicts will have acquired some physical complaints. If such an addict in Kentucky found a physician who would prescribe narcotics for the physical complaint, the narcotics agents did not question the need."[39] Here are two examples:

Case 45: "Subject's father had tuberculosis, and became addicted to narcotics about the turn of the century. His mother became addicted so she could keep going, to take care of her husband. When the subject was 9 years old, the family physician began giving him narcotics for asthma. He continued using them until his death."[40] This patient's original addiction occurred before passage of the Harrison Act. Following passage of the act, and following the mother's death, the physician cut off his supply and left him addicted but without narcotics. The subject scrounged for narcotics in various ways. He was admitted to Lexington for "cure" seven times in seven years. "Then he developed tuberculosis, and found a physician who prescribed for him to the time of death."[41]

Case 179 was given an opiate after an injury. "He had never before experienced the rest, relaxation and general feeling of well-being [see Chapter 2 on opiates as tranquilizers] which followed drug use. When his original supply ran out, he went to another physician for more. . . . Next, he made contact with sellers of morphine, and bought much of his narcotics on the illicit market. . . . Finally, when he was in his late sixties, a physician began prescribing narcotics regularly enough to maintain him on about five grains [300 milligrams] of morphine per day." [42]

Other old-time Kentucky doctors did not wait until an addict was in his sixties to supply legal opiates. An outstanding example was a rural physician whom Dr. O'Donnell calls Dr. Smith. As other doctors in Dr. Smith's county died or decided (following passage of the Harrison Act) to give up prescribing opiates for addicted patients, their patients gravitated to Dr. Smith, who "professed to believe that after an addict has used narcotics for a number of years, abstinence is dangerous to life." [43] Eventually Dr. Smith "inherited" some 20 addicts who had previously received their narcotics from other physicians. He at first sent youthful addicts to a state hospital to be "cured," but when he saw them promptly relapse, he concluded that cure was impossible and added these young addicts to his list for opiate prescriptions. He was also prepared to prescribe for local residents after their return from Lexington. In all, he dispensed in his prime some 500 grains (30,000 milligrams) of morphine per week—equivalent to 1,000 or 1,500 New York City "bags." [44] Narcotics agents, aware of his practices, went over his records repeatedly but never brought charges against him. When interviewed for the O'Donnell study, Dr. Smith was nearing retirement and had only two addicted patients left; since the other physicians in the county had given up dispensing narcotics to addicts, no one knew what would happen to these patients if they outlived Dr. Smith.

Did this maintenance of addicts on legal opiates exist only in Kentucky, or was it more general? When asked this question following publication of his report, Dr. O'Donnell replied:

My impression very strongly is that the practice in Kentucky did not differ from that throughout the Southern states. I personally knew at the Lexington Hospital individual addicts from all over the South, maintained by physicians, in what appeared to be the same pattern as I observed in Kentucky. Up to a few years ago, I also saw occasionally drug enforcement officers at the state level—again in Southern states—all of whom estimated that their states had from 200 to 400 or 500 elderly addicts * maintained by physicians, against whom they had no idea of taking any action.

---

* This indicates that far more addicts were being maintained on legal opiates in the Southern states than in the whole of Britain.

My personal belief is that it has been, and probably continues to be, a general practice throughout the South to ignore the physician, provided a) he is prescribing for only one or a few addicts, b) these are elderly or obviously ill, so that there is at least some slight pretext for the prescribing, c) the physician clearly is not making any appreciable amount of money from his prescriptions, and d) the amounts prescribed would not allow the addicts who receive the prescription to divert any appreciable amount of drugs to other addicts.

My guess has been that enforcement agents ignore such cases both because they see little harm in them, and because it would be difficult to get a local jury to convict such physicians.*

I have much less information on non-Southern states, but my guess has been that the same considerations would lead to the same practices in them. In my occasional contacts with enforcement officers, in such places as New York and Philadelphia, they expressed much the same attitudes as did the Southern officers.[45]

There is some suggestion in the Kentucky report that economic and social status played a role in determining whether an addict could secure his opiates legally or had to patronize the heroin black market. If the addict were the kind of person the physician wanted as a patient, and if he paid his bills, he was more likely to get legal morphine. Much the same may be true elsewhere. In New York City in the 1960s, it will be recalled, Dr. Marie Nyswander reported: "I've yet to see a well-to-do addict arrested." [46] Even Commissioner Anslinger himself, it will also be recalled, was willing to arrange a morphine supply for the chairman of a Congressional committee.

How well did the Kentucky addicts do while they were being maintained on legal opiates by their personal physicians? Overall, Dr. O'Donnell was not too favorably impressed, but he did cite some exceptions.

Fourteen of the addicts in his sample, for example, were physicians. "The practice of the addicted physician often deteriorated (but not always—some addicted physicians were described as 'the best doctor in town')." [47]

In three cases Dr. O'Donnell compared life on illegal opiates with life on legally prescribed opiates—to the credit of legally prescribed opiates. "In all three, an improvement in work pattern followed the securing of a stable legal source [of drugs]. This can be interpreted as suggesting that the change in source of narcotics caused or permitted the improvement in employment." [48] In other cases, however, addicts were unemployed or poorly employed on illicit heroin and remained unemployed or poorly employed on legally prescribed opiates—suggesting that legal opiates are not a panacea.

* The Federal Bureau of Narcotics may also have been loath to have the constitutionality of the federal narcotics laws tested in cases such as this.

In one respect, however, Dr. O'Donnell is enthusiastic about legal opiate prescription—and the data fully support his enthusiasm. This concerns the relation of legal opiates to crime. Former Federal Narcotics Commissioner Anslinger, Dr. O'Donnell notes, insisted that drug addiction *per se* "causes a relentless destruction of character and releases criminal tendencies." [49] The O'Donnell data, in contrast, indicate that addicts maintained on legal opiates lead law-abiding lives; crime is associated not with opiates but with the need to acquire opiates illegally.

Specifically, among 45 male addicts who received their opiates legally from a physician, 41 were never convicted of a crime during the entire course of their addiction. Among 82 male addicts who secured all or almost all of their drugs illegally, in contrast, 59 were convicted of crimes —and the majority of them were multiple offenders. Fourteen were convicted six or more times. [50] Many of the addicts who secured their drugs illegally, moreover, supported themselves through daily crime—committing enormous numbers of offenses for which they were *not* convicted.

The data [Dr. O'Donnell states] . . . confirm the generally accepted conclusion that drug use *per se* does not cause crimes. The subjects who received drugs from a physician were using as much narcotics as others, and in recent years probably more, since their drugs were not diluted like illicit heroin. . . . Yet only a few of them have a record of arrests, and there is much less indication for them than for others of undetected offenses.

. . . In this sample, addicts with a stable legal source of narcotics were unlikely to acquire a criminal record, while those who bought most of their drugs on the illicit market were likely to acquire one. . . . If stable and legal sources of narcotics had been available to more subjects in this sample, they would have committed fewer crimes. [51]

Dr. O'Donnell cautiously adds, however, that this may not apply to *all* addicts. Merely supplying legal opiates to a professional criminal will not necessarily cause him to change his profession. The justification for supplying legal narcotics in such cases is much the same as the justification for supplying insulin to a professional criminal with diabetes.

One more aspect of the narcotics problem in Kentucky deserves brief mention. During the period under study, Dr. O'Donnell states, the Kentucky black market for opiates slowly withered away. For a considerable period of years after World War II, there was simply no place in Kentucky where an addict could go to buy illicit heroin. There were no "pushers" because there weren't enough customers.

No doubt many factors contributed to this welcome development. But surely the substantial proportion of addicts maintained on legal opiates by their physicians was one of the factors which made heroin peddling unprofitable and contributed to the gradual disappearance of the black market.

During the 1950s and even more in the 1960s, as the older opiate-prescribing doctors died off and younger doctors with a deeply ingrained distrust of addicts took their place, addicts found it harder and harder to secure a legal opiate source. And late in the 1960s, after the completion of Dr. O'Donnell's book, black-market opiates returned to Kentucky.

A tentative conclusion. If this Consumers Union Report were appearing in 1965, we would unhesitatingly join the late Police Chief August Vollmer, the New York Academy of Medicine, the Council on Mental Health of the American Medical Association, the Joint Committee on Narcotic Drugs of the American Medical Association and American Bar Association, President Kennedy's Advisory Commission on Narcotic and Drug Abuse, the *Wall Street Journal,* the New York *Times,* and others quoted earlier in urging that planning begin forthwith for establishing a system of supplying morphine or heroin or both to addicts, under legal auspices, on at least a small-scale experimental basis. In taking such a stand, we would have emphasized the following factors.

• Addicts themselves are far better off on low-cost, legal, medicinal opiates than on exorbitantly priced, adulterated, and contaminated street heroin.

• Society is far better off when addicts are on legal rather than exorbitantly priced illegal opiates.

• With addicts on legal opiates, law-enforcement agencies, courts, and prisons could concentrate on offenders who supply opiates to nonaddicts.

• It is economically disastrous and morally indefensible to permit the American system of heroin distribution to continue to flourish and enrich itself—without even trying to find an alternative.

• Even though serious flaws in the new system of distribution might develop, the new system could not possibly be worse than the existing heroin black market.

Since 1965, however, a new factor has entered the scene—the "methadone maintenance program" for the treatment of heroin addiction. We shall next consider methadone maintenance, and return later, in our Conclusions and Recommendations (Part X), to the question of dispensing heroin to addicts.

14.

Enter methadone maintenance

Dr. Vincent P. Dole, specialist in metabolic diseases at the Rockefeller University, came to an interest in heroin addiction through his studies of obesity, which in some respects might be considered addiction to food. During the 1950s, when most experts were saying that obesity results from overeating and that people get fat because they eat too much and "lack the will power" to cut down, he launched at the Rockefeller Institute (now the Rockefeller University) a series of studies of metabolism in obese people. He soon discovered that many obese people metabolize food quite differently from other people. His technique was to hospitalize obese patients for substantial periods, place them on a scientifically formulated diet, and study their metabolic processes before, during, and after weight reduction. Dr. Dole's work, along with that of Dr. Jean Mayer at Harvard and of others at other centers, has profoundly altered scientific views on obesity. No longer is "weakness of will" an accepted cause.

The craving of his obese patients for food struck Dr. Dole quite early in his obesity research as remarkably reminiscent of a cigarette smoker's craving for cigarettes—or a narcotics addict's craving for narcotics. The tendency of obese patients to relapse after dieting also resembled the tendency of cigarette smokers and heroin addicts to relapse even after prolonged periods of abstinence. His obesity studies led Dr. Dole to conclude that, far from being due to weakness of will, relapses among some obese patients have a metabolic, biochemical origin.

In 1962, Dr. Dole began planning a similar metabolic study of heroin. His initial step, of course, was to review the existing scientific studies. He found a substantial medical literature, both in English and in other languages—but one very serious gap. Almost all of the American studies concerned opiates in the test tube, or in laboratory animals, or in non-addicted volunteers, or imprisoned addicts. American physicians in general had divorced themselves from the problems of *the addict in the street* ever since the early waves of physician arrests under the Harrison Narcotic Act. Both the Stevenson study of British Columbia addicts and the O'Donnell report on Kentucky addicts were unpublished. The most significant published account of addiction under American street conditions that Dr. Dole could find was a book by Dr. Marie Nyswander, a psychiatrist, entitled *The Drug Addict as a Patient*.

A graduate of Sarah Lawrence and of the Cornell University Medical

School, Marie Nyswander had been commissioned a lieutenant (junior grade) in the navy late in World War II, assigned to the Public Health Service, and posted at the United States Public Health Service hospital for addicts in Lexington. Her experience with addicts there led her, unlike many psychiatrists, to accept addicts as patients when she entered private practice. In 1957, in a New York City storefront, she had launched a service project for addicts, with a team of New York psychiatrists and psychoanalysts offering their services to the city's addicts. Thus Dr. Nyswander had had experience with multiple approaches to the treatment of addiction—the Lexington approach, her own approach as a therapist with addicted patients, that of her storefront project, and the efforts of other psychotherapists and psychoanalysts.* She recognized that none of them accomplished very much. Like so many others during the 1950s and 1960s, she was thus eventually forced to the conclusion that maintaining addicts on legal opiates was the only feasible solution. She was beginning to think about risking her reputation, and perhaps even her freedom, by launching private research—a narcotics-dispensing clinic of her own, using her personal funds—at just the time when Dr. Dole turned his attention from obesity to heroin addiction.

Dr. Dole read *The Drug Addict as a Patient,* and in October 1963 invited Dr. Nyswander to the Rockefeller Institute for a conference. Early in 1964, he invited her to join his new research project. (In 1965 they were married.) The two made a very nearly ideal team. Dr. Dole knew nothing about addicts, and Dr. Nyswander knew little about the complexities of biochemistry and human metabolism; each brought to the project precisely what the other lacked.

As in the case of his earlier obesity project, Dr. Dole's first step was to bring into the Rockefeller Hospital sufferers from the disease he was studying. "The first patient," Dr. Nyswander later recalled, "was a 34-year-old single male of Italian extraction, and the second, a 21-year-old male of Irish background. Both had a history of drug use for eight years, had spent several years in prison for possession of drugs and theft, and had made numerous efforts to get off drugs by detoxification in voluntary hospitals and in the federal hospital in Lexington. . . . Both patients had tried psychotherapy." [2] Both were still "hooked," and were delighted to participate in a project in which they were to receive narcotics without having to steal and evade the police.

---

* Dr. Nyswander, though she had not herself taken opiates, also had a clear *personal* insight into the nature of addiction, craving, and relapse after "cure." In 1960 she stopped smoking cigarettes. "The craving for cigarettes," she later reported, "exists as an entity, separate from pleasure. Nor did the craving diminish with time. After six months, I'd still have dreams in which I'd surreptitiously cop a cigarette. . . . If it's this hard to stop smoking, think what it must be to stop heroin." [1] After eight months of abstinence, Dr. Nyswander relapsed and started smoking again.

Both were started on small doses of morphine, a quarter of a grain (15 milligrams) four times a day. As in the obesity project, which began with patients being allowed to eat as much as they wanted, these patients were allowed to increase their doses as they pleased; within three weeks they were requesting and getting eight shots totaling 600 milligrams (10 grains) a day. Morphine became their whole lives. "Much of the time they sat passively, in bathrobes, in front of a television set. They didn't respond to any of the other activities offered them. They just sat there, waiting for the next shot." In this sense they were good patients; "they cooperated beautifully and honestly" [3] in the many metabolic tests to which Dr. Dole subjected them. But they demonstrated the major problem faced by all morphine-dispensing and heroin-dispensing programs—the problem of dosage. In this respect, indeed, they closely resembled the obese patients in the earlier Dole study.

In Britain, in Kentucky, and in other places where legal opiates are dispensed, the dosage problem takes several forms. If a physician gives an addict less than he wants, the addict may obtain more from a second physician, or may buy additional drugs on the street. If the physician gives the addict as much as he asks for, the addict may share his large dose with others, or sell a part. The problem is solved in various ways. After staying for a time on a given dose—even an enormous dose—an addict becomes "tolerant" to that dose, and functions quite well on it; this no doubt would have happened to the two Dole-Nyswander patients if the work with them had continued. Some patients, moreover, are able and willing to stabilize themselves on quite moderate doses. Still others "bounce" up and down. In the case of their first two patients, however, Drs. Dole and Nyswander were not really trying to solve the American heroin problem; they were only seeking to determine the metabolic pathways that morphine follows inside the human body. When the metabolic tests on morphine were completed, their plan called for detoxifying and then discharging the two addicts. Indeed, Federal Bureau of Narcotics regulations required this.

The approved technique of detoxification in most hospitals today was developed in Lexington during the 1950s. The first step consists in transferring the patient from morphine or heroin to methadone, a synthetic narcotic developed by the Germans during World War II. The daily methadone dose is then progressively reduced over a period of ten days or so until a zero dose is reached. Most authorities agree that this methadone detoxification treatment is preferable to direct withdrawal from morphine or heroin because, even though it takes longer, it reduces the suffering. Drs. Dole and Nyswander placed their patients on methadone as a step toward withdrawal. Instead of reducing the methadone immediately, however, they decided to keep the patients on high doses of methadone for a considerable period while the same metabolic tests were rerun. Thus they would be able to compare morphine and methadone metabolism in the same patients.

While the patients were on methadone, however, surprising changes began to occur. "The older addict began to paint industriously and his paintings were good," Dr. Nyswander later told Nat Hentoff of the *New Yorker*. "The younger started urging us to let him get his high-school-equivalency diploma. We sent them both off to school, outside the hospital grounds, and they continued to live at the hospital." [4] They also continued to take their methadone daily. So far as Dr. Dole and Dr. Nyswander could see, they had become normal, well-adjusted, effectively functioning human beings—to all intents and purposes *cured* of their craving for an illegal drug.

When the same results were procured with the next four "hard-core" addicts placed on methadone maintenance, Dr. Dole went to see Commissioner of Hospitals Ray E. Trussell, the New York City official most fully informed about narcotics problems. It was Dr. Trussell who had closed down the disastrous Riverside Hospital program and had established the voluntary detoxification program at Manhattan General. He now became the godfather of the Dole-Nyswander program as well.

"Dr. Dole came to see me at the Department of Hospitals, and he had six pieces of paper with him," Dr. Trussell later recalled. "Each was a summary protocol on each of six patients on whom he had demonstrated with Dr. Nyswander his breakthrough on how to apply methadone in such a way as to . . . allow an individual, after a brief period at the hospital, to start doing something about his life and become a self-sustaining member of society.

"Dr. Dole just wanted six beds, and all we had was about 20,000! We were very glad to accommodate him. We arranged for Dr. Dole to go to Manhattan General . . . and he replicated there, together with Dr. Nyswander, the same findings." [5]

In addition to housing the new program, Dr. Trussell found money to finance it. "The mayor [Robert F. Wagner] gave me $80,000 one day on a car ride," he recalled in 1969, "and Dr. Perkins gave me $300,000 of Mental Health money and the Deputy Mayor gave me $1 million of anti-poverty money because addicts are certainly impoverished and we put together a budget and took a calculated risk that this program would go."* [7]

---

* Manhattan General Hospital was subsequently taken over by a voluntary hospital complex, the Beth Israel Medical Center, and it became the Morris J. Bernstein Institute of Beth Israel—today one of the world's leading centers of narcotics addiction research. Dr. Trussell, by coincidence, is now General Director of Beth Israel, and the former Manhattan General unit on East Eighteenth Street is his pride and joy. "We admit approximately 9,000 admissions a year for detoxification alone," he told

During the years since 1964, methadone maintenance has continued to work. One of the first two Dole-Nyswander patients—the twenty-one-year-old Irish addict, "hooked" on heroin at the age of fourteen, a school dropout at fifteen, twice imprisoned for narcotics violations—earned his high-school-equivalency diploma while on methadone. He also earned a full college scholarship. Still on methadone, he graduated from college with a degree in aeronautical engineering. "He . . . has a full-time job now," Dr. Dole told the United States House of Representatives Select Committee on Crime on June 29, 1970; and at the age of twenty-eight, after six years on methadone, he "is going to night school to get a master's degree." [8]

The other initial patient followed a quite different path. Like many young people today, he had no interest in climbing onto the career escalator and "making a success." He has been described as "a quiet introspective fellow who has intermittent jobs and is active in the groups concerned with social reforms." [9] In January 1971 he was still taking his methadone daily, and "having no problems with drugs or alcohol." [10]

Dr. Dole recently commented on these two cases and countless others: "The interesting thing about methadone treatment is that it permits people to become whatever they potentially are. Whereas addicts, under the pressure of drug abuse and drug-seeking look very much the same, when they are freed from this slavery they differentiate and become part of the spectrum of humanity." [11]

The second patient illustrates another highly significant fact about methadone. After he had been taking it for five years, this patient— then thirty-nine—decided he no longer needed the drug and left the program after tapering off his daily methadone dose. He had then been abstinent from heroin for five years; he was fully rehabilitated; he did not associate with addicts—so why continue to take methadone?

Alas, as in other cases, the postwithdrawal anxiety, depression, and craving returned as soon as he discontinued methadone treatment—a craving, not for methadone, but for *heroin*. He relapsed. Readmitted to the Dole-Nyswander program, he went back on daily methadone and, Dr. Dole reports, "has had no problem since." [12]

---

the Second National Conference on Methadone Treatment in October 1969. "We have a lovely new waiting room with a separate nice entrance off Eighteenth Street exclusively for patients coming into the hospital for one of our three classes of addiction services. [It is] the hospital with a welcome sign on the mat for addicts." [6] Most of the early work on methadone maintenance was carried out here; the world's pioneer methadone maintenance program is still under way here; and satellite methadone maintenance clinics have been established under Beth Israel's auspices in other parts of the city.

15.

How well does methadone maintenance work?

The number of patients on the Dole-Nyswander program increased from 6 when Dr. Dole first discussed the program with Dr. Trussell early in 1965 to 1,866 on October 31, 1969.[1] During the following year, the number almost doubled—to 3,485 on October 31, 1970.[2] By then there were 42 centers in New York City, plus 4 in Westchester County, distributing methadone to patients under the Dole-Nyswander aegis.[3] In addition, there were numerous city, state, and private methadone maintenance programs in the New York area, and a number of physicians were prescribing methadone maintenance for their private patients. The discussion below concerns primarily the 3,485 patients attending the 46 Dole-Nyswander clinics, since the data available on these patients are among the most complete and most reliable in the entire history of addiction treatment programs.

At Dr. Dole's request, Dr. Trussell arranged for the establishment of an independent "evaluation unit" in the Columbia University School of Public Health. This unit is not responsible to Dr. Dole but to an independent committee, which includes a number of the country's outstanding authorities on narcotics addiction and on drug research. Dr. Henry Brill, New York State Associate Commissioner of Mental Health and chairman of the American Medical Association Committee on Narcotic Drugs, was selected as chairman of the evaluation committee. A few years before, following a study of narcotics addiction policies in Great Britain, Dr. Brill had published a report declaring that American addicts should *not* be supplied with drugs. Another member appointed to the committee, Dr. Donald B. Louria, was also at the time of his appointment an outspoken opponent of maintenance programs. As operating chief of the evaluation unit, Dr. Frances Rowe Gearing was selected—a public-health authority widely known for her independence of mind and judgment. Thus the cards were stacked against overoptimism in several ways—by selecting as the evaluation center the same school of public health that had revealed the zero success rate of the Riverside program, by selecting an evaluation chairman opposed to maintenance programs, and by providing that the evaluation unit should assemble data independently, in addition to reviewing the data supplied by Dr. Dole. Data collection and the publication of interim reports were to proceed simultaneously with the experiment, so that failure would not be discovered too late, after many millions had been spent—as in the case of the Riverside and New York State programs.

Dr. Gearing reported on the Dole-Nyswander patients at three methadone maintenance conferences held in New York in 1968, 1969, and 1970; Dr. Dole also reported at each of these conferences. The details below are based on all six reports.

Among the first 2,325 patients admitted to the Dole-Nyswander program after January 1964, all but 459 were still on daily methadone in October 1969—a dropout rate of 20 percent.[4] By October 1970, admissions had increased to a total of 4,376—but the dropout rate remained 20 percent.[5] Thus the methadone maintenance "success rate" might from one point of view be considered 80 percent.

It is important to note, however, that in this and other methadone maintenance programs, methadone *per se* is successful in 100 percent of all cases, or virtually 100 percent, if success is defined as it is for other drugs. Insulin, for example, lowers the blood sugar level in very nearly 100 percent of all diabetes patients. Methadone similarly relieves the craving for heroin in all or substantially all heroin addicts.

There is another sense, however, in which methadone is not quite that successful. The parallel with insulin will explain this discrepancy. If a significant proportion of diabetics were to try insulin for a while and thereafter refuse to take it any longer, we would conclude that the drug was a *therapeutic* failure in such cases even though it was a pharmacological success. Applying this standard to the Dole-Nyswander program, the success rate is about 97 percent; only 3 percent of those entering the program drop out *voluntarily*.[6] (The reasons for higher voluntary dropout rates in less successful methadone maintenance programs are discussed in Chapter 18.)

One percent died,[7] and might also be deemed failures. When it is recalled, however, that these were all hard-core addicts, who had in the past injected heroin daily for years, that 75 percent of them had damaged livers before coming on the program, and that they suffered on admission to the program from the many other health handicaps, reviewed earlier, common to poverty-stricken addicts dependent on high-cost, adulterated, and contaminated heroin, the deaths must be attributed at least in part to the sequelae of being a heroin addict rather than to methadone failure. In many or most fatal cases it would be reasonable to conclude that death ensued because methadone came too late. These were like the casualties occurring in a war after a truce had been agreed to—or like the diabetics who continued to die prematurely for several years after insulin became available in 1923.

A third standard of success which might be set is *abstinence from heroin.* This standard, in turn, depends on whether abstinence is defined absolutely or relatively. Addicts on the program who use any drug to excess—alcohol, barbiturates, amphetamines, opiates—are subject to involuntary discharge. Not one of the addicts on the program was discharged for *heroin* abuse. Fewer than one percent of addicts on methadone use heroin regularly.[8]

This does not mean, of course, that few addicts take heroin at any time after beginning methadone maintenance. When told that methadone blocks the heroin effect—that a shot of heroin will have no effect on them—many simply don't believe it until they try it out. "Many patients have made sporadic attempts to use heroin again, especially during the first six months of treatment," [9] Dr. Dole explains. Specifically, among patients whose urine was tested three times a week—using a test sensitive enough to identify any narcotic taken since the previous test—55 percent showed "clean urine" on every test for the whole first year.*[10] An additional 30 percent showed only a few "dirty urines," usually during their first weeks or months on the program when they were testing the blockade effects. The remaining 15 percent "continued to use heroin intermittently (e.g., on weekends) even though the euphoric effect was blocked. These tended to be isolated schizoid individuals who were unable to find new friends or participate in ordinary activities." [11] If these "occasional" or "weekend" users be deemed failures—perhaps partial failures would be a better term—the methadone maintenance program was 85 percent successful.

Yet another criterion of methadone maintenance is living a law-abiding life, which may seem a curious standard for a form of medical therapy. Many of the Dole-Nyswander patients were criminals *before* they became addicted; to expect methadone to curb their criminality as well as their addiction seems like asking too much of any medical therapy. Yet that is precisely what happened.

"Drug-related crime has been sharply reduced by the blockade of narcotic drug hunger," Dr. Dole reported in 1968.

Prior to treatment 91% of the patients had been in jail, and all of them had been more or less continuously involved in criminal activities. Many of them had simply alternated between jail and the slum neighborhoods of New York City. The crimes committed by these patients prior to treatment had resulted in at least 4,500 convictions (for felonies, misdemeanors and offenses), a rate of 52 convictions per 100 man-years of addiction. The figure is obviously a minimum estimate of their pretreatment criminal activity since convictions measure only the number of times an addict has had the misfortune to be caught. For every

---

* This was the first narcotic addiction program in which "success" was evaluated with the help of effective urine tests.

conviction, the usual addict has committed hundreds of criminal acts for which he was not apprehended.

Since entering the treatment program, 88% of patients show arrest-free records. The remainder have had difficulties with the law. Some of these individuals, however, were arrested merely on suspicion, on charges such as loitering, or by inclusion in a group arrest. In such cases, if the charges were subsequently dismissed, the episode has not been considered a criminal offense in our statistics. The remainder, 5.6% of the patients, were [found] guilty of criminal offenses, and were convicted. In all, there have been 51 convictions in 880 man-years of treatment experience (a rate of 5.8 convictions per 100 man years).[12]

The vast bulk of the offenses committed while on methadone maintenance were misdemeanors and other minor offenses rather than felonies.

These Dole findings were independently confirmed by Dr. Gearing's evaluation unit. In her study the *arrest* records (including arrests not followed by conviction) of the addicts on methadone maintenance were compared with the arrest records of other addicts, of the same age and ethnic group, who came to the Morris J. Bernstein Institute during the same month—but received only detoxification instead of methadone maintenance. The comparison is shown in Figure 3; note that the 101 addicts on the methadone maintenance program for more than twenty-four months had an arrest record very close to zero.

In Dr. Gearing's 1969 report, arrest rates had fallen from 6 per 100 man-years the first year on methadone to 3 per 100 man-years the second year on methadone, and to 2 per 100 man-years the third year.[13] This latter rate—one arrest every 50 years—is lower than the rate (about one arrest every 40 years) for the United States population as a whole, including babes in arms and the aged.

At the 1970 conference, Dr. Gearing's report showed a further improvement; arrests for those staying a fourth year on methadone were only about one per 100 man-years. Figure 4 compares the arrest records of patients on the methadone maintenance program (MMP) with arrests among the "contrast group" of addicts not placed on methadone. The chart summarizes 5,557 man-years of experience on methadone maintenance.

The only possible conclusion is that the overwhelming majority of patients on the Dole-Nyswander program, after years as criminals on heroin, lead a law-abiding life on methadone maintenance—and the longer they stay on methadone, the more law-abiding they become.

An even more stringent measure of success is the ability to function effectively in the community: to attend school and get passing grades, to keep house for a family, or to work at a productive job. Here again, the addicts admitted to the methadone maintenance program had many

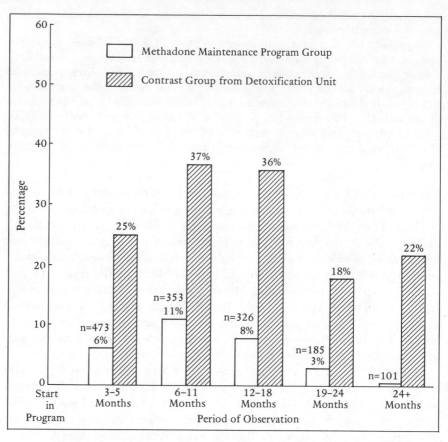

FIGURE 3. Arrests for 544 Men in Methadone Maintenance Program Three Months or Longer as of March 31, 1968, and Contrast Group according to Length of Observation[14]

strikes against them. Exorbitantly priced black-market heroin had disrupted their home lives. Few had finished high school; few had any training or special skills; Past employment records were poor. At the time of admission to the program, only 15 percent of 723 male addicts had jobs. That a methadone maintenance program should make them employable or educable seemed a most unlikely possibility.

Yet, once again, that is precisely what happened. Within three months of starting methadone maintenance, more than half of the male addicts were productively employed or attending school. After a year the proportion rose to nearly two-thirds. Figure 5 shows changes in employment and in socially acceptable—that is, arrest-free—behavior over a forty-two-month period.

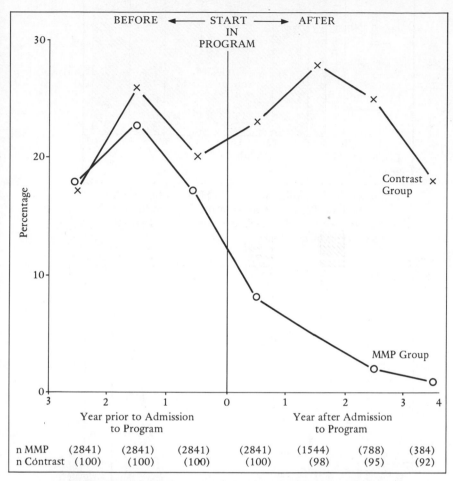

FIGURE 4. Arrests for 2841 Men in Methadone Maintenance Program
Three Months or Longer as of March 31, 1970, and Contrast Group
by Months of Observation[15]

This record, moreover, was not just the result of early enthusiasm.
As the program ended its fifth year, the failure ratio remained low,
as shown in Figure 6.

"The greatest surprise has been [this] high rate of social productivity,
as defined by stable employment and responsible behavior," Dr. Dole
reported in 1968. He was prompt to add, however, that "this, of course,
cannot be attributed to the medication, which merely blocks drug hunger
and narcotic drug effects. The fact that the majority of patients have
become productive citizens testifies, in part, to the devotion of the staff

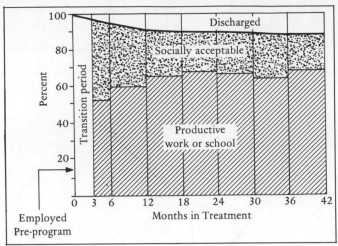

FIGURE 5. Rehabilitation of 723 Male Addicts under Methadone Treatment, as Measured by Productive Employment and Crime-free Status, over a Period of Forty-two Months[16]

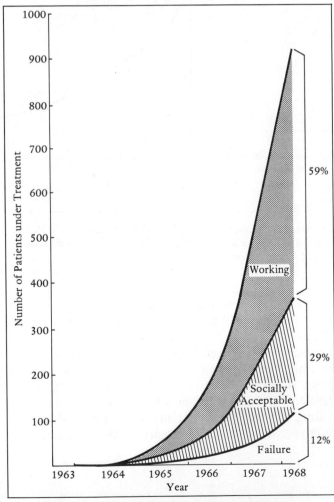

FIGURE 6. Growth of the Methadone Maintenance Treatment Program[17]

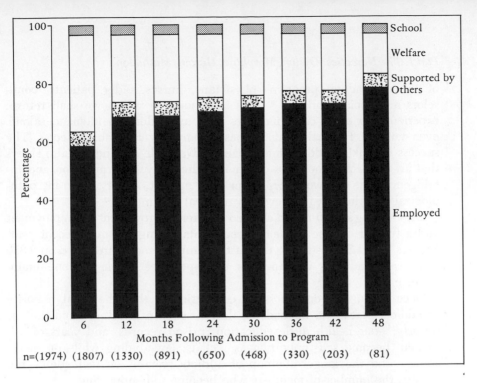

FIGURE 7. Employment Status and School Attendance for 1974 Men in Methadone Maintenance Three Months or Longer as of March 31, 1970[18]

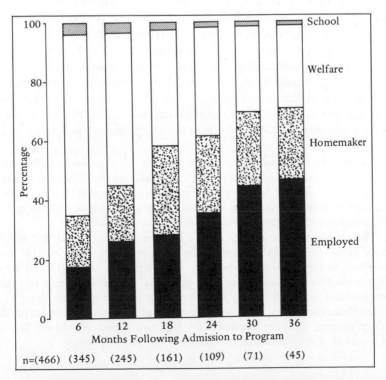

FIGURE 8. Employment Status and School Attendance for 466 Women in Methadone Maintenance Three Months or Longer as of March 31, 1970[19]

of the methadone program—physicians, nurses, older patients, counselors and social workers." [20] This is a point to which we shall return; experience in other cities indicates that methadone maintenance alone, even without full-scale staffing, has remarkably favorable effects. "The success in making addicts into citizens," Dr. Dole continued, "also shows that an apparently hopeless criminal addict may have ambition and intelligence that can work for, rather than against, society when his pathological drug hunger is relieved by medical treatment." [21]

Dr. Gearing's 1970 report showed further improvement in employment and a further decline in welfare recipients during the most recent year. Figures 7 and 8, illustrating this further improvement, are based on 2,880 man-years and 721 woman-years of experience on methadone maintenance.

Once again, the only possible conclusion is that the great majority of addicts placed on methadone, despite such preexisting handicaps as poverty, poor health, little education, prison records, and years of addiction, become self-supporting as well as law-abiding while on methadone—and the longer a group of addicts remains on methadone, the greater the number of members who become self-supporting.

The 1969–1970 employment record of these ex-addicts is particularly impressive because it occurred during a period of high and rising nationwide unemployment, when even nonaddicts had trouble finding and holding jobs. The record would no doubt have been substantially better had New York City enjoyed full employment. The proportion of methadone maintenance patients on welfare in 1970 was probably only a little higher than the proportion among their neighbors, of the same ethnic group and socioeconomic status, who had never touched heroin.

The employment record of methadone maintenance patients was also remarkable in the face of a systematic discrimination against them. Attention was called to this discrimination in 1971 by Ronald Bayer of New York's Greenwich House methadone maintenance program:

Among the well-publicized consequences of the methadone maintenance approach to heroin addiction is that it allows former addicts to secure regular employment. In the course of the past year, however, it has become clear through numerous reports by methadone patients that a disturbing pattern of job discrimination against former addicts exists in New York.

The problem is particularly serious because three of the largest employers in New York—the Transit Authority, the Telephone Company and the Post Office —refuse to hire methadone patients. This situation is aggravated by the fact that these three organizations have generally provided a point of entry to the employment market for many young people who lack special training.

Such discriminatory activity has exceedingly negative effects upon the methadone patient, not only financially (though this aspect should not be minimized in a period of job scarcity) but in terms of his own self-image.

Efforts to work through the Mayor's office have proven unproductive with one bureaucratic hand passing the buck to the next. At stake is the human dignity of those who have for so long lived lives of degradation and who are now striving to save themselves.

If the city and state are serious about the rehabilitation of former addicts, it is imperative that firm action be taken against both public and private employers who are guilty of discriminatory activity.[22]

In testimony before the House Select Committee on Crime on April 27, 1971, Dr. Frances R. Gearing explained how jobs are secured for methadone patients despite this initial prejudice against them: ". . . It is like getting the first olive out of the bottle. Getting the first man on methadone maintenance employed in a particular industry or group is the tough one. Once they have accepted the first one and they find out that he is a useful citizen, then getting other people into that [industry] is a simpler job." [23]

The patients in the Dole-Nyswander program—at least until recently— were a selected group in several respects. Obviously psychotic addicts were excluded—but, as noted earlier, there are very few of them. An attempt was made to exclude patients with multiple drug problems— those using both heroin and alcohol, for example—but despite this effort, patients with multiple drug problems did get in. The chief element in selection was the fact that most patients had to remain on a waiting list for many months before acceptance in the program—but a subsequent comparison of waiting-list patients with patients who were promptly admitted showed no significant difference in success rates. Addicts were accepted only at their own request, not on referral from courts and law-enforcement agencies, the theory being that no one should be forced to accept treatment. But many of the addicts who "volunteered" were in fact just one step ahead of the police. Applicants with criminal charges pending against them were accepted in large number, provided they applied personally rather than being referred by judge, prosecutor, or the police. The restrictions on patients admitted were set initially in 1965 when the program was tentative and experimental. Some restrictions were maintained to ensure comparability of statistics from year to year, while others have since been relaxed. As shown below, the results in methadone maintenance programs without admission restrictions do not differ greatly from the Dole-Nyswander results.

To many readers, the results of methadone maintenance may seem bizarre and inherently incredible. How can an addicting narcotic such as methadone accomplish such transformations?

The answer is, of course, that methadone by itself does not accomplish this—just as heroin by itself does not transform honest men and women into thieves and prostitutes. The American heroin black market demands

$20 a day or so from each addict—and disaster results from this demand. Addicts who fail to meet it are cut off from their heroin supply; hence every addict meets it if he can. The Dole-Nyswander system of methadone maintenance, in contrast, expects that addicts lead reasonably law-abiding lives and get jobs or return to school. Most addicts find it far easier and more satisfactory to meet the expectations of a methadone maintenance program than the demands of the heroin black market; hence most refrain from crime and get jobs.

Heroin addicts who abstain from heroin without going on methadone maintenance, it will be recalled, run about a 50–50 risk of becoming alcoholics or barbiturate addicts. Methadone maintenance greatly lessens but does not wholly eliminate this risk. About 10 percent of the patients on methadone maintenance, Dr. Gearing reports, "continue to present problems with abuse of amphetamines and barbiturates, and . . . ten percent demonstrate chronic alcoholism.*

"These two problems account for the majority of failures in rehabilitation of patients in the program." [24]

What *kinds* of patients do well on methadone maintenance? The answer appears to be *all* kinds. Efforts to identify particular kinds of patients who do exceptionally well or exceptionally poorly on methadone maintenance have been notably unsuccessful. The tabulation below, for example, shows the varying rates of success by sex, color, age, education, and other characteristics—with "success" defined as ability to stay on the Dole-Nyswander program without interruption for two years or longer. The success rate varies from group to group only within narrow limits —from 70 percent to 90 percent.

Proportion of Patients Who Remain on Dole-Nyswander Methadone Maintenance Program without Interruption for Two Years or Longer

80 percent of males

80 percent of females

82 percent of white patients

81 percent of Puerto Rican patients

77 percent of black patients

86 percent of males under 25 when admitted

76 percent of males over 34 when admitted

* Methadone, in short, does not block alcohol or barbiturate effects in the way in which it blocks heroin effects. The development of a drug like methadone, which would prove equally safe and effective against alcohol, or barbiturate addiction, or cigarette smoking, or other addictions, and which would satisfy the craving these drugs produce in addicts, would surely rank among the major triumphs of modern medical science. Yet only trivial efforts are being made to find such drugs.

70 percent of females under 25 when admitted

81 percent of females over 34 when admitted

85 percent of those with two criminal convictions or fewer

72 percent of those with three or more convictions

86 percent of those with intact marriages

79 percent of others

79 percent of high-school graduates

80 percent of nongraduates

79 percent of those addicted before age 21

80 percent of those addicted after 21

83 percent of those not multiple drug abusers

77 percent of multiple drug abusers

82 percent of those without history of alcohol abuse

75 percent of those with history of alcohol abuse

88 percent of those legally employed on admission

77 percent of those not legally employed on admission

90 percent of those on heroin five years or less

77 percent of those on heroin more than five years [25]

When two or more criteria are combined, it is true, more striking differences appear. Using computer techniques, Drs. Carl D. Chambers and Dean V. Babst of the New York State Addiction Control Commission, with Dr. Alan Warner of Dr. Dole's staff, were able to discover that an addict who was law-abiding before admission to the program *and* who had no alcohol problem had a 95.8 percent chance of staying on the program two years, while a patient with seven or more criminal convictions on his record before admission *and* no employment skill to market had only a 55.6 percent chance. But even the latter patient was far from hopeless. ". . . Ancillary services should be marshalled and focused toward the buffering against these attributes," the three researchers concluded.[26] Instead of being barred from the program, these high-risk patients should be admitted and provided with added vocational training and other services.

Finally, all of the figures above refer to success or failure following a single admission to the program. Many patients who are expelled from the program or who leave it voluntarily return and do well the second or third time around. This trend can be expected to continue. Thus in the long run, when successes on subsequent admissions are included in the figures, the success rates may be expected to improve on those here presented.

It is sometimes alleged that while methadone maintenance may be good for society—cutting down on thefts and other crime—it leaves the poor addict himself still an addict. Patients on methadone and the staffs of maintenance clinics interviewed in the course of research for this Consumers Union Report expressed a very different view. They stressed the benefits to the individual addict and his family—the general improvement in health, the reconciliations with parents, the marriages restored, the revolutionary effects on children when one or both parents switch from heroin to methadone, the sense of achievement, the end of the need to prostitute oneself to secure heroin money, the money available for the simple pleasures of life instead of for heroin—and above all the methadone patient's secure feeling that he is no longer a hunted criminal. They perceived the benefits to society at large as merely incidental to these and many other benefits to the addicts themselves.

16.

Methadone side effects

No medication produces only a single desired effect. Patients on methadone maintenance report a wide range of side effects, especially during the early weeks or months when their daily dose of methadone is being stabilized.

In New Orleans, for example, Dr. William A. Bloom, Jr., of the Tulane University School of Medicine, and an associate, Dr. Brian T. Butcher, gave 209 patients on methadone maintenance a checklist of 33 assorted symptoms ranging from runny nose to loss of appetite, and asked them to check any from which they suffered. As might be expected, this highly suggestive procedure produced a bumper crop of reported symptoms.[1]

Symptom	Percentage of Patients Reporting
Weight gain	80
Constipation	70
Increased intake of fluids	63
Delayed ejaculation	60
Increased use of alcohol	40
Increased frequency of urination	37
Numbness of hands and feet	32
Hallucinations	17

Dr. Avram Goldstein of Stanford University carried out a similar study of side effects in 206 methadone maintenance patients. This study [2] also revealed numerous side effects—but led to rather reassuring conclusions.

"Almost without exception," Dr. Goldstein reported, "the body symptoms complained of on methadone were present prior to starting on the program, when the patient was using heroin. Most of these improved on methadone, so that despite the natural tendency to blame all troubles on the drug one happens to be taking, it is difficult to classify them as side effects." Examples of symptoms reported before methadone which showed improvement while on methadone were headache, joint pains, hiccups, diarrhea, loss of libido, nervousness, runny nose, difficulty urinating, and unhappiness.

Some other complaints, Dr. Goldstein continued, were actually due to inadequate methadone dosage during the build-up period. They occurred principally in the evening, eight hours or longer after methadone.

"Symptoms that fall into this category comprise the constellation recognized by addicts as 'feeling sick,' including insomnia, nausea and vomiting, muscle pains, and anorexia [lack of appetite]." Those symptoms were relieved as the dose was gradually increased.

Excessive sweating was a common complaint among Dr. Goldstein's California patients. "It was present to some degree in three-fourths of the patients before methadone and in moderate or severe form in ten to fifteen percent. By the third month [on methadone] it had become worse in 43 percent of the patients and better in about 30 percent, remaining unchanged in the remainder. There was no dose relationship." Other methadone side effects, Dr. Goldstein added whimsically, were "dramatic reductions in the frequency of theft and the amounts expended for heroin."

Contrary to Dr. Bloom's findings, Dr. Goldstein found that "excessive use of alcohol remained unchanged as compared with premethadone use (about 20 percent of patients), as did the use of amphetamines (5 to 10 percent), and marijuana (about 45 percent)." Use of barbiturates declined from 20 percent before methadone to 6 percent while on methadone.

The most important point about these and other side effects, however, is that—in New Orleans, in California, in New York, and in other programs as well—they only rarely lead a patient to discontinue methadone. In the Goldstein sample, for example, only five out of 206 patients left the program voluntarily, and several of these dropped out because they were leaving the area.[3]

Some opponents of methadone maintenance have alleged that it is part of a genocide conspiracy against the black race—designed to render black males impotent and both males and females sterile. Because these charges are quite widely believed in some black communities, they deserve the most thorough consideration. The relevant data follow.

Menstrual function. In New York City's Beth Israel program, 82 out of 83 women addicts of childbearing age menstruated normally after conversion to methadone—"usually within one to two months." [4]

Among 15 women on the West Philadelphia methadone maintenance program, 8 did not menstruate at all while on heroin. Seven out of the 8 began to menstruate again when converted from black-market heroin to methadone maintenance.[5] Here and in most of the comparisons that follow, however, it must be remembered that other changes in life-style accompanied the conversion. Just as heroin *per se* was probably not responsible for all of the preconversion problems, so methadone *per se* cannot be credited with all the postconversion improvements.

Only 4 of the 15 women in the West Philadelphia study had regular menstrual periods while on heroin; 12 of the 15 had regular menstrual periods on methadone maintenance. Of the 3 exceptions, one had periods longer than normal, one had periods shorter than normal, and one did not menstruate.[6] Such variations are to be expected, of course, in any group of women. The high rate of improvement suggests that while heroin addiction and its accompanying life-style (often including prostitution) may impair menstrual function, permanent damage is rare.

Female sexual function. The 15 women in the West Philadelphia study were asked to rate (1) their sex drive, (2) their sex activity, and (3) their enjoyment of sex while on heroin and after conversion to methadone. Only 4 of the 15 women reported normal sex drive on heroin; this increased to 10 after conversion. Eleven women reported below-average sex activity on heroin, as compared with 5 after conversion to methadone. Five reported normal enjoyment of sex on heroin; this rose to 8 after conversion.[7] Sexual complaints, it should here be recalled, are also frequent among nonaddicted women.

Likelihood of pregnancy. Increased likelihood of pregnancy is almost universally reported as a side effect among female heroin addicts who convert to methadone—though whether this is a pharmacological result of the switch from heroin to methadone or of the accompanying change in life-style remains in doubt. The pregnancies are sometimes unwanted. Typical is this statement of Dr. Bloom: "The rate of pregnancy in our New Orleans methadone programs has been as high as 20 percent during the past year. Female patients of childbearing age appear to be more fertile once they are stabilized on methadone. They should be informed of this, and where appropriate, be offered birth control information or measures." [8]

Outcome of pregnancy. During the first few years of methadone maintenance, the question of possible damage to the fetus in pregnancy was often raised. The question can now be answered decisively. The rate of congenital malformations among babies born to mothers taking high doses of methadone both before and during pregnancy does not differ significantly from the rate to be expected among nonaddicted mothers of the same age, color, and socioeconomic status.[9]

The course of pregnancy among women on methadone is generally uneventful, with few complications. Birth complications are also what might be expected in a comparable nonaddicted group.

Careful evaluation of the babies at birth, performed at several centers, reveals only two deviations from what would be expected. The Beth Israel findings in 19 babies is typical of the findings generally.

First, while few of the Beth Israel babies born to mothers on methadone maintenance were in fact premature—born too soon—one-third of them had the low birth weight (under 2,500 grams) typical of premature babies. This is, of course, a handicap. The proportion of low-birth-weight babies is about the same as among babies born to mothers on heroin.[10] How much the heroin and methadone contribute to the problem, however, remains in doubt. Low birth weight is also a characteristic of babies born to mothers who smoke heavily—and almost all of these mothers were heavy smokers. Low birth weight is also frequent among the poor, the black, and those otherwise socially handicapped; almost all of these mothers were in one or more of these categories.

The other condition frequently found in babies born to mothers on methadone was hyperirritability—the pattern often mistakenly called "withdrawal symptoms." In the Beth Israel series, 8 of the 19 methadone babies were born completely free of such symptoms and 6 more had symptoms too mild to require medication. Five babies had moderate symptoms requiring medication. None had severe symptoms.[11] This was a better record than for Beth Israel babies whose mothers were heroin addicts *not* on methadone. As noted earlier, this hyperirritability may be related to low birth weight—or to factors wholly unrelated to opiates.

Development following birth. Dr. Saul Blatman, the Beth Israel pediatrician in charge of infant care for babies born to addicted mothers and to mothers on methadone maintenance, presented at the Third National Conference on Methadone Treatment the first follow-up report on the postnatal development of methadone babies. The report covered 14 children from four and a half to forty-two months of age.

Each child seen by us has been found to be developing physically within normal limits without exception. Psychometrics performed during these visits using the Knobloch–Modified Gesell Test or the Bayley Scales of Infant Development showed the following overall range: A normal or average test for 11 of the 14 babies; a below average test, as far as development of intelligence is concerned, in one baby; and a high normal or high average intelligence in one baby. One normal baby, who is average in all other respects, showed poor language development at ages 23 and 33 months. Overall, the impression is that this group compares favorably with other children of similar age.[12]

Male sexual function. The evidence to date suggests (though it does not yet prove) that methadone, like heroin, has a modestly depressant effect on male sexual function in some cases. The evidence is much more convincing that many males converted from street heroin to methadone maintenance enjoy a significant *improvement* in sexual function.

The best data so far were presented at the Third National Conference on Methadone Treatment by Dr. Paul Cushman, Jr., of St. Luke's Hospital in New York City, who studied thoroughly 20 male patients aged twenty-four to fifty-two, maintained on methadone for from ten months to five years. Only 7 of these 20 men reported that they were consistently potent while on street heroin. After conversion to methadone, in contrast, 16 of the 20 reported normal potency. The number reporting normal libido rose from 7 on street heroin to 17 on methadone maintenance. Delayed ejaculation was frequent both while on heroin and after conversion to methadone maintenance—though some patients reported normal ejaculation time on heroin, some on methadone, and some on both.[13]

The cause of depressed sexual function was apparently not hormonal. Testosterone levels and luteinizing hormone (LH) levels were both within normal limits in all 20 cases.[14] Dr. Cushman summed up:

. . . Some patients on methadone had some sexual difficulties remaining [but] 50 percent reverted [to normal] within the first month and an additional 25 percent within the first year; another ten percent within 18 months. Nevertheless, there were 10 percent with continuing sexual problems apparently not present during heroin use. In addition, there were another 10 percent who experienced transient disturbance in sexual function during initiation of methadone treatment not present during heroin addiction.[15]

The data here reviewed clearly demonstrate that methadone is a drug poorly suited to serve the purposes of a "genocide conspiracy" against black heroin users. Conversion from street heroin to methadone maintenance actually improves sexual function, both male and female, in a large proportion of cases—and notably increases the likelihood of normal pregnancy and normal birth.

Pain and methadone maintenance. Astonishing findings concerning pain were reported at the Third National Conference on Methadone Treatment by Dr. Morton I. Davidson of Beth Israel Medical Center, findings based on experience with several thousand methadone patients.

These patients are able to be managed in a relatively routine fashion. Perception of pain has been *no* problem. There never has been a problem of masking symptomatology. They have experienced dental problems and perceive pain normally. . . .

When it comes to relieving pain, we have had experience with the use of superimposed narcotics such as morphine or Demerol. These have been successful. Patients have been relieved of their pain. The explanation for this has not been worked out. . . .

We have had patients who have undergone surgery varying from abdominal to orthopedic surgery to chest surgery. The patients have been managed with no particular difficulty regarding anesthesia.[16]

Overdose. Like aspirin and other drugs, methadone should not be left lying around within reach of small children. The usual maintenance dose, if taken by a child, may be fatal unless proper treatment is instituted.

A few cases have been reported of children attracted to the "orange juice" in the family refrigerator who have died of the methadone it contained. Some methadone maintenance programs therefore require that patients who take home methadone mixed with a soft drink must carry and store it in a locked box. Dr. Dole has developed, and a pharmaceutical company is marketing, a methadone tablet that is not readily injectable, need not be mixed with a soft drink, and need not be refrigerated. The new tablets are now in use in many programs, and are expected to reduce the risk of methadone overdose in children.

Fortunately, the antidote for methadone overdose is simple and readily available in hospital emergency rooms—a *series* of injections of the same narcotic antagonist, nalorphine (Nalline), used for treating overdose of other opiates. Nalorphine produces almost immediate relief. A few methadone overdose deaths have been reported, however, in children given only one injection of nalorphine. The antagonist works like magic—but its effect lasts only for a few hours, while the methadone effect may persist for a day or more. After the first nalorphine dose wears off, the child may again fall into a life-threatening methadone coma. Hence, the hospital staff must keep the child under continuous observation, and repeat the nalorphine injection whenever signs of lethargy occur.

In 1970 and 1971, some deaths among addicts on methadone were attributed to "methadone overdose." As in the case of so-called "heroin overdose" deaths, however, these fatalities followed moderate rather than excessive doses of the narcotic. Hopefully, solution of the Syndrome X mystery will solve these methadone "overdose" deaths too (see Chapter 12).

17.

Why methadone maintenance works

The two major reasons for the success of methadone maintenance are surely no secret. Methadone is legal; hence the addict who enters a methadone maintenance program casts off his role of hated and hunted criminal when he downs his first methadone tablet or glass of methadone-spiked orange drink. And methadone is cheap. The cost of the usual dose —100 milligrams per day—is ten cents. It is supplied the addict either free or (in some programs with ancillary services outside New York) for $10 to $14 per week.

If morphine or heroin were legally dispensed at low cost, the same two advantages would be equally well achieved. Thus in those two respects the favorable results of methadone maintenance cannot be attributed solely to the methadone.

Like morphine and heroin, methadone is a narcotic and therefore, by definition, an addicting drug. This fact is often cited as a disadvantage. Indeed, newspapers, politicians, and even some physicians have expressed the hope that a nonaddicting drug for the treatment of heroin addiction can be found.

This hope, however, is based on a misunderstanding. One main advantage of methadone is that it *is* addicting. For an addicting drug, it will be recalled, is one that an addict continues to take day after day and year after year.

In fact, several nonaddicting drugs for the treatment of heroin addiction have already been tried out. Among them are the narcotic antagonists; cyclazocine and nalaxone are examples. An addict who injects heroin while on one of these drugs perceives no effect. Thus the antagonists, like methadone, are "blocking agents." But they are inferior to methadone in at least two other major respects.

First, they do not assuage the postaddiction syndrome—the anxiety, depression, and craving that recur for months and perhaps years after the last shot of heroin. The contrast with methadone is readily visible. A psychiatrist who has had experience with both methadone and antagonist maintenance programs contrasts "the relaxed, jovial atmosphere of a methadone ward," where patients are free of the postaddiction syndrome, with "the tension, frustration, and anxiety that characterize a cyclazocine ward." [1] Clearly methadone is in this respect a far more hopeful base for building social rehabilitation.

The other major difference is that since the antagonists are not addicting, a patient can stop taking them at will.* Most patients do stop taking them—and then promptly return to black-market heroin. The greater success of methadone results in considerable part from the fact that it is an addicting drug.

In 1971, despite the earlier failures of narcotic antagonists,† interest was renewed in these drugs as a potential "cure for addiction." A massive research program was proposed for an improved antagonist, or for an improved way of administering those currently available. It was suggested, for example, that a long-term supply or "depot" of an antagonist might be implanted somewhere in the addict's body, surrounded by a membrane that would release the drug at the desired rate continuously over a period of a month or even six months. If such a long-acting material were available, it was argued, addicts could be *required* to take it at suitable intervals, under penalty of imprisonment. Hence, it was said, such a drug might solve the addiction problem, even if addicts didn't like the drug.

What the large-scale use of a long-acting narcotic antagonist would in fact produce, however, is a horde of men, women, and adolescents assailed by anxiety and depression, with a continuing craving for heroin— and no way to assuage their distress (except, perhaps, via alcoholism). Is this the "cure" society seeks for today's narcotics addicts? ‡

Despite the shortcomings of the narcotic antagonists as a "cure for addiction," further research into these drugs could prove valuable. For the central facts of addiction—the withdrawal syndrome followed by the postaddiction syndrome—are still little understood. The study of narcotic antagonists is quite likely to throw further light on the mystery of why some drugs merely block the heroin effect while others—notably methadone—both block the heroin effect and relieve the depression, anxiety, and craving for heroin.

* Dr. William R. Martin, chairman of the Addiction Research Center at Lexington, and the scientist who first proposed use of narcotic antagonists in the treatment of heroin addiction, reported (1971): "Patients learned that by skipping doses they could experience the euphorogenic action of [taking] heroin the day following the last dose of cyclazocine." [2]

† The most recent study of cyclazocine, reported in the *International Journal of the Addictions* [3] in 1971, indicates that of 186 addicts offered cyclazocine, 33 accepted, of whom 11 were believed to be abstinent twenty months later. The study suggests, but does not prove, that the few patients who accept cyclazocine do significantly better than similar patients who attempt abstinence without cyclazocine.

‡ The civil-liberties implications of requiring the taking of a drug that not only perpetuates anxiety, depression, and craving but also blocks relief of that syndrome for prolonged periods deserves fuller consideration than was given the subject during the 1971 discussions of long-acting narcotics antagonists.

An ethical consideration is also involved in the use of long-acting narcotic antagonists: why is it *wrong* to provide an addict with an addicting drug such as methadone— that is, one that carries a built-in pharmacological compulsion for continued use—but *right* to use legal compulsion, even imprisonment, to force continued use of a non-addicting drug?

It is unfortunate, of course, that patients must continue to take methadone year after year, just as it is unfortunate that diabetics must continue to take insulin or some other diabetes drug year after year. But the heroin addict's need for continuing medication is *not* the result of methadone; it arises out of his initial addiction to heroin. Methadone relieves the patient of the life-shattering effects of that need.

A patient on methadone maintenance is commonly thought to be addicted to methadone* and might therefore be called a methadone addict. The term "methadone addict" is seriously misleading, however, since— as we have seen—the patient on methadone maintenance does not resemble in the least the popular stereotype of the addict. He neither acts like an addict nor thinks of himself as an addict. To avoid confusion, the terms *heroin addict* and *methadone patient* have become standard usage, and are used throughout this Report.

If being legal and being cheap were methadone's only advantages, one would expect methadone maintenance to be neither better nor worse than morphine maintenance or heroin maintenance. But in four other significant respects, methadone is distinctly superior to either morphine or heroin as a maintenance drug. The first of these advantages is that methadone is fully effective when taken by mouth.[5] Thus the whole long, tragic list of infections spread by injection needles is eliminated at one fell swoop. Infections due to morphine and heroin injection can be minimized by dispensing them in sterile ampules with nonreusable needles, but the oral drug is obviously a further improvement.

Second, methadone is a *long-acting* drug. An adequate oral dose in the morning keeps the user on a relatively even keel until the next morning.†[6] Stabilized methadone patients do not "bounce" from "sick" (incipient withdrawal symptoms) to "nodding" (excessively tranquilized). Addicts on morphine or heroin, in contrast, must "shoot up" several times a day, and many of them bounce.

Third, some addicts, as noted above, have a tendency to escalate their doses of morphine or heroin. Once stabilized on an adequate daily dose of methadone, in contrast, patients are content to remain on that dose year after year;[7] some even ask to have the dose reduced. Thus the main problem of morphine and heroin maintenance programs—the dosage problem—is readily resolved.

* Dr. Marie Nyswander disputes this common view. She points out that a methadone maintenance patient who discontinues methadone does not develop a craving for methadone and does not go looking for methadone. Instead, his craving for *heroin* returns and he goes looking for heroin. Hence, he is not, in common parlance, addicted to methadone. He is an ex-heroin addict who is relieved of his heroin addiction so long as he takes his methadone.[4]

† An even longer-acting drug related to methadone—acetyl-alpha-methadol—is said to be effective for three days or longer and may ultimately replace methadone as a maintenance drug.

Methadone's fourth advantage is that it *blocks* the heroin effect.[8] A patient stabilized on an adequate daily dose of methadone who shoots heroin discovers to his own amazement that it has no effect—that he has wasted his money. The higher the methadone maintenance dose, the larger a dose of heroin is thus blocked. The methadone dose can be set at whatever level is necessary to block the largest heroin dose a patient is likely to secure.* There is nothing mysterious about this blocking effect; it is just a special case of cross-tolerance. Any opiate or synthetic narcotic, in a given dose, will block the effects of any other opiate or synthetic narcotic given in a substantially smaller dose. The Dole-Nyswander program merely makes use of this well-known relationship among opiate and synthetic narcotics to discourage the use of heroin while on methadone.

No "high" or "bang" or "rush" is experienced when methadone is taken by mouth in regular daily doses. Indeed, nothing whatever is experienced except the taste of the orange drink in which methadone is dissolved. To demonstrate this, Drs. Dole and Nyswander occasionally gave patients who came in for their daily dose of methadone a placebo instead. The patients couldn't tell the difference. Not until hours later, when withdrawal symptoms began to appear, did they realize that they had not received methadone. When methadone is mainlined, however, some people get much the same reaction that some people get from heroin. This is one reason why methadone for maintenance use is dispensed in a hard-to-inject, soft-drink or tablet form in the United States. In Britain, physicians are permitted to prescribe—and some do—injectable methadone for addicts.

Finally, methadone staves off not only the acute effects of withdrawal from heroin—a fact long known—but the postaddiction syndrome of anxiety, depression, and craving as well, year after year. On methadone the patient no longer thinks constantly about heroin, or dreams of it, or shapes his whole life to ensure a continuing supply. He no longer engages compulsively in "drug-seeking behavior." He is, quite soon after going on methadone, freed of the heroin incubus. In this sense, he is "cured."

These advantages of methadone, however, should not be interpreted as criticisms of legalized heroin or morphine maintenance, as practiced in Britain today and in Kentucky earlier, for example. While the latter are no doubt inferior to methadone maintenance in the respects described above, they are still a vast improvement over the American heroin black market.

* In Britain, where large doses of unadulterated medicinal heroin are available, much larger doses of methadone are dispensed than in the United States—up to 400 milligrams per day, for example, as compared with the usual 100 milligrams daily here.[9]

18.

Methadone maintenance spreads

At the 1968 methadone maintenance conference, reports were heard from programs in Chicago and Philadelphia as well as New York.[1] By the 1969 conference, at least 23 cities were known to have methadone maintenance programs—some of them several programs. Reports were again heard from Chicago, Philadelphia, and New York, along with Minneapolis, St. Louis, Baltimore, New Haven, New Orleans, Miami, and Vancouver.[2] At the 1970 conference, Washington, D.C., San Francisco, and other cities also reported.[3] The discussion that follows is based in part on these reports, and in part on visits paid to methadone maintenance programs in New Haven, Baltimore, New Orleans, San Francisco, Portland (Oregon), Vancouver, Chicago, and London in the course of research for this Consumers Union Report.

Several programs outside New York started when a courageous local physician heard about the Dole-Nyswander program and decided to give it a try on his own personal responsibility. Dr. Emmett P. Davis, a Baltimore physician with a private practice primarily in pediatrics, started the first Baltimore program in this way; his program is now under the aegis of a private agency, Man Alive, Inc., set up for the purpose.[4] Several other Baltimore programs are now in operation, one administered by Johns Hopkins.

In Minneapolis, too, the first methadone program was launched as a private undertaking by an internist in private practice, Dr. Robert A. Maslansky. By the time he had 39 patients on the program, however, he found he had too little time left for his regular practice. Accordingly, he stopped further private enrollments, and launched a second program under the auspices of Mount Sinai Hospital in Minneapolis. A third program was later established in that city.[5]

In New Orleans it was a municipal judge, Andrew Bucaro, who spearheaded methadone maintenance. Judge Bucaro, like many others on the bench, grew weary and angry at the steady parade of addicts passing before him—few of them for the first or even the second time. When he heard about methadone maintenance, he began phoning physicians in a search for one who would try it in New Orleans. After eight consecutive rebuffs, he reached Dr. James T. Nix, who already had one patient on methadone in his private clinic.[6] The two Nix clinics now have more than 160 New Orleans patients coming in for methadone daily, and six other methadone maintenance clinics (including one for women run by a Catholic nun) are now operating. By the fall of 1970 the eight New Orleans clinics were treating about 1,200 patients.[7]

The pioneer methadone-dispensing physicians, as might be expected, faced some community opposition; they were, after all, dispensing an addicting drug to addicts. Several programs reported repeated visits from federal, state, and local narcotics agents, and a few were closed down; but nobody was criminally prosecuted. Dr. Nix in New Orleans notified his county medical society on March 7, 1968, that he was going to open a methadone maintenance clinic—and received the following ultimatum in reply six days later:

It was the unanimous opinion of the Board of Directors of this Society that it would be wise, particularly from an ethical standpoint, for you to disband this clinic.

Please let me hear from you by March 23, 1968, as to your intention in this matter; i.e., do you plan on continuing the clinic or has it been disbanded?[8]

Dr. Nix bravely continued his clinic, and no further action was taken by the county medical society.

Dr. Maslansky in Minneapolis reported several difficulties. The three programs there, he noted, "have not gone without some official criticism. . . . Our legal preoccupations in each clinic have been formidable from the beginning."[9] The clinics were warned by law-enforcement officers that the Harrison Narcotic Act (Section 151–392) "provides criminal action against . . . those who would issue a prescription to an addict for the purposes of providing the user with narcotics sufficient to keep him comfortable. . . ."[10] The sponsors of the programs refused to be intimidated, however, and no prosecution under Section 151–392 was initiated.

Dr. Maslansky was also called to account before the Minnesota Board of Medical Examiners. His license to practice medicine was clearly at stake. "I lost 20 pounds, that's all I can say," he told the 1969 methadone conference. At the beginning of his hearing Dr. Maslansky felt that the board members "thought they were dealing with either somebody perniciously involved . . . for the simple [purpose] of making money out of it, or, even worse, [with] a benighted do-gooder."[11] After Dr. Maslansky had addressed the board for ten or fifteen minutes, however, he recalled, "I could see that they had melted somewhat, and after the full presentation, in fact, the Board came around full circle and simply asked me how they could be of some help to me. In fact, since then they have been immeasurably helpful in getting the entire thing off the ground."[12] Similar changes in attitude, once methadone maintenance has been adequately explained, have been reported in other cities.

Everywhere the new programs were faced with expressions of concern that doses of methadone might be diverted from the maintenance program to the black market. Some methadone has been diverted, and some will no doubt be diverted in the future, despite intensive efforts to prevent such diversion. But the diversion problem must be viewed in proper scale. The American black market is currently supplying addicts with an estimated 250 to 375 million heroin "fixes" per year. The diversion of even tens of thousands of doses of methadone to that market would thus add barely a drop to the ocean of illegal narcotics already available.

"It is true occasionally," Dr. Trussell remarked at the 1969 methadone conference, "that one of our 1,300 patients will give one of his friends one of his bottles of methadone in orange juice. I do not worry about this because the same fellow could go 300 yards in almost any direction and get all the heroin he wanted." [13]

Some of the programs outside New York offer, along with the methadone, routine health care plus a wide range of individual psychiatric services, group psychotherapy, social work, employment counseling, legal aid, and rehabilitation services, much on the Dole-Nyswander pattern. In all probability these auxiliary services are useful and effective, and raise a clinic's success rate. What amazes visitors to less comprehensive programs, however, are the relatively good results achieved merely with methadone plus the limited kind of counseling that may occur when an addict comes in for his dose. Drs. Dole and Nyswander themselves have recently set up a small-scale experimental unit in which methadone is dispensed with a minimum of auxiliary services; when the results from this unit are later compared with the results in full-service units serving comparable groups of addicts, more light will be thrown on the value of and need for full auxiliary services.

Since the cost of the methadone itself is trivial—ten cents per day—the cost of a program depends primarily on the range of such auxiliary services. Dr. Dole estimated in 1970 that a budget for comprehensive treatment, including not only methadone but all of the auxiliary services, costs $1,500 the first year, $1,000 the second year, and $500 a year thereafter. This, of course, is only a fraction of what it costs to imprison an addict— and an even smaller fraction of what society loses through each addict who maintains his addiction through crime.

The programs that lack broad auxiliary services are cheaper. The Man Alive program in Baltimore and the Nix Clinic program in New Orleans, for example, originally operated on $500 or $600 per patient per year, including first-year patients. (In Baltimore, and elsewhere, volunteers helped keep down the cost of staffing.) Both the New Orleans and Baltimore programs, moreover, were very nearly self-supporting; the patients themselves paid $10 or $11 a week for the service. In Maryland, methadone maintenance programs are now chargeable to Medicaid, like other accepted forms of medical care, and Man Alive, Inc., now receives a substantial state grant for its operations.[14]

Ultimately it should prove safe and feasible to make methadone available on prescription, like insulin or any other maintenance medicine, at a daily cost of ten cents—$36.50 per year—a price that the user himself can readily pay.

In New Orleans, the methadone maintenance program for women addicts administered by Sister David serves imprisoned addicts. Each day the police paddy wagon brings the women prisoners to the clinic and takes them back again. On the day of their release from prison, they are already fully stabilized methadone maintenance patients, freed of their craving for heroin and blockaded against heroin effects.

Most programs take both wives and husbands, and a substantial portion of the addicts on some programs are couples.

Many of the successful methadone maintenance programs across the country rely heavily on addicts themselves for two major roles. One is the counseling of patients newly admitted to the program. An addict fresh off the street isn't likely to believe much of what a doctor or nurse tells him— but he gets the message promptly from another addict. Second, the patients fully rehabilitated on the program are indispensable in keeping a sharp eye open for potential abuses. Rehabilitated addicts have an enormous stake in the long-run success of the program, and will protect it in every way possible. An addict newly admitted often looks for "angles"; he can easily fool the doctors, but he can hardly fool his fellow addicts who have long since learned all the tricks. Dr. Jerome H. Jaffe commented on this at the 1969 methadone maintenance conference:

At least in Chicago, if somebody comes in and takes something, we know exactly who he is and where he hangs out. He's going to have 300 enemies in our program who have very few compunctions about letting him know that he's jeopardizing the entire program, and their way of demonstrating their displeasure with him may be much more severe than anything the courts can do.[15]

Dr. Herbert D. Kleber, director of the New Haven program, commented similarly:

The patients feel a great sense of loyalty to the program and feel very strongly that each individual in a program is responsible not only for himself but for every other individual in the program, and therefore if someone messes up, that is a threat not only to himself—the possibility that he can go back to jail—but to everyone else in the program.[16]

Not all programs achieve this high morale. The impression gained on visits to methadone clinics was that the ones which fail to make use of patients in their day-to-day operation have lower patient morale and are less successful.

Relations between the methadone maintenance programs and the police are usually tense in the beginning; police officials understandably wonder what the world is coming to when doctors dispense addicting narcotics to addicts, free of charge or at low cost. But the police, too, change their minds when they see the results of methadone maintenance. Dr. William A. Bloom of the Tulane University School of Medicine methadone maintenance program cites an example.

We invited the police to refer to us the worst addicts they knew of, just to see what happens, and the result of this, we think, has been [our] single best selling point, because the police and the addicts on the street . . . know each other—they work the same hours. . . .[17]

The police soon learned that the majority of [patients on methadone] no longer have new tracks [needle marks] and can prove a legal source of employment and they know we've got a good product.[18]

Among the most significant of the addiction treatment programs currently under way outside New York is one sponsored by the Illinois Department of Mental Health. Like most other states, Illinois until a few years ago spent little or nothing on addicts, beyond the costs of arresting, convicting, and imprisoning them. Unlike California and New York State, it thus had no vested interests in existing programs, and no vast annual expenditures to maintain ineffective programs. In 1965, Illinois established a Narcotic Advisory Council, and in 1967 that council set up a wide range of addiction services, all under a common administration *but in competition with one another.*[19] The director until 1971 was Dr. Jerome H. Jaffe of the University of Chicago–Pritzker School of Medicine.

Among the Illinois programs were a methadone maintenance program with auxiliary rehabilitation services, a methadone maintenance program without auxiliary services, a detoxification program, a program using other drugs (such as cyclazocine), a drug-free program using group psychotherapy and other psychological approaches, and a "therapeutic community" program modeled on Synanon and Daytop. Addicts were assigned *at random* to these programs. A further control was provided by addicts on the waiting list who received no services whatever. Thus each type of program could demonstrate its worth, or lack of worth, on patients all drawn from the same pool.

In addition to replicating the Dole-Nyswander methadone results in New York City, the Illinois program has pioneered a number of ingenious variations on the Dole-Nyswander theme. One of these variations consisted in taking types of patients specifically excluded from the New York program—such as criminal offenders assigned to the program by the courts as an alternative to imprisonment. Some of these court cases were put on methadone; others received group therapy and other rehabilitation procedures without methadone. Dr. Jaffe summed up the preliminary results at the October 1969 methadone maintenance conference: "We can only say that the [court referrals] assigned to methadone . . . do as well as people who volunteer. . . . They do . . . considerably better than [court referrals] who are randomly assigned to non-methadone programs." [20]

While the Illinois findings are still preliminary, they almost all point to methadone maintenance as the keystone in any comprehensive program for narcotics addicts. Dr. Jaffe was asked about this at the October 1969 meeting:

Dr. Paul H. Blachly (Portland, Oregon): ". . . I would like to ask Dr. Jaffe . . . given a fixed amount of money, what would be the best way to [use it] most effectively?"

Dr. Jaffe: "I think our data indicates unequivocally . . . if I had dollars to spread around in my town . . . we would be expanding our methadone program without any question."

Dr. Blachly: "How much of that will go into rehabilitation if you have to make the choice between more drug and more rehabilitation?"

Dr. Jaffe: "Every time I'm presented with an absolute choice, more will go into the drug. Fortunately I think our community is rational and mature enough to recognize that every dollar they invest in the program as a whole is going to save them money in terms of the cost to the community and the rehabilitation of people who are now able to function. So that for the time being our expansion is limited only by our capacity to train and orient and to work out effective working relationships with other programs. When money becomes a problem I will tell you now that it will go into the provision of adequate amounts of drug rather than elaborate rehabilitation programs." [21]

Dr. Jaffe was also asked what proportion of all addicts were likely to accept a methadone program.

"At present," he replied, "we have had applications from 1,500, approximately, of the known . . . 6,000 heroin users, in Chicago; and [about] 80 percent . . . prefer some form of methadone program. So that those people seem to have an uncanny notion of what is good for them. . . ." [22] Those dragooned into treatment by court edict as well as those who volunteered preferred the methadone program and did well on it. Only 3 percent of the addicts expressed a preference for a "therapeutic community" experience of the Synanon or Daytop type. [23]

The Tulane Medical School methadone maintenance program in New Orleans takes addicts over eighteen years of age who have been addicted to narcotics for at least six months. Some of the other programs throughout the country set a minimum age of twenty-one for methadone maintenance, and a minimum period of addiction of two, three, or even four years. Dr. Blachly of Portland, and others, however, question the wisdom of these limitations. The prognosis for the teen-age addict is so dismal, they say, and the likelihood of continuing addiction so high, that they favor making methadone available even to quite young addicts, and even after a relatively brief period of addiction. There have been suggestions, however, that newly addicted teen-age addicts who are still on their "heroin honeymoon" and have not yet experienced the woes of long-term addiction may do less well on methadone.

The Dole-Nyswander program has had patients as young as nineteen-and-a-half. In addition, a few younger teen-agers, some as young as sixteen, are being maintained on methadone experimentally; all were addicted to heroin at least two years before being accepted for methadone maintenance. Withholding methadone maintenance because of age "is a real dilemma," Dr. Dole told the 1969 methadone conference. "We have had parents and ministers come to us and . . . say, 'Does this boy have to go to jail and suffer two more years of addiction which he already is in? He's been in jail.' So I think that the answer as of today is that if a person is unmistakably an addict with an uncontrollable daily heroin habit and already into and on his way into more trouble for two years, then he is sufficiently into it to justify methadone treatment." [24]

Age is one of two major methadone issues on which there is as yet no consensus. The other concerns the length of time an addict must remain on methadone.

Dr. Dole in New York City has had the broadest experience in "weaning" patients from methadone. In a number of cases, he reports, patients who have been on his program with complete success for periods as long as five years have asked to be "tapered off" so that they can live drug-free thereafter. These patients have long since severed their ties with the underworld. They have renounced a life of crime. They may have steady jobs, good homes, warm relations with spouse and children. They no longer have a craving. Why should they continue the nuisance of going to a clinic and swallowing an orange drink spiked with methadone?

By the end of 1969, Dr. Dole had had experience with 562 patients who were weaned from methadone. The *pharmacological* results were consistent in all cases. "It is easy to reduce the methadone dose down to about 50 milligrams per day. Drug hunger is still controlled. . . . If you then continue to reduce the dose to somewhere between 20 and 40 milligrams per day, the person will begin to experience a return of the old heroin hunger, not hunger for methadone but [for] heroin." [25] This return of the post-addiction syndrome (anxiety, depression, and craving) is parallel to that of the addict who serves five years drug-free in a prison—yet heads for the nearest black market soon after his release.

The renewed craving for heroin, Dr. Dole concedes, is not uniform;

some feel it more acutely than others—but they all feel it, including "the people who have been thoroughly rehabilitated." [26]

This finding is of great theoretical as well as practical importance. Heroin relapse after prolonged abstinence is generally attributed, as we have seen, to social or psychological factors. The addict, it is said, returns to his old addicted buddies and therefore relapses. He sees others "shooting" and therefore relapses. He loses his job or wife or girl friend and therefore relapses. Dr. Dole's observation is that the addict's craving (and drug-seeking behavior) returns even though he has cut himself off from his old neighborhood and his old associations, and has built a whole new satisfying life free of heroin. The craving, he is therefore convinced, is a biochemical phenomenon rather than a psychological urge. "The thought that a social rehabilitation might cure a metabolic disease I think can be well disproven by the experience we have had to date." [27]

Dr. Dole does *not* deny that a few patients now on methadone might hereafter live completely abstinent. A few people, after all, can permanently kick the heroin habit *without* methadone at all. "But this, I can say quite flatly, will be a minority," [28] Dr. Dole concludes. Most heroin addicts on methadone, like most diabetics on insulin or other antidiabetes drugs, he believes, will have to continue to take the drug for the rest of their lives or until something even better than methadone is discovered. Those who do give up methadone—including those fully rehabilitated—experience a return of the postaddiction syndrome followed by drug-seeking behavior and relapse in a high proportion of cases. Then, somewhat sheepishly, many of them come back to methadone maintenance again.

Dr. Jaffe, on the basis of the more limited Illinois experience, is not quite so sure about the inability of methadone patients to live drug-free. Some Illinois patients ask to be weaned from methadone after only a few months. A substantial proportion of those who are weaned, Dr. Jaffe concedes, relapse to heroin as in New York. But a few have made it thus far—and the Illinois research program includes several efforts to develop ways to help them make it.

Sometimes there are excellent reasons for *not* weaning a patient from methadone. A striking example is cited by Dr. Gerald E. Davidson of the Harvard Medical School, director of the Chestnut Hill Clinic, a psychiatric clinic with a large methadone maintenance program, and medical director of Elan, a drug-free therapeutic community.

"One of my patients," Dr. Davidson reports, "is a boy from the most self-consciously 'best' suburb of Boston. He comes from a broken family, dropped out of high school, and had been in difficulty for some time. He was carried on methadone for a while, and I said to him one day: 'Phil, how about quitting?' He said: 'Look, doc, I spent two years in a mental hospital diagnosed as a schizophrenic, and then I found dope—first heroin and then methadone. Since I've been on dope I finished high school and got a scholarship to art school. I'm only a junior but I'm teaching courses and I've got faculty status and my work has been winning prizes all over the place. I'll be damned if I quit now.' "

Addicts, like other patients, Dr. Davidson comments, "frequently know what is good for them. They frequently know better than doctors and other wise, helpful, well-intentioned people. . . ." He continues, "I have repeatedly seen many young people—and adults, too—who, on comparatively small doses of methadone, tell me they feel normal, are able to work, are able to live with their families and to carry on a normal life. Otherwise they are what we call borderline . . . personalities, who cannot tolerate any kind of frustration, who cannot really maintain a job, who tend to act out with some kind of violence—whether verbal, physical or in some other way—whenever they're frustrated, and who, in general, are quite unsuccessful in life. Many of these people do extremely well on methadone." [29]

Not all of the other methadone maintenance programs enjoy the Dole-Nyswander success rates, and a few are clearly failures. In no program, however, is a high failure rate due to the methadone *per se*. Methadone elsewhere, as in the Dole-Nyswander program, is pharmacologically effective: it relieves the addict of his craving for heroin.

In some cases, low success rates* are due to the attitudes of the staffs of methadone maintenance programs. One program, for example, lost more than half its patients in the first twenty-four weeks. Investigation revealed that the staff was nagging and hounding the patients and in general treating them as if they were criminals. The patients, not unnaturally, walked out. When the staff is all white and middle-class, and the patients are not, there is greater likelihood that friction between staff and patients will lower the success rate. Using methadone patients themselves to help operate the program raises morale noticeably.

Senator Harold Hughes of Iowa pointed out one way in which a program can be sabotaged.

We had a very small methadone withdrawal program running [in Des Moines]. There had been nothing prior to this at all but apparently the police infiltrated the withdrawal program and put men in the withdrawal room as patients in order to gain confidential information from the addicts. This blew the program clear out of the water, and now there is not a heroin addict that would come for treatment to anyone in the city. The addicts are back on the streets having to steal $100, $200, $300 a day to maintain their heroin habit.

---

* That is, low as compared with the Dole-Nyswander program. No methadone maintenance program approaches the tragic failure rates of the nonmethadone programs described in Chapter 10.

We all support the police, and we all support everything we can do to cut back the importation of heroin and opium, getting the suppliers and distributors. We can have a health program trying to get people off the streets but as long as we use them as an infiltrative organism of the vice squad they will be unsuccessful.[30]

A clear light is thrown on the problems of methadone maintenance failures by a follow-up study of 95 patients who left one of the eight New Orleans methadone maintenance programs. This study,[31] by Richard G. Adams and William C. Capel in collaboration with Drs. William A. Bloom and Gordon T. Stewart, is the first of its kind to be published; it demonstrates how much a methadone maintenance program (or any other program) can learn from studying its own failures.

The study was undertaken because of what seemed like an excessively high failure rate; of 264 patients admitted to the program between November 1968 and February 4, 1970, 95 (35 percent) had dropped out by the end of the fifteen-month period. On analysis, however, it appeared that the failures were fewer than appeared.

Seventeen of the 95 dropouts, for example, had transferred to other methadone maintenance programs and could hardly be deemed failures. Seven other dropouts later returned to the program. One dropout was in a hospital with tuberculosis, one was a soldier in Vietnam, and three were dead. Five claimed that they left the program because they wanted to live drug-free, and three or four of these appeared to be making it; they "seem to have dropped out of the drug scene, are working, and are not associating with present or former clinic members." Several left soon after starting on methadone—one after being on the program only two days. One, married and with nine children, seemed to be doing very well (he had held the same job for seven years), even though he was back on heroin. Thus, the actual failure rate was closer to 20 percent.

Fifty-eight dropouts were interviewed and asked, "Why did you drop out of the program?"

One reason often given was that the patients didn't like a particular "straw boss"—a fellow-patient "who was given authority by the clinic operators to keep the peace, enforce rules, and maintain order, to see that no weapons, narcotics, or contraband drugs were brought, consumed or sold on the premises, and to perform a variety of other chores. This man had a reputation of being dangerous and powerful but also of being a stoolie for the police and of jacking or stealing from addicts themselves. He is therefore both feared and disliked." Complaints against him fell into five categories: "(1) ratting to the program directors, resulting in disciplinary action; (2) ratting to the police; (3) access to and illicit sale of methadone; (4) threats of bodily harm to extort loans; and (5) general abuse of authority." One of the patients who dropped out explained: "He is a rat for the police. He borrows money and then threatens you if you ask for it. He had access to the methadone and sold it—I even bought some. I would like to go back on that program but not until he leaves."

In all, 17 patients cited this man as at least one of their reasons for dropping out. The remarkable finding of the study, however, was the fact that so many patients stayed in the program *despite* the presence of such a character in a position of authority—a tribute, surely, to the holding power of methadone.

The situation in this clinic might be considered an argument against placing patients in positions of authority in a methadone maintenance program. Quite the reverse, however, is actually the case. If patients had been accepted as part of the therapeutic team at the beginning of this program, the administration would have been warned in advance against placing such a man in a position of power—or his abuses would have come to light far earlier. It was *absence* of patient cooperation in the clinic's management (with the exception of this one patient) which made such abuses possible.

Twenty-eight percent of the dropouts interviewed also cited as a reason their "difficulty in paying for methadone." This reason seems highly implausible on the face of it. The clinic charged only $10 a week for methadone. Every addict on the list had been spending far more than that—often ten or twenty times that much—for black-market heroin. The New Orleans report, however, indicates that there is a difference:

. . . Whereas they feel little compunction about stealing to support a heroin habit, heroin addicts do not want to steal to support the methadone habit. One of the dropouts, now in prison, explained it this way: "It is one thing to get money hustling for smack [heroin] but when you are on methadone you want to stop hustling and get a job . . . then the money is hard to get."

One possible solution, of course, is to discontinue clinic fees altogether. Another is to waive the fee for unemployed patients and other hardship cases.

"Difficulty in seeing a doctor" was complained of by 17 percent of the dropouts interviewed. "Uncertain doctors' hours, long waits, 'come back next week,' and other delays finally led several to abandon the program." Fourteen percent complained of "arrogance, lack of understanding, 'police type' attitude, and airs of superiority." One patient summed up this type of complaint: "You are supposed to act the way they think a junkie should act."[32]

In the light of such findings, even a 35 percent dropout rate seems readily understandable, and the reforms required to lower the dropout rate are clearly visible. Consumers Union strongly recommends that every methadone maintenance clinic—but especially those with dropout rates higher than that of the Dole-Nyswander program—conduct such follow-up studies periodically to find out what is wrong.

A cause of relatively high failure rates in some areas is antimethadone propaganda aimed at methadone patients, designed to turn them against the program. Some of this propaganda is well-meaning; it comes from people who believe that addiction is curable and that a patient on methadone is still an addict. "Be a man and kick the methadone" is the message. Some of the propaganda, however, is less well motivated. Patients are told that methadone gets into the bones and rots them, or destroys sexual function, or harms users in other ways. Black methadone patients, as noted above, are told that methadone is "white man's medicine," part of a genocide conspiracy. There is reason to believe that heroin traffickers, among others, are active in spreading such antimethadone rumors, for an obvious reason: every patient on methadone means one less customer for illicit heroin.

In several cities visited in the course of research for this Consumers Union Report, the chief source of antimethadone propaganda was not the heroin traffickers but the staffs of therapeutic communities and other treatment facilities, usually ex-addicts themselves. They are unquestionably well-intentioned, and they believe quite fervently that methadone is part of the "opiate evil." Their sincerity earns them a strong influence on community sentiment. Listeners feel an instinctive sympathy for these ex-addicts who have "made it the hard way." Yet the policy they recommend is disastrous, for as we have shown, the therapeutic communities can at best salvage a few—while methadone is already salvaging tens of thousands. As a methadone program becomes well established in a community, and as the success of its patients becomes visible in the neighborhood, the effectiveness of antimethadone propaganda campaigns tends to taper off.

Another cause of relatively high failure rates is lack of skill in helping addicts through the difficult first weeks or months on methadone. If the early doses are too small, the addict experiences discomfort and thinks he has been lied to about methadone. If escalation is too rapid, side effects occur—including, as noted above, a temporary diminution of sexual potency. Patients experiencing either of these kinds of effects need not only dosage adjustment but also guidance and counsel from informants they trust—preferably ex-addicts who have "made it" on methadone and who can honestly assure them that most of the unwanted effects are temporary.

The quality of life of the addict while still on heroin may also be a factor affecting failure rates. The chief advantage of methadone, after all, is that it "gets the monkey off the back" of the addict. Among addicts who are leading reasonably satisfactory lives on morphine or heroin (as in Dr. O'Donnell's Kentucky study), the relative advantages of methadone may be fewer and the program therefore less successful. Recently addicted adolescents in particular may not appreciate the full advantages of methadone maintenance because they have not yet experienced the full miseries of street addiction.

Finally, it should be noted that each program in effect sets its own failure rate. Few patients give up methadone maintenance voluntarily; most patients who leave are involuntarily terminated for repeated violation of the program's rules. An excessively punitive discharge policy, especially for addicts new to the program, is thus inevitably reflected in a high failure rate.

This is hardly an exhaustive catalogue of reasons why some methadone maintenance programs do less well than others. In each case of less than optimal success rates, a local study is called for to identify the reasons—and correct them. In general, however, the dice are loaded in favor of a high success rate for every methadone maintenance program, for each program is in competition with black-market heroin and its attendant prices and hazards. Any methadone maintenance program that cannot win customers away from *that* competition must be doing something terribly wrong.

19.

The future of methadone maintenance

By December 1971, the number of American addicts on methadone maintenance was estimated at 25,000—and may have been considerably higher. Federal, state, and local plans, public and private, in various stages of realization, moreover, called for an increase to 50,000 or more within the next year or so.

The rate of growth, interestingly enough, was *nowhere* limited by the availability of addicts eager to enter a methadone maintenance program. It was limited in part by the lack of funds to finance such programs, in part by the lack of trained staff to man them, and in large part by lethargy —the lack of enough public officials and private citizens willing to invest the effort needed to get programs started or expanded.

As late as the fall of 1971, no city had reported a capacity to supply methadone to all addict applicants. All cities had waiting lists. Hence it is impossible to estimate what proportion of addicts will accept methadone maintenance voluntarily. The number of addicts eager for methadone maintenance tends to grow as the programs grow and as news of their advantages spreads. Heroin addicts, as we have noted, are not mentally retarded. They recognize a good buy when they are offered one.

Recent British experience casts some light on the proportion of addicts who can voluntarily be converted to methadone maintenance or to other alternatives to heroin. As of December 31, 1970, the 1,430 men and women receiving narcotic drugs on Britain's National Health Service were distributed as follows:

732 on methadone alone *
140 on heroin alone
241 on methadone and heroin
 91 on morphine alone
 70 on pethidine (known in the United States as
    meperidine or Demerol) alone
 40 on dipipanone alone
 28 on dextromoramide alone
 39 on heroin and cocaine
 49 on other drugs or drug combinations [1]

* British patients on methadone, as noted earlier, can obtain injectable methadone and injection equipment. Many (not all) do in fact inject their methadone. This British policy, which seems strange and objectionable to many Americans, seems quite natural in Britain.

The fact that more than half of all the addicts known to the United Kingdom Home Office are being maintained on methadone alone is of particular significance, for any one of those 732 methadone patients can at any time decide to go back to heroin and have a legal right to get it, free of charge and of medicinal strength and purity—along with free sterile disposable injection equipment.

The British figures are significant in another respect: within the next few years, British authorities will be able to evaluate and compare the various maintenance drugs now in use there. Thus, for the first time, reliable data will be available on the relative advantages of methadone, heroin, morphine, and other maintenance drugs and drug combinations, taken orally or injected, in a country where all are legal and all are free of charge.

Within the next few years—and perhaps much sooner—at least some American cities will be offering methadone maintenance on a large enough scale to supply all voluntary applicants. At that point a further question will arise: what shall be done about addicts who stay on black-market heroin despite vacancies in a nearby methadone maintenance program?

From time to time, politicians and others who have not done their homework, and who fail to understand the narcotics problem, offer the same old answer to this question: *pass another law.* During the 1970 political campaign in New York State, for example, a candidate running for the office of New York State attorney general demanded a law for the "compulsory transfer of patients from dependence on heroin to dependence on methadone." [2]

The laws already in effect in New York State and in the United States provide long terms of imprisonment for the mere possession of heroin— indeed, for the possession of a hypodermic needle with which heroin might be injected. Other Draconian provisions of existing law have been reviewed in earlier chapters. These laws, of course, *already* serve to force heroin addicts to enter methadone maintenance programs—unless they want to risk the dire penalties specified. Adding another narcotics law and another penalty to the many already on the books will hardly increase the existing legal pressure on addicts to switch to methadone maintenance.

It is also frequently proposed that experimental *heroin* maintenance programs be set up in addition to methadone maintenance programs. These proposals are discussed in our Conclusions and Recommendations below (see Part X).

The chief peril of methadone maintenance for the future lies not in the pharmacological properties of the drug or in its abuse by addicts or others, but in the ways it may be misused by politicians and institutions. Let us explain.

The heroin addict today is a serf of the heroin black market. When he goes on methadone maintenance, he becomes a potential serf of whoever controls the methadone program. This is not the fault of methadone, of course; it is the result of his becoming addicted to heroin in the first place. Whether on heroin or methadone, the addict must dance to whatever tune the piper plays.

Most existing methadone maintenance programs play a sensible tune. They expect essentially three things of an addict: that he not get arrested, that he find and hold a job if he possibly can, and that he limit his consumption of alcohol, barbiturates, and other drugs as well as of heroin. The vast majority of patients comply. A patient is involuntarily discharged from the program, as noted earlier, only when repeated violations make it clear that methadone maintenance is doing the patient no good.

Let us suppose, however, that methadone maintenance programs drift into the hands of agencies with other goals. One example is a police department, which might use a methadone maintenance program as a recruiting center for stool pigeons, or witnesses. Leaders of the black community are particularly concerned that the power of those who control methadone maintenance may be misused to repress black organizations and aspirations. These are not idle imaginings. In at least one city, patients on methadone maintenance have already been organized to vote for a political candidate who promised to support a continuation of their supply. In a number of other cities, methadone maintenance programs are deeply enmeshed in local politics.

Probation and parole departments have been establishing or planning to establish methadone maintenance programs in several states and cities —and police departments may be next. The patient on methadone maintenance who must placate a police officer, or a probation or parole officer empowered both to return him to prison and to cut off his methadone, is in a vise with two turnscrews.

A thoughtful review of this problem was presented at the Third National Conference on Methadone Treatment (1970) by Dr. Robert G. Newman, director of the New York City Health Department's Methadone Maintenance Treatment Program. "It is my conviction," Dr. Newman stated, "that the abuse and misuse of addiction treatment programs poses at least as great a threat to our patients as does the abuse of illicit drugs." Then he went on to explain:

Many proponents of methadone treatment dismiss as ridiculous the assertion by some militant groups that the program is a means by which the establishment can control (their word is enslave) certain communities. While I do not believe that this danger is an imminent one, I do agree that it is a very real potential threat. It is entirely conceivable to me that applicants might some day be rejected, or patients discharged, on the basis of political and/or antisocial behavior ("antisocial," of course, to be defined by those in power). The likelihood of such medical blackmail is increased by the intermingling of medical and social goals which certain programs set for themselves. We emphasize that, along with the medication which we dispense, we encourage the use of the supportive services which are offered to help the patient in his efforts to become rehabilitated, to lead a socially acceptable and productive life. Providing such assistance to those who want it is a responsibility we should accept in treating "the whole patient." On the other hand, what if the patient does not want to be rehabilitated, and does not seek to adopt what we feel is a desirable pattern of behavior? Perhaps a patient wishes to spend the rest of his life collecting welfare payments instead of working; perhaps he is a highly successful and well-adjusted numbers-runner; perhaps he is a member of an extremist group (right or left makes no difference) who feels his calling in life is to make bombs in cellars, or attack policemen, or burn synagogues. How will the professional staff relate to such a patient who, despite his antisocial life-style, abstains from all drug use, reports punctually and regularly to the clinic for his medication, and whose activities in no way pose a threat to the treatment unit itself? Even more pertinent to the topic of this paper, how much latitude will the staff be permitted in resolving the conflict when the employer is the government?

My questions are obviously rhetorical. I believe that medical care should not be withheld except for strictly medical reasons, or when the care of other patients is compromised. An orthopedist would not refuse to set a broken ankle even if he knew the injury was incurred in the course of a burglary, and even though he were thoroughly convinced that, once healed, the patient would promptly return to his work. An epileptic is not refused his Dilantin because the physician disagrees with his political activities. Similarly, though we offer a comprehensive program for our methadone patients, and encourage them to utilize what is available, we should not present our services on an all-or-none basis. To do so would be analogous to a doctor withholding insulin from a diabetic because the patient refuses simultaneous help in controlling his obesity.

Hopefully, most health workers share this view, and will defend it against all pressures which might arise to compromise what they should accept as the primary role: serving their patients.[3]

No absolute protection from the abuse of methadone maintenance programs by those who control them is possible. A young man or woman who doesn't want to fall into the clutches of a corrupt methadone maintenance program can best protect himself by staying away from heroin in the first place. Consumers Union does offer three suggestions, however, for minimizing the likelihood that future methadone maintenance programs will be misused for political, social, police, or other extraneous ends.

First, ultimate policy control of the programs as well as day-by-day supervision must be securely lodged in *medical* rather than political, probation, parole, or police hands. This principle is not observed today in a number of cities. Cities and states where politicians control methadone maintenance programs should begin planning now to transfer them to medical auspices—before a local political scandal threatens the whole methadone program. This is particularly true of some programs in New York City and State (but not of the Dole-Nyswander program, which is under firm medical control).

Second, as Dr. Newman of the New York City program has suggested, the regulations governing expulsion from a methadone maintenance program should be spelled out in specific and objective terms, so that patients are not left at the mercy of the staff or the institution. In his own program, Dr. Newman reports, "conditions for discharge unequivocally preclude the use of this medical treatment as a means of coercing social conformity among our patients." [4] In some cities, politicians are already using their influence to get patients into a crowded methadone maintenance program; in the absence of objective criteria for discharge it is only one small step further for a politician to threaten to have a patient expelled from a program—or, indeed, to have him expelled.

Third, every large city and every state should aim for *multiplicity* of independent and competing maintenance programs rather than one monolithic source of methadone. If one program becomes corrupt and seeks to manipulate its patients for political or other ends, patients should be free to transfer to another.

The role of the physician in private practice is also important here. Indeed, the private practitioner should play several roles in the future of methadone maintenance. For example, he is the only feasible source of supply in villages and towns where there are too few addicts to warrant a full-scale methadone maintenance program.

The physician in private practice is also essential as a safeguard against the manipulation of patients on organized programs. If the only local program in a city harbors a grudge against a patient and threatens to cut off his methadone supply because of his political views, or because he participates in protest meetings, or for any other reason, the patient's only alternatives are to surrender or find another source of supply. The availability of methadone from physicians in private practice is thus a major protection for the patient on a public program.

Dr. Newman implicitly recognized this role of the private practitioner in his statement to the Third National Conference on Methadone Treatment: ". . . We are already exploring ways by which private practitioners can be involved in the management of patients enrolled in the [New York City] program. In so doing, we are trying to anticipate the day when this form of therapy can be safely and effectively transferred from government to the private sector. As the acceptability and availability of methadone maintenance becomes more widespread, its potential use in exerting social control will lessen." [5]

There are also cogent arguments *against* letting physicians in private practice prescribe or dispense methadone for addicts. One objection is that they lack the ancillary services useful for rehabilitation. This is true; but as noted above, many patients do well on methadone without ancillary services.

A second objection raised is that a few physicians in private practice may abuse their privilege and prescribe methadone indiscriminately. Here a distinction must be made. One major purpose of methadone maintenance is to woo addicts away from the heroin black market. If a physician accomplishes this by prescribing methadone to addicts, he should surely be encouraged. Indeed, the prescription of methadone by easygoing physicians practicing in the slums or suburbs may attract some addicts who won't patronize an organized, regimented clinic—and may thus help solve the heroin problem. If an addict prefers to get his methadone this way, why shouldn't he? Members of minority ethnic groups, or middle-class white adolescents, may be much more likely to go to a physician affiliated with their own group, or sympathetic to it, rather than to a clinic which they perceive as hostile.

The possibility that a corrupt physician might prescribe addicting doses of methadone to a *nonaddict,* of course, raises a different problem—but not a particularly frightening one. Such a physician can today prescribe addicting doses of morphine to a nonaddict, if he wants to run the risk of imprisonment. No new hazard is introduced by permitting him to prescribe methadone instead, subject to the same risk of imprisonment. Any physician found to be overprescribing or prescribing to nonaddicts, whether the drug is morphine or methadone, should of course be promptly called to account.

In sum, Consumers Union recommends that the major burden of supplying methadone maintenance to heroin addicts be borne by a multiplicity of organized clinics, under firm medical rather than political control, offering a wide range of medical, legal, employment, and counseling services along with the methadone—and with explicitly stated regulations governing discharge from the program. It also recommends, however, that physicians in private practice be authorized to prescribe methadone for maintenance purposes—in part to meet the needs of addicts who cannot conveniently get to the organized clinics, or who perceive the local clinics as alien and hostile, and in part to serve as standby sources of methadone maintenance for patients who may be improperly manipulated or discriminated against in the organized clinic setting.

Finally, a word about perspective. As methadone maintenance programs continue to expand, we can expect all kinds of unfortunate methadone "incidents" to occur and to fill newspaper headlines. If methadone is left lying around carelessly some children may get hold of it, and they will die of it—just as children get hold of aspirin left lying around, and die of it. Some methadone patients may share their methadone with friends or sell some on the black market. Some methadone patients, like other people, may commit murder, theft, and prostitution, and all manner of other offenses—and when caught, they are going to be identified in the press as methadone patients. Every once in a while a newspaper reporter is going to disguise himself as an addict and get drugs from a clinic (as reporters did in 1920, and as a New York *Times* reporter did in 1971 [6]). Editorial writers, politicians, and others, in the future as in the past, are going to seize on such incidents to urge an end to methadone maintenance. Or they are going to demand unreasonable restraints on methadone maintenance programs—restraints that will in effect sabotage the programs and diminish their usefulness.*

It was attacks like these which discredited the opiate-dispensing clinics in the 1920s (see Chapter 13). A repetition of that experience, with methadone maintenance discredited as the result of a series of trivial but sensational scandals, is still a possibility in some cities.

When incidents discrediting methadone maintenance generate headlines in your community, as they almost certainly will, we suggest that you ask yourself a simple question. Whatever the shortcomings of methadone maintenance, and whatever the mistakes made by your local maintenance programs, do you really prefer the old-fashioned American black-market system of heroin distribution?

---

* A simple example, among many, is the rule governing how often a patient must come personally to the clinic for his methadone, often at great cost in time and inconvenience. Clinics uniformly require that patients come in daily at first, until their reliability has been established, and drink their whole glassful with a nurse watching to make sure they don't take some of it home with them to give away or sell. After a while, patients come in every other day, and those who demonstrate their trustworthiness are in some clinics eventually permitted to take home a whole week's supply. The rule usually works because addicts who must come in daily know that when they prove reliable, they will be permitted to come in at less frequent intervals. Occasionally, however, a patient with a week's supply may take pity on some heroin addict who is currently broke and suffering the torture of withdrawal, and who still has months ahead on a waiting list before he will be admitted to the methadone program himself. Or the patient may be broke and sell a little methadone to an addict. If the addict happens to be a stool pigeon, the methadone patient may be arrested for violating the narcotics laws, and the newspapers may demand that other patients no longer be allowed to take methadone home with them. This in effect sabotages the maintenance program and further buttresses the heroin black market.

20.

Heroin on the youth drug scene— and in Vietnam

During 1970 and 1971, the mass media carried news of two new and distressing opiate trends. A growing number of white, middle-class young people, in suburbs as well as inner cities, were said to be mainlining heroin. And United States military personnel—primarily in Vietnam, but also at duty stations in the United States and throughout the world—were similarly said to be sniffing, smoking, or mainlining heroin in substantial numbers.

It was still much too early, as this Consumers Union Report was nearing completion, to evaluate these two new phenomena in detail, to ascertain their causes with precision, or to put forward specific policies for handling them. A few central points, however, can be established with reasonable confidence. Let us review the two new patterns of heroin use in turn.

Heroin among middle-class white young people. How common is heroin use in comfortable residential areas and suburbs? Nobody knows.*

Anecdotal evidence indicated that by 1971, heroin had become the most popular illicit drug (except for marijuana) among young people in at least a few suburbs. How many suburbs? Which suburbs? No one knew or could find out. Indeed, the only reliable source of information concerning heroin on the youth drug scene came from the free clinics and other indigenous institutions (see Chapter 65)—institutions to which youthful heroin users naturally turned when they realized that they were "hooked." These institutions could report only that heroin addiction was rapidly rising in certain neighborhoods.

One very distressing aspect of heroin's spread to the suburbs was that it seemed to signal a crumbling of the long-standing dividing line between heroin and the other drugs, licit and illicit. That line had been recognized and accepted by almost all middle-class white young people through all the years from 1914 till late in the 1960s. Young people might risk alcohol, nicotine, marijuana, hashish, LSD, and a variety of other

---

* President Nixon's Message to Congress, June 17, 1971, stated: "Even now, there are no precise national statistics on drug use and drug addiction in the United States, the rate at which drug use is increasing, or where and how this increase is taking place. Most of what we think we know is extrapolated from those few states and cities where the dimensions of the problem have forced closer attention, including the maintenance of statistics."

drugs—but heroin? Certainly not—except, of course, for some poverty-stricken denizens of inner cities and a few others.

This breakdown of the barrier against heroin use was at least in part, it should now be apparent, the natural and inevitable result of the official United States antidrug stance, which linked many illicit drugs—even marijuana—to heroin in antidrug pronouncements. Thus, marijuana was defined as a narcotic in many laws. The same penalties were decreed against the possession or sale of marijuana as against the possession or sale of heroin. Authorities mistakenly spoke of "marijuana addicts." The often-repeated slogan, "Marijuana leads to heroin," further obscured the distinction between the two drugs. At the same time, the distinction between injecting a drug and swallowing, sniffing, or smoking it was also blurred; antidrug propaganda concealed the fact that sniffing, swallowing, or smoking a drug is much safer than mainlining it. As a result, the indigenous institutions report, many naïve young people eventually responded to the propaganda and accepted the view that heroin mainlining must not be very different from marijuana-smoking, or "acid-dropping," or other accepted forms of illicit drug use.

Most people who begin to experiment with an addicting drug assume that *they* are going to be exceptions—*they* are not going to get hooked. The antidrug campaigns to which young people were exposed during the 1960s gave them a further assurance: even if they did get hooked on heroin, the propaganda insisted, there were highly effective therapeutic communities and other treatment facilities where they could be cured—"rehabilitated." For some young people the message received was, why worry about getting hooked? Addiction is only temporary.

There was no reason for young people to doubt these officially sponsored assurances that heroin addiction is curable. If even the schools, with their known hostility toward drugs and especially toward heroin, were interrupting classes for assemblies at which "ex-addicts," after a few months of abstinence, assured young people that they had been able to quit with a little help, why should the message be doubted? What possible reason could adults have to mislead young people in this respect?

What possible reason indeed? Surely when the history of the drug crisis of the 1960s is utimately written, the story of the parade of young ex-addicts brought to school assemblies to demonstrate that heroin addiction is curable will rank among the most bizarre of the decade's drug phenomena.

After the public was informed, during the summer of 1971, of widespread heroin addiction among the United States armed forces in Vietnam and elsewhere, the same reassurances were reiterated. Public officials from the President of the United States down announced that everything possible would be done to "rehabilitate" (which to most people meant "cure") addicts in uniform.* Once again, the mistaken view that heroin addiction is really a short-term problem, treatable by public institutions, was publicized to the entire country.

Perhaps these three errors of public policy—the repeated equating of marijuana and other popular drugs with heroin, the failure to explain the difference between eating, sniffing, or smoking a drug and mainlining it, and the insistence that heroin addiction is temporary and curable—do not constitute an exhaustive explanation of why the long-effective barrier against heroin in middle-class white communities crumbled late in the 1960s. A few years hence, perhaps, in retrospect, it may be possible to identify additional ways in which official drug policies and other factors breached the barrier that formerly separated heroin from other drugs.

Marijuana laws and policies, like heroin laws and policies, also appear to have contributed in several ways to increased use of heroin (see Part VIII).

First, laws and law-enforcement policies tended to force marijuana into underground channels of distribution—including some of the same channels which were distributing heroin.

Second, by making marijuana scarce at particular times in particular places, law-enforcement drives caused marijuana smokers to look around for substitute drugs. Sometimes the substitute they found was heroin (see table on Page 442).

Third, the illegal status of marijuana caused students and other young people to set up their own informal channels of marijuana distribution. These same informal channels were at least occasionally used also for the distribution of low-cost heroin after 1969, and perhaps earlier. Half a dozen youthful users, for example, might send one of their number down to Mexico, where heroin is cheap, for a month's or two-months' supply. Or cheap, highly potent Mexican heroin might be picked up on the American side of the border in California, Arizona, or Texas. Again, very potent heroin was coming in from Vietnam and from other points in Asia through "informal channels"; this low-priced Asian heroin, too, was being

* President Nixon's Message to Congress on June 17, 1971, for example, contained such statements as these:

"*Rehabilitation: A New Priority.* . . . I am asking the Congress for a total of $105 million in addition to funds already contained in my 1972 budget to be used solely for the treatment and rehabilitation of drug-addicted individuals. . . . The nature of drug addiction, and the peculiar aspects of the present problem as it involves veterans [of the Vietnam war], make it imperative that rehabilitation procedures be undertaken immediately. . . . In order to expedite the rehabilitation program of Vietnam veterans, I have ordered the immediate establishment of . . . immediate rehabilitation efforts to be taken in Vietnam. . . . The Department of Defense will provide rehabilitation programs to all servicemen being returned for discharge who want this help, and we will be requesting legislation to permit the military services to retain for treatment any individual due for discharge who is a narcotic addict. All of our servicemen must be accorded the right to rehabilitation."

informally distributed at a fraction of the price charged by the traditional black market.

The availability of low-priced heroin through informal channels extending into middle-class white communities had a series of effects. Since the pioneer suburban heroin users were getting their drug at moderate cost, they did not suffer the degradation typical of traditional "junkies." Often they continued in school or in their usual patterns of life. They themselves and their friends thus became convinced that it is possible to take heroin without experiencing the pauperization and criminalization typical of inner-city junkies. In short, they were on their "heroin honeymoon"—at cut rates. The relative innocuousness of heroin under these circumstances confirmed the view stressed by official drug propaganda that heroin and marijuana hazards are pretty much the same. As for the risk of getting "hooked," they could readily (they thought) get cured or rehabilitated if that happened. That, as noted above, was what even the President of the United States was assuring them. It is hardly surprising, under these circumstances, that heroin use spread. Indeed, it is surprising that use did not explode on an even grander scale.

But the honeymoon did not last. Informal channels of distribution work for marijuana; since it is not addicting, a temporary local marijuana famine is at worst an inconvenience. The unreliability of informal *heroin* channels—an unreliability that became more acute as law-enforcement agencies gradually learned how to harry these new suppliers—proved a much more serious matter. Young addicts found themselves undergoing withdrawal when their informal supplies were cut off—with no place to turn for heroin but to the established, traditional, high-priced "jugglers" or "pushers." When their funds were exhausted, they turned to the free clinics and other indigenous institutions to which they had been accustomed to turn for help with their nonheroin problems (see Part IX).

The Haight-Ashbury Medical Clinic in San Francisco has documented this trend. It opened a special section for heroin addicts in November 1967, and by November 1969 it had seen nearly 1,000 heroin users, almost all of whom were addicted. (Since national drug styles tend to be set first in the Haight-Ashbury, the increased use of heroin surfaced there a little earlier than in most other communities.) Of the addicts served by the clinic, about 25 percent (classed as "old-style junkies") had first used heroin before January 1964; about 20 percent (classed as "transitional junkies") first used heroin between then and January 1967; and the remaining 55 percent or so were "new junkies," who began to use heroin after January 1967.[1]

The preponderance of "new junkies," of course, was influenced largely by the fact that the Haight-Ashbury Medical Clinic was familiar to and trusted by this newly addicted group; old-style junkies were less likely to register there for help. Hence the figures tend to exaggerate the ratio of new-style to old-style addicts. But neither the figures nor Figure 9 below exaggerates the extent to which heroin addiction is a relatively new phenomenon among the young, predominantly white population served by the Haight-Ashbury Medical Clinic.

Staff members at the Haight-Ashbury Medical Clinic hoped at first that the "new junkies," since they differed from the "old-style junkies" in age, race, education, duration of addiction, and many other characteristics, would prove easier to cure. But, as noted in Chapter 10, this hope has not to date been fulfilled. "New junkies" offered detoxification and other clinic services relapsed at roughly the same high rate as "old-style junkies." [2]

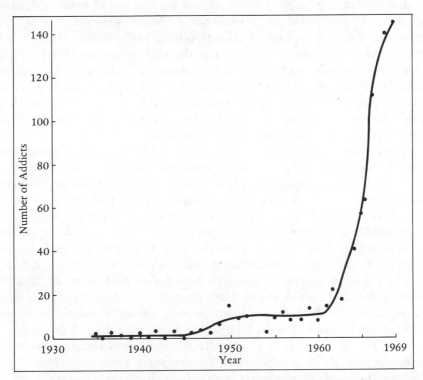

FIGURE 9. First Use of Heroin by Addicts Attending Haight-Ashbury Medical Clinic in the years 1967–1969 [3]

In 1970, accordingly, California's clinics serving the youthful drug-using population applied for permission to try methadone maintenance with these "new junkies." Approval was delayed by state authorities; it was not until 1971 that methadone maintenance became available in California on more than a trivial scale—and it is therefore still too early to determine whether methadone maintenance works as well with the "new junkies" as it has been working elsewhere with the "old-style junkies."

Heroin addiction in the armed forces. During the spring of 1971, the mass media carried the unwelcome news that heroin addiction was rife among American enlisted men in Vietnam, and perhaps also at other United States military bases at home and overseas. "The figure on heroin users most often heard here," one newspaper reported from Saigon in May 1971, "is about 10 to 15 percent of the lower-ranking enlisted men . . . as many as 37,000 men. Some officers working in the drug suppression field, however, say that their estimates go as high as 25 percent, or more than 60,000 enlisted men." [4] Later reports put the rate of heroin addiction at about 14 percent of the servicemen in South Vietnam; if true, this represented one of the highest addiction rates in the history of the opiate drugs. It was probable, however, that the high figures included servicemen who had only used heroin a few times and who were not yet addicted,* or that the figures were inflated in other ways. Subsequent estimates placed the addiction rate as low as 4.5 percent. Even so, there could be no doubt that the country faced a major problem of heroin addiction among American military personnel.

Since American forces in Vietnam were subjected, before going overseas, to the same antidrug propaganda as other young civilians, it is probable that this propaganda played the same role in breaking down the taboo against heroin among them as among young civilians back home. In addition, military drug policy on marijuana in Vietnam unwittingly triggered the shift from marijuana (which GI's had been smoking earlier) to heroin after July 1970. This is made clear in two reports [6] by Dr. Norman E. Zinberg, a psychoanalyst and professor of education at Clark University, who toured Vietnam in September 1971 on a fact-finding mission for the United States Department of Defense and the Drug Abuse Council—the latter a private agency set up to encourage reason and common sense in United States drug laws, policies, and attitudes.

". . . The Army itself is universally credited with causing the swing to heroin through its own blunder: the campaign against marijuana," Dr. Zinberg states. Military officials in Vietnam discovered the wide use of marijuana among their troops in 1968.

* Among 1,000 returnees passing through the Oakland (California) Army Terminal for release from service, for example, 930 voluntarily filled out an anonymous questionnaire concerning drug use. Of the 930, 16 percent admitted having used heroin at least once during the preceding 30 days; just under 10 percent said they had used it 11 or more times during that period, and 4.2 percent reported having used it 30 times or more during the month. [5]

True to the American activist tradition, as soon as a problem was identified, a full-fledged assault to stamp it out got under way. Radio and TV spots proclaimed the evils of marijuana and indicated that a smoker could . . . damage . . . [his] brain and become psychotic. . . . "Drug-education lectures," repeating the scare stories about grass [marijuana], became compulsory. In an all-out drive, the Army repeatedly searched billets, sent out officers to sniff for the weed in barracks and secluded fields, and even trained marijuana-sensitive dogs. . . .

It was a very efficient campaign. Marijuana is relatively bulky, and the smoke is detectable by smell. In one week there were 1,000 arrests for possession. Much official satisfaction was expressed in press releases which indicated that "the" drug problem in Vietnam was being brought under control. The Army had not yet learned, and has not yet learned, that you don't get something for nothing.[7]

The aftermath of the army's antimarijuana campaign, Dr. Zinberg continues, was disastrous: "Human ingenuity being what it is—and the desire for an intoxicant in Vietnam being what it was—many soldiers simply switched [to heroin]. Once it appeared, medical officials and commanding officers realized that they had acquired a far more serious problem." One commanding officer told Dr. Zinberg: "If it would get them to give up the hard stuff, I would buy all the marijuana and hashish in the Delta as a present." [8]

That an antimarijuana campaign can increase the use of heroin, documented by Dr. Zinberg in Vietnam, is of course relevant also to United States civilian antimarijuana campaigns. This is a topic to which we shall return in Part VIII.

The military response to the new drug peril was readily predictable. "The Army is presently engaged in the same type of all-out campaign against heroin despite the results of the marijuana campaign . . .," Dr. Zinberg reported in December 1971. "Its hard-sell education program again presents false information and exaggerated facts that contradict what the men know from their own experience. The very intensity of the campaign rouses their suspicions. ('What do they really want?' was a question I heard again and again. . . .)" [9]

The army's all-out campaign against Vietnam heroin failed to curtail the supply of heroin, of course, just as similar civilian law-enforcement campaigns have failed in the United States. What law enforcement achieved, in Vietnam as in the United States, was an increase in the price of heroin. Gloria Emerson explained why, in a dispatch from Camp Crescenz, South Vietnam, appearing in the New York *Times* for September 12, 1971. Heroin had been cheap and plentiful for a battalion stationed there, Miss Emerson reported, until a new commander, Major John O'Brien, took over. Major O'Brien found on his arrival that he himself could buy heroin all around at a trivial price—$2 or $3 for a whole vial (250 milligrams). In a series of raids he confiscated 409 vials of heroin, 40 syringes, three water pipes for smoking heroin, and two boxes of morphine. He built new barbed-wire fences around the base to keep out smugglers, arrested traffickers, sought helicopter coverage of the base at night to discourage smuggling, and tightened security in numerous other ways. Major O'Brien himself told Miss Emerson the result: "The price has gone up now because it's harder to get." Vials formerly available at $2 or $3 were now priced at $12.[10] (They would cost about $125 at New York City street prices.)

It was natural, of course, for Major O'Brien and others to conclude that the key to the heroin outbreak was the low cost and ready availability of heroin in Vietnam—but this was far too simplistic an analysis. In Thailand, which he also visited, Dr. Zinberg found very little heroin used by GI's—"although the supply is even more abundant and cheaper than in Vietnam." [11] A drug which attracts one clientele under one set of circumstances may attract a quite different clientele—or none at all— under different circumstances.

Once the results of the antimarijuana drive in Vietnam—the switch to heroin—became apparent, Dr. Zinberg notes, "the campaign against marijuana relaxed so that it is now on the market and much used by GI's once again." [12] But by then it was too late; "the social barrier" [13] against heroin, in Dr. Zinberg's phrase, had been broken—and for users actually addicted to heroin, of course, marijuana was no longer an acceptable alternative.

The early United States military experience with heroin in Vietnam confirms in several other respects the view of heroin expressed in this Consumers Union Report. For example, we have scrupulously refrained from attributing heroin use to personality defects or to the moral shortcomings of heroin users. We have ignored reports suggesting that the American civilian heroin addict has the kind of personality that "cannot function in society at all. He is an anti-social, bitter, 'loner.'" [14]

Dr. Zinberg comments on this point: "Some of the heroin users in Vietnam follow this pattern, but the larger group is made up of men who are like everybody's next-door neighbor. They come from small towns in the midwest or south; their personalities are not unusual; they have had slight previous experience with drugs; they are in good physical condition; they represent all ethnic and educational groups about equally." [15]

Dr. Zinberg also asks the question: if the army's antiheroin drive were to succeed, and heroin were to become unavailable to GI's, to what drug would they next turn? The evidence reviewed in Chapter 10 above suggests that for many, perhaps most, heroin users, skid-row alcoholism would be the ultimate outcome.

We noted above that most nineteenth-century opiate addicts either took their drug by mouth, or smoked them; mainlining heroin became the dominant form of narcotic use only when repressive measures and the resulting high prices made less damaging routes of administration too costly. Dr. Zinberg and others report precisely the same phenomenon in Vietnam. With high-quality heroin exceedingly cheap before the army's antiheroin drive, some 90 to 95 percent of all GI users sniffed ("snorted") the drug or inserted a little in a cigarette and smoked it. Some [16] even took it orally; "I saw one young man who had just returned to base after 13 days in the field pour a vial of heroin (approximately 250 milligrams) into a large shot of vodka and drink it," Dr. Zinberg reports.[17] After the army's antiheroin campaign raised prices, however, such prodigality was no longer economically feasible; mainlining therefore increased in popularity. "The increase in intravenous use," Dr. Zinberg comments, "suggests that perhaps as a result of the Army's righteous efforts to stamp out heroin entirely, the drug scene has turned nastier, with potentially unpleasant consequences. When a widely used drug suddenly becomes difficult to obtain, users will conserve their supplies for the greatest effect." [18] In sum, the United States military in Vietnam reenacted on a more modest scale in 1970 and 1971 the changes in opiate use (described earlier) which the United States as a whole had experienced following passage of the Harrison Narcotic Act in 1914.

Much anxiety was expressed, when the facts about military heroin addiction became publicly known in mid-1971, concerning the fate of GI heroin addicts when they returned to the United States—and concerning the effect of their return on the civilian drug scene. The popular reaction to the problem was prompt and unequivocal: *We must cure them, rehabilitate them.* In response to this demand, and to the realities of the situation, the Nixon administration announced a variety of measures—rehabilitation centers in Vietnam and at other military bases, an expanded Veterans Administration addict-rehabilitation program, expanded federal assistance for civilian treatment centers to which addicted veterans could go after discharge, and so on. We have reviewed in Chapter 10 the failure of such programs throughout the past century.

Even if the government's new treatment programs should prove somewhat more successful than the old ones, moreover, they could hardly be expected to prove 100 percent effective—and few people, in the fall of 1971, were looking far enough ahead to face the question on the horizon: what is going to happen to the addicted Vietnam, and other, veterans who go through the new rehabilitation programs and *don't* get cured? Are they to be arrested and imprisoned for the possession of heroin, for the possession of hypodermic needles and other injection paraphernalia, for sharing heroin with one another, and for other heroin-associated crimes? Are they to be left at the mercy of the American heroin black market? Are they to be forced to pay $20 for a nickel's worth of heroin— with all of the human suffering and deterioration that that price level entails?

A British visitor in 1922, it will be recalled, commented in amazement on how "in the United States of America a drug addict is regarded as a malefactor"—even in the case of addicted "soldiers who were gassed and otherwise maimed in the Great War [World War I]" [19] and whose addiction arose as a result. Whether, after subjecting them to unsuccessful cures or "rehabilitation programs," the country will make the same tragic and cruel mistake with uncured Vietnam veterans that it made half a century earlier with addicted World War I veterans remained in doubt at the end of 1971.

Fortunately, there was an alternative: methadone maintenance.

Part II

Caffeine

Caffeine, one of a class of chemicals known as the xanthines, is still
prescribed occasionally by physicians. Xanthines (caffeine, theobromine,
theophylline) can in varying degrees cause central nervous system
stimulation and cardiac stimulation; they also act as mild diuretics.
Combined with other drugs, caffeine is sometimes used for headache,
particularly migraine, and in some "pain remedies" (for example,
A-P-C capsules). Nonmedically, caffeine is the most widely used central
nervous system stimulant, popular in the form of coffee, tea, cocoa
(which also contains theobromine), and "cola" drinks. Heavy users of these
beverages report tolerance (including cross-tolerance among the
xanthine beverages), physical dependence with withdrawal symptoms,
and craving.

21.

Early history

In Part I, we dealt with the most hated and feared of all drugs—heroin and other narcotics. In subsequent sections, we shall consider other widely publicized drugs that are today considered responsible for the "drug problem." People tend to categorize these and other drugs in various ways—as "licit" or "illicit," as "good" or "bad"—and some drugs are treated as if they were not drugs at all. As we shall show, however, the boundaries of those categories have little objective justification; they vary from generation to generation and from country to country.

In this Consumers Union Report, accordingly, we have sought to provide an overview of psychoactive drugs in general—especially those that, licitly or illicitly, are subject to recreational, nonmedicinal use. Caffeine, nicotine, and alcohol are considered as fully and as objectively as their importance in our culture warrants—without regard for their current legal status as "licit" or their popular status as "nondrugs."

A sound history of drugs in our culture must begin with the era of the great fifteenth- and sixteenth-century European explorers. American schoolchildren learn that Christopher Columbus and countless others set sail across unknown seas in search of the treasures of the Indies—gold and spices. And, the school books might have added, drugs. For the civilized residents of western Europe in Columbus's time were very poor in mind-affecting substances: no coffee, no tea, no tobacco, little opium, no LSD-like drugs, little or no marijuana, no cocaine-like stimulants, and no sedatives or intoxicants except alcohol. As a result, Europeans had to make use of alcohol in a variety of ways—as a social beverage, a before-meals apéritif, a thirst-quenching beverage during meals, an after-dinner drink, an evening drink, a nightcap, a tranquilizer, a sedative, a religious offering, an anesthetic, a deliriant, and a means of getting drunk. Alcohol thus permeated every aspect of European culture, and still does.

Wherever they went, however, the European explorers from Columbus on found other mind-affecting drugs, and brought them home with them.* Tobacco was discovered on Columbus's first voyage. Cocaine was found in large areas of South America. Caffeine and LSD-like drugs were found scattered all over the world. During the next two centuries, the Europeans

---

* The Arctic was an exception. Dr. Andrew T. Weil said (1970): "Every culture throughout history has made use of chemicals to alter consciousness—except the Eskimos, who had to wait for the white man to bring them alcohol, since they could not grow anything." [1]

not only adopted nicotine and caffeine but spread them everywhere. They also imported opium. In a remarkably short space of time, western Europe was converted from an alcohol-only culture to a multidrug culture.

European explorers, travelers, and traders found caffeine in many forms:

• *Coffee* was found and brought back to Europe from Arabia and Turkey; it had spread to these and other Near Eastern and North African regions from Ethiopia.

• *Tea* was brought back from China.

• The *kola nut* was found in common use in West Africa, and was later introduced into cola drinks as a source of caffeine.

• The *cocoa* tree was found in Mexico, the West Indies, and much of Central and South America. Chocolate from this tree was the favorite beverage of the Emperor Montezuma; it was said that 50 pitchersful a day were prepared for his use. This drink was soon popular throughout the world.

• The *ilex* plant, source of the caffeine drink known as *maté* or Paraguayan tea, was found in Brazil and elsewhere in the American tropics; this tea is still drunk in the United States as yerba maté, and in parts of South America it rivals coffee and tea in popularity.

• *Cassina*—also known as yaupon, as the Christmas berry tree, and as the North American tea plant—was found in common use as the source of a caffeine beverage among Indians from Virginia to Florida and west along the Gulf coast to the Rio Grande. It was reported at the time that "none [of] the Indians but their great Men and Captains, who have been famous for their great Exploits of War and Noble Actions, are admitted to the use of this noble Bevaridge." [2] White settlers in these regions prepared a tea known as the "Black Drink," "Black Drought," or dahoon, from the same plant; they also let the leaves ferment to produce a drink containing both alcohol and caffeine.

During the Civil War, when the South was under blockade so that supplies of coffee and tea were cut off, cassina again became a popular beverage in the Confederacy. During and after World War I, when coffee prices soared, Congress and the United States Department of Agriculture launched projects to popularize cassina as a substitute source of caffeine; cassina-flavored ice cream and cassina soft drinks as well as cassina teas were marketed. [3]

The introduction of caffeine drinks into countries that had not previously known them—like the introduction of other exotic drugs such as nicotine and marijuana—aroused a sense of deep moral outrage and evoked efforts to repress the new drug. The Mohammedans of Arabia, for example, first used the newly introduced coffee to help them stay awake during prolonged religious vigils. This "use as a devotional anti-soporific stirred up fierce opposition on the part of the strictly orthodox and conservative section of the priests. Coffee by them was held to be an intoxicating beverage, and therefore prohibited by the Koran, and severe penalties were threatened to those addicted to its use." [4] An early Arabian writer summed up: "The sale of coffee has been forbidden. The vessels used for this beverage . . . have been broken to pieces. The dealers in coffee have received the bastinado, and have undergone other ill-treatment without even a plausible excuse; they were punished by loss of their money. The husks of the plant . . . have been more than once devoted to the flames, and in several instances persons making use of it . . . have been severely handled." [5] "Notwithstanding threats of divine retribution and other devices," however, "the coffee-drinking habit spread among the Arabian Mohammedans, and the growth of coffee and its use as a national beverage became as inseparably connected with Arabia as tea is with China." [6]

Dr. Robert S. de Ropp notes that when coffee was introduced into Egypt in the sixteenth century, "the 'coffee bugaboo' . . . caused almost as much fuss as the 'marijuana bugaboo' in [the] contemporary United States. Sale of coffee was prohibited; wherever stocks of coffee were found they were burned. . . . All this fuss only had the result of interesting more people in the brew and its use spread rapidly." [7]

In Europe, too, coffee became a popular drink despite (or perhaps because of) efforts at repression and medical warnings.

Medical opposition to coffee continued into the twentieth century. A typical medical attack can be found in *Morphinism and Narcomanias from Other Drugs* (1902) by T. D. Crothers, M.D., superintendent of the Walnut Lodge Hospital in Connecticut, editor of the *Journal of Inebriety*, and professor of nervous and mental diseases at the New York School of Clinical Medicine. Dr. Crothers classed coffee addiction with morphinism and alcoholism. "In some extreme cases delusional states of a grandiose character appear; rarely violent or destructive, but usually of a reckless, unthinking variety. Associated with these are suspicions of wrong and injustice from others; also extravagant credulity and skepticism." [8] One case of coffee psychosis he cited concerned "a prominent general in a noted battle in the Civil War; after drinking several cups of coffee he appeared on the front of the line, exposing himself with great reckless-ness, shouting and waving his hat as if in a delirium, giving orders and swearing in the most extraordinary manner. He was supposed to be intoxicated. Afterward it was found that he had used nothing but coffee." [9] Another of Dr. Crothers's charges against coffee resembles an accusation currently levied against marijuana: "Often coffee drinkers, finding the drug to be unpleasant, turn to other narcotics, of which opium and alcohol are most common." [10]

A similar view of the evils of caffeine drinks can be found in *A System of Medicine* (1909), edited by Sir T. Clifford Allbutt, K.C.B., M.A., M.D., Ll.D., D. Sc., F.R.C.P., F.R.S., F.L.S., F.S.A., Regius Professor of Physic (Internal Medicine) in the University of Cambridge, England, and by Humphrey Davy Rolleston, M.A., M.D., F.R.C.P. The chapter on "Opium Poisoning and Other Intoxications" in this textbook, used in American as well as British medical schools, was by Sir Clifford and Dr. Walter Ernest Dixon, professor of materia medica and pharmacology, King's College, London—one of the foremost pharmacologists of his generation.

We have seen several well-marked cases of coffee excess . . . [Sir Clifford and Dr. Dixon reported]. The sufferer is tremulous, and loses his self-command; he is subject to fits of agitation and depression; he loses color and has a haggard appearance. The appetite falls off, and symptoms of gastric catarrh may be manifested. The heart also suffers; it palpitates, or it intermits. As with other such agents, a renewed dose of the poison gives temporary relief, but at the cost of future misery. [11]

Tea, Sir Clifford and Dr. Dixon found, is in some respects even worse; it produces "a strange and extreme degree of physical depression. . . . A grievous sinking may seize upon a sufferer. . . . The speech may become vague and weak. By miseries such as these, the best years of life may be spoilt."* [13]

---

* Sir Clifford's and Dr. Dixon's views on coffee and tea may be contrasted with their statement that "opium is used, rightly or wrongly, in many oriental countries, not as an idle or vicious indulgence, but as a reasonable aid in the work of life. A patient of one of us took a grain [60 milligrams] of opium in a pill every morning and every evening for the last fifteen years of a long, laborious, and distinguished career. A man of great force of character, concerned in affairs of weight and of national importance, and of stainless character, he persisted in this habit, as being one which gave him no conscious gratification or diversion, but which toned and strengthened him for his deliberations and engagements." [12]

22.

Recent findings

To many, the above indictments will seem incredible—nothing more than quaint ramblings of puritanical physicians of an earlier, unenlightened generation. Yet, caffeine *can* be a dangerous drug. Contemporary scientists echo several of the early allegations made against caffeine. A reliable summary of current scientific opinion can be found in the 1970 edition of Goodman and Gilman's textbook, *The Pharmacological Basis of Therapeutics*. There Dr. J. Murdoch Ritchie reviews both the desirable and hazardous effects of the caffeine found in coffee, tea, cocoa, cola drinks, and other popular beverages.

The desirable effects are remarkably similar to those of cocaine and the amphetamines, to be reviewed in Part V:

Caffeine stimulates all portions of the [cerebral] cortex. Its main action is to produce a more rapid and clearer flow of thought, and to allay drowsiness and fatigue. After taking caffeine one is capable of a greater sustained intellectual effort and a more perfect association of ideas. There is also a keener appreciation of sensory stimuli, and reaction time to them is appreciably diminished. This accounts for the hyperesthesia, sometimes unpleasant, which some people experience after drinking too much coffee. In addition, motor activity is increased; typists, for example, work faster and with fewer errors. However, recently acquired motor skill in a task involving delicate muscular coordination and accurate timing may . . . be adversely affected. These effects may be brought on by the administration of 150 to 250 milligrams of caffeine, the amount contained in one or two cups of coffee or tea.[1]

In addition to its effects on the cerebral cortex and other portions of the central nervous system, caffeine in modest doses (a few cupfuls of coffee or tea) affects the heart rate, heart rhythm, blood vessel diameter, coronary circulation, blood pressure, urination, and other physiological functions. The secretion of gastric acids is stimulated, a matter of concern in connection with peptic ulcers. "A number of investigators have shown," Dr. Ritchie writes,

that the administration of caffeine to animals in large single doses, in smaller repeated daily doses, or by intramuscular injection in beeswax results in pathological changes in the gastrointestinal tract and ulcer formation. . . . The significance of experimental peptic ulcers produced in this way has been questioned because of the high doses used. However, in view of the responsiveness of the human gastric mucosa to caffeine, cognizance must be taken of the ubiquitous use of coffee and cola beverages in the pathogenesis of peptic ulcer, and in management of the ulcer patient.[2]

Coffee also markedly affects the human metabolic rate. "Numerous investigators have reported that the ingestion of 0.5 gram of caffeine [three or four cups of coffee] may increase the basal metabolic rate an average of 10 percent and occasionally 25 percent." [3]

A typical case history of a victim of caffeinism, similar to the cases described in 1909 by Sir Clifford Allbutt and Dr. Dixon, was reported in the *Journal of the American Medical Association* in 1967 by Dr. Hobart A. Reimann of the Hahnemann Medical College and Hospital in Philadelphia. The patient, a thirty-nine-year-old housewife and waitress, had run a low-grade fever for six months, with occasional flushing and chilliness, insomnia, irritability, and lack of appetite; she had lost 20 pounds in the course of this mysterious illness and now weighed only 107 pounds. When antibiotics failed to bring down her fever, she was admitted to the hospital for further diagnostic tests. Except for a finding of albumin in her urine, however, laboratory tests were all negative—and throughout her five days in the hospital her temperature remained normal.

"On further inquiry," the case report continued, "the patient stated that she . . . smoked a pack or more of cigarettes and drank from 15 to 18 cups of brewed coffee from 8 a.m. until 4 p.m. when she left home for work." [4] Careful temperature measurements after she left the hospital and started drinking 15 to 18 cups of coffee daily again showed that her temperature rose daily to a peak at 4 P.M., and declined again each day when she started work at 5 P.M., interrupting her daily coffee-drinking. Warned that coffee might be producing her symptoms, she gave up the beverage altogether. Thereafter her temperature remained normal, her appetite improved, her insomnia lessened, and she began to regain her lost weight. "The patient declined a request to resume the former high intake of coffee to see if fever again appeared." [5]

Caffeinism, Dr. Reimann noted in conclusion, "is said to be current among intellectual workers, actresses, waitresses, nocturnal employees, and long-distance automobile drivers. Illness otherwise unexplained may be caused by excessive ingestion of the xanthine alkaloids, including those in coffee, tea, cocoa, and those in some popular [cola] beverages." [6]

Some readers may seek to distinguish their own use of coffee from the objectionable use of mind-affecting drugs by other people on the ground that they drink coffee only because they enjoy the taste—not as a mind-affecting stimulant. A detailed study of this alleged motivation difference was published in 1969 by Drs. Avram Goldstein and Sophia Kaizer of the Department of Pharmacology, Stanford University School of Medicine.

Drs. Goldstein and Kaizer distributed a questionnaire to all of the housewives in a housing project for married graduate students; 239 of the 250 questionnaire recipients (96 percent) responded. The coffee-drinking habits reported by the 239 young women were distributed as follows:[7]

Amount of coffee	Percentage drinking
None	23
1 or 2 cups daily	20
3 or 4 cups	27
5 or more cups	26
Unknown	4
	100

Even those who drank only one or two cups of coffee a day almost invariably drank a cup in the morning. When asked *why* they drank coffee in the morning, the vast majority (72 percent) give the usual answers suggesting that coffee is a nondrug: they "enjoyed it" or they "liked the taste." A remarkable number, however, gave additional answers indicating a concomitant awareness of a stimulant drug effect:[8]

Reason	Percentage
Helps you wake up	46
Gets you going in the morning	42
Gives you a "lift"	28
Stimulates you	24
Gives you energy	21

Nearly a third of these young housewives, moreover, frankly recognized that they were *dependent* on their morning coffee; they said that they drink it because they "feel the need for it."

A special subgroup of the morning coffee drinkers consisted of 25 housewives who drank coffee *before* breakfast. This group was particularly aware of the drug effect of the coffee; 80 percent reported that it "helps you wake up," 56 percent that it "gives you a lift," and 44 percent that it "stimulates you." In this group, moreover, 60 percent reported that they drink coffee in the morning because they "feel the need for it." [9]

The housewives were also asked what would happen if they skipped their morning coffee. Here a remarkable difference arose between the light users (one or two cups daily) and the moderate and heavy users (three or more cups daily). Drs. Goldstein and Kaizer report: "Among the moderate and heavy users (especially the latter) in contrast to the light users, an array of symptoms that may fairly be described as a withdrawal syndrome is revealed: headache, irritability, inability to work effectively, nervousness, restlessness, and (curiously) lethargy." [10]

To check the questionnaire responses, Drs. Goldstein and Kaizer invited some of the housewives to participate in a controlled experiment.[11] Eighteen non-coffee drinkers and 38 drinkers of five or more cups a day were each supplied with nine coded vials containing specially compounded instant coffee. They were told to use one vial each morning in preparing their morning cup. The coffee prepared with the various vials could not be distinguished either by appearance or by taste; but three of the vials contained 300 milligrams of caffeine (the equivalent of two or three cups of brewed coffee), three contained 150 milligrams, and three contained no caffeine at all. The subjects were asked to score their moods in various respects before drinking the morning cup and again at half-hour intervals for the subsequent two hours. The 9,240 mood scores thus secured were analyzed with the aid of a computer.[12]

The results strikingly confirmed the women's earlier questionnaire responses. The five-or-more-cups-a-day users felt less alert, less active, less content, more sleepy, and more irritable before their morning coffee. On days when they drank caffeine-free coffee, they continued to feel that way throughout the next two hours; and they felt increasingly jittery, nervous, and shaky as the caffeineless hours dragged by. On days when their morning cups contained caffeine, however, these withdrawal symptoms were dramatically relieved. They also reported fewer headaches on caffeine mornings. The favorable effects were more marked with the 300 milligram dose than when the morning cup contained only 150 milligrams of caffeine.[13]

The effects were reversed among the participants who did not ordinarily drink coffee. These housewives reported an increase in *unpleasant* stimulant effects such as jitteriness and nervousness, plus more gastrointestinal complaints on caffeine mornings.[14] Since this study was double-blind —neither the housewives nor the experimenters knew until after the scoring was completed whether a particular housewife on a particular day had received 300 milligrams, 150 milligrams, or no caffeine at all— the study clearly demonstrated the specific drug effects of one or two cups of coffee. If there ever was any doubt that caffeine as consumed in the United States, a cupful or two of coffee at a time, is a mind-affecting drug, those doubts were put to rest by the Goldstein-Kaizer study.

Many coffee drinkers who think of caffeine as a nondrug when they themselves drink it recognize that it is a drug in another context—they forbid coffee and tea to their children. Thus caffeine is often the first forbidden drug for which children yearn (and which they may imbibe in secret when they get a chance). The taboo against caffeine for children, moreover, is curiously inconsistent. For while refusing them coffee and tea, many parents make available, and even encourage children to drink, cola beverages that also contain significant amounts of caffeine. More remarkable still, hot chocolate and cocoa are widely accepted as specific children's beverages—despite the fact that they contain significant quantities of caffeine.

Is caffeine addicting? Opinions vary, depending on one's definition of addiction. One feature of heroin addiction, it will be recalled, is *tolerance*, the gradual fading of effects as the same dose is taken daily. "An appreciable degree of tolerance may develop to certain effects of the xanthines," Dr. Ritchie reports in Goodman and Gilman's textbook, "especially the diuretic and vasodilator actions. Cross-tolerance between the members of the group also occurs," [15] as it does among the various narcotics.

Another feature of heroin addiction is the withdrawal syndrome or *physical dependence*. Caffeine unquestionably produces withdrawal effects at some dosage levels. "There is no doubt that the excitation of the CNS [central nervous system] produced by large amounts of caffeine is followed by depression," Dr. Ritchie writes. "There has been considerable controversy, however, as to whether this is also true after the mild physiological stimulation produced by the small amounts contained in the average cup of tea or coffee." [16] The 1969 Goldstein-Kaizer findings demonstrate that physical dependence does occur on five or more cups of coffee a day.

Like the amphetamines, the barbiturates, and alcohol, caffeine produces the most marked adverse effects when taken to excess. "Overindulgence in xanthine beverages," Dr. Ritchie notes, "may lead to a condition which might be considered one of chronic poisoning. Central nervous stimulation results in restlessness and disturbed sleep; myocardial stimulation is reflected in cardiac irregularities, especially premature systoles [irregularities of heart rhythm], and in palpitation and tachycardia [rapid heart rate]. The essential oils of coffee may cause some gastrointestinal irritation, and diarrhea is a common symptom. The high tannin content of tea, on the other hand, is apt to cause constipation." [17]

When taken in very large doses, moreover, caffeine is a potent poison. "A fatal dose of caffeine given to an animal," Dr. Ritchie reports, "produces convulsions because of the central stimulating effect. Early in the poisoning, these are epileptiform in nature; as the action of the drug on the spinal cord becomes manifest, strychnine-like convulsions may appear. Death results from respiratory failure." [18] The fatal caffeine dose in man is estimated at 10 grams (70 to 100 cups of coffee).

Even a single gram of caffeine (7 to 10 cups of coffee) produces acute toxic effects. "Insomnia, restlessness, and excitement are the early symptoms," Dr. Ritchie notes, "which may progress to mild delirium"—such as that reported by Dr. Crothers for the Civil War general. "Sensory disturbances such as ringing in the ears and flashes of light are common. The muscles become tense and tremulous. Tachycardia and extrasystoles are frequent, and respiration is quickened." [19]

These effects may seem irrelevant to the ordinary coffee drinker, who is rarely tempted to drink seven cups, much less a hundred cups, at a sitting. But here another popular American custom must be borne in mind. Caffeine in tablet form is readily available without a prescription at drugstores and some supermarkets throughout the country. Sold under such trade names as *NoDoz*, it comes in 100 milligram tablets priced at 69 cents for fifteen tablets, more or less. Many Americans use caffeine in this concentrated form. How many, and how much of it they take at a time, is unknown—but ten tablets contain a gram of caffeine, enough to produce the symptoms of acute toxicity described above.

A remarkable case of the adverse effects of caffeine tablets taken in excess was reported in 1936, in the *New England Journal of Medicine*, by Drs. Margaret C. McManamy and Purcell G. Schube. The patient in this case began taking a grain and a half of caffeine citrate (equivalent to 45 milligrams of pure caffeine) three times a day during the fall and winter of 1935, on the advice of a hospital intern. This overcame the "persistent fatigue and exhaustion which had lasted for three years and which was interfering with her working efficiency."* But she also "became nervous, restless, and could not sleep at night. For her insomnia she was given phenobarbital." [20]

In February 1936, in order to pep herself up for a party, she took several of the grain-and-a-half caffeine citrate tablets. "Shortly afterward she became silly, elated, and euphoric. As hours passed she consumed more and more of the tablets until before the party started she had taken the contents of the box—forty tablets, sixty grains," equivalent to 1,800 milligrams of pure caffeine. "She became confused, disoriented, excited, restless and violent, shouted and screamed and began to throw things about her room." Despite her deep religious feelings, "she became exceedingly profane. Finally she collapsed and was removed to a general hospital." The staff there, ignorant of her caffeine "binge," diagnosed her condition as "psychoneurosis, anxiety type, with a hysterical episode."

Five weeks later she again took an entire box of the caffeine citrate tablets and was admitted to the general hospital in "an irrational state varying from wild, manic screaming, kicking and biting, to muttering semi-stupor." Again the role of caffeine was overlooked. A consultation was held. The verdict: "Hysteria without question." When she failed to improve and remained wildly manic for several days, she was transferred

---

* A decade or two later, amphetamine rather than caffeine would very probably have been prescribed for those complaints (see Part V).

to a psychiatric hospital, where she was at first kept tied to a bed. After almost two months in the hospital, during which she slowly recovered, a mild relapse occurred. "Investigation showed that she was drinking coffee, four cups a day." At this point, suspicion for the first time turned to caffeine. "Coffee and tea were removed from her vicinity and soon she again became entirely normal, and was dismissed from the hospital." [21]

When we examine the behavioral effects of large doses of caffeine in animal experimentation, even more shocking findings must be noted. Several research teams have reported, for example, that rats fed massive doses of caffeine become aggressive and launch physical attacks against other rats. More remarkable still, a caffeine-crazed rat may bite and mutilate himself. "Automutilation was so acute and intense in some rats that the animals died from hemorrhagic shock." [22]

Some readers may here be moved to protest that the bizarre behavior of rats fed massive doses of caffeine is irrelevant to the problems of human coffee drinkers, who are not very likely to bite themselves to death. Let us promptly and wholeheartedly agree. There is a lesson to be learned, nevertheless, from these rat reports. If the drug producing this effect in rats were marijuana, or LSD, or amphetamine, the report would no doubt have made headlines throughout the country. One of the distorting effects of categorizing drugs as "good," "bad," and "nondrugs" is to protect the "nondrugs" such as caffeine from warranted criticism while subjecting the illicit drugs to widely publicized attacks—regardless of the relevance of the data to the human condition.

Thus we come to the coffee paradox—the question of how a drug so fraught with *potential* hazard can be consumed in the United States at the rate of more than a hundred billion doses a year (see Chapter 61) without doing intolerable damage—and without arousing the kind of hostility, legal repression, and social condemnation aroused by the illicit drugs.

The answer is quite simple. Coffee, tea, cocoa, and the cola drinks have been *domesticated*. Caffeine has been incorporated into our way of life in a manner that minimizes (though it does not altogether eliminate) the hazards inherent in caffeine use. Instead of its being classified as an illicit drug, thereby grossly amplifying caffeine's potential for harm, ways to make caffeine safer have been searched for and found.

In the first place, people generally take caffeine in forms so diluted as to make it highly unlikely that excessive doses—more than 300 or 400 milligrams at a sitting—will be ingested. The contrast here with alcohol is noteworthy. Whiskey, gin, and other distilled beverages, in contrast to light wines and beer, increase the likelihood that excessive amounts of alcohol will be ingested.

Again, coffee is customarily served with cream or milk, which may at least partially protect the lining of the stomach from the irritation the coffee might otherwise produce. Society's failure to take similar steps with respect to nicotine—by encouraging the chewing of tobacco, for example, instead of tobacco smoking, thus minimizing the hazard of lung cancer— will be discussed in Part III.

People have also developed the custom of drinking coffee and tea *after* a meal—further protection for the stomach lining. Cocktails, in contrast, are usually drunk *before* a meal, increasing the inherent hazards.

By keeping coffee legal, society has avoided extortionate black-market prices that might otherwise bankrupt coffee drinkers and lead them into lives of crime. And coffee drinkers are not stigmatized as criminals, driven into a deviant subculture with all that criminalization entails.

That other drugs now deemed illicit might be similarly domesticated, with a similar reduction in the damage they wreak on individuals and on society, is a possibility readers may wish to keep in mind as they read the chapters that follow.

Part III

Nicotine

Nicotine no longer has medicinal uses. Taken in tobacco—cigarette, cigar, pipe, chewing, and snuff—its effects are variable; it can act as a stimulant, depressant, or tranquilizer. Tobacco is one of the most physiologically damaging substances used by man. When smoked in cigarettes it is the chief cause of lung cancer. Tobacco is also a factor in other cancers, in coronary artery disease, in emphysema of the lungs, and in other diseases. Since nicotine is one of the most perniciously addicting drugs in common use, most tobacco users are "hooked" and, in effect, *locked* to the damaging effects of the tobacco.

Part III

Neuroses

23.

Tobacco

Columbus and other early explorers who followed him were amazed to meet Indians who carried rolls of dried leaves that they set afire—and who then "drank the smoke" that emerged from the rolls. Other Indians carried pipes in which they burned the same leaves, and from which they similarly "drank" the smoke.

The Indians knew, of course, the strange power that these leaves had over them. When two sixteenth-century English sea captains persuaded three Indians to accompany them to London, the Indians, "unable to give up their habit of smoking, brought supplies of tobacco with them." [1]

Sailors aboard the early exploring vessels also tried this curious, mind-affecting smoke, and found that they liked it. Then as today, nicotine produced a unique combination of effects: at moments when stimulation is needed, smokers perceive the smoke as stimulating, and when they feel anxious, they perceive the smoke as tranquilizing. Like the Indians who taught them to smoke, moreover, the early sailors promptly learned another fact about tobacco: after they had smoked for a while, they had to go on smoking several times a day, day after day, or they fell prey to a miserable craving that only tobacco could satisfy. The tobacco did not have to be smoked; the Indians knew (and the sailors learned) that the craving is assuaged when tobacco is chewed, or taken as snuff—ground to a powder and inhaled. But it had to be *tobacco* leaves—no other substances would relieve the craving. Accordingly, when the sailors returned home they carried abundant supplies of tobacco—and seeds—with them. They also carried leaves and seeds when they embarked on subsequent expeditions to other parts of the world. Within a few decades, they had spread the tobacco plant—and tobacco addiction—literally around the world.

Magellan's crew smoked tobacco, and left seeds in the Philippines and other ports of call. The Dutch brought tobacco to the Hottentots; the Portuguese brought it to the Polynesians.* Soon, wherever sailors went —in Asia, Africa, even Australia—they found tobacco awaiting them. The natives tended the plants, and learned to smoke the leaves them-

---

* Jerome E. Brooks wrote (1952): "All along the sea routes . . . wherever they had trading posts, the Portuguese began the limited planting of tobacco. Before the end of the sixteenth century they had developed these small farms to a point where they could be assured of enough tobacco to meet their personal needs, for gifts, and for barter. By the beginning of the seventeenth century these farms had, in many places, become plantations, often under native control." [2]

selves. A failure of the tobacco crop became a local disaster. Early sailors, approaching the island of Nias in the Malay Archipelago, were greeted with cries: "Faniso Toca'!" and "Faniso sabe'!"—that is, "Tobacco, sir, strong tobacco," and "We die, sir, if we have no tobacco!"[3]

Settlers in the Americas, like visitors, learned to smoke. Bishop Bartolomé de las Casas reported as early as 1527 that the Spanish settlers on the island of Hispaniola (Haiti) smoked cigars like the Indians. "When reproached for such a disgusting habit," he added, "they replied that they found it impossible to give it up."[4]

As tobacco smoking spread through England, the demand often exceeded the supply, and prices then soared. London tobacco shops were equipped with balances; the buyer placed silver coins in one pan and might receive in the other pan, ounce for ounce, only as much tobacco as he gave silver. The high price, however, did not curb demand. In 1610 an English observer noted: "Many a young nobleman's estate is altogether spent and scattered to nothing in smoke. This befalls in a shameful and beastly fashion, in that a man's estate runs out through his nose,* and he wastes whole days, even years, in drinking of tobacco; men smoke even in bed."[5]

The addicting nature of tobacco was noted at about the same time by Sir Francis Bacon, who wrote: "The use of tobacco is growing greatly and conquers men with a certain secret pleasure, so that those who have once become accustomed thereto can later hardly be restrained therefrom."[6]

By 1614, despite the high price of tobacco in London, its use had spread even to the very poor. One observer reported: "There is not so base a groome, that commes into an Alehouse to call for his pot, but he must have his pipe of tobacco, for it is a commoditie that is nowe as vendible in every Taverne, Inne, and Alehouse, as eyther Wine, Ale, or Beare, and for Apothicaries Shops, Grosers Shops, Chaundlers Shops, they are (almost) never without company, that from morning till night are still taking of Tobacco. . . ."[7] The number of tobacco shops in London in 1614 was estimated at 7,000.[8]

In the Americas, the addiction of the Indians to tobacco raised problems for the Catholic Church. The Indians insisted on smoking even in church, as they had been accustomed to do in their own places of worship. "As early as 1575," we are told, "a Mexican [Church] Council issued an order forbidding the use of tobacco in the churches throughout the whole of Spanish America. Soon, however, the missionary priests from Europe themselves became so addicted to the habit that it was found necessary to make laws to prevent them from smoking or taking [tobacco] snuff during any part of the Mass or the Divine Office."[9]

---

* Sixteenth-century Englishmen, like many American Indians, customarily exhaled the smoke through the nose.

By the mid-seventeenth century, tobacco had spread through central Europe, where its addicting nature was clearly visible. In Bohemia in 1662, it was reported, "the common people are so given up to the abuse that they imagine they cannot live without several pipes of tobacco a day—thus squandering in these necessitous times the pennies they need for their daily bread." [10] And from Nuremberg in 1661: "Many a one becomes so used to the stuff that he cannot be parted from it neither day nor night." [11] At Karlsruhe at about the same time there is mention of "the smoking fellows of Northern Germany who live only to smoke and who cannot live without it. . . ." [12] And from Austria in 1677: "For although tobacco be not necessary for the sustenance of man, yet have matters gone so far that many are of a mind that they would rather lack bread than tobacco." [13]

In Africa at the same time, the story was remarkably similar:

West Coast Africans had developed such a taste for the kind of tobacco brought them by the Portuguese that they clearly preferred to transact business only with these whites. A good part of the business lay in the capture of inland Negroes for the slave trade. Prices for slaves became fairly standardized; a Negro trader in Guinea, for instance, would be paid six or seven rolls of Brazil tobacco (each weighing seventy-five pounds) for the delivery of another Negro into servitude. The use of tobacco was never more corrupted—nor did it ever bring a greater price. Hottentots in the Cape Colony were so eager for tobacco, almost any kind, that the commodity was a major item in the sale of the land which established the Colony in 1652. Poor, ignorant natives continued to part with their land and valuable articles for comparatively small quantities of the new sedative to which they had wholly succumbed. For a piece of roll tobacco they willingly sold their splendid steers, the measure of the animal from horns to extended tail being equal to a single length of twisted leaf.[14]

Where tobacco smoking was taboo, as in churches, tobacco snuff was inhaled instead—but this also proved addicting. The Princess Elizabeth Charlotte of Orleans made this point clearly in a letter to her sister early in the eighteenth century:

Our King likes [snuff] no more than I do, but all his children and grand-children take to it, without caring for displeasing the King. It is better to take no snuff at all than a little; for it is certain that he who takes a little will soon take much, and that is why they call it "the enchanted herb," for those who take it are so taken by it that they cannot go without it; so take care of yourself, dear Louise! [15]

Pope Urban VIII issued a formal bull against tobacco, sealed with the Fisherman's Ring, in 1642, and Pope Innocent X issued another in 1650 [16]

—but clergy as well as laymen continued to smoke.* Bavaria prohibited tobacco in 1652, Saxony in 1653, Zurich in 1667,[18] and so on across Europe—but the states, like the Church, proved powerless to stem the drug. The Sultan Murad IV decreed the death penalty for smoking tobacco in Constantinople in 1633.

Whenever the Sultan went on his travels or on a military expedition his halting-places were always distinguished by a terrible increase in the number of executions. Even on the battlefield he was fond of surprising men in the act of smoking, when he would punish them by beheading, hanging, quartering, or crushing their hands and feet and leaving them helpless between the lines. . . . Nevertheless, in spite of all the horrors of this persecution and the insane cruelties inflicted by the Sultan, whose blood-lust seemed to increase with age, the passion for smoking still persisted. . . . Even the fear of death was of no avail with the passionate devotees of the habit.[19]

The first of the Romanoff czars, Michael Feodorovitch, similarly prohibited smoking, under dire penalties, in 1634. "Offenders are usually sentenced to slitting of the nostrils, the bastinado, or the knout," a visitor to Moscow noted.[20] Yet, in 1698, smokers in Moscow would pay far more for tobacco than English smokers—"and if they want money, they will struck their cloaths for it, to the very shirt." [21]

The case of Japan is for several reasons of special interest. Though Marco Polo had brought rumors about Zipangu (Japan) home with him, no European actually saw that land until about 1542, when a Chinese pirate vessel with several Portuguese seamen on board was driven off course by a storm and forced to take shelter in a Japanese harbor. The shipwrecked Portuguese, of course, had their tobacco with them—and thus Japan learned about smoking. Other Portuguese followed, bringing more tobacco. "Japanese accounts still exist," Count Corti writes, "describing how the Portuguese merchants and seamen . . . taught the inhabitants of Kiushiu to smoke. By 1595 the habit was well established." [22] An edict prohibiting smoking followed in 1603.

As no notice was taken of this edict, still severer measures were taken in 1607 and 1609, by which the cultivation of tobacco was made a penal offence. Finally, in 1612, Jeyasu decreed that the property of any man detected in selling tobacco should be handed over to his accuser, and anyone arresting a man conveying tobacco on a pack-horse might take both horse and tobacco for his own. Yet in spite of all attempts at repression smoking became so general that in 1615 even the officers in attendance on the Shôgun—at that time residing

---

* By 1725 even the Pope was forced to capitulate. Louis Lewin wrote (1924): "Benedict XIII, who himself liked to take snuff, annulled all edicts . . . in order to avoid the scandalous spectacle of dignitaries of the church hastening out in order to take a few clandestine whiffs in some corner away from spying eyes." [17]

at Yeddo, the modern Tokio—had acquired the habit. The result was a sterner warning, to the effect that anyone in the army caught smoking was liable to have his property confiscated. In 1616 the penalties were made still more severe: to a sentence of imprisonment a fine was added, in many cases equivalent to an increase of from thirty to fifty days on the original term. But it was all of no avail; the custom spread rapidly in every direction; until, as we read in an Imperial poem of the time, many smokers were to be found even in the Mikado's palace. Finally even the princes who were responsible for the prohibition took to smoking, and the great land-owners and rulers of the Daimios, the military and feudal aristocracy, who were all devotees of the habit, were glad to let the laws fall into abeyance. In 1625 permission was given to cultivate and plant tobacco, except in ricefields and vegetable gardens. By 1639 tobacco had taken its place in polite Japanese society as an accompaniment to the ceremonial cup of tea offered to a guest.[23]

From those days until today, it is most important to note, no country that has ever learned to use tobacco has given up the practice.* More remarkable still, no other substance has been found through the centuries since 1492 that can take the place of tobacco. Tobacco smokers who learn to smoke opium or marijuana go right on smoking tobacco in addition—clear evidence, surely, that it is *something in the tobacco* rather than the act of smoking which underlies the addiction.

---

* The one apparent exception is England, where tobacco *smoking* went out of style for a time during the eighteenth century. The exception is only apparent, however, for eighteenth-century Englishmen continued to get their regular nicotine dosage by inhaling snuff. Edward H. Pinto wrote (1961): Snuff-taking "does not seem to have made great progress in challenging the supremacy of smoking, even in Court circles, until snuff-taking William and Mary came to the throne in 1689 . . . and by the time of Anne (1702), another confirmed snuff taker, it is related that scarcely a man of rank but carried the insidious dust about him. . . . Queen Charlotte, though only seventeen when she married George III, was such a confirmed snuff taker that she was known as 'Snuffy Charlotte.'" Use by the common people of Britain began in 1702 when the British fleet "captured from the Spanish, near Cadiz, several thousand barrels of choice Spanish snuff, and near Vigo a further cargo of Havana snuff, intended for the Spanish market. This vast quantity . . . was sold at the English seaports at a very low price, the proceeds being prize money for the benefit of the sailors and officers. Thus was the general snuff habit born in Britain." [24]

Snuff is still taken there—and in the United States, where some 25,000,000 pounds are consumed per year. A January 1971 press release of the Smokeless Tobacco Council reports: "The headmistress of a young ladies' seminary in the Midwest was puzzled recently by the fact that so many of her students had given up smoking. On investigation, she found out why: Being unable to smoke except at specified times of the day, and in the one room of the school set aside for it, the girls had discovered a really wonderful and beautifully simple substitute: They'd begun using snuff!" [25]

24.

The case of Dr. Sigmund Freud

Through the centuries since Columbus, countless millions of smokers the world over have tried to stop smoking. Some have succeeded, many have failed. One of those who failed was Dr. Sigmund Freud. The account of his failure that follows is drawn from the three-volume biography of Freud by Dr. Ernest Jones,[1] himself a psychoanalyst and one of Freud's closest associates.

In 1894, when Freud was thirty-eight, Dr. Jones reports, his best friend, Dr. Wilhelm Fleiss, informed Freud that his heart arrhythmia was due to smoking, and ordered him to stop. Freud tried to stop, or to cut down his cigar ration, but failed. "He was always a heavy smoker—twenty cigars a day were his usual allowance," Dr. Jones writes. "In the correspondence [between Freud and Fleiss] there are many references to this attempt to diminish or even abolish the habit, mainly on Fleiss's advice. But it was one respect in which even Fleiss's influence was ineffective."[2]

Freud did stop for a time at one point, but his subsequent depression and other withdrawal symptoms proved unbearable. He described these symptoms vividly:

Soon after giving up smoking there were tolerable days. . . . Then there came suddenly a severe affection of the heart, worse than I ever had when smoking. . . . And with it an oppression of mood in which images of dying and farewell scenes replaced the more usual fantasies. . . . The organic disturbances have lessened in the last couple of days; the hypo-manic mood continues. . . . It is annoying for a doctor who has to be concerned all day long with neurosis not to know whether he is suffering from a justifiable or a hypochondriacal depression.[3]

Within seven weeks, Freud was smoking again.

On a later occasion, Freud stopped smoking for fourteen very long months. "Then he resumed," Dr. Jones reports, "the torture being beyond human power to bear."[4]

More than fifteen years later, at the age of fifty-five, Freud was still smoking twenty cigars a day—and still struggling against his addiction. In a letter to Dr. Jones he remarked on "the sudden intolerance of [my heart] for tobacco."[5]

Four years later he wrote to Dr. Karl Abraham that his passion for smoking hindered his psychoanalytic studies. Yet he kept on smoking.

In February 1923, at the age of sixty-seven, Freud noted sores on his right palate and jaw that failed to heal. They were cancers. An operation was performed—the first of thirty-three operations for cancer of the jaw and oral cavity which he endured during the sixteen remaining years of his life. "I am still out of work and cannot swallow," he wrote shortly after this first operation. "Smoking is accused as the etiology of this tissue rebellion." [6] Yet he continued to smoke.

In addition to his series of cancers and cancer operations, all in the oral area, Freud now suffered attacks of "tobacco angina" whenever he smoked. He tried partially denicotinized cigars, but even these produced anginal pains and other heart symptoms. Yet he continued to smoke.

At seventy-three, Freud was ordered to retire to a sanitarium for his heart condition. He made an immediate recovery—"not through any therapeutic miracle," he wrote, "but through an act of autonomy." [7] This act of autonomy was, of course, a firm decision to stop smoking. And Freud did stop—for twenty-three days. Then he started smoking one cigar a day. Then two. Then three or four. . . .

In 1936, at the age of seventy-nine, and in the midst of his endless series of mouth and jaw operations for cancer, Freud had more heart trouble. "It was evidently exacerbated by nicotine," Dr. Jones writes, "since it was relieved as soon as he stopped smoking." [8] His jaw had by then been entirely removed and an artificial jaw substituted; he was in almost constant pain; often he could not speak and sometimes he could not chew or swallow. Yet at the age of eighty-one, Freud was still smoking what Dr. Jones, his close friend at this period, calls "an endless series of cigars." [9]

Freud died of cancer in 1939, at the age of eighty-three. His efforts over a forty-five-year period to stop smoking, his repeated inability to stop, his suffering when he tried to stop, and the persistence of his craving and suffering even after fourteen continuous months of abstinence—a "torture . . . beyond human power to bear"—make him the tragic prototype of tobacco addiction.

All smokers who try to stop smoking do not, of course, suffer the anguish Freud suffered. Even some chain cigarette smokers who have smoked two packs or more a day for many years are able to stop when they decide the time has come. In retrospect at least, some of these ex-smokers report that "breaking the habit" was easy, or was difficult for only a few days or weeks. But Freud's case was far from unique. Indeed, we shall cite evidence below which suggests that the great majority of smokers are, like Freud, unable to stop smoking. Even those most highly motivated to stop, moreover, are among the failures. Sufferers from Buerger's disease are a startling case in point.

Buerger's disease is a condition in which the blood vessels, especially those supplying the legs, are constricted so that circulation is impaired whenever nicotine enters the bloodstream. If a patient with this condition continues to smoke, gangrene may eventually set in. First a few toes may have to be amputated, then the foot at the ankle, then the leg at the knee, and ultimately at the hip. Somewhere along this gruesome progression gangrene may also attack the other leg. Patients are strongly advised that if they will only stop smoking, it is virtually certain that the otherwise inexorable march of gangrene up the legs will be curbed. Yet surgeons report that it is not at all uncommon to find a patient with Buerger's disease vigorously puffing away in his hospital bed following a second or third amputation operation. Much the same is true of patients who suffer a heart attack, or stroke, or the onset of high blood pressure. These patients have a life-and-death incentive to abstain—yet many go right on smoking.

Chest specialists similarly tell of men and women with progressive emphysema, whose breathing becomes increasingly difficult until eventually death occurs from respiratory failure. Even during the last months of their ordeal, when they must breathe oxygen intermittently instead of air, some of them go right on alternating cigarette smoke and oxygen. These and other lines of evidence have led Dr. Vincent P. Dole of the Rockefeller University, a leading authority on heroin addiction (see Part I), to conclude: "Cigarette smoking is a true addiction. The confirmed smoker acts under a compulsion which is quite comparable to that of the heroin user." [10]

Confirmation of Dr. Dole's conclusion comes from Synanon, the therapeutic community for heroin addicts and others (see Chapter 10). Prior to May 1970, the New York *Times* reported in 1971,[11] almost all Synanon residents were heavy cigarette smokers. Since Synanon supplied food, clothing, and all other necessities, including cigarettes, to its residents without charge, the cost to the community was high—almost $200,000 a year for cigarettes for 1,400 residents.

In May 1970, Charles E. Dederich, founder and head of Synanon, decided not only to stop supplying cigarettes without charge but also to ban smoking on Synanon property altogether. In addition to the saving in money, Dederich was motivated by the fact that an X ray of his own chest showed cloudy areas in the lungs, and that some 200 young people under fifteen living in the seven Synanon centers were learning to smoke there.

A New York *Times* reporter visited Synanon in May 1971, on the first anniversary of the smoking ban.

"Once the decision was made," he stated, "smoking became the No. 1 crime for the community and was punishable by shaved heads or eventual expulsion." Dederich, himself an inveterate smoker, was among those who quit smoking.

It wasn't easy, for Dederich and for many of the others. "I couldn't have stopped without the help of my colleagues," Dederich was quoted as saying.

The most common reactions reported were depression, irritability, and weight gains ranging from seven to thirty pounds. After a year, the reporter stated, "most of the trauma of withdrawal is over. The majority say the thought of a cigarette is rare, although some admit to an 'occasional urge' or fluctuating weight."

Those who felt that the urge had receded, however, were the successes —and not all of those who tried succeeded. "About 100 people left during the six-month period following the ban and chose possible readdiction to drugs outside Synanon to life without cigarettes," the *Times* added.

"With most drugs," one Synanon resident explained, "you get over the symptoms in a few days, a week at most. But with tobacco, we've noticed them for at least six months." Another, who had personally "kicked" both heroin and tobacco, made a comparison of the two even more startling than Dr. Dole's:

It was much easier to quit heroin than cigarettes.[12]

Many ex-heroin addicts, it will be recalled, become alcoholics or suffer other distressing postaddiction misfortunes. No exhaustive study has been made of the problems of ex-cigarette smokers; but at the May 1971 meeting of the American Psychiatric Association, two psychiatrists from the Silver Hill Foundation in New Canaan, Connecticut—Drs. John S. Tamerin, director of research, and Charles P. Neumann, medical director— presented some relevant data on "Casualties of the Anti-Smoking Campaign." [13]

Drs. Tamerin and Neumann divided the casualties into major and minor. "Among the major casualties," they reported, "are cases of paranoid psychosis and violence following precipitous cessation of smoking." Such major casualties are probably rare.

Minor casualties include "the pansymptomatic individual with a history of repeated failure who again fails in an attempt to quit smoking, producing intensified feelings of worthlessness." As an example, Drs. Tamerin and Neumann presented the case of "an obviously neurotic nurse's aide" who participated in a Silver Hill Foundation group-therapy program designed to help cigarette smokers quit.

She was under much pressure from her family to quit smoking but had been unsuccessful in repeated attempts to quit on her own, and prior involvement with other cessation programs had failed. . . . After several meetings in which others in the group announced they had stopped smoking, this woman claimed that she, too, had stopped completely. It was later discovered that she was still smoking, but concealing it within the group. She did, however, admit to extreme anxiety associated with attempting to quit and was given tranquilizers to assist her briefly during the withdrawal phase. She continued to be anxious and reported a voracious and indiscriminate appetite, even finding herself devouring leftovers from patients' plates. This unfortunate experience was clearly producing guilt and shame, and anger at a program that was supposed to be helping her. Eventually she did admit that she was sneaking cigarettes. It became apparent that she was not a candidate, at least at this time in her life, for the program, and it was suggested that she withdraw. Furthermore, in order to prevent the emergence of even more severe psychopathology, she was given brief supportive psychotherapy. In the therapy, a particular effort was made to help her feel that her continued smoking did not mean that she was deficient, inadequate, or inferior to those who had been able to quit.[14]

Drs. Tamerin and Neumann comment at some length on what they call "a new species created by the antismoking campaign—the hidden smoker.

Like their predecessors, the hidden drinkers, they have been pressured into a pattern of secrecy and deception. This syndrome is now being encountered among individuals who may acknowledge the validity of the data on smoking and disease and promise to stop—and do, for a while. Eventually the need to smoke returns. The individual, however, feels too guilty to reinitiate the habit at home. Consequently, he may smoke at work while denying at home that he smokes at all. This lie may eventually reach such proportions that his coworkers, attending a social function in his home, are pressured into collusion with him. This pattern, of course, must be humiliating to the smoker himself and highly uncomfortable for the other people who are drawn into this new form of marital deception.

Equally unfortunate variants of this species are those individuals who work for organizations which have become heavily committed to and identified with the antismoking campaign. Such individuals may even be members of the higher echelon. However, if they are totally unable to stop smoking, they may be excluded from many organizational functions because of the group's concern about the negative public reaction. Such individuals are, of course, under enormous pressure to stop smoking and their inability to do so fills them with feelings of guilt, shame, and anger. Certain of these individuals may be able to curtail their smoking in public, but they are unable to stop completely and it is not unusual to hear reports of those who still sneak smokes in bathrooms and empty offices. One might suggest that an organizational attitude or policy which in any way fostered this type of behavior regression might benefit from constructive reexamination.[15]

Among the other "frequently observed consequences of cessation," Drs. Tamerin and Neumann continue, are "compulsive overeating, an impairment of intellectual integrative capacity, social discomfort, anxiety, depression or even depersonalization."

Drs. Tamerin and Neumann do not, of course, suggest that antismoking campaigns be terminated in order to prevent such casualties.* Rather,

---

* Dr. Daniel Horn, director of the National Clearinghouse for Smoking and Health, estimates that no more than 10 or 15 percent of smokers are better off continuing to smoke rather than risking the deleterious psychological consequences of quitting.[16]

they recommend "awareness of the psychodynamic and pharmacologic importance of cigarettes to smokers, and cautious use of 'hard sell' approaches which may induce guilt or shame."

Approaches that "attempt to stimulate guilt via the implicit statement, 'See what you are doing to your family,' or shame via the implication 'There is something inferior or defective about you if you can't stop' may backfire," the two psychiatrists warn. "The unfortunate consequence of guilt- and shame-inducing approaches is that they may overwhelm the ego rather than informing, assisting, and strengthening it. The result of such approaches—reflected in some of the case material presented—is to leave the smoker afraid, ashamed, and guilt-ridden but weakened as he reaches for another cigarette to soothe those painful feelings." [17]

25.

Nicotine as an addicting drug

What is it in tobacco that produces the craving? The answer is well-known: nicotine.*

The first modern scientific evidence for this conclusion appeared in the English medical journal *Lancet* in 1942. Dr. Lennox Johnston there reported that he had given small injections of nicotine solution to 35 volunteers, including himself. "Smokers almost invariably thought the sensation pleasant," Dr. Johnston declared, "and, given an adequate dose, were disinclined to smoke for a time thereafter. . . . After a course of 80 injections of nicotine, an injection was preferred to a cigarette." If the nicotine injections were abruptly discontinued, craving arose. Dr. Johnston found that in satisfying this craving, one milligram of injected nicotine was roughly the equivalent of smoking one cigarette. He concluded that "smoking tobacco is essentially a means of administering nicotine, just as smoking opium is a means of administering morphine."[2]

Further evidence for the importance of the nicotine in the cigarette came in 1945, in an experiment undertaken by Drs. J. K. Finnegan, P. S. Larson, and H. B. Haag of the Medical College of Virginia. They secured from the United States Department of Agriculture a batch of a newly developed strain of tobacco specifically bred to contain very little nicotine—much less than the low-nicotine brands now on the market. They added nicotine to half of the batch to bring it up to the usual nicotine level. Then they had both halves of the batch made up into cigarettes identical in all respects except for the nicotine content. The question they sought to answer was the obvious one: would smokers accept the low-nicotine cigarettes?

Twenty-four regular smokers, aged twenty-two to fifty, all of them inhalers, participated in the experiment. All of them were given all the cigarettes they wanted, in carton lots. The first cartons handed out contained cigarettes with the usual amount of nicotine. Then, without their knowledge, the smokers were abruptly switched to cartons of the low-nicotine cigarettes—and after they had smoked four or more cartons of them, they were switched back again without warning.

* Dr. M. A. Hamilton Russell wrote (1971): "If it were not for the nicotine in tobacco smoke people would be little more inclined to smoke cigarettes than they are to blow bubbles or light sparklers."[1]

Six of the 24 smokers did not miss the nicotine. They "experienced no change in physical or mental tranquility during their period on low-nicotine cigarettes." [3] These six were clearly *not* addicted to nicotine. One of them, incidentally, was the heaviest smoker of all, consuming three packs a day both before and during the experiment.

Six others experienced "a vague lack in the satisfaction they normally derived from smoking."

Three "definitely missed the nicotine but became adapted to the change in one to two weeks."

Nine participants "definitely missed the nicotine and continued to do so throughout the period (approximately one month). The symptoms experienced by the latter two groups for the most part took the form of varying degrees of heightened irritableness, decreased ability to concentrate on mental tasks, a feeling of inner hunger or emptiness . . . in short, virtually the same symptoms experienced by many individuals on stopping smoking."

Some of the smokers in the last group, Dr. Finnegan and his associates added, "just could not take it." Despite the fact that they had promised to smoke only the cigarettes supplied to them by the pharmacologists, and despite the fact that they could smoke as many of these as they pleased, whenever they pleased, they "admitted to interspersing a few cigarettes of ordinary nicotine content during their period on low-nicotine cigarettes." [4]

In a Swedish study reported in 1959, Drs. B. Ejrup and P. A. Wikander gave subjects increasing injections of nicotine over a ten-day period. The subjects felt satisfied and saturated; they either took only a few puffs of a cigarette from time to time or gave up smoking entirely on the days when they received injections. [5]

All of these studies had certain flaws in design. In 1967, however, Drs. B. R. Lucchesi, C. R. Schuster, and G. S. Emley reported a very nearly flawless experiment at the University of Michigan Medical School that produced parallel results. Each subject participating in this experiment spent six hours a day for fifteen consecutive days in a soundproof, air-conditioned isolation booth with a needle in an arm vein. He could read or smoke or engage in other quiet activities as he chose. On some days, ordinary salt water was fed into the vein through the needle; on other days a nicotine solution was fed in. The nicotine solution was so dilute that a subject could not tell the difference between it and the salt water. More important, the subjects did not know that the experiment had anything to do with smoking or with nicotine. They simply knew that there was an ashtray handy, so they could smoke if they pleased.

On days when salt water was injected, the subjects smoked an average of 10.1 cigarettes per six-hour session. On nicotine-injection days, they smoked only 7.3 cigarettes [6]—and they left significantly longer butts.* [7] The injected nicotine had markedly diminished their internal demand for cigarette nicotine.

Dr. C. D. Frith of the Institute of Psychiatry, London University, England, reported somewhat similar results in 1971.[8] The nine male subjects in his sample, all of them accustomed to smoke more than 15 cigarettes a day, were given low-nicotine cigarettes on some days, moderate-nicotine cigarettes on other days, and high-nicotine cigarettes on the remaining days. The more nicotine in the cigarettes, the longer the time elapsed between one puff and the next. The more nicotine in the cigarettes, the longer it took to smoke one cigarette. The more nicotine in the cigarettes, the fewer cigarettes were smoked per day. All three of these relationships point to the same conclusion: the smoker smokes to get nicotine, and regulates his smoking to assure the desired nicotine dosage, puff by puff, minute by minute, and day by day.

The same year, Dr. B. L. Levinson and three associates, of Harvard University, reported on an experiment involving efforts to "taper off" cigarette smokers by permitting them to smoke fewer and fewer cigarettes per day over a twelve-week period. "The greatest difficulty in further smoking reduction occurred at the 12–14 cigarettes per day level . . . ," the study noted. "It was hypothesized that . . . further reduction is inhibited by the manifestation of withdrawal symptoms caused by some physiological addiction." [9]

The view here presented—that cigarette smoking is for most smokers an addiction to the drug nicotine—has a small but growing body of proponents in the United States. Scientists in other parts of the world, too, are increasingly accepting this view. In Britain, indeed, the nicotine-addiction view of smoking has now been espoused by the Addiction Research Unit (ARU) of the Institute of Psychiatry, London—a unit initially established to study heroin addiction.

"We can no longer afford to regard cigarette smoking as a 'minor vice, ' " Dr. M. A. Hamilton Russell of the ARU reported in 1971. "It is neither minor nor a vice, but a psychological disorder of a particularly refractory nature and all the evidence places it fair and square in the category of the dependence disorders." By "dependence disorder," Dr. Hamilton Russell means (as shown below) very nearly what this Consumers Union Report means by "addiction." He then continues: "It is the belief that all dependence disorders may be in some way related, and that cigarette dependence is an important member of this group, that has

* The longer butt length as well as the fewer cigarettes smoked meant a significant reduction in nicotine consumption. For the cigarette itself acts as a filter; much of the nicotine in the early puffs of smoke remains in the cigarette and only reaches the smoker in the later puffs.

prompted the Addiction Research Unit . . . to add cigarette smoking to its field of study." [10] We shall cite a number of additional ARU conclusions in the discussion that follows.

One hallmark of an addicting substance is the fact that users seek it *continuously,* day after day. If they can take it or leave it—take it on some days and not be bothered by lack of it on other days—they are not in fact addicted. Judged by this standard, nicotine is clearly addicting; the number of smokers who fail to smoke every day (except among children just learning to smoke) is very small. The typical pattern of nicotine use, moreover, is not only daily but *hourly.* Nearly four male smokers out of five and more than three female smokers out of five consume 15 or more cigarettes a day—roughly one or more per waking hour. Here are the figures, from a 1966 United States Public Health Service survey of a cross-section of the adult American population.[11]

	PERCENTAGE	
Number of cigarettes per day	*Males*	*Females*
0 through 4	6.0	10.9
5 through 14	15.3	26.9
15 through 24	43.9	45.2
25 through 34	19.8	9.2
35 through 44	11.0	6.3
45 through 54	2.1	0.8
55 plus	1.7	0.6
No answer	0.2	0.1

No other substance known to man is used with such remarkable frequency. Even caffeine ranks a poor second.

Dr. Hamilton Russell of the ARU has a physiological explanation for this hourly-or-oftener pattern of use:

Certainly the level of nicotine in the brain is crucial for the highly dependent smoker. The blood-brain barrier is no barrier to nicotine. On the basis of animal studies it is probable that nicotine is present in the brain . . . within a minute or two of beginning to smoke, but by 20–30 minutes after completing the cigarette most of this nicotine has left the brain for other organs (e.g., liver, kidneys, stomach). This is just about the period when the dependent smoker needs another cigarette. The smoking pattern of the dependent smoker who inhales a cigarette every 30 minutes of his waking life [a pack and a half a day] is such as to ensure the maintenance of a high level of nicotine in his brain.[12]

Dr. Hamilton Russell also notes: "It is far easier to become dependent on cigarettes than on alcohol or barbiturates. Most users of alcohol or sleeping tablets are able to limit themselves to intermittent use and to tolerate periods free of the chemical effect. If dependence occurs it is usually in a setting of psychological or social difficulty. Not so with cigarettes; intermittent or occasional use is a rarity—about 2 percent of smokers." [13]

In the discussion of heroin in Part I, it was noted that nobody knows how many casual "weekend users" end up as heroin addicts and how many escape addiction. Dr. Hamilton Russell does provide statistics of this kind with respect to nicotine. "It requires no more than three or four casual cigarettes during adolescence," he reports, "virtually to ensure that a person will eventually become a regular dependent smoker." [14] And again: "If we bear in mind that only 15 percent of adolescents who smoke more than one cigarette avoid becoming regular smokers and that only about 15 percent of smokers stop before the age of 60, it becomes apparent that of those who smoke more than one cigarette during adolescence, some 70 percent continue smoking for the next 40 years." [15]

Dr. Hamilton Russell then goes on to explain this remarkable long-term effect of a few early smoking experiences: "The first few cigarettes are almost invariably unpleasant." Hence an adolescent may try one cigarette, decide he doesn't like it, and never smoke again. But if, despite the unpleasant side effects, he goes on to smoke a second and then a third and fourth, "tolerance soon develops to the unpleasant side-effects and skill is quickly acquired to limit the intake of smoke to a comfortable level, thus lowering the threshold for further attempts. Herein lies a possible cause of the virtual inevitability of escalation after only a few cigarettes. With curiosity satisfied by the first cigarette, the act is likely to be repeated only if the physical discomfort is outweighed by the psychological or social rewards. If these motives are sufficient to cause smoking to be repeated in the face of unpleasant side-effects, there is little chance that smoking will not continue as these side-effects rapidly disappear." [16] Once the threshold—the third or fourth cigarette—has been crossed, few turn back.

In Part I, we noted the widespread but mistaken belief that heroin addiction can be cured—by sending addicts to Synanon, or to Daytop, or to prison, or to one of the California, New York State, or federal rehabilitation centers. The unwillingness to recognize tobacco as a truly addicting drug runs even deeper. Many people, for example, do not recognize tobacco as a drug at all. They still see smoking as a "bad habit," to be given up like fingernail-biting or thumb-sucking. In an effort to demonstrate that nicotine is not addicting, three arguments are commonly offered.

First, it is alleged that the withdrawal of nicotine does not produce withdrawal symptoms; hence there is no *physical dependence* on nicotine. A 1966 study by the American Institutes of Research, made under a grant from the United States Public Health Service, demolishes this allegation. Among smokers deprived of their drug, the study indicates, 59 percent of males and 61 percent of females report drowsiness; 41 percent of males and 47 percent of females report headaches; 27 percent of males and 38 percent of females report digestive disturbances; and so on. In general, females report more symptoms than males. The table below supplies details.

Symptoms during smoking withdrawal	PERCENTAGE	
	Males [17]	*Females* [18]
Nervousness	65	77
Drowsiness	59	61
Anxiety	53	58
Lightheadedness	44	32
Headaches	41	47
Energy loss	39	52
Fatigue	38	42
Constipation or diarrhea	27	38
Insomnia	29	32
Dizziness	26	25
Sweating	18	10
Cramps	16	23
Tremor	15	15
Palpitations	12	21

Dr. Peter H. Knapp and his associates at the Boston University School of Medicine have directly observed and measured withdrawal signs and symptoms under double-blind conditions—and have shown that it is nicotine rather than some other smoke ingredient which is responsible for at least some of them.[19]

Dr. Hamilton Russell of the ARU adds that the *craving* for nicotine, too, may in fact be a physiological withdrawal symptom. "Psychological processes are mediated by physiological events. Intense subjective craving, so long regarded by the unsympathetic as 'merely psychological,' may well be governed by physiological adaptive mechanisms in the hypothalamic reward system which are no less 'physical' than the similar mechanisms . . . responsible for many of the classical phenomena of opiate withdrawal."[20] And Dr. Hamilton Russell states: "Most smokers only continue smoking because they cannot easily stop. . . . If he smokes at all, the most stable well-adjusted person sooner or later becomes a regular dependent user (or misuser)—in other words, he is hooked."[21] Or, in the terminology of this Report, he is addicted.

A second argument seeking to distinguish cigarette smoking from true addiction alleges that smokers do not become *tolerant* to nicotine. This argument is equally fallacious. The youthful smoker begins with a few puffs. He is soon able to tolerate most of a cigarette. As his tolerance rises, he may smoke two cigarettes the same day, and then three, leaving shorter and shorter butts. If he exceeds his tolerance, he suffers signs of acute toxicity—pallor, sweating, nausea, perhaps vomiting, and so on. In due course, as tolerance rises further, he may reach ten or even fifteen cigarettes a day—a level that might have proved disastrous earlier in his smoking career. Eventually he levels off at a pack a day or more.

Dr. Hamilton Russell of the ARU adds some fascinating physiological details:

Before he can enjoy inhaling deeply, the novice must acquire a degree of tolerance to the local irritation and autonomic side-effects of smoking. Some tolerance is quickly acquired but it usually takes 2 or 3 years before the smoking pattern is such as to enable a high nicotine intake. A different aspect of tolerance is revealed by studies of urinary nicotine excretion, which have shown that non-smokers excrete as unchanged nicotine a greater portion of a given dose than do smokers. This suggests that in smokers recurrent exposure to nicotine may induce enzyme changes that are responsible for the altered nicotine kinetics. Thus there is evidence that, in addition to psychological dependence, most cigarette smokers fulfill the criteria for physiological dependence [addiction], namely tolerance and physical withdrawal effects.[22]

The third effort to distinguish cigarette use from addiction alleges that cigarette use does not lead to antisocial behavior. As shown in Part I, however, it is not heroin addiction but the limited availability and high cost of black-market heroin which leads to antisocial behavior among heroin addicts. Much the same is true with respect to nicotine addiction. When the supply of cigarettes is curtailed, cigarette smokers behave remarkably like heroin addicts. Following World War II, for example, the tobacco ration in Germany was cut to two packs per month for men and one pack per month for women. Dr. F. I. Arntzen of the Research Center for Psychodiagnosis in Münster, Germany, questioned hundreds of Germans during this cigarette famine, and reported his findings in the *American Journal of Psychology* in 1948.

"Up to a point," Dr. Arntzen noted,

the majority of the habitual smokers preferred to do without food even under extreme conditions of nutrition rather than to forego tobacco. Thus, when food rations in prisoner-of-war camps were down to 900–1000 calories, smokers were still willing to barter their food rations for tobacco. Of 300 German civilians questioned, 256 had obtained tobacco at the black market, 37 had bought tobacco and food, and only 5 had bought food but no tobacco. Many housewives who were smokers bartered fat and sugar for cigarettes. In disregard of considerations of personal dignity, conventional decorum, and esthetic-hygienic feelings, cigarette butts were picked up out of the street dirt by people who, on their own statements, would in any other circumstances have felt disgust at such contact. Smokers also condescended to beg for tobacco, but not for other things. . . .

In reports on subjective impressions, 80 percent of those questioned declared that it felt worse to do without nicotine than without alcohol.* [23]

The German experience after World War II suggests an explanation of why we Americans in recent generations have lost awareness of the addicting nature of nicotine. People become acutely aware of an addiction only when their supply is cut off. The Indians before Columbus knew that tobacco was addicting because their supply was precarious; † and the same was true of the sixteenth-century mariners. In the twentieth century, in contrast, warehouses and channels of distribution have been organized so that cigarettes are conveniently and continuously available; it is seldom necessary to "walk a mile for a Camel." Only when the supply is cut off—as, for example, when someone decides to give up smoking—does the smoker become acutely aware of the craving. Even then, because of the devastating implications of being addicted to a drug, he tends to deny being addicted—even though the intensity of the craving causes him to violate his resolution and start smoking again.

The data from "smoking clinics" tend to confirm the view that cigarette smoking is an addiction. These clinics offer groups of men or women who want to stop smoking many kinds of aid and encouragement. In 1970, Professor William A. Hunt, psychologist at Loyola University in Chicago, and Professor Joseph D. Matarazzo of the Department of Medical Psychology, University of Oregon School of Medicine, reviewed the relapse rates among attenders at seventeen clinics where "valid and reliable" follow-up studies had been made. The combined relapse rate of these seventeen studies for smokers who successfully stopped smoking is graphically portrayed in Figure 10. At the end of forty-eight months, more than 80 percent of those who had successfully stopped were smoking again. Even among those abstinent for an entire year, one-third or more relapsed during the next three years. Professors Hunt and Matarazzo comment that

* Reports of women who are willing to prostitute themselves for a carton of cigarettes, and of men who trade stolen goods for cigarettes, are also common during and after wars.

† The question, indeed, may even be raised whether nicotine addiction was a factor in converting hunting and fishing tribes to agriculture. Perhaps tobacco culture came first, to assure a continuing supply. Tribes thus tied to their tobacco fields and unable to migrate to fresh hunting grounds would next have to cultivate corn, beans, or other nutrient crops in order to maintain themselves in their newly fixed abodes.

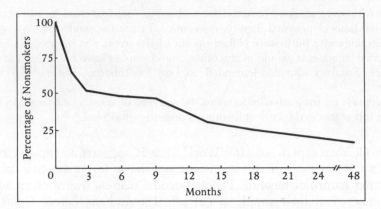

FIGURE 10. Abstemious Behavior as a Function of Time after Successful Therapy at Seventeen "Smoking Clinics"[25]

the shape of the curve shown in Figure 10 is quite similar to the shape of the curve portraying relapse among heroin addicts.[25]

Note that the 20 percent success rate at the end of the fourth year does not apply to those who *entered* the seventeen clinics; it applies only to those who *successfully stopped* during therapy. Failures in the course of therapy are excluded.

26.

Cigarettes — and the 1964 Report of the Surgeon General's Advisory Committee

From 1492 to about 1910, tobacco was commonly smoked in cigars and pipes, inhaled as snuff, and chewed. Leaf-wrapped cigarettes—miniature cigars—were known to the American Indians before Columbus landed; and cigarettes with paper wrappers were available at least as early as the eighteenth century. But the cigarette as it is known today was first marketed in quantity toward the end of the nineteenth century. Not until the first quarter of the twentieth century did the cigarette become the most popular way of securing an hourly nicotine dose (see Figure 11).

Many factors contributed to this meteoric rise in popularity of the cigarette, including improved cigarette paper, automatic manufacturing machinery that lowered the price, and intensive nationwide advertising campaigns for the new cigarette brands. But the major factor was the appearance of a new type of tobacco—known variously as "bright," "flue-cured," or "Virginia"—which made cigarette smoke more readily *inhalable*. Cigarettes made of the new tobacco were called *mild* ("not a cough in a carload") because the smoke could be drawn deep into the lungs. The size of the new cigarettes was also admirably adapted to the nicotine dose most people prefer. It was therefore easier for women and children to *learn* to smoke cigarettes; the likelihood of nicotine overdose among novices, with such acute toxic side effects as pallor, sweating, nausea, vomiting, and even loss of consciousness (fainting), was minimized.

The explosive increase in cigarette smoking after 1910 can also be attributed in part to the public-health campaigns of that era against the *chewing* of tobacco and its inevitable accompaniment, the cuspidor. The sputum of tobacco chewers, according to repeated public-health warnings, spreads tuberculosis and perhaps other diseases. Most of those who gave up tobacco chewing no doubt turned instead to cigarette smoking. The ashtray replaced the cuspidor, and lung cancer replaced tuberculosis as the major lung disease.

Perhaps because of their attractiveness to children and women, the new "mild" cigarettes aroused renewed hostility against nicotine. Beginning in the early 1900s, new anticigarette leagues, patterned on the politically potent antisaloon leagues, were founded and flourished both nationally and locally. Smoking by women and children was particularly

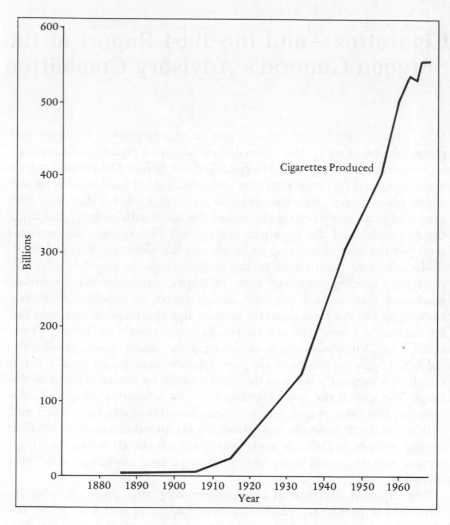

FIGURE 11. Production of Cigarettes, 1880 to 1968[2]

assailed. This view was taken even by many confirmed pipe and cigar smokers—including Thomas A. Edison, himself addicted to cigars. In 1914 Edison wrote a widely publicized letter to Henry Ford alleging that unlike cigar smoke, the smoke from a paper-wrapped cigarette "has a violent action in the nerve centers, producing degeneration of the cells of the brain, which is quite rapid among boys. Unlike most narcotics, this degeneration is permanent and uncontrollable. I employ no person who smokes cigarettes." [2]

Buttressed by such authoritative statements from respected public figures, the anticigarette campaigns were remarkably successful among lawmakers. By 1921—the year after alcohol prohibition—fourteen states had enacted cigarette prohibition, and ninety-two anticigarette bills were under consideration in twenty-eight state legislatures. The campaigns were not as effective, however, among cigarette smokers. Men, women, and children went right on smoking (as in the realms of the czar, the sultan, and the mikado centuries before), and in 1927 the last of the state-wide cigarette prohibition laws was repealed.[3] Only laws against sales to minors remained.

Examples of these laws are cited below. All of these laws were in effect in the early 1960s, and some may indeed remain in effect today.

A Florida law made it illegal for anyone under the age of twenty-one to smoke cigarettes. It was also illegal in Florida to provide anyone under twenty-one with a cigarette, a cigarette wrapper, or a substitute; a twenty-year-old caught in possession of a cigarette could be hauled into court and compelled to testify concerning its source.

In Georgia, Kansas, West Virginia, and perhaps other states, the legal age for smoking was also twenty-one. In Idaho, incredible as it may seem, the minimum cigarette age for men was twenty-one, but girls could smoke at eighteen.

In Maine an *offer* to sell cigarettes to a minor was punishable. In Florida it was unlawful to advise or counsel anyone under twenty-one to smoke. In Massachusetts snuff and cigars were forbidden to young people under sixteen; the ban against cigarettes continued until eighteen. In North Dakota it was unlawful to permit minors to gather in a public place to use tobacco. In Pennsylvania, a minor who refused to divulge the source of cigarettes or cigarette paper could be fined, imprisoned, or certified to the juvenile court; refusal to serve as an informer against his cigarette supplier also made a child a criminal in South Carolina.

These laws led, of course, to ridicule and contempt on the part of law-defying young people.

If the anticigarette laws had been effective, one might view them from a different perspective. But here are the cigarette production figures during the decades when anticigarette campaigns were at their height and anticigarette laws were mushrooming in the state legislatures:

Years	Cigarettes per Year (Billions) [a]
1900–1909	4.2
1910–1919	24.3
1920–1929	80.0 [5]

[a] The comparable 1970 figure was 583 billion.[4]

As we shall show in Parts VII and VIII, the laws and campaigns of the 1960s against LSD and marijuana helped to popularize those drugs. In retrospect, it seems reasonable to conclude that the anticigarette laws and campaigns earlier in the century were similarly among the significant factors popularizing the cigarette. The prohibition served as a lure.

Thomas Edison was no doubt wrong in alleging that cigarettes permanently damage the cells of the brain—but he was right in his view that cigarettes are more damaging than pipes or cigars. In part at least, this is because cigarette smoke is usually inhaled deep into the lungs. Some cigarette smokers do not inhale the smoke, while some cigar and pipe smokers do inhale. In general, however, the conversion to cigarette smoking meant a phenomenal increase in smoke inhalation.

Evidence of the added hazard this introduced was soon forthcoming. In 1921, for example, Dr. Moses Barron reported that there had been only four cases of death from lung cancer found among 3,399 autopsies performed at the University of Minnesota from 1899 through 1918. Between 1919 and July 1921, in contrast, there were nine lung-cancer deaths in 1,033 autopsies—an 800 percent increase.* [7] In 1927, Dr. F. E. Tylecote reported in the British medical journal *Lancet* that almost every patient with lung cancer he had seen was a regular smoker, usually of cigarettes.[8] Thereafter confirmatory evidence accumulated rapidly, and lung cancer among smokers reached epidemic proportions.

Conclusive evidence that cigarette-smoking is by far the most important cause of lung cancer, and is also a major factor in deaths from coronary heart disease, chronic bronchitis, emphysema, and other diseases, was collected during the 1950s and 1960s in a brilliant series of large-scale studies conducted by Dr. E. Cuyler Hammond and his associates of the American Cancer Society. The ACS studies also revealed greatly increased illness rates among smokers and a notable shortening of life expectancy; cigarettes were more damaging in many of these respects than cigars or pipes. Finally, and of the utmost importance, the ACS studies established the fact that *ex-smokers* live longer than smokers, and that the longer they go without smoking, the closer their life expectancy approaches the life expectancy of those who have never smoked.

Recent studies have also shown that cigarette smoking during pregnancy adds to the hazards of the unborn baby. An English and an American researcher, C. M. Fletcher and Daniel Horn, summarized the evidence in a 1970 World Health Organization publication, "Smoking and Health":

There is now clear evidence from seven large independent surveys that the babies born to women who smoke during pregnancy are, on the average,

---

* By 1952, the rate at the University of Minnesota had risen to 264 lung-cancer deaths in 8,332 autopsies—almost a 3,000 percent increase over the pre-1919 rate.[6]

150–240 grams lighter than those of non-smokers and that smokers have two or three times as many premature babies [defined as babies weighing less than 2,500 grams]. By their first birthday, these small babies have caught up with and are as heavy as those of non-smoking mothers.

Recent studies of over 8,000 pregnancies have, however, shown that the risk to the fetus from a mother's smoking may be more serious than this, for the babies of mothers who smoked during pregnancy were about twice as likely to be aborted, to be stillborn, or to die soon after birth as the babies of non-smoking mothers. The risk to babies of mothers with pre-eclamptic toxemia was increased if the mother smoked. In one study it was calculated that one in five of babies lost would have been saved if their mothers had not smoked.[9]

The data incriminating cigarette smoking as a health hazard were reviewed in a report of the Royal College of Physicians of London in 1962, and in the *Consumers Union Report on Smoking and the Public Interest* in 1963. These reports, however, reached only hundreds of thousands of people; publicity was relatively limited in the mass media.

On January 11, 1964, a turning point was reached. The *Report of the Surgeon General's Advisory Committee on Smoking and Health,* published amid unprecedented worldwide fanfare in the mass media, convinced even most smokers that cigarette smoking shortens human life, causes lung cancer and other forms of cancer, and exacerbates heart disease, emphysema, bronchitis, and a number of other illnesses—gravely increasing the risk of dying of them.

For a brief few weeks, this report had a major nationwide impact. Within a few days after its publication, some chain supermarkets announced that cigarette sales had fallen 20 to 25 percent. In Iowa, where the impact of the report was most noticeable, tax officials reported that the number of taxed packages fell 31.7 percent in February 1964, the month after the report was issued. Nationally, the drop in taxed packages was between 15 and 20 percent. The true impact of the report was much greater than even these figures suggest. For casual smokers (of less than a pack a day) were more likely to stop smoking than heavy smokers (two packs or more a day). Thus a 20 percent decline in number of *cigarettes* smoked may have represented a 25 or even 30 percent decline in number of *smokers still smoking.*[10]

But the curtailment was short-lived; what has been called "the Great Forswearing" of January and February 1964 was followed by the "Great Relapse" of March—further evidence that in the twentieth century, as in the sixteenth, nicotine remained an addicting drug. Within a few months cigarette consumption was back almost to pre-1964 levels.

The failure of the *Report of the Surgeon General's Advisory Committee* to curtail cigarette smoking more than briefly was naturally a disappointment, but health agencies did not despair. The United States Public Health Service, the American Cancer Society, and countless other national and local agencies launched campaigns with three major and related goals: to inform people that cigarette smoking is dangerous, to persuade people to stop smoking, and to help those who were having trouble in stopping. The possibility that nicotine, for a large percentage of users, might be an addicting drug—the possibility that many people might not be able to stop, even though they wanted to, decided to, and tried to— was not given serious consideration. It was during the same years 1964- 1970, it will be recalled, that the public was similarly being assured that heroin addiction is curable.

Judged by their effect on *attitudes*, the antismoking campaigns launched following the 1964 *Report of the Surgeon General's Advisory Committee* were notably successful. A survey conducted by the United States Public Health Service in 1966 revealed the following attitudes among a nation- wide cross section of males *who were current cigarette smokers*: [11]

71.3 percent agreed that smoking is harmful to health.

67.3 percent disagreed with the statement that cigarettes do more good to a person than harm.

59.5 percent hoped that their children would never smoke.

57.7 percent agreed that cigarette smoking is a cause of lung cancer.

56.3 percent disagreed with the statement: "The chances of getting lung cancer from smoking cigarettes are so small that it's foolish to worry about it."

54.6 percent agreed that smoking is a dirty habit.

44.9 percent agreed that there is something *morally* wrong with smoking cigarettes.

43.1 percent agreed that cigarette smoking is a cause of emphysema and chronic bronchitis.

33.4 percent agreed that cigarette smoking is a cause of coronary heart disease.

Among women who were currently smoking cigarettes, and among non- smokers, the percentages decrying cigarettes were even higher on every one of those questions.*

These figures, clearly, are a tribute to the effectiveness of the anti- smoking campaigns. Even many confirmed cigarette smokers were per- suaded by the campaigns that smoking is a dirty habit, harmful to health and morally reprehensible. But the prevalence of negative attitudes to- ward smoking among smokers, unfortunately, had little effect on their actual smoking. Here are the cigarette consumption figures.[13]

---

* Also noteworthy was an increase in support for cigarette prohibition. In 1964 and again in 1966, only 23 percent of respondents in a National Clearinghouse for Smoking and Health survey agreed with the statement, "The selling of cigarettes should be stopped completely." In a 1970 survey, 38 percent of respondents agreed with this prohibitionist position.[12]

Year	Number of cigarettes smoked (in billions)	Daily per capita consumption (aged 18 and over)
1958	449.8	10.8 cigarettes
1959	467.4	11.2 cigarettes
1960	484.4	11.4 cigarettes
1961	502.7	11.7 cigarettes
1962	508.4	11.7 cigarettes
1963	523.9	11.9 cigarettes
1964	511.2	11.5 cigarettes
1965	528.7	11.7 cigarettes
1966	541.2	11.8 cigarettes
1967	549.2	11.7 cigarettes
1968	545.6	11.5 cigarettes
1969	528.9	10.8 cigarettes
1970	542.0	11.0 cigarettes

In short, the number of cigarettes consumed in 1970 was up 3.4 percent since 1963, while *per capita* consumption was down 7.6 percent.

The increase in cigarette consumption, moreover, occurred despite an increase of more than 40 percent in retail cigarette prices between 1964 and 1970.[14] Retail expenditures for cigarettes increased from an estimated $7.2 billion in 1964 to an estimated $10.5 billion in 1970.[15] Thus despite the anticigarette campaigns and despite the increased awareness of smoking hazards, Americans were spending 45 percent more for cigarettes in 1970 than in 1964.

The *Report of the Surgeon General's Advisory Committee* and the subsequent anticigarette campaigns did have one major effect, however. Vast numbers of smokers turned from plain to filter-tip cigarettes and from high-tar-high-nicotine to low-tar-low-nicotine brands. While the data are not conclusive, it seems probable that the increase in number of cigarettes smoked *per smoker* was related to this switch; some smokers no doubt increased their daily cigarette quota to compensate for the smaller amount of nicotine in each cigarette. Other smokers no doubt compensated by taking more puffs on each cigarette and leaving shorter butts.

In the eighteenth century, Charles Lamb described his own addiction to nicotine in striking language:

> For thy sake, tobacco, I
> Would do anything but die.

The current evidence indicates that Lamb seriously understated the case.

Meanwhile, what of the effects of current public health anticigarette campaigns on children and young people? A 1970 survey made for the

American Cancer Society by Lieberman Research, Inc., shows that, as in the case of adults, the campaigns—including the anticigarette TV commercials of 1968-1970—were enormously effective in molding the attitudes of young people toward cigarettes.

The Lieberman study covered a nationwide cross section of young people aged thirteen through eighteen, both smokers and nonsmokers. More than two-thirds of these teen-agers (70 percent of the nonsmokers and 66 percent of the smokers) recalled anticigarette presentations to which they had been exposed in school.[16] More than half had seen anticigarette educational films and posters. Almost all of them had seen the powerful anticigarette messages then being aired on television; indeed, the teen-agers in the sample reported having seen an average of 8.9 anticigarette television spots during the previous four weeks.[17]

The vast majority of these teen-agers, moreover, were convinced by what they had seen and heard. When asked whether cigarette smoking causes cancer, for example, 86 percent of the teen-age nonsmokers and 65 percent of the teen-age smokers agreed that it did.[18] Similarly, 71 percent of the teen-age nonsmokers and 66 percent of the smokers agreed it was "definitely or probably true" that cigarette smoking triples the likelihood of a heart attack.[19]

As in the case of adults, however, a firm conviction that smoking causes cancer and heart attacks had very little effect on teen-age smoking habits. "When children enter their teen-age years," the 1970 survey noted, "the rate of cigarette smoking is relatively low. By the time they reach the end of their teen-age years, the rate of cigarette smoking is not far from the rate for the general adult population." [20]

Two surveys made for the National Clearinghouse for Smoking and Health, a unit of the United States Public Health Service, suggest that during the years from 1968 to 1970, the proportion of teen-agers recruited to cigarette smoking was actually *increasing** Here are the figures.

---

* The 1970 Lieberman Report also revealed that more than half of all teen-agers who smoke had their first cigarettes by the age of twelve and 85 percent had smoked before the age of fifteen.[21]

Age at First Cigarette	Percentage of Total Who Ever Had Smoked
8 years or under	14
9–10 years	14
11–12 years	27
13–14 years	30
15–16 years	12
17–18 years	2
Don't know or no answer	1
	100

PERCENTAGE SMOKING

Year	Boys	Girls
1968	14.7	8.4
1970	18.5	11.9 [22]

Why do boys and girls convinced that cigarette smoking causes cancer and heart attacks nevertheless start smoking cigarettes? One answer fairly leaps from the pages of the Lieberman survey. The single most important fact about smoking has been kept a secret from them. *They have not been told that nicotine is an addicting drug.* As a result, most of them think that they will smoke for a while and then stop. Indeed, among the teen-age smokers in the Lieberman survey, only 21 percent thought it "very likely" that they would still be smoking five years hence; and an additional 27 percent thought it only "fairly likely." [23] *The majority confidently expected to stop in five years or less.*

The thought that many smokers *can't* stop seems not to have occurred to these teen-agers. They believed not only the campaigns stressing smoking as a cause of cancer and heart attacks, but also the campaigns insisting that it is possible to stop smoking if you "make up your mind" to stop. So why not smoke for a few years and then swear off? That in effect was the majority view among the teen-agers in the Lieberman sample.

The campaigns do not, of course, tell children that it is *easy* to stop smoking. They suggest that it requires considerable effort of will and perhaps some suffering. As noted in Part I, this is precisely the kind of challenge that attracts young people. A majority of the teen-age smokers in the Lieberman sample envisioned themselves as confronting that challenge a few years hence, and winning.

The role of cigarette advertising in exacerbating the problem of nicotine addiction is difficult to evaluate. Smoking does not depend on advertising. In Italy, where all cigarette advertising has been banned, there has been little change in cigarette consumption.[24] People who already smoke go right on smoking, largely because they are addicted to nicotine.

But why do young people *start* smoking? Here the answer is more complex. Fifteen-year-olds start in part because their elders smoke and in part because other teen-agers smoke. But it seems highly likely that cigarette advertising—which associates smoking with youth and music and joy and sex—is an auxiliary factor, perhaps a quite potent one.

For almost all of these children, of course, smoking was illegal; for many of them, smoking a cigarette was their first experience with an illicit drug.

It may be, of course, that a ban on all cigarette advertising would have little or no immediate effect on the recruiting of youthful new smokers; the *other* factors may be sufficient to maintain recruiting at present levels even in the absence of advertising. But no other methods of discouraging young people from beginning to smoke offer any likelihood of success so long as cigarette advertising remains licit.

The view here presented—that cigarette smoking is an addiction to the drug nicotine, that the overwhelming majority of those who smoke more than a few cigarettes become addicted, and that relatively few addicts quit permanently—seems to fly in the face of common sense. Some readers of this Report, for example, have no doubt quit smoking themselves— perhaps with relatively little difficulty. Most readers no doubt know personally quite a few individuals who have quit. And most people, especially in 1970 and 1971, read repeated newspaper stories announcing that millions of cigarette smokers had quit smoking—stories emanating in large part from the National Clearinghouse for Smoking and Health. Surely, some readers may feel, the case for the addicting nature of cigarette smoking is being exaggerated in this Consumers Union Report.

Since United States statistics concerning ex-smokers are currently in dispute, let us start with a British view.

"In the 10-year period 1958–68," Dr. Hamilton Russell of the Addiction Research Unit notes,

there was little change in smoking prevalence among men in the United Kingdom—about 69 percent were smokers, 15 percent ex-smokers, and 16 percent had never smoked. In such a sample the ex-smokers form 18 percent of the smokers and ex-smokers combined. . . . Using the 1968 statistics for women, a similar figure is obtained. Thus some 18 percent of smokers have stopped smoking and become ex-smokers. This so-called natural discontinuance of smoking tends to occur after the age of 30 and rises further with increasing age. The average daily cigarette consumption also tends to drop quite sharply after the age of sixty. The ex-smoker status, however, is not a stable one and many relapse to regular smoking. This relapse rate is related to the duration of the ex-smoker status. Among ex-smokers [who have abstained for less than one year] 37 percent relapse within two years compared with 19 percent of those [who have abstained for one to two years] and 5 percent of those [who have abstained for more than two years]. There is therefore a sizeable turnover, with regular smokers discontinuing only to relapse later. The evidence suggests that in the present social climate of this country [Britain] it is unlikely that more than 15 percent of people who smoke regularly undergo natural discontinuance to permanent ex-smoker status before the age of 60. Furthermore, this situation has not changed appreciably over the past ten years.[25]

This analysis of ex-smoker statistics should serve to warn against excessive optimism when superficially impressive figures are publicized. A headline announcing that a substantial percentage of all smokers have quit, for example, must be viewed with extreme caution. If the same percentage of all smokers had also quit ten years ago, the progress made against smoking is clearly *nil.*

Dr. Hamilton Russell's analysis also explains the instinctive common-sense error in judgment people make when they decide that the war against cigarettes must be going well because they see around them so many former smokers who have quit. If they had looked around them a decade ago, they would also have noted many ex-smokers.

Data concerning current smokers, nonsmokers, and ex-smokers in the United States are available from the National Center for Health Statistics, a unit in the United States Public Health Service.

	Percentage 1955*	Percentage 1966*	Percentage 1968
Current smokers	41.8	40.6	38.5
Never smoked	50.9	47.6	48.0
Ex-smokers	7.3	11.8	13.5 [26]

* There were minor changes in data-gathering methods between 1955 and 1966, but not enough to impair the comparability of the figures.

The above figures do not suggest a major victory over nicotine between 1955 and 1968. They are subject, however, to an important qualification. The surveys on which they are based asked each respondent to reply not only for himself but also for other members of the same household. It is easy for a respondent to report accurately who in his household smokes and who does not smoke; but in such a survey ex-smokers are sometimes reported as having "never smoked." Two 1970 surveys, one by the National Clearinghouse for Smoking and Health and the other by the Social Research Group of George Washington University, asked each respondent to report only for himself. As a result, the number of ex-smokers is larger than in the statistics cited above, while the number of current smokers remains about the same.

	Percentage— National Clearinghouse for Smoking and Health, 1970	Percentage— Social Research Group, 1970
Current smokers	36.2	38
Never smoked	40.3	39
Ex-smokers	23.5 [27]	22 [28]

The "ex-smoker" figures in these two studies seem to offer a ray of hope. But this apparent increase in ex-smokers since 1955 is not balanced by a decrease in current smokers; the ex-smokers in the 1970 surveys seem to come mostly from the "never smoked" category in the earlier surveys. Little comfort can be drawn from the fact that the proportion of current smokers in the country has declined from 41 to 42 percent in 1955 to 36 or 38 percent in 1970.

27.

A program for the future

It is possible to argue, of course, that all is going well on the cigarette front. The number of cigarettes smoked per capita is down a little, the number of smokers is down a little, the number of ex-smokers is up, perhaps substantially, and the number of cigarettes smoked is not rising very rapidly. If the antismoking campaigns are just continued on the present pattern, stressing voluntary abstinence, the figures may continue to improve.

It is also possible to argue, however, that sooner or later, however reluctantly, society may have to face the bankruptcy of anticigarette programs based on voluntary abstinence—that is, on a denial that cigarettes are addicting. If there are still tens of millions of cigarette smokers a generation hence, including millions of fresh teen-age recruits, along with tens of thousands of lung-cancer deaths annually and hundreds of thousands of premature deaths from cardiovascular disease, chronic bronchitis, and emphysema, all cigarette-associated, despite increasing unanimity of agreement among smokers themselves that smoking is a major health menace, even those who deny that cigarette smoking is an addiction to nicotine may have to concede, however reluctantly, that the time is ripe for a change in national policy. (Some readers may even conclude that the time is already overripe.)

Without prejudging the issue of *when* public health policies toward cigarette smoking should change, let us explore for a moment three *directions* that a new policy might take when and if the time comes to recognize openly and officially that cigarette smoking is an addiction and that voluntary abstinence is not the solution.

First, efforts should be made to popularize ways of delivering frequent doses of nicotine to addicts without filling their lungs with smoke, or to minimize smoke delivery to the lungs. This will reduce or eliminate the lung-cancer hazard. Here are some of the ways in which this might be accomplished:

- Develop a short cigarette with *high* nicotine content, capable of delivering a maximum of nicotine to the bloodstream with a minimum of smoke to the lungs.
- Convert smokers from cigarettes to cigars or pipes.
- Develop a cigarette with noninhalable smoke.

Degree of
Inhalation

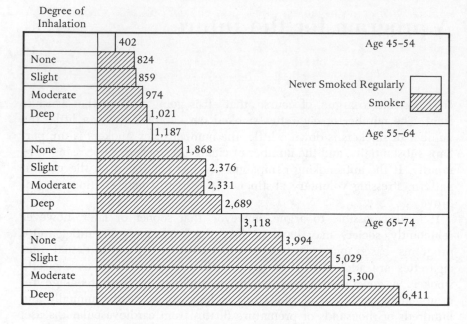

FIGURE 12. Death Rates by Degree of Inhalation, Male Smokers and
Nonsmokers, per 100,000 Person-Years[1]

- Develop smoke-free ways of delivering nicotine to the lungs—for example, nicotine inhalers.
- Popularize chewing tobacco and snuff.
- Develop ways of taking nicotine by mouth, perhaps in pill form. (Dr. Murray Jarvik of the Albert Einstein College of Medicine in New York is currently exploring this possibility, with a grant from the American Cancer Society. In Sweden, trials of a nicotine chewing gum are under way.)

The results that can be expected from keeping cigarette smoke *out of the lungs,* even among smokers who continue to smoke, are quite impressive. The overall death rate per 100,000 person-years among male smokers aged forty-five to fifty-four falls from 1,021 among those who inhale deeply to 824 among those who do not inhale at all. Between the ages of sixty-five and seventy-four, the drop is even more impressive— from 6,411 among those who inhale deeply to 3,994 among those who do not inhale at all. Figure 12 gives the details.

Keeping carcinogenic smoke out of the lungs, however, is only a partial solution. Switching to cigars, pipes, and chewing tobacco does not eliminate the risk of cancers of the oral cavity. Moreover, the bulk of the damage suffered by smokers is due to diseases of the heart and circulatory system—and it is the nicotine itself that has adverse effects on the heart. The second direction in which future policy must move, accordingly, is to find a *nicotine substitute.*

Such a substance should have no adverse effects (or significantly less disastrous effects), on the heart or other organs, but should satisfy the craving for nicotine.

Can such a substance be found?

The odds in favor are good. Literally scores of nicotine "congeners"— molecules closely related to nicotine chemically—are known; and many of these are also known to have no effects on heart action. What is not known is which of them will satisfy the nicotine craving.

With scores of chemical candidates for the role of a safe nicotine substitute already available, and with additional scores or perhaps hundreds waiting to be synthesized by chemists, why are no tests of these nicotine congeners being run? The answer appears to be essentially a moral one.

Few Americans recognize that nicotine is an addicting drug. Most people, therefore, feel that smokers should stop smoking voluntarily— that is, by an "effort of will"—rather than depending on a "chemical crutch," a nicotine substitute. The attitude toward nicotine thus parallels the attitude of some who oppose the methadone treatment for heroin addiction (see Part I), arguing that heroin addicts should stop by an "effort of will."

This is perhaps a worthy moral stand. But it has not, to date, proved successful. For while highly moral efforts have for seven years been concentrated on persuading smokers to stop smoking, and teaching them how to stop smoking, smokers have gone right on smoking—more than 500 billion cigarettes per year—and from 250,000 to 300,000 smokers a year go right on dying prematurely as a result of their smoking.

A third fresh direction for anticigarette public-health campaigns to take is to *tell people the facts about nicotine addiction.* It should be shocking to the conscience of the country that such facts have been kept a secret from young people.

Messages about nicotine *addiction* should be woven into the school curriculum. When children first study American Indians, they should learn that Indians were so addicted to tobacco that they could not do without it. When children learn the routes of the great explorers, they should be informed that the mariners were so addicted to tobacco they had to take supplies with them, and planted tobacco seeds along their routes. The sad plight of nicotine addicts cut off from their supplies—"Tobacco, sir, strong tobacco," and "We die, sir, if we have no tobacco!"—should be understood at a very early age. Full meaning should be restored to the word "addicting," which anticigarette and antiheroin campaigns have debased to the role of a paper tiger.

Part IV

Alcohol, the Barbiturates, the Tranquilizers, and other Sedatives and Hypnotics

Though traditionally classified as a depressant, alcohol actually has a wide spectrum of apparently contradictory effects. At various dose levels and phases of the drinking cycle it may depress or stimulate, tranquilize or agitate. It may release inhibitions or put the drinker to sleep. Medically, alcohol was long prescribed as a tonic, a sedative, and a soporific, but its traditional role in medicine has now been taken over largely by the barbiturates, minor tranquilizers, and other sedatives and hypnotics.

Among the barbiturates are the "long-acting," such as phenobarbital, and the "short-acting," such as pentobarbital (Nembutal) and secobarbital (Seconal). As shown in Chapter 29, alcohol is very similar in effect to a short-acting barbiturate. ("Short-acting" means both that the drug's effects set in sooner and more abruptly and that they wear off sooner.)

The minor tranquilizers resemble the barbiturates in some respects and differ in others (see below); included among them are meprobamate (Miltown, Equanil), chlordiazepoxide (Librium), and diazepam (Valium). Also classified as sedatives and hypnotics are glutethimide (Doriden), ethchlorvynol (Placidyl), chloral hydrate, and others.

As used nonmedically in our society, alcohol is taken occasionally and in moderation with few undesirable side effects by the great majority of users. Its potential for harm, however—mental and physical—makes alcohol one of the most dangerous of all drugs to those who get drunk, to those who become addicted, and to those about them. An estimated 10 to 12 percent of all drinkers are alcoholics or "problem drinkers"; the number of alcoholics—that is, alcohol addicts—is estimated to total five million people. As with other addicting drugs, no user can foresee whether or when he will become addicted to alcohol.

Moderate use of long-acting barbiturates appears to carry less risk of addiction than use of short-acting barbiturates or alcohol. The minor tranquilizers and some of the other sedatives and hypnotics also carry the hazard of addiction to lesser degrees. The use of virtually all of these drugs can produce symptoms like those of alcohol drunkenness—nausea, incoordination, loss of inhibitions, violence, etc. The best-known withdrawal symptom is the "hangover," experienced at times by even moderate users of these drugs; convulsions, delirium tremens, and even death are among the risks shared by addicts following abrupt withdrawal.

28.

The barbiturates for sleep and for sedation

Two of the most common afflictions for which human beings through the centuries have sought relief in drugs are anxiety and insomnia. During much of the nineteenth century, the opiates were prescribed to relieve those symptoms; but they were addicting. The bromide salts were also often used to induce sleep or "calm the nerves"; but they gradually lost popularity because of the risk of chronic bromide poisoning. Chloral hydrate and paraldehyde, both quite effective as sedatives and hypnotics (sleeping potions), have an objectionable taste and smell. Thus many conservative physicians, even after the turn of the century, continued to prescribe alcohol as the sedative and hypnotic of choice—a glass of wine in midmorning and midafternoon, perhaps, plus the traditional nightcap to induce sleep.

But a growing number of patients in need of sedatives and hypnotics were also ardent "teetotalers," who had "taken the pledge" of total abstinence from intoxicating beverages. Other patients didn't like the taste or smell of alcohol. Still others tended to take more alcohol than prescribed. Hence, despite the wide range of sedatives and hypnotics available at the end of the nineteenth century, the search for a better drug continued. It was in the course of this search that two German scientists, von Mering and Fischer, synthesized a new chemical called barbital, a derivative of barbituric acid.

Tested on both animals and humans, barbital seemed to have precisely the desired qualities. When a patient complaining of insomnia, for example, was given a capsule containing a moderate dose of barbital and told that it would facilitate sleep, the patient promptly fell asleep. Nervous, anxious patients given much smaller doses for daytime use and told the drug would "calm their nerves" found that it did. In 1903 barbital was introduced into general medical practice under the trade name Veronal—and soon became very popular.

A second barbituric acid derivative, phenobarbital, was introduced under the trade name Luminal in 1912. More than 2,500 other barbiturates were subsequently synthesized, and some fifty of them were accepted for medical use—as sedatives, as sleeping pills, and for other purposes. Long-acting barbiturates were developed for daytime sedation; short-acting barbiturates followed for prompt sedation and for inducing sleep without delay.[1] Combinations were also introduced—a short-acting bar-biturate to put you to sleep combined with a long-acting one to keep you asleep.

These new drugs seemed to have notable advantages over their pred-ecessors, including alcohol. They were odorless and tasteless. Precise quantities could be dispensed in capsule or tablet form. When barbitu-rates were taken as directed, in small doses for sedation and moderate doses for sleep, few side effects were noted. True, the short-acting bar-biturates carried some risk of addiction, but there was no evidence that the long-acting barbiturates were addicting. After taking small daily doses for weeks or even months, a patient could discontinue without discomfort—much as most people can take a daily alcohol cocktail or nightcap without becoming addicted. It was hardly surprising, therefore, that the barbiturates became so popular among physicians and patients alike. By the end of the 1930s an estimated *billion* grains were being taken each year in the United States alone.[2]

The barbiturates remain exceedingly useful today. "Phenobarbital is one of our mainstays in the treatment of epilepsy and is almost irreplace-able for this purpose," a professor of internal medicine wrote in 1971. "Phenobarbital and . . . Librium [chlordiazepoxide, a tranquilizer] in small doses are extremely valuable in the management of high blood pressure, peptic ulcer, and anxiety. The majority of people who are given these drugs (it must be nearly 99.9 percent) never develop any dependence on them, so that in a relative sense they are quite safe."*[4] Short-acting barbiturates, such as secobarbital and pentobarbital, he added, are another matter.

---

* Dr. Jerome H. Jaffe wrote (1970): "It has been found that 0.2 grams of pentobarbi-tal [a short-acting barbiturate] per day can be ingested over many months without the development of any tolerance or physical dependence."[3]

29.

Alcohol and barbiturates:
Two ways of getting drunk

While the enormous usefulness of the barbiturates cannot be questioned, evidence increasingly accumulated during the 1930s and 1940s to indicate that, when misused, they are not so great an improvement over alcohol as had at first been supposed. Indeed, they resemble alcohol in almost all respects. You can get drunk on barbiturates (especially the short-acting kinds) as on alcohol. You can become addicted to barbiturates (especially the short-acting kinds) as to alcohol. A barbiturate addict suffers much the same delirium tremens when withdrawn from barbiturates as an alcoholic withdrawn from alcohol. And abrupt withdrawal may in both cases prove fatal. The parallel between the short-acting barbiturates and alcohol is particularly close, for alcohol is also a short-acting drug. (A long-acting alcohol might be a safer drug.)

Among the several studies establishing the parallel between the barbiturates and alcohol, one small-scale experiment conducted at the United States Public Health Service Hospital in Lexington, Kentucky, is of special interest because of the many details it provides. Dr. Harris Isbell and his associates at Lexington isolated in a hospital research ward five prisoner volunteers serving sentences for narcotic law violations. The five were closely observed for a preliminary period, and subjected to a battery of neurological and psychological tests. Then each patient was given a large dose of a barbiturate.

The result was "a marked degree of intoxication," [1] which resembled alcohol intoxication in almost all respects. In a word, the five men became dead drunk. "All patients had difficulty in thinking and deterioration in their ability in performing the psychologic tests." They also showed neurological signs of alcohol intoxication, such as tremors and incoordination.[2]

As in the case with alcohol drunks, the reactions of the five patients drunk on barbiturates were far from uniform. Three of them passed out cold; the other two did not. Before passing out, two patients "became garrulous, boisterous, and silly"—the familiar behavior of many alcohol drunks. Two others became quiet and depressed, as also happens on alcohol. Just as an alcohol drunk often tries to pretend he is sober, moreover, these two "made desperate efforts to suppress signs of intoxication." The fifth patient, though he received as large a dose as the others, appeared to be little affected. In all cases, "signs of intoxication began to diminish within two hours after the drug was administered, and after four to five hours all clinical evidence of intoxication had disappeared." The patients slept poorly that night, however, and "on the subsequent day they were nervous and tremulous and complained of anorexia [loss of appetite] and headache. They compared these [withdrawal] symptoms to a 'hangover' after an alcoholic debauch."

Having thus demonstrated that a barbiturate drunk is precisely like an alcohol drunk, including the subsequent hangover, Dr. Isbell and his associates next went on to reproduce by means of barbiturates all of the phases of *chronic* alcoholism. Each morning for more than three months, the five men were given a small "eye-opener" dose of a barbiturate before breakfast. Larger doses were then administered through the day—at 9 A.M. and at 2, 7, and 11 P.M.—much as some chronic alcoholics drink through the day. "Generally, the signs of intoxication were minimal early in the morning and increased throughout the day," the Isbell report noted, "reaching maximum intensity after the 11 P.M. dose" [3]—a finding equally common among some alcoholics.

"They neglected their appearance, became unkempt and dirty, did not shave, bathed infrequently, and allowed their living quarters to become filthy. They were content to wear clothes soiled with food which they had spilled. All patients were confused and had difficulty in performing simple tasks or in playing cards or dominoes."

During the preliminary drug-free period of the experiment, the five men had become good friends and had developed a spirit of camaraderie among themselves. While drunk on barbiturates, in contrast, they became "irritable and quarrelsome. They cursed one another, and at times even fought"—all traits of the alcohol drunk.

At any cocktail party, one drunk may behave affectionately and garrulously while another becomes morose and a third becomes combative. Among these barbiturate drunks, too, "the effects on mood varied from day to day and from patient to patient. S-1, though occasionally euphoric, garrulous, and pleasant, was usually depressed, complained of various aches and pains, and continually sought increases in medication, although he was so intoxicated that he frequently could not walk." [4] Bartenders, of course, are familiar with the similar behavior of the drunk who, though barely able to stagger to the bar, pleads for just one more drink. Also like an alcoholic, patient S-1 "would weep over his wasted life and the state of his family."

Alcoholics often "swear off"—until it's time for the next drink; S-1 was like that, too. He "frequently asked to be released from the experiment, but would always change his mind within thirty minutes after missing a dose." [5] In a word, he was addicted.

Patient P-3 was "frequently elated, hyperactive, and garrulous. At other times he was depressed, quiet and withdrawn and talked of the joys of death, but when pressed denied suicidal intentions. He continually attempted to obtain increases in medication. Although he always got along well with other patients when not intoxicated, he became involved in three fights and in a considerable number of cursing matches while taking pentobarbital." [6]

Patient A-5, in contrast, "became even quieter and more withdrawn than he was before. . . . He sometimes spent days alone in his room and came out only for meals. . . . He had vague paranoid ideas"—like many alcoholics—"and stated the belief that the other patients did not like him and that the attendants were showing favor to them. He could not play dominoes without becoming involved in altercations. Some evidence suggestive of homosexual trends appeared. . . . He frequently made confused attempts to obtain increases in medication and seemed, as did S-1 and P-3, to be motivated by a desire to become completely unconscious." [7]

The remaining two patients "showed less pronounced changes in behavior. They continued to maintain good relationships with the other patients and with the attendants, and their personal appearance deteriorated less. . . The general picture in both these men was that of a person who was drunk and enjoyed it." Psychological and neurological test results closely paralleled the results of tests on chronic alcoholics; the neurological signs increased throughout the day, so that by 11 P.M. "all the patients would be staggering and unable to walk except by sliding along the walls. In spite of close supervision, they occasionally fell and were injured." [8] Similar falls and injuries are frequent among alcoholics. "The patients also tended to be more boisterous and quarrelsome at night, and most fights occurred at that time. . . . Great care had to be exercised to prevent patients from smoking in bed and setting fires"—a major hazard also among alcoholics.

As in the case of alcoholics, the amount of barbiturate needed to keep these barbiturate addicts drunk "varied widely from subject to subject." [9]

It was following withdrawal of barbiturate, however, that the parallel between that drug and alcohol was most impressively demonstrated. When an alcoholic who has been continuously drunk for days or weeks is abruptly deprived of his alcohol, he goes through a series of well-defined stages. At first he seems to be sobering up normally. Then anxiety and weakness set in, along with a gross tremor—"the shakes." The patient eats little but vomits often. A more dangerous stage follows, characterized by "rum fits"—convulsions like those seen in epilepsy. Then comes delirium tremens—a life-threatening condition characterized by delusions, hallucinations, and other signs of psychosis as well as physical signs (such as profuse sweating and, in some cases, high fever). These five barbiturate addicts went through precisely this sequence of changes when their drug was withdrawn.

Dr. Isbell and his associates, of course, had had long experience with morphine and heroin addicts at the Public Health Service Hospital in Lexington. They were therefore in a position to compare these barbiturate phenomena with the comparable opiate phenomena.

The manifestations of chronic barbiturate intoxication are, in most ways, much more serious than those of addiction to morphine [they noted]. Morphine causes much less impairment of mental ability and emotional control and produces no motor incoordination. Furthermore, such impairment as does occur becomes less as tolerance to morphine develops, and withdrawal of morphine is much less dangerous than is withdrawal of barbiturates.[10]

The Isbell group also compared the barbiturates and alcohol. "It is obvious," they concluded, "that chronic barbiturate intoxication is a dangerous and undesirable condition, which is very similar to chronic alcoholism"; and they added, "The similarity of the barbiturate withdrawal syndrome to alcoholic delirium tremens is striking." [11] Readers were left to draw the two corollaries for themselves—that alcoholism is in most respects much more serious than morphine addiction; and that withdrawal of alcohol is even more dangerous than morphine withdrawal.

Current scientific opinion confirms the findings of earlier decades. Thus Dr. Jerome H. Jaffe notes in Goodman and Gilman's textbook (1970):

. . . The subjective effects of barbiturates and sedatives . . . are similar to those of alcohol. [As with alcohol], the effects vary considerably with the dose, the situation, and the personality of the user. . . . The patterns of abuse are as varied as those for alcohol and range from infrequent sprees of gross intoxication, lasting a few days, to the prolonged, compulsive, daily use of huge quantities and a preoccupation with securing and maintaining adequate supplies.[12]

In addition to this evidence demonstrating the parallel between barbiturates and alcohol, there is even more startling evidence to indicate that these two substances are in fact producing many of the *same* effects —that the barbiturates might be labeled a "solid alcohol" and alcohol classed as a "liquid barbiturate." A man who drinks increasing quantities of alcohol, for example, becomes tolerant to alcohol effects—but he simultaneously develops cross-tolerance for barbiturate effects as well, and can tolerate an enormous dose of a barbiturate the very first time he tries the drug. The same is true in reverse; as the barbiturate addict increases his dose, he simultaneously achieves cross-tolerance for alcohol as well as barbiturates, and can take enormous doses. Some alcoholics under pressure to give up alcohol do give it up completely, without any of the usual suffering, "shakes," "rum fits," and delirium tremens—by substituting barbiturates for alcohol. (Some who make the changeover report that they prefer the barbiturates.) Many addicts use alcohol and barbiturates interchangeably, depending on which is cheaper or more conveniently available at the moment. Many use the two drugs at the same time. Simultaneous use is dangerous, however; for with either drug, there is only a narrow margin between the maximum dose that an addict can manage and the lethal dose—and it is harder to gauge the dose when both drugs are taken together.

Finally, the barbiturate effect of alcohol and the alcohol effect of the barbiturates is demonstrated during delirium tremens; either drug can *relieve* delirium tremens, whether caused by the same drug or by its twin. Indeed, one of the standard treatments for alcohol delirium tremens is to place the patient on intoxicating doses of a barbiturate, and then slowly to taper off the dosage. Drugs of another closely related group, the minor tranquilizers, are also now used for this purpose.

There are also significant practical differences between alcohol and the barbiturates. The latter are less likely to lead to serious malnutrition and accompanying neurological damage (see below), and are less damaging to the gastrointestinal system. Alcohol in the form of light wines and beer is less concentrated, so that the imbibing of a moderate series of doses can be spread over a period of time. An overdose of alcohol is toxic and sometimes lethal; but it is much easier to pop a whole handful of pills than to down a quart of whiskey. Hence, death from barbiturate overdose (or from a combination of alcohol and barbiturate), either accidental or with suicidal intent, is more common. Despite these and other differences, some in favor of alcohol and some the barbiturates, the close parallel between these drugs might be expected to lead to similar moral attitudes toward them—and to similar laws and national policies.

In fact, however, society takes a very different stance with respect to these twin drugs. Alcohol is treated as a nondrug; it is on sale in multidose bottles at some 40,000 liquor stores and in countless other outlets as well; it is freely sold to those "of age," in saloons, taverns, cocktail lounges, nightclubs, roadhouses, and even ordinary family restaurants; and more than $250,000,000 a year is spent on advertising alcohol. The barbiturates, in contrast, are legally salable only on prescription in pharmacies; other sales are severely punishable criminal offenses. It is a curious fact, indeed, that Americans today are bombarded with advertising urging them to buy a liquid that, if secured without a prescription in tablet or capsule form, could lead to imprisonment for both seller and buyer.

30.

Popularizing the barbiturates as "thrill pills"

The first major campaign against nonmedical barbiturate use was launched in 1942, with an article in a magazine called *Hygeia* (subsequently renamed *Today's Health*), published for the lay public by the American Medical Association. The article was called "1,250,000,000 Doses a Year." A second *Hygeia* article, "Waco Was a Barbiturate Hotspot," followed in June 1945—and similar articles have appeared through the decades since then in *Hygeia* and *Today's Health*. Their main message was to warn people away from barbiturates unless they were secured on prescription from a personal physician. Other magazines followed the *Hygeia* line; thus *Collier's* ran an article, "Thrill Pills Can Ruin You," in April 1949. States began passing laws against nonprescription barbiturates; arrests engendered newspaper headlines, and for the first time a black market in barbiturates became profitable. Agents of the United States Food and Drug Administration began to suppress nonprescribed barbiturates—generating more publicity. By the end of the 1940s, a nation that had for decades used barbiturates sensibly, to go to sleep or to calm the nerves, had been persuaded that the drugs were "thrill pills." What might have been anticipated did in fact occur. Some people who would never for the world have taken a sedative or a sleeping pill now began getting drunk on the new "thrill pills." For them the warnings served as lures; illicit barbiturate use increased from year to year. Throughout the 1950s and 1960s, the relatively harmless sleeping tablets of the 1930s played their new role as one of the major illicit American drugs.

At first the illicit barbiturate users were mostly adults; children and adolescents tended to prefer stimulants to depressants. By the 1960s, however, even young children had heard the news that you can get roaring drunk on "barbs," and had succumbed to the lure. "Especially during the past year," Dr. Sidney Cohen told the Subcommittee on Juvenile Delinquency of the United States Senate Judiciary Committee on September 17, 1969, "young people, some in the pre-teen age group, have become involved." [1] The fact that barbiturates were available in many family medicine cabinets as well as on the black market no doubt facilitated this trend. Dr. Cohen cited a survey indicating that at one college, 24 percent of students had used barbiturates—though in almost all cases only sporadically. "There is now no generation gap in the abuse of barbiturates," Dr.

Cohen concluded. Production in 1969, he indicated, would total ten billion doses, up 800 percent from 1942, when the antibarbiturate campaign was launched—"enough to provide each man, woman, and child in this land with 50. At least half of this supply gets into the illicit market." * 2

The American experience with barbiturates after 1940—the explosion of illicit barbiturate use following warnings, publicity, restrictive laws, and punitive arrests—should have taught society a lesson. Yet during the 1960s the same policies were followed with respect to LSD and marijuana—with much the same results, but on an even larger scale.

An elementary conclusion seems warranted. The more often the warning lure is presented, the direr the prophecies of doom, and the more emotion-laden the tone of the message, the greater the likelihood of popularizing the drug under attack.

---

* Though enormous, the ten billion doses of barbiturates, licit and illicit, were of course only a modest fraction of the number of comparable doses of alcohol consumed per year.

31.

The nonbarbiturate sedatives and the minor tranquilizers

As the barbiturates came under frequent attack following 1941, and as the market for them soared, efforts were naturally revived to find additional drugs that might compete for that flourishing market.

One result of this search was the introduction into medical practice of a variety of prescription sedatives and sleeping pills bearing such trade names as Doriden, Placidyl, and Noludar. Advertisements in the medical journals urged physicians to prescribe these drugs precisely because they were nonbarbiturates. In fact, however, these newer sedatives and hypnotics belong, pharmacologically if not chemically, to the same class of drugs as alcohol and the barbiturates. You can get drunk on them; you can become addicted to them; and you can suffer delirium tremens when they are withdrawn. The parallel can be seen in this excerpt from the Placidyl "product information" material prepared for physicians by the manufacturer, Abbott Laboratories:

Patients who are taking PLACIDYL or other [central nervous system]-acting drugs should be cautioned about the possible combined exaggerated effects with alcohol, barbiturates, tranquilizers or other central nervous system depressants [that] might result in blurring of vision, paralysis of accommodation and profound hypnosis.

Patients also should be cautioned concerning driving a motor vehicle, operating machinery, or other hazardous operations requiring alertness shortly after taking PLACIDYL.

PLACIDYL should be administered with caution [to] patients with suicidal tendencies and large quantities of the drug should not be prescribed.

Psychological and Physical Dependence: PLACIDYL, LIKE OTHER SEDATIVE-HYPNOTIC DRUGS, HAS THE POTENTIAL . . . FOR THE DEVELOPMENT OF PSYCHOLOGICAL AND PHYSICAL DEPENDENCE. INSTANCES OF SEVERE WITHDRAWAL SYMPTOMS, INCLUDING CONVULSIONS AND [DELIRIUM] CLINICALLY SIMILAR TO THOSE SEEN WITH BARBITURATES, HAVE BEEN REPORTED IN PATIENTS TAKING REGULAR DOSES AS LOW AS 1000 MG. PER DAY OVER A PERIOD OF TIME WHEN THE DRUG WAS SUDDENLY DISCONTINUED. [Capitals in original.]

In view of the potential of PLACIDYL (ethchlorvynol) for inducing dependence, prolonged administration of the drug is not recommended.

Patients, particularly those known to be addiction-prone, or those who are likely to increase dosage of PLACIDYL on their own initiative, should be observed for evidence of signs or symptoms which may indicate possible early withdrawal or abstinence symptoms. Signs and symptoms associated with withdrawal and abstinence include unusual anxiety, tremor, ataxia [muscular incoordination], slurring of speech, memory loss, perceptual distortions, irritability, agitation and delirium. Other less well defined signs and symptoms, not necessarily due to withdrawal and abstinence[,] may include anorexia, nausea, or vomiting, weakness, dizziness, sweating, muscle twitching and weight loss. Abrupt discontinuance of PLACIDYL following prolonged overdosage may result in convulsions and [delirium].

Treatment of a patient who manifests withdrawal symptoms from PLACIDYL abuse involves readministration of the drug to approximate the same level of chronic intoxication which existed before the abrupt discontinuance. . . . A gradual, stepwise reduction of dosage may then be made over a period of days or weeks. The patient must be hospitalized or closely observed and gives general supportive care as indicated.

PRECAUTIONS: . . . Patients who respond unpredictably to barbiturates or alcohol, or who exhibit excitement and release of inhibitions in association with such agents may also react in this way to PLACIDYL.

Rarely, patients may exhibit symptoms suggestive of an unusual susceptibility to the drug: prolonged hypnosis, profound muscular weakness, excitement, hysteria, or syncope [fainting] without marked hypotension.

In occasional patients the drug appears to be absorbed very rapidly and may produce transient giddiness or ataxia. Should this occur, a glass of milk or other food should be given with subsequent doses of the drug, or the drug discontinued.

ADVERSE REACTIONS: Hypotension [low blood pressure], nausea or vomiting, gastric upset, aftertaste, blurring of vision, dizziness, facial numbness, and allergic reaction typified by urticaria [hives] have been reported following PLACIDYL (ethchlorvynol) administration. Mild "hangover" and symptoms of mild excitation have occurred in some patients. . . .[1]

In addition to these nonbarbiturate sedatives, a second new class of drugs has been introduced in an effort to capture some of the vast barbiturate market. These drugs are the minor tranquilizers,* of which meprobamate (marketed as Miltown and as Equanil) was the first and remains the best known. Other well-known minor tranquilizers are chlordiazepoxide (Librium) and diazepam (Valium).

These tranquilizers have effects so similar to those of the barbiturates that for a number of years experienced clinicians refused to recognize any real difference; and even today the distinction is difficult to establish. Thus Dr. Murray E. Jarvik states in Goodman and Gilman's textbook (1970):

* The "minor tranquilizers" are so called to distinguish them from the drugs used in the treatment of schizophrenia and other psychoses—the "major tranquilizers" such as chlorpromazine. The major tranquilizers are not used nonmedically, and are therefore not considered in this Report.

The pharmacological effects of meprobamate are very similar to those of the barbiturates. Indeed, in clinical usage it is difficult, if not impossible, to differentiate between the two drugs. Only by careful pharmacological analysis can certain distinctions be discerned.[2]

The major difference is that a dose of a minor tranquilizer sufficient to calm anxiety seems to produce a little less sleepiness and interference with motor activities than does a dose of a barbiturate equally effective against anxiety. In other respects, the differences are hardly noteworthy. "The withdrawal syndrome following abrupt discontinuance of high doses of meprobamate resembles that following barbiturate withdrawal," Dr. Jarvik notes.[3]

According to *The Medical Letter* (1969), "Librium and Valium are effective sedatives, but, except in potentially suicidal patients, it is still not clear that they have any important advantage over the barbiturates."[4] In 1971, *The Medical Letter* added, "When anxiety is severe or interferes with everyday pursuits and relationships, a sedative drug such as a barbiturate, chlordiazepoxide [Librium], diazepam [Valium], or meprobamate is a useful adjunct to psychotherapy. . . ."[5]

The hazards of Valium are set forth in the "product information" supplied to physicians by the manufacturer, Roche Laboratories, reading in part as follows:

WARNINGS: . . . As is true of most preparations containing central nervous system-acting drugs, patients receiving . . . Valium (diazepam) should be cautioned against engaging in hazardous occupations requiring complete mental alertness such as operating machinery or driving a motor vehicle. . . .

Since Valium (diazepam) has a central nervous system depressant effect, patients should be advised against the simultaneous ingestion of alcohol and other central nervous system depressant drugs. . . .

Physical and Psychological Dependence: Withdrawal symptoms (similar in character to those noted with barbiturates and alcohol) have occurred following abrupt discontinuance of diazepam (convulsions, tremor, abdominal and muscle cramps, vomiting and sweating). These were usually limited to those patients who had received excessive doses over an extended period of time. Particularly addiction-prone individuals (such as drug addicts or alcoholics) should be under careful surveillance when receiving diazepam. . . .

ADVERSE REACTIONS: . . . Side effects most commonly reported were drowsiness, fatigue and ataxia. Infrequently encountered were confusion, constipation, depression, diplopia [double vision], dysarthria [stammering], headache, hypotension, incontinence, jaundice, changes in libido, nausea . . . slurred speech, tremor . . . vertigo [dizziness] and blurred vision. . . .[6]

—in short, much the same side effects as those produced by alcohol, the barbiturates, and the nonbarbiturate depressants.

The risks associated with Placidyl and Valium are cited here only as examples; virtually all prescription drugs carry lists of "contraindications," "precautions," "warnings," and "adverse reactions." Those hazards of prescription drugs should be borne in mind when the hazards of black-market drugs such as LSD (Part VII) and marijuana (Part VIII) are evaluated. Consideration might also be given to requiring comparable warnings on packages of and in advertisements for alcoholic beverages and tobacco products.

To round out the picture, let us return for just a moment to the pre-barbiturate sedatives, chloral hydrate and paraldehyde. These, too, it has now been established, can produce drunkenness, addiction, and delirium tremens hardly distinguishable from those produced by alcohol, the barbiturates, the nonbarbiturate sedatives, and the minor tranquilizers.[7]

Thus the wheel comes full circle.

32.

Should alcohol be prohibited?

Heroin, LSD, and marijuana are prohibited in the United States today, in part on the ground that they are dangerous and in part on the ground that they serve no useful medical purpose. The prohibition of the barbiturates, the nonbarbiturate depressants, and the minor tranquilizers—despite their potential hazards—is rarely suggested even by antidrug extremists; their unquestioned importance as medicines stands in the way. But what about alcohol? Should it not be banned on the same grounds that heroin, LSD, and marijuana are prohibited?

Let us put aside the weighty arguments *against* alcohol prohibition, and try to consider seriously for the moment the arguments in its favor.

Alcohol addiction is second only to nicotine addiction in incidence and prevalence in the United States today. A conservative estimate is that five million Americans are alcoholics, but figures of as high as seven to nine million alcoholics and "problem drinkers" are also cited.[1] Alcohol addicts are unable to refrain from their drug even though they decide to, want to, and try to quit drinking alcohol; those who succeed for a time remain in imminent danger of relapse.* To the millions of alcohol addicts must be added millions of "spree drinkers" who are not addicted but who get roaring drunk from time to time. Alcohol prohibition, if enacted and effectively enforced, would keep these addicts and drunks away from their drug; and it would prevent new cohorts of young people from becoming addicted—or so it might be logically argued.

* It is commonly supposed that alcohol addicts, like narcotics addicts, are weak-willed and that it is their weakness of will that led them to become—and to remain—addicts. The evidence is superficially plausible: even though two people may drink alcohol (or take barbiturates) in precisely the same pattern, it is said, only one of them may become addicted. The difference between the two may not be in strength of will, however; it is at least equally plausible to hypothesize a difference in enzymes or in other biochemical factors distinguishing the metabolism of alcohol in the addict and in the similarly exposed nonaddict. Nobody really knows. The preponderance of the evidence currently available favors the view that the difference lies in the childhood of the two drinkers, in their social environment, and in the stresses to which they are exposed as adults. But, as noted with respect to narcotics (see Chapter 10), most researchers through the decades have been *looking* for psychological and sociological evidence; it is hardly surprising (or convincing) that that is what they have found. If as much research, energy, and ingenuity were devoted to the search for biochemical factors, the preponderance of evidence might soon shift to the biochemical explanation. There has recently been a small increase in biochemical studies of alcoholism, but it is still too early to review or evaluate the findings here.

Alcohol addiction, unlike morphine addiction, is utterly destructive to the human mind. Among 70,000 first admissions of males to state mental hospitals in 1964, for example, more than 15,000 (22 percent) were given a diagnosis of alcoholism at the time of admission. Among female mental hospital admissions, the proportion with an alcoholism diagnosis was 5.6 percent. "In nine states, alcoholic disorders lead all other diagnoses in mental hospital admissions. Maryland, for example, reports that 40 percent of all male admissions are for alcoholism." [2] The remarkable absence of *narcotics* addicts among mental hospital admissions was noted in Part I.

Alcohol is similarly destructive of the human body. "The impact of problem drinkers on the medical-surgical wards of general hospitals is illustrated by a study in which the extent of drinking problems among 100 consecutive male admissions to a general hospital was determined. No preselection was made in terms of the diagnosis of the patients, and the hospital did not have a psychiatric service. The admitting physicians identified twelve of the 100 men as problem drinkers, and seventeen additional cases of probable alcoholism were uncovered by the researcher, making a total of 29 percent." [3]

Whether alcohol is solely responsible for this damage to mind and body, or whether defective nutrition also plays a role, has long been debated. Alcohol contains calories; indeed, a heavy drinker may consume half or more of his caloric needs in the form of alcohol. The result is to reduce quite drastically his consumption of proteins, vitamins, and other essential nutrients. The informed consensus is that the two effects march hand in hand; irreversible brain and liver damage, for example, is less severe in the alcoholic who maintains adequate nutrition—but it can occur all the same.* Making alcohol unavailable would thus contribute enormously to physical as well as mental health.

Alcohol is also by a wide margin the biggest law-enforcement problem in the United States today. "In 1965, out of close to five million arrests in the United States for all offenses, over 1,535,000 were for public drunkenness (31 percent). In addition, there were over 250,000 arrests for driving while intoxicated. Another 490,000 individuals were charged with disorderly conduct, which some communities use in lieu of the public drunkenness charge. Thus at least 40 percent of all arrests are for being drunk in a public place or being under the influence while driving. . . . Many persons arrested for public drunkenness are no more intoxicated than countless other individuals who escape arrest because they are not exposed and vulnerable to police detection as are skid row men. The public

* Proposals to fortify alcoholic beverages with vitamins—especially the B vitamins—have occasionally been made, but have been rejected on the ground that doing this might encourage drinking. Hence neurological and liver damage continues to be needlessly frequent among alcoholics.

is more likely to insist on the police removing the unshaven, toothless, poorly clothed men than an equally drunk visiting business man." * [5]

Homicide is also an alcohol-related crime. A 1954 Ohio study revealed that 43 percent of those who committed homicide had been drinking.[6] A Texas study the following year indicated that 28.5 percent of all homicides took place in bars, cocktail lounges, and other public places where liquor was served.[7] More remarkable still, drinking increases the likelihood that a man or woman will be a *victim* of homicide. A 1951 Baltimore report indicated that 69 percent of homicide victims had been drinking.[8] Among 588 Philadelphia homicides, according to a careful study by Dr. M. E. Wolfgang in 1958, alcohol was *absent* from both killer and victim in only 36 percent of the cases. In 9 percent of the cases, alcohol was found only in the corpse of the victim; in 11 percent it was found only in the bloodstream of the killer—and in 44 percent of the cases, both killer and victim had been drinking.† [9]

The Wolfgang report on Philadelphia homicides also revealed that alcohol is associated with specific *methods* of homicide; thus 72 percent of the stabbings involved the presence of alcohol, as compared with 69 percent of the beatings, 55 percent of the shootings, and only 45 percent of the "miscellaneous" methods.

"On the basis of the present data," Dr. Richard H. Blum—who assembled the figures above—concludes, "one can say that there is a strong link between alcohol and homicide and that the presumption is that alcohol plays a causal role as one of the necessary and precipitating elements for violence. Such a role is in keeping with the most probable effects of alcohol as a depressant of inhibition control centers in the brain—leading to release of impulses." [10]

In sum, the total of alcohol-related arrests reaches 55 percent of all arrests.[11] Surely it makes more sense, alcohol prohibitionists might argue, to ban the drug itself rather than to arrest millions of users of the drug *after* they have committed murder or lesser offenses.

Alcohol is a significant factor in the "battered child syndrome." In a high proportion of cases in which a parent beats his young child so severely that hospitalization is required or that death ensues, the parent is drunk at the time.

The relationship between alcohol and suicide is also very close. A 1962 Washington State study, for example, showed that 23 percent of suicide attempts were made by persons who were known to be alcoholics and 31 percent of the successful suicides were known to be committed by alco-

* In 1966, New York City police stopped arresting for drunkenness, with no perceptible effects—except to free the police (and courts and jails) for other kinds of crimes.[4]

† In the Isbell study (see Chapter 29), it will be recalled, four of the five experimental subjects, though peaceful and friendly when sober, quarreled and fought when drunk.

holics.[12] The true figures, the investigators warned, were almost certainly higher. Other studies report similar findings—and also indicate that many suicides were drinking or drunk *at the time of the act.* Dr. Karl Menninger and other psychiatrists have suggested, indeed, that alcoholism is itself a form of "chronic suicide." No one knows how many cases of death from acute and chronic alcoholism are in fact suicides, with alcohol as the deliberately chosen means of rapidly or slowly achieving death. Nor is it possible to estimate the number of suicides among drunken drivers who are found dead at the wheel following a crash. But most drivers found dead at the wheel have been drinking.

"Coroners' reports on levels of blood alcohol found in autopsies reveal high concentrations . . . in fatal accident victims," Dr. Blum notes. "Among drivers rated as probably responsible for their accidents, 73 percent had been drinking to some extent whereas only 26 percent of the similarly exposed (site-matched controls) * had been drinking. Forty-six percent of the accident responsible group had blood alcohol concentrations in the very high 0.25 percent and over range. In contrast, not a single one of the drivers in the large control group had a concentration in this range." [13] In another study, 50 percent of the fatally injured drivers had blood alcohol levels of 0.15 percent or more at the time of death.[14] Among fifty pedestrians dying within six hours after an automobile accident in yet another study, 74 percent had been drinking, as compared with 33 percent of the controls sampled at the same accident site. One-third of those killed had blood alcohol levels greater than 0.15 percent— as compared with only one-sixteenth of the controls.[15] "It appears clear," Dr. Blum concludes, "that drinking is a factor not only in driver accidents but also in pedestrian (victim) fatalities." [16]

The possibility remains, of course, that alcohol in small amounts— insufficient to impair driving skills—may actually prevent some accidents as a result of its calming effect. But on balance, alcohol almost certainly causes far more accidents, and far more fatal accidents, than it prevents.

Alcohol drinking leads in some cases to narcotic addiction. "In Western society," Dr. Jaffe wrote in Goodman and Gilman's textbook (1965), "individuals who later become addicts invariably have experiences with alcohol prior to using opiates. A considerable number of such persons also experimented first with marijuana, amphetamines, barbiturates, and tranquilizers. Such agents seem to serve the function of alerting the individual to the fact that substances exist which may be able to alter feelings of inner tension." [17] In addition, as noted in Part I, many narcotic addicts first turn to heroin in order to escape the ravages of alcoholism.

Many people worry about the effects of drugs taken during pregnancy,

---

* In a site-matched control study, the blood alcohol level of the drivers responsible for accidents is compared with the level in other drivers, randomly selected from among those present in the same vicinity at the same time.

but *alcohol* consumed during pregnancy is rarely included in this concern. Does alcohol pass through the placenta, and if so, does it damage unborn babies? It is shocking indeed to have to report that no one really knows; few studies have been made. The probability is that alcohol does pass through the placenta; and that if taken by a pregnant woman in large quantities over long periods it is unlikely to do the fetus any good.

An opponent of alcohol prohibition might argue that alcohol, after all, is drunk by adults; drugs such as marijuana and LSD are more in need of prohibition because high-school and college-age students use them. But the facts do not bear this out. A survey published in the September 1971 issue of *Playboy* magazine found alcohol rather than marijuana to be the drug of choice among college students by a vote of two to one. Even in high schools where marijuana and LSD are readily available and in common use, surveys indicate that alcohol remains the chief drug problem. High-school students not only drink alcohol; they get roaring, stinking drunk on it. They vomit. They "black out" (forget what has happened). And they pass out cold. A further discussion of alcohol and marijuana use among high-school and college students will be found in the discussion of marijuana in Part VIII.

One of the most powerful arguments in favor of alcohol prohibition is rarely advanced—that it is useless to prohibit other drugs, even heroin, so long as alcohol remains freely available. Many heroin addicts deprived of heroin promptly turn to alcohol instead and become alcoholics (see Part I). Many marijuana smokers whose marijuana supply is cut off increase their alcohol consumption (see table on Page 442). Many barbiturate addicts also turn to alcohol—and the same is presumably true of the users of other drugs as well. Thus, banning other drugs accomplishes little of value; it simply increases the number of those who turn to alcohol (or increases the amount they drink). Until people are willing to enforce alcohol prohibition, this argument therefore concludes, they are simply wasting their efforts in trying to enforce heroin prohibition, marijuana prohibition, and other drug prohibitions.

This discussion hardly exhausts the arguments for alcohol prohibition, but it is perhaps sufficient to demonstrate the inherent logic of such a proposal. From the humanitarian as well as the societal point of view, for the benefit of drinkers and potential drinkers as well as teetotalers, for the benefit of ex-heroin addicts and users of other drugs, and especially for the benefit of young people, alcohol should be promptly prohibited—except for one consideration.

33.

Why alcohol should not be prohibited

In contrast to the many logical arguments in favor of alcohol prohibition, the one decisive argument *against* such a measure is purely pragmatic: prohibition doesn't work. It should work, but it doesn't.

The evidence, of course, was accumulated during the thirteen-year period 1920–1933. The arguments in favor of prohibition before 1920 were overwhelming. The Eighteenth (Prohibition) Amendment passed both houses of Congress by the required two-thirds majority in December 1917, and was ratified by the required three-fourths of the forty-eight state legislatures a bare thirteen months later. After experiencing alcohol prohibition for thirteen years, however, the nation rebelled. The Twenty-first (Prohibition Repeal) Amendment passed both houses of Congress by the required two-thirds majority in February 1933—and this time it took less than ten months to secure ratification by three-fourths of the forty-eight state legislatures.

Alcohol prohibition was *not* repealed because people decided that alcohol was a harmless drug. On the contrary, the United States learned during Prohibition, even more than in prior decades, the true horrors of the drug. What brought about Repeal was the slowly dawning awareness that alcohol prohibition wasn't working.

Alcohol remained available during Prohibition. People still got drunk, still became alcoholics, still suffered delirium tremens. Drunken drivers remained a frequent menace on the highways. Drunks continued to commit suicide, to kill others, and to be killed by others. They continued to beat their own children, sometimes fatally. The courts, jails, hospitals, and mental hospitals were still filled with drunks. In some respects and in some parts of the country, perhaps, the situation was a little better during Prohibition—but in other respects it was unquestionably worse.

Instead of consuming alcoholic beverages manufactured under the safeguards of state and federal standards, for example, people now drank "rotgut," some of it adulterated, some of it contaminated. The use of methyl alcohol, a poison, because ethyl alcohol was unavailable or too costly, led to blindness and death; "ginger jake," an adulterant found in bootleg beverages, produced paralysis and death.[1] The disreputable saloon was replaced by the even less savory speakeasy. There was a shift from relatively mild light wines and beers to hard liquors—less bulky and therefore less hazardous to manufacture, transport, and sell on the black market. Young people—and especially respectable young women, who rarely got drunk in public before 1920—now staggered out of speakeasies and reeled down the streets. There were legal closing hours for saloons; the speakeasies stayed open night and day. Organized crime syndicates took control of alcohol distribution, establishing power bases that (it is alleged) still survive. Marijuana, a drug previously little used in the United States, was first popularized during the period of alcohol Prohibition (see Part VIII); and ether was also imbibed (see Chapter 43). The use of other drugs increased, too; coffee consumption, for example, soared from 9 pounds per capita in 1919 to 12.9 pounds in 1920.[2] The list is long and could be lengthened—but we need not belabor the obvious.

During the early years of alcohol Prohibition, it was argued that all that was wrong was lack of effective law enforcement. So enforcement budgets were increased, more Prohibition agents were hired, arrests were facilitated by giving agents more power, penalties were escalated. Prohibition still didn't work.

The United States thus learned its lesson—with respect to alcohol. More remarkable, the mere memory of Prohibition, forty years after Repeal, is still so repellent that no proposal to revive it would be taken seriously. Since alcohol is treated as a nondrug, however, the relevance of the lesson to other drug prohibitions has been overlooked.

The Twenty-first (Repeal) Amendment left power in the states to retain statewide alcohol prohibition—and made it a federal offense to ship alcoholic beverages into a dry state. Statewide alcohol prohibition, however, failed like national prohibition. State after state repealed its statewide alcohol prohibition laws; Mississippi's, in 1966, was the last to go.

In summary, far more would be gained by making alcohol unavailable than by making any other drug unavailable. Yet the United States, after a thirteen-year trial, resolutely turned its face against alcohol prohibition. Society recognized that prohibition does not in fact prohibit, and that it brings in its wake additional adverse effects.

All of the drugs discussed in this Part, including alcohol, have important medicinal or social uses. All are subject to the same kinds of misuse. Establishing a social policy designed to maximize the benefits and to minimize the damage done by these drugs is a challenge for the future. But the first step toward that goal is surely apparent today: to make known the simple fact that the widely publicized perils of the barbiturates are in fact the perils of alcohol—and that the other drugs in this class are not without hazard. When the United States eventually arrives at a sound policy for any of these drugs, this policy will almost certainly be a consistent policy for all of them. And society will seek to minimize for all of them what we have characterized in this Report as "the lure of the warning."

Part V

Coca Leaves, Cocaine, the Amphetamines, "Speed"—and Cocaine Again

Cocaine, a drug extracted from the leaves of the South American coca plant, is a stimulant of the central nervous system that produces euphoria (a sense of well-being). It still has some medicinal uses in anesthesiology, but has for the most part been superseded by synthetic drugs.

The *amphetamines* are a large group of synthetic drugs with marked cocainelike effects but are longer-acting than cocaine. Examples are dextroamphetamine (Dexedrine), methamphetamine (Methedrlne, Desoxyn), and amphetamine itself (Benzedrine). The amphetamines are widely used to stave off sleepiness among those who work (or play) long hours, and are popular as "diet drugs" and as antidepressants.

Tolerance to the effects of both cocaine and the amphetamines sometimes sets in; hence there is a tendency among some who use the drugs nonmedically to escalate the dosage. Though usually taken orally, these drugs are injected intravenously by "speed freaks." Excessive doses, especially if taken intravenously, produce hyperactivity, paranoid thinking, other psychotic symptoms, and (occasionally) violent behavior. Both cocaine and the amphetamines are addicting to some people under some circumstances.

Other central nervous system stimulants that differ from the amphetamines chemically but resemble them in numerous pharmacological respects include phenmetrazine (Preludin), diethylpropion (Tenuate, Tepanil), and methylphenidate (Ritalin); they are often prescribed as antidepressants and as "diet drugs." These drugs and the amphetamines should not be confused with drugs prescribed as antidepressants that do *not* stimulate the central nervous system, such as imipramine hydrochloride (Tofranil) and amitriptyline (Elavil), which are rarely used nonmedically and therefore are not covered in this Report.

Part V

Coca Leaves, Cocaine, the Amphetamines, Speed — and Cocaine Again

34.

Coca leaves

When the Spanish *conquistadores*, early in the sixteenth century, first encountered the empire of the Incas,* they found that the Emperor himself —the Inca—controlled the use of a remarkable drug contained in the leaves of a mountain shrub now known as *Erythroxylon coca*. When these leaves were chewed, euphoria and other desirable effects soon followed. "Among the highest rewards the Inca could give," Dr. Hector P. Blejer explained in the *Canadian Medical Association Journal* for September 25, 1965, "was the right to chew the coca leaf, which was prized far above the richest presents of silver or gold."[1] Priests and supplicants were allowed to approach the Altar of the Inca only if they had coca leaf in their mouths. "Even at the moment of death it was, and still is, believed by the natives that, if the moribund person was able to perceive the taste of the coca leaves pressed against his mouth, his soul would go to paradise."[2] A plentiful supply of the divine drug was buried with each Inca nobleman.

The *conquistadores* took over the Inca's coca leaves along with his empire. Although superstitiously afraid to use the drug themselves, they "gave coca freely to the Indians to control them, and hold them more tightly as virtual slaves. Under the effects of the coca leaf the Indians worked harder, longer, and with less food [coca, like amphetamine, is a potent appetite suppressant]. . . . It also helped them, perhaps, to endure, and forget, and even escape their misery."[3]

The Spaniards supported their empire by taxing the Indians heavily; "ironically, some of these taxes had to be paid in coca leaves, a commodity in which the administration had a very profitable turnover."[4]

Meanwhile, high in the Andes Mountains, where the coca shrub has been cultivated since time immemorial, natives beyond the reach of the Spanish occupation continued to chew coca leaves, as no doubt they had chewed them before the days of the Incas, and as they continue to chew them today. Far from suffering disaster, they have managed through the centuries to survive the rigors of an incredibly harsh mountain environment, to the continuing amazement of European visitors. Nor do the Andean leaf-chewers appear to become addicted; on moving down to ordinary altitudes, many of them give up their coca without apparent hardship. †

* The portion of South America that today comprises Peru, Bolivia, Ecuador, and parts of Chile and Colombia.

† Dr. Jerome H. Jaffe wrote (1965): "It is reported that two million Peruvians who live in the Andean highlands, or 90 percent of the adult male population, consume . . .

Nineteenth-century European and American scientists, naturally enough, took an interest in this potent drug. "All trustworthy travelers agree," an American physician, Dr. J. L. Corning, wrote in 1886, "that the most noticeable effect . . . consists in a marvelous invigoration of the strength, both mental and physical. The native is enabled to undertake the most difficult and prolonged marches with little other sustenance." A large dose, however, Dr. Corning added, "produces a species of intoxication, accompanied by sensations of lively satisfaction as well as hallucinations of various kinds." [6]

The chewing of coca leaves, for some unknown reason, never became popular either in Europe or North America. Various drinks made from the coca leaf, however, were introduced into Europe—notably "Mariani's wine," a red wine or elixir containing coca, manufactured during the nineteenth century by a Corsican, Signor Angelo Mariani. "Among his clients," Dr. Blejer notes, "were Gounod, Massenet, and Pope Leo XIII, who for years was supported in his ascetic retirement by Mariani's product." [7] Just as caffeine helped pious Mohammedans stay awake during prolonged religious rituals, so coca helped Christian ascetics withstand the pangs of hunger during prolonged fasts.

In the United States, a resident of Atlanta, Georgia, named John Styth Pemberton, introduced a product similar to Mariani's wine in 1885. Pemberton had previously been marketing patent medicines such as Triplex Liver Pills and Globe of Flower Cough Syrup. The registered trademark for his new product was *French Wine Coca—Ideal Nerve and Tonic Stimulant.* The next year, he added yet another coca product, a syrup that he called Coca-Cola.* The "Cola" in the name indicated the presence of an extract of kola nut—an African product that contains about 2 percent caffeine. That year, Pemberton is said to have sold twenty-five gallons of the syrup. At various times it was advertised as "a remarkable therapeutic agent" and as a "sovereign remedy" for a long list of ailments, including melancholy and (curiously) insomnia.

Coca-Cola became one of the chief targets of Dr. Harvey Wiley in his drive to have a Pure Food and Drug Law enacted (see Chapter 7). By 1906, when the law was passed, Pemberton's successors as makers of Coca-Cola had switched from ordinary coca leaves to decocainized coca leaves, but caffeine was still included in the formula. In 1909, Dr. Wiley, as head of the Bureau of Food and Drugs, initiated a famous case entitled

---

cocaine . . . in the form of coca leaves. In view of the fact that many of these highlanders, who have chewed coca leaves for years, abandon the practice when transferred to a lower altitude, it does not seem appropriate to call this use of cocaine an addiction." [5]

* These and other Coca-Cola facts are taken from E. J. Kahn's book, *The Big Drink: the Story of Coca-Cola* (New York: Random House, 1960).

United States v. Forty Barrels and Twenty Kegs of Coca-Cola. The company was charged with adulteration (because the Pure Food Act prohibited adding caffeine to a product) and misbranding (because, it was charged, Coca-Cola contained no coca and little cola). After dragging through the courts for nine years, and following Dr. Wiley's retirement from the government, the Coca-Cola Company agreed to make certain changes in its manufacturing process; in exchange for paying all legal costs, the company was allowed to reclaim its barrels and kegs. (As reported in the January 1971 issue of *Consumer Reports,* Consumers Union laboratory tests confirmed the presence of caffeine in Coca-Cola and in Pepsi-Cola.)

The Harrison Narcotic Act of 1914 mistakenly classed coca products as *narcotics;* and since 1914 coca leaves have been subject to the same penalties as opium, morphine, and heroin. The American coca-leaf interests, however, were powerful enough to secure a special clause in the Harrison Act exempting *decocainized* coca leaves—just as the proprietary opiate interests were able to secure a clause in the act exempting patent medicines containing small amounts of opium, morphine, and heroin.

A search of the medical literature has turned up little data to indicate that the chewing of coca leaves or the imbibing of beverages containing small amounts of coca is more damaging to mind or body than the drinking of coffee or tea.* Nor are the physiological and psychological effects notably different; both coca and caffeine are primarily stimulants of the central nervous system.

---

* A leading American authority on drugs of plant origin used by primitive peoples—Professor Richard Evans Schultes, Director of the Botanical Museum of Harvard University—reports that during his plant explorations in the Amazon Valley he chewed coca leaves daily for eight years, did not become addicted, and suffered no apparent physical harm from the custom.[8]

35.

Cocaine

The chief active ingredient in coca leaves, the alkaloid cocaine, was isolated in pure form in 1844.[1] Little use was made of it in Europe, however, until 1883, when a German army physician, Dr. Theodor Aschenbrandt, secured a supply of pure cocaine from the pharmaceutical firm of Merck and issued it to Bavarian soldiers during their autumn maneuvers. He reported beneficial effects on their ability to endure fatigue.[2]

Among those who read Dr. Aschenbrandt's account with fascination was a poverty-stricken twenty-eight-year-old Viennese neurologist, Dr. Sigmund Freud (whose subsequent ordeal with nicotine was recounted in Chapter 24). Young Freud at the time was suffering from depression, chronic fatigue, and other neurotic symptoms. "I have been reading about cocaine, the essential constituent of coca leaves, which some Indian tribes chew to enable them to resist privations and hardships," Freud wrote to his fiancée, Martha Bernays, on April 21, 1884. "I am procuring some myself and will try it with cases of heart disease and also of nervous exhaustion. . . ." [3] The account of Freud's experiences which follows is drawn largely from the three-volume *Life and Work of Sigmund Freud*, by Ernest Jones.

Freud "tried the effect of a twentieth of a gram [50 milligrams] and found it turned the bad mood he was in into cheerfulness, giving him the feeling of having dined well 'so that there is nothing at all one need bother about,' but without robbing him of any energy for exercise or work." [4]

In addition to taking cocaine himself, Freud offered some to his friend and associate, Dr. Ernst von Fleischl-Marxow, who was suffering from an exceedingly painful disease of the nervous system (which was later to prove fatal), and who was addicted to morphine. Freud also prescribed cocaine for a patient with gastric catarrh. The initial results in all three cases were favorable. Freud decided cocaine was "a magical drug," and he wrote his fiancée, Martha:

If it goes well I will write an essay on it and I expect it will win its place in therapeutics by the side of morphium and superior to it. I have other hopes and intentions about it. I take very small doses of it regularly against depression and against indigestion, and with the most brilliant success. . . . In short it is only now that I feel I am a doctor, since I have helped one patient and hope to help more. If things go on in this way we need have no concern about being able to come together and to stay in Vienna.[5]

Freud even sent some of his precious cocaine to Martha, "to make her strong and give her cheeks a red color." Indeed, Dr. Jones writes, "he pressed it on his friends and colleagues, both for themselves and their patients; he gave it to his sisters. In short, looked at from the vantage point of our present knowledge, he was rapidly becoming a public menace."[6]

In a subsequent letter to Martha, Freud wrote more on his personal experience with cocaine:

Woe to you, my Princess, when I come. I will kiss you quite red and feed you till you are plump. And if you are froward you shall see who is the stronger, a gentle little girl who doesn't eat enough or a big wild man *who has cocaine in his body.* [Italics in original.] In my last severe depression I took coca again and a small dose lifted me to the heights in a wonderful fashion. I am just now busy collecting the literature for a song of praise to this magical substance.[7]

Freud's haste in publishing his findings may astonish twentieth-century readers. On April 21, 1884, he was still only planning to secure some cocaine. On June 18, his essay was completed; and the "Song of Praise" to cocaine was published in the July 1884 issue of the *Centralblatt für die gesammte Therapie.*

This essay, Dr. Jones writes, had "a tone that never recurred in Freud's writings, a remarkable combination of objectivity with a personal warmth as if he were in love with the content itself. He used expressions uncommon in a scientific paper such as 'the most gorgeous excitement' that animals display after an injection of cocaine, and administering an 'offering' of it rather than a 'dose'; he heatedly rebuffed the 'slander' that had been published about this precious drug. This artistic presentation must have contributed much to the interest the essay aroused in Viennese and other medical circles. . . . He even gave an account of the religious observances connected with its use, and mentioned the mythical saga of how Manco Capac, the Royal Son of the Sun-God, had sent it as 'a gift from the gods to satisfy the hungry, forify the weary, and make the unfortunate forget their sorrows.' "[8]

More to the point, Freud described in detail the effects of small doses of cocaine on his own depression. These included "exhilaration and lasting euphoria, which in no way differs from the normal euphoria of the healthy person. . . . You perceive an increase of self-control and possess more vitality and capacity for work. . . . In other words, you are simply normal, and it is soon hard to believe that you are under the influence of any drug. . . . Long intensive mental or physical work is performed without any fatigue. . . . This result is enjoyed without any of the unpleasant after-effects that follow exhilaration brought about by alcohol. . . . Absolutely no craving for the further use of cocaine appears after the first, or even after repeated taking of the drug; one feels rather a certain curious aversion to it." [9] Cocaine, Freud concluded, was useful for "those functional states comprised under the name neurasthenia" [10]—Freud at this time had diagnosed his own depressions as neurasthenic—as well as for indigestion and for the withdrawal of morphine.

Freud also sought to inject cocaine directly into the area of a nerve to block intractable pain. In this he failed, but others succeeded;* and until better agents became available, cocaine was often used as local anesthesia for surgery.

Some of Freud's findings on cocaine as a psychoactive drug were amply confirmed by subsequent research. "The subjective effects of cocaine include an elevation of mood that often reaches proportions of euphoric excitement," Dr. Jaffe reported in Goodman and Gilman's textbook (1965). "It produces a marked decrease in hunger, an indifference to pain, and is reputed to be the most potent antifatigue agent known. The user enjoys a feeling of great muscular strength and increased mental capacity and greatly overestimates his capabilities. The euphoria is accompanied by generalized sympathetic stimulation. As is the case with amphetamine, a disturbed personality is not a prerequisite for cocaine-induced euphoria, and the drug is quite effective in relatively normal personalities." [11]

Freud's experience, however, proved to be only part of the story. In July 1885, a German authority on morphine addiction named Erlenmeyer launched the first of a series of attacks on cocaine as an addicting drug. In January 1886 Freud's friend Obersteiner, who had at first favored cocaine, reported that it produced severe mental disturbances similar to those seen in delirium tremens. Other attacks soon followed; and Freud himself was subjected to "grave reproaches." [12] Freud continued to praise cocaine as late as July 1887, when he published a final defense of the drug. But soon thereafter he discontinued all use of it both personally and professionally. Despite the fact that he had been taking cocaine periodically over a three-year span, he appears to have had no difficulty in stopping. His abandonment of cocaine was no doubt influenced in large part by the experience of Dr. von Fleischl-Marxow, the patient with whom Freud had shared his initial gram of cocaine.

Fleischl suffered from multiple tumors of various peripheral nerves— neuromata—which gave him excruciating pain. He took morphine for this pain. At first Freud's cocaine proved a welcome substitute for the morphine—but Fleischl found it necessary to escalate his cocaine dose.

* Among those who succeeded, as noted in Chapter 5, was the young American surgeon, Dr. W. S. Halsted.

After a year on cocaine he was taking a full gram of it daily—twenty times the dose Freud himself took from time to time. Indeed, Freud noted, Fleischl had spent $428 for a three-month supply of cocaine, an enormous sum in Vienna in those days. On June 8, 1885, Dr. Jones adds, "Freud wrote that the frightful doses had harmed Fleischl greatly and, although he kept sending Martha cocaine, he warned her against acquiring the habit." Thereafter Fleischl developed a full-fledged cocaine psychosis, "with white snakes creeping over his skin." [13] Freud and other physician friends nursed Fleischl faithfully, often throughout the long nights, but to little avail. In June 1885 Freud estimated that Fleischl could live six more months at most; he actually survived for six more pain-wracked years.

Nor was Fleischl's experience unique; subsequent observations were to reveal that repeated use of large doses of cocaine produces a characteristic paranoid psychosis in all or almost all users, and that the tendency to overuse is widespread. A peculiar characteristic of this psychosis is "formication"—the hallucination that ants, or insects, or (as in Fleischl's case) snakes, are crawling along the skin or under it.

Why was Freud, unlike his friend Fleischl, able to use modest doses of cocaine—30 to 50 milligrams injected under the skin—from time to time for three years without developing either a craving for the drug or a need to escalate the dose? At least three alternative explanations are available. Dr. Jones, a psychoanalyst, believed that it requires an "addictive personality" to establish an addiction; lacking an addictive personality, he declares, Freud did not become a cocaine addict. (He did, however, become addicted to cigars, as described in Chapter 24.) The other two explanations are pharmacological.

One holds that there must be some biochemical difference—perhaps a difference in enzymes—between people like Freud who can take a particular addicting drug without becoming addicted and people like Fleischl who escalate the dose and become addicted. This hypothetical difference in enzymes may (or may not) be hereditary. The third explanation relates the addiction (or lack of it) to dosages and frequency of use. Because Freud took cocaine only occasionally, according to this theory, he had no need to escalate his dose. And because he did not escalate the dose, he did not become addicted. Some other explanation, of course, may ultimately prove true.

By 1890, the addicting and psychosis-producing nature of cocaine was well understood in medical circles; yet for another twenty years it does not appear to have occurred to many people to demand a *law* against the drug.* In the United States, cocaine was widely used not only in

---

* Dr. Charles B. Towns wrote (1912): "When an overseer in the South will deliberately put cocaine into the rations of his Negro laborers in order to get more work

Coca-Cola but also in "tonics" and other patent medicines, including very popular "catarrh cures"—for, like the amphetamines, cocaine has the effect of reducing mucous membrane swelling and thus enlarging the nasal and bronchial passages. This property no doubt first gave users the idea of *sniffing* cocaine, a common form of cocaine use even today. "Most of the cases of the cocaine habit have been admittedly created by the so-called catarrh cures," Dr. Charles B. Towns wrote in *Century Magazine* in 1912, "and these contain only two to four percent of cocaine.* In the end, the snuffer of catarrh powders comes to demand undiluted cocaine." [15]

Cocaine addiction differs from opiate addiction, and from alcohol and barbiturate addiction, in at least two respects. A cocaine user, even after prolonged use of large doses, does not, if deprived of his drug, suffer from a dramatic withdrawal crisis like alcoholic delirium tremens or like the opiate withdrawal syndrome. The *physical* effects of cocaine withdrawal are minor. This has led many authorities, mistakenly, to classify cocaine as a nonaddicting drug. However, cocaine withdrawal is characterized by a profound psychological manifestation—*depression*—for which cocaine itself appears to the user to be the only remedy; cocaine addiction in this respect resembles tobacco addiction more closely than it resembles opiate addiction or alcoholism. The compulsion to resume cocaine is very strong.

Moreover, cocaine addiction can lead to a severe psychosis *while the user is still on the drug*. This is in contradistinction to the opiate withdrawal syndrome and to the delirium tremens of alcoholism or barbituarate addiction, which set in hours or days *after* the drug is withdrawn.

Decades ago, cocaine users discovered that a mixture of cocaine and morphine or heroin relieves the excess agitation and tension produced by large doses of pure cocaine. The users of morphine and heroin similarly discovered that the mixture increases both the "bang" or "rush" or "flash" and the mood elevation produced by their favorite drug. The combination came to be known as the "speedball," and it has long been popular among some addicts in Britain, the United States, and elsewhere.

Since 1914, the possession, sale, and giving away of cocaine have been subject to the same dire federal penalties as those governing morphine and heroin; and most state laws similarly identify cocaine as a "narcotic."

During the 1940s, 1950s, and most of the 1960s, the smuggling of cocaine into the United States was curtailed and the black market in cocaine was

---

out of them to meet a sudden emergency, it is time to have some policy of accounting for the sale of a drug like cocaine." [14]

* "Street cocaine" sold on the New York black market in 1970 was reported to contain about 6 percent pure cocaine.

relatively small. The reduced use of cocaine, however, can hardly be attributed, even in part, to law-enforcement efforts. Rather it was the result of pharmacological research. Cocaine was replaced by a new group of synthetic drugs, the amphetamines, which were available far more cheaply than cocaine after 1932, and which had certain other advantages over the natural imported product. Late in the 1960s, when narcotics law-enforcement agencies began cracking down heavily on the amphetamine black market, cocaine smuggling and cocaine use enjoyed a renaissance.

36.

The amphetamines

The drug now known as amphetamine was first synthesized in 1887;[1] but medical uses were not noted until 1927, when its effectiveness in raising blood pressure was discovered, as well as its effects in enlarging the nasal and bronchial passages and in stimulating the central nervous system. The drug was accordingly marketed in 1932, under the trade name Benzedrine.[2] In 1935, its effectiveness as a stimulant led physicians to try it, with excellent results, against a rare but serious disease, narcolepsy, the victims of which fall asleep repeatedly.

Other amphetamines, and other uses for these drugs, soon followed. In 1937 the discovery was made that the amphetamines have a paradoxical effect on some children whose functioning is impaired by an inability to concentrate. Instead of making them even more jittery, as might be expected, the amphetamines calm many of these children and notably improve their concentration and performance.

By the end of 1971, at least 31 amphetamine preparations (including amphetamine-sedative, amphetamine-tranquilizer, and amphetamine-analgesic combinations) were being distributed by 15 pharmaceutical companies.[3]

The more scientists learned about these new drugs, the closer the parallel with cocaine appeared. The following description of the psychic effects of a modest dose of amphetamine, written by Drs. Ian P. Innes and Mark Nickerson in Goodman and Gilman's textbook (1970), may be compared with Sigmund Freud's description of the effects of cocaine (see Chapter 35):

> The main results of an oral dose . . . are as follows: wakefulness, alertness, and a decreased sense of fatigue; elevation of mood, with increased initiative, confidence, and ability to concentrate; often elation and euphoria; increase in motor and speech activity. Performance of only simple mental tasks is improved; and, although more work may be accomplished, the number of errors is not necessarily decreased. Physical performance, for example, in athletics, is improved. These effects are not invariable, and may be reversed by overdosage or repeated usage.[4]

Large doses of cocaine, it will be recalled, are followed by depression. Precisely the same proved true of the amphetamines: "Prolonged use or large doses are nearly always followed by mental depression and fatigue.

Many individuals given amphetamine experience headache, palpitation, dizziness, vasomotor disturbances, agitation, confusion, dysphoria, apprehension, delirium, or fatigue." [5]

Cocaine, it will also be recalled, first came into common use after a German army physician issued it to Bavarian soldiers. During World War II, the American, British, German, and Japanese armed forces similarly issued amphetamines to their men to counteract fatigue, elevate mood, and heighten endurance. In at least two respects, the amphetamines proved superior to cocaine. First, they can be taken orally in tablet form; cocaine is poorly absorbed from the gastrointestinal tract and is therefore usually either injected under the skin or into a vein, or else sniffed. Second, the amphetamines taken orally have a much longer duration of effectiveness—seven hours or so—while cocaine must be taken at more frequent intervals for a sustained effect.

After World War II, many physicians prescribed the amphetamines routinely for depression. In many cases they proved worthless or even harmful. In certain cases, however, they proved helpful during the depressive phase of a manic-depressive psychosis; and in certain cases patients unable to concentrate on their work, because of the kind of "neurasthenic" depression and fatigue from which Sigmund Freud suffered, reported that the drug elevated their mood just enough to enable them to work effectively—as cocaine had aided Freud.

Just as cocaine and heroin users learned that a combination of the two drugs (the speedball) provided results superior to either drug taken alone, so some psychiatrists and pharmacologists concluded on the basis of clinical experience that a combination of an amphetamine and a barbiturate or tranquilizer secured improved effects in some cases of depression. This superiority has not been fully established through adequately controlled, double-blind tests, in which neither the physician who administers the drug nor the patient taking it knows whether medication or an inert substance (placebo) is being taken. Nevertheless, Dexamyl and other combinations of this kind are still commonly prescribed by physicians, not only against chronic fatigue and against depression but also as supposed aids to dieting.

Do amphetamine users escalate their doses, as is so often the case with cocaine users? Not always. A small daily dose of an amphetamine, for example, may continue to be effective for years for narcolepsy and among those children for whom the drug has a calming effect. Some patients who occasionally use an amphetamine for fatigue or depression report that the same modest dose remains effective year after year. Other users escalate their dose rapidly to enormous levels—swallowing whole handfuls of amphetamine tablets instead of only one or two. The eventual outcome is often an amphetamine psychosis very similar to the cocaine psychosis from which Fleischl suffered—even to the feeling of ants, insects, or snakes crawling over or under the skin.

Side by side with the expansion of the legal market for prescribed amphetamines after World War II, a modest black market in the drugs also grew up. Early black-market patrons included in particular truck drivers trying to maintain schedules which called for long over-the-road hauls without adequate rest periods. Soon truck stops along the main transcontinental routes dispensed amphetamines as well as coffee and caffeine tablets (see Chapter 22) to help the drivers stay awake. Students, who had long used caffeine tablets, now turned instead to these new amphetamine "pep pills" when cramming for exams. The use of amphetamines by athletes and by businessmen (and their secretaries) was reported as early as 1940.[6]

Periodic law-enforcement drives to curb black-market amphetamines proved ineffectual, or perhaps even counterproductive; for the publicity surrounding the arrests served to advertise the product—and the arrests, by increasing the risk and therefore the price, served to attract additional entrepreneurs. When amphetamines were hard to get from other sources, users purchased Benzedrine inhalers, broke them open, and ingested the substantial quantities of amphetamine found inside. Later the Benzedrine inhalers were withdrawn from the market; they were replaced by inhalers that do not contain amphetamine.

Cocaine users also turned to the black market for amphetamines, and used them much as they had formerly used cocaine. The cost of the amphetamines is trivial—as little as 75 cents per thousand tablets at wholesale, even during the 1960s. Thus peddlers could sell black-market amphetamines at a fraction of the cost of imported cocaine and still make a substantial profit. The "speedball" of the 1960s contained heroin and an amphetamine rather than heroin and cocaine.

In 1965, amendments to the federal food-and-drug laws were passed, designed to curb the black market in amphetamines as well as in barbiturates and other psychoactive drugs. The amendments did indeed make it harder to divert legally manufactured amphetamines into the black market. A second effect, however, was to stimulate greatly the illegal manufacture of amphetamines in kitchens and garages within the United States. This is a topic to which we shall return.

37.

Enter the "speed freak"

Amphetamines taken orally can be used in excess with unfortunate results; but enormous quantities of oral amphetamines were consumed in the United States during the 1940s and 1950s with apparently little misuse. As late as 1963, indeed, the American Medical Association's Council on Drugs, while recognizing the possibility of misuse, reported that "at this time compulsive abuse of the amphetamines constitutes . . . a small problem [in the United States]." [1] Much the same finding was reported from Sweden (see Chapter 39).

The intravenous injection of large doses of amphetamines, in contrast, is among the most disastrous forms of drug use yet devised. The early history of amphetamine mainlining has been explored by a California criminologist and authority on illicit drug use, Dr. Roger C. Smith, in an unpublished study he made available for this Report. Dr. Smith is now director of Marin Open House, a comprehensive center for drug and other problems in San Rafael, California. The Smith study was a part of the San Francisco Amphetamine Research Project, financed by the National Institute of Mental Health and launched by Dr. Smith in May 1968, in cooperation with the Haight-Ashbury Medical Clinic in San Francisco. Much of this chapter is drawn from Dr. Smith's study, "The Marketplace of Speed: Violence and Compulsive Methamphetamine Abuse," and from a report by a California psychiatrist, Dr. John C. Kramer, entitled "Introduction to Amphetamine Abuse," published in the *Journal of Psychedelic Drugs* in 1969. Dr. Kramer began his amphetamine research while he was on the staff of the California Rehabilitation Center in Corona, California—a center in which "speed freaks" as well as heroin addicts are incarcerated; he is at this writing on the faculty of the University of California at Irvine and on the staff of Dr. Jerome H. Jaffe's Special Action Office for Drug Abuse Prevention in Washington, D.C.

The earliest reference to the intravenous use of amphetamines that Dr. Smith was able to unearth concerned groups of American servicemen stationed in Korea and Japan during the early 1950s.[2] These men were said to have learned to mix amphetamines—then nicknamed "splash"— with heroin and to inject the combination. This was, in effect, the traditional "speedball," with amphetamine substituted for cocaine. Servicemen brought the custom home with them after the Korean War. No doubt other small groups also learned to mainline amphetamine, alone or with heroin, during the 1950s; but no public furor was raised against the practice—and it did not spread alarmingly—until the 1960s.

Sigmund Freud's first dispensing of cocaine to a patient, it will be recalled, was to help his pain-wracked friend, Fleischl-Marxow, get along without morphine. During the late 1950s, in the San Francisco Bay Area, a number of physicians prescribed amphetamine injections for the same purpose—or allegedly for the same purpose.

Dr. Smith reports there is little doubt that *some* Bay Area physicians were sincere in this use of amphetamines as a treatment for heroin addiction. They were nevertheless arrested for supplying drugs to heroin addicts. Other California physicians, it appears, were less conscientious. Some of them, for example, prescribed Methedrine (methamphetamine) "for heroin addiction" without even examining patients to see if they had needle marks. One Methedrine user told Dr. Smith:

Then there was a doctor . . . who would write anything for anybody at anytime and he was making $7 a visit and on the day we went down there he wrote almost 400 prescriptions at $7 a head. So you can imagine how much money he was making. He made $2,800 that one day and they used to make caravans down there and even from [Los Angeles] to his place. You'd get within two blocks of his office and you'd start seeing people you knew from all over.[3]

One heroin addict reported that for $6 or $7 he could get from one physician a prescription for 100 Methedrine ampules—plus hypodermic needles and sedatives. He could then sell enough of the ampules at $1 or $1.50 apiece to make a living. "In many instances," Dr. Smith adds, "heroin addicts who had formerly engaged in burglary, bad checks, credit cards, or a variety of other 'hustles,' began to make money exclusively by sales of Methedrine."[4] It was at about this time, in the early 1960s, that Methedrine came to be known as "speed"—perhaps an allusion to its use in the traditional "speedball." More recently, "speed" has come to refer to *any* amphetamine which is injected intravenously.

In addition to the "scrip-writer" physicians described above, some San Francisco pharmacies began selling injectable amphetamines without a prescription, or on the basis of crudely forged prescriptions, or on a telephoned "prescription" from a user posing as a physician. Federal, state, and local law-enforcement agencies cracked down on such practices in 1962 and 1963; physicians and pharmacists alike were convicted of law violations, accompanied by widespread publicity. Thus the delights of amphetamine mainlining, previously known primarily to heroin addicts, became a matter of common knowledge and general interest.

When the injectable amphetamine scandal broke publicly in 1962, and federal and state agents descended on the manufacturers, Abbott withdrew Desoxyn ampules from the market. In July 1963, Burroughs Well-come similarly withdrew Methedrine ampules from distribution through retail pharmacies, but continued to make them available to hospitals as an adjunct to surgical anesthesia and for other essential uses. Withdrawal of legal supplies meeting FDA standards of purity for injectable products marked a turn for the worse. The black market next secured nonsterile am-phetamines at trivial cost in vast quantity from large chemical manu-facturing companies which shipped in bulk. The infection rate among addicts no doubt rose when these nonsterile products took the place of FDA-approved ampules.

The 1962 crackdown on legal sources of amphetamines also triggered the emergence of illicit factories, called "speed labs," where speed was manufactured. "According to many of the users interviewed during the course of this study," Dr. Smith reports, " 'speed labs' began to operate as early as 1962, and by 1963 several labs were in operation in the San Francisco Bay Area. Because of the shortage of speed in other cities on the West Coast [a shortage caused by the withdrawal of Burroughs Wellcome and Abbott ampules and by the crackdown on physicians and pharmacies], the manufacture and distribution of speed became an extremely profitable enterprise, and opened up new sources of revenue within the San Francisco drug scene." [5] The further history of these labs will be reviewed in Chapter 40.*

By 1965 or 1966, the full impact of speed mainlining became visible. A report entitled "Amphetamine Abuse: Pattern and Effects of High Doses Taken Internally," by Drs. John C. Kramer, Vitezslav Fischman, and Don C. Littlefield in the *Journal of the American Medical Association* for July 31, 1967, outlined the problem—and Dr. Kramer's 1969 paper, cited above, supplied later details.

The first use of intravenous amphetamine, Dr. Kramer notes, is "an ecstatic experience," and the user's first thought is, "Where has this been all my life?" Dr. Kramer goes on, "The experience somehow differs from the effects of oral amphetamines not only quantitatively but also quali-tatively." After this first experience, the user mainlines intermittently for a time; "doses probably equivalent to twenty to forty milligrams per

---

* The 1965 amendments to the federal drug laws, by requiring manufacturers and wholesalers to keep records of all shipments, made it more difficult to divert legal amphetamines to the black market. This served to protect the "speed labs" from low-price legal competition and enabled them to raise prices. American black-market operators got around the new law, however, by placing large orders for legal ampheta-mines to be sent to addresses in Mexico; they then smuggled the American ampheta-mines back into the United States. (The same dodge had been used by morphine traffickers during the first years after passage of the Harrison Act of 1914.) When law-enforcement officers at length caught up with this practice, excessive shipments to Mexico were curbed. This further protected the black-market speed labs in the United States from competition.

injection may be taken once or a very few times over a day or two. Days or weeks may intervene between sprees. Gradually the sprees become longer and the intervening periods shorter; doses become higher and injections more frequent." [6] The sequence recalls Dr. von Fleischl-Marxow's experience with cocaine in Vienna in the 1880s. "After a period of several months," Dr. Kramer continues, "the final pattern is reached in which the user (now called a 'speed-freak') injects his drug many times a day, each dose in the hundreds of milligrams, and remains awake continuously for three to six days, getting gradually more tense, tremulous and paranoid as the 'run' progresses. The runs are interrupted by bouts of very profound sleep (called 'crashing') which last a day or two. Shortly after waking . . . the drug is again injected and a new run starts. The periods of continuous wakefulness may be prolonged to weeks if the user attempts to sleep even as little as an hour a day." [7]

Dr. Kramer cautions against the simplistic view that anyone who once shoots amphetamine intravenously inevitably follows this pattern of escalation. "There are individuals who have tried it once or several times and have chosen not to continue." [8] Nevertheless, the tendency to progress to compulsive use is very strong.

The desired effects of speed-injecting, Dr. Kramer continues, "are extremely vulnerable to the impingement of tolerance. It takes ever more drug to recreate this chemical nirvana. It is the desire to re-experience the flash and the desire to remain euphoric, and to avoid the fatigue and the depression of the 'coming down,' which drives the users to persist and necessarily to increase their dose and frequency of injection. And it is this persistence of use and these large doses which bring on all the other effects of these drugs." [9]

Dr. Roger C. Smith here adds a highly significant fact about the intravenous-amphetamine euphoria. Many young people in our culture are brought up with a seriously damaged self-image. The methods of discipline imposed upon them as children, or other factors, convince them of their own inherent worthlessness, though they may mask this sense of worthlessness with bravado. "Many of the young people who are currently involved in the speed scene," Dr. Smith notes, "report that they were initially attracted to the drug because of the instant improvement noted in self-image. Many suffered from feelings of inferiority and lack of self-worth, which manifested itself in chronic, and often debilitating, depression.

"Many [of these young people with damaged self-images] had experimented with a variety of depressants, including heroin, barbiturates, and alcohol, but found that this only increased their feelings of depression and self-deprecation. The alleviation of depression brought about by the use of speed may well be the key factor in determining why *some* individuals progress from occasional to compulsive use of the drug" [10]— though Dr. Smith also emphasizes that other factors may come into play as well.

In any event, Dr. Kramer points out, the improvement of self-image and relief from depression is purchased at a very high price if intravenous amphetamines are the mode of relief. Whether or not small oral doses of amphetamine are effective aids to dieting, the large doses taken during speed "runs" produce profound anorexia (lack of appetite). "Users uniformly lose weight during periods of abuse. Appetite suppression may be so profound that users may find the very act of swallowing difficult." [11] Some users force themselves to take small amounts of highly nutritious foods or beverages, or inject themselves with vitamins and dietary supplements. Upon awakening after a prolonged speed run, a user may eat large amounts. But even so, "undernutrition and malnutrition result, and undoubtedly complicate all the other effects of high dose amphetamine use." [12]

Sleep deprivation similarly exacerbates and complicates the direct pharmacological effects of the drug. "The observation that many of the physical and psychological symptoms are largely dissipated after sleeping for a day or two suggests that the insomnia alone is a major contributor to the syndrome," Dr. Kramer notes. But, he adds, "the fact that some symptoms persist after weeks or months of abstinence indicates that sleep deprivation is not alone responsible. Considering that the usual pattern seen during well-established high dose abuse is of three to six days of wakefulness followed by one or two days of sleep, . . . users spend about one-fourth of their time in sleep, about the same proportion as non-users only distributed differently." [13]

A paranoid psychosis, similar to the cocaine psychosis, is the almost inevitable result of long-term, high-dose, intravenous speed injection. This psychosis "can be precipitated by either a single large dose or by chronic moderate doses," [14] Dr. Kramer adds.

Typical features of the speed psychosis include feelings of persecution, feelings that people are talking about you behind your back (delusions of reference), and feelings of omnipotence.* Unlike paranoid schizophrenics,

---

* The formication hallucination first noted by Freud's friend Fleischl—that is, imaginary snakes or insects crawling on or under the skin—also characterizes the speed psychosis. Speed freaks call them "crank bugs," Dr. Roger C. Smith reports. "It is common to see speed freaks with open running sores or scabs on their faces or arms as a result of picking or cutting out these hallucinated crank bugs." He quotes an experienced twenty-four-year-old speed freak on the subject: "It's just that when you're shooting speed constantly you start to feel like there's bugs going around under your skin and you know they're not there, but you pick at them anyway. . . . Once in a while you'll see a little black spot and you'll watch it for ten minutes to see if it moves. If it doesn't move it isn't alive. You can feel them on your skin. I'm always trying to pick them out of my eyebrows." [15]

however, "speed freaks" are usually aware that these feelings are drug-induced; that is, they retain insight. "High-dose intravenous users of amphetamines generally accept that they will sooner or later experience paranoia. Aware of this, they are usually able to discount for it." Nevertheless, Dr. Kramer adds, "when drug use has become very intense or toward the end of a long run even a well-practiced intellectual awareness may fail and the user may respond to his delusional system." [16] Dr. Kramer cites others as believing that the drug merely brings into the open pre-existing paranoid tendencies. On the basis of his own experience with a large number of high-dose users, Dr. Kramer expresses the opinion, which he agrees is not testable, that despite differences in vulnerability to the paranoid effect, "anyone given a large enough dose over a long enough time will become psychotic." [17]

Dr. Smith cites numerous examples of this paranoia of the speed freak. "Each user has several entertaining stories relating to something which he did in order to protect himself from the police or secret agents whom he suspected were about to arrest him. In some instances the individual will lock himself in a room and refuse to come out, will arm himself with a knife or gun, or may, on rare occasions, actually assault a suspected informant or policeman. Tales of such activity have now become an integral part of the lore of the speed scene. . . ." [18] The fact that the speed scene is actually heavily infiltrated with informers and narcotics officers does nothing, of course, to dispel this paranoia.

The paranoid behavior of the speed freak may at times look superficially like murderous aggression. Dr. Smith quotes a "veteran" of the speed scene on this point:

It happens quite often by mistake where somebody's all jacked up and has been for say a week, maybe two or three weeks, and somebody burns [cheats] them, they may go crash for a day or so to get their head back together somewhat, and when they get up they don't remember too much what the person looked like or who the person was, they're just out running around. I've seen people who are running around on the streets with a gun under their jacket, and they run up behind somebody and say ". . . that looks like him—long blond hair. We got you." and then "Sorry, wrong one" and go on down the street and on to the next guy with long blond hair and stop him.[19]

An even greater hazard of violence, Dr. Smith adds, accompanies the mainlining of amphetamines along with barbiturates:

In the course of our research, we have interviewed numerous individuals who regularly combine speed with barbiturates, boiled down and injected intravenously, who have exhibited highly irrational, often violent behavior. Barbiturates are commonly used to terminate the speed run and induce sleep, although they are sometimes used intermittently as the drug of choice. Even the most committed speed user agrees that individuals shooting [short-acting] barbiturates (sometimes as much as 10 Seconals per injection) are the most dangerous and irrational individuals in the drug scene. The barbiturates produce a state of disinhibition similar to alcohol intoxication, with slurred speech, staggering, and often, surliness and aggressiveness which can easily be escalated to physical violence, particularly when used in combination with speed.[20]

In support of this view, Dr. Smith quotes a drug user's description of one of his friends:

He's a very nice person, and extremely generous; however, when he gets all jacked up and he is wired [stimulated with speed] and is doing reds [Seconals], then he is in trouble. Because pretty quick he's got a shot gun and everybody else has got a shot gun. I've seen him out in front of . . . the freeway entrance herding the hitch-hikers away because he's paranoid of them. At four o'clock in the afternoon, with a full length shot gun, he's screaming "move on, you can't stand there, move on." That's just the way he gets.[21]

Another user adds: "Barbs make you want to get out on the street and start kicking asses. Speed gives you the energy to get up and do it." [22]

Contrary to a widespread impression, Dr. Smith goes on to explain, the confirmed *heroin* addict is a highly skilled individual. "It is his skill as a 'hustler' which economically sustains the heroin marketplace." [23] It is the speed freak who is in fact unskilled and poorly adapted to the drug scene.

He is generally white, essentially middle-class in terms of education, family background and attitudes, and totally lacking in the kind of criminal skills which are essential to survival in a criminal environment. As critical as his lack of criminal skills is his failure to understand the values and norms traditionally associated with criminally oriented groups or subcultures. These values and norms are often antithetical to those of conventional society, but nonetheless they serve approximately the same function, namely, to offer guidance to participants and to control behavior which would be harmful to the group as a whole. . . .

While there is a backlog of experience and tradition which the heroin addict in neighborhoods of high use can draw on, there is nothing similar in the speed culture, which emerged in its present form in late 1967, and is still undergoing rapid changes. Since there is little dependence on legitimate business for the exchange of merchandise for money, and very little integration with other illegal enterprises as one traditionally finds in heroin cultures, the "hustling" which does take place is sporadic, unskilled and predatory in nature, often directed toward fellow users and dealers, and only occasionally does it involve others outside the scene.

The speed freak is, in many ways, an outcast in a society of outcasts. He is regarded as a fool by heroin addicts, as insane and violent by those using the psychedelics or marijuana, and as a "bust" by non-drug-using hustlers.[24]

Coming from a middle-class background, the speed freak attempts initially to support himself by "legitimate" means, "such as panhandling, selling underground newspapers, or working." But speed tends to incapacitate him for both legitimate employment and "hustling":

> The compulsive speed user is usually incapable of hustles which demand composure, since he is highly agitated, suspicious and fearful that at any moment he may be detected, or the drug effect may leave him so paranoid that he would not take advantage of opportunities because they appear "too easy" or a "setup." Because of his compulsive verbalization, hyperactivity, emaciated physical state and bizarre demeanor, few businessmen will accept checks or credit cards from him. In our experience, many "speed freaks" who have attempted to pass bad checks have become panicked at a request for identification, convinced that his intended victim suspects him and will report him to police. In several instances, users have presented a check and immediately fled.
>   Because of the style of life which most compulsive users are involved in, their demeanor is overtly suspicious. While most heroin addicts can operate without fear of detection because of the drug effect, the speed user fits the popular stereotype of a "dope fiend." [25]

Cut off in these ways from both licit and illicit employment, Dr. Smith continues, the speed freak survives by sponging on others and by dealing in drugs. Lacking skills and standards, he cheats. And the victims of his cheating are generally speed freaks like himself, paranoid like himself, on the verge of violence like himself. The violence that ultimately emerges—a high level of violence, including rape, mayhem, homicide—arises when the direct drug effect, the paranoia, occurs in a chaotic community where almost everybody is simultaneously engaged in sponging on everybody else, cheating everybody else—and suspecting everybody else. This is the scene that leads even confirmed drug users to conclude that "speed is the worst."

Contrary to a popular belief, however, speed—even in enormous doses —very rarely kills. Dr. Smith, for example, cites one case in which a speed freak injected 15,000 milligrams of the drug—15 full grams—in a twenty-four-hour period without acute illness. For neophytes, it has been stated, "death has followed rapid injection of 120 mg"; but "doses of 400 to 500 milligrams have been survived." [26] "Very few deaths have been recorded in which overdose of amphetamines has been causal," [27] Dr. Kramer declares.

That even massive doses of speed rarely kill is surely a tribute to the inherent toughness of the human body. That the human mind can ultimately recover even from prolonged amphetamine paranoia is an equal tribute to its toughness—yet that appears to be the case.

"What has been most striking in our experience," Dr. Kramer declares —and Dr. Smith agrees—"has been the slow but rather complete recovery of users who, according to their own descriptions and that of others, had become rather thoroughly disorganized and paranoid prior to their detention."[28] The more florid symptoms fade within a few days or weeks. "Some confusion, some memory loss, and some delusional ideas may remain for perhaps six to twelve months. After that time, though there may be some residual symptoms, they are slight, and not disabling, and are noticed primarily by the (now abstinent) user himself. Most commonly, ex-users report slightly greater difficulty in remembering."[29]

Following full or almost full recovery, curiously enough, ex-users also report a personality change that they deem favorable. Many of them, it will be recalled, were depressed, withdrawn, silent, and lacking in self-esteem before turning to speed. "As a group they describe being more open and talkative than they had been prior to their use of amphetamines. They like the result and declare with certainty that it is due to their experience with amphetamines."[30]

"Anyone concerned with the welfare of amphetamine users," Dr. Kramer goes on to stress, "and the users themselves, should recognize that most, if not all, can recover from even the most profound intellectual disorganization and psychosis given six months or a year of abstinence."[31] This message, in addition to being true, is of considerably more public-health significance than the false popular slogan, "Speed kills."

The problem is how to achieve prolonged abstinence. Many speed users, like most of the heroin users, Dr. Smith notes, have tried repeatedly to stop by a conscious act of will. Few succeed. Their withdrawal misery is too great. "Many users who attempt abstinence find it difficult because of the fatigue which results, extreme at first, gradually diminishing but persistent, perhaps for months,"[32] Dr. Kramer adds.

Abstinence is often forced on a speed freak by a prison sentence, or by incarceration under a so-called civil commitment program, or by commitment to a mental hospital.

"No data has yet been collected to indicate the long-term value of such enforced abstinence," Dr. Kramer concedes; but on the basis of his own experience on the staff of the California Rehabilitation Center he is highly skeptical. "Certainly, many who have been incarcerated have returned to their drug use upon release."[33] Thus the revolving-door pattern so familiar to heroin addicts may be the future of speed freaks as well. A person genuinely concerned for the welfare of speed freaks, Dr. Kramer sadly notes, is "in a bind. Users do not readily volunteer for care, but commitment programs offer little besides enforced abstinence. Should the user be permitted to live in the limbo of his drug or forced into the limbo of an institution? Can voluntary programs be devised which are sufficiently useful and attractive that users will seek them out and persist in their program? Can commitment programs be devised which do not resemble slightly benign prisons? Or, do we just let the user seek heaven or hell on his own terms while the community offers help only on its own terms?" [34] Dr. Kramer poses these questions; neither he nor Dr. Roger C. Smith nor we have any glib answers to offer. Drug-scene participants themselves, however, may currently be finding answers (see Chapter 42).

38.

How speed was popularized

The damage done by heroin, as demonstrated in Part I, is largely traceable to antinarcotics laws and policies and to the heroin black market that has grown up under the shelter of those laws and policies. The damage done by LSD, as we shall also see, is in large part a function of laws and attitudes. This is certainly *not* true of the speed phenomenon. Unlike the heroin and the LSD cases, it is large intravenous doses of the drug itself that have devastating effects in the case of speed. But laws and policies were certainly responsible in considerable part for *popularizing* speed.

One instance of this, the antispeed campaign launched by the United States Food and Drug Administration in 1962 and 1963, has already been cited. It was the publicity accompanying this campaign that alerted a whole generation of young people to the perils (and pleasures) of speed. As in other cases described earlier and to be described in subsequent chapters, the peril became the lure.

A somewhat different process helped to popularize speed following San Francisco's 1967 "Summer of Love." That summer many thousands of adolescents took off for the Haight-Ashbury district, the center of the "hippie movement," where marijuana and LSD were freely available. This migration, and others like it, will be discussed at length in Part IX. There was relatively little speed, and little violence, that first summer.* The sheer size of the immigration, however, overwhelmed the LSD-using "flower people" who had established the Haight-Ashbury subculture. In increasing numbers, they moved into the hills. Their places were taken by young people looking, not for love and mind-expansion, but for drug "kicks." Marijuana and LSD faded into the background; speed took over. New times, new customs, new participants, new needs, new wants—and a new drug to meet those needs and wants.

The conversion to speed was facilitated, moreover, by the antimarijuana and anti-LSD campaigns being waged at the time. The "LSD chromosome scare," to be discussed in Part VII, was a central feature of this campaign. Many young people heeded the warnings with which the newspapers, magazines, and radio and TV programs were flooded, and gave up LSD. In its place they turned to speed. The change was for the worse.

Users of marijuana and LSD recognized and publicized the overwhelm-

* By September 1967, however, one-third of 413 residents of the Haight-Ashbury area had injected amphetamines intravenously at least once.[1]

[291]

ing hazards of speed in an unsuccessful attempt to turn the tide. Thus the poet Allen Ginsberg, the author of "Howl," remarked in an interview in the Los Angeles *Free Press,* an underground newspaper: "Let's issue a general declaration to all the underground community, *contra speedamos ex cathedra.* Speed is antisocial, paranoid making, it's a drag, bad for your body, bad for your mind, generally speaking, in the long run uncreative and it's a plague in the whole dope industry. All the nice gentle dope fiends are getting screwed up by the real horror monster Frankenstein speed freaks who are going around stealing and bad mouthing everybody." [2] This quote from Ginsberg was widely publicized throughout the underground press. Timothy Leary, the Beatles, and the Mothers of Invention also warned against speed.[3] The overground press, however, continued to rail against LSD—and marijuana.

Police and narcotics officials, too, must bear some of the responsibility. Their main concern at the time was certainly marijuana and LSD, the traditional "hippie" drugs. While they searched for caches of those drugs, speed took over. A seventeen-year-old girl whose friends had used speed remarked: "Some police officers we interviewed said pot was deadly and addictive! When kids try it and see it's all a lie they figure the stuff about speed is false, too." [4]

Two psychiatrists, Drs. James R. Allen and Louis Jolyon West, and a medical student, Joshua Kaufman, after a study of adolescents who ran away to the Haight-Ashbury in the summer of 1967, made the same point in more general terms: "The horrible reactions to marijuana predicted by various authorities were virtually never seen. The runaways generally took this to mean that all the widely advertised dangers of drugs were establishment lies. This further alienated them from the social structure and made them more willing to experiment with all sorts of chemicals." [5]

Even the warning, "Speed kills," may have played its subtle role in popularizing speed. The 1970 *Interim Report* of Canada's Commission of Inquiry into the Non-Medical Use of Drugs (popularly known as the Le Dain Commission) comments on this possibility:

Some "speed" users who inject almost suicidal doses of methamphetamine into their veins without any regard for their safety and health, may actually be trying to test the truth of the youth slogan "Speed Kills". The role of the doomed person who is at once a martyr sacrificing himself, a hero braving the confrontation with certain destruction and a gambler playing dice with death, is a role which seems to have a strong seductive pull for some young people who are morbidly hungry for compassion, admiration and excitement. For these individuals the slogan "Speed Kills", may, paradoxically, carry more attractive than deterrent power—and thus may not serve the purpose for which it is being promoted.[6]

Sound public policy, the speed phenomenon suggests, would dictate telling young people the truth. They should be informed, for example, that speed, though it very rarely kills, is far more damaging than marijuana. But most drug propaganda campaigns try to keep this a secret— for it may also reveal to young people that marijuana is far less damaging than speed.

We shall return to this theme—the many ways in which laws, policies, and propaganda campaigns serve to encourage a shift from less dangerous to more dangerous drugs—in subsequent chapters of this Report.

39.

The Swedish experience

During the past few years, the American public has been warned of what happened to amphetamines in Sweden. Sweden, we have been told, was so blind to the hazards of the amphetamines that in 1965 these drugs were made available free of charge on the Swedish health plan. The results were 10,000 or 20,000 amphetamine "abusers" springing up practically overnight in a small country of 7,000,000. Now (the story goes) Sweden has banned amphetamines altogether, even on prescription. The Nixon administration's 1969–1970 drug bill proposed that the United States also prohibit amphetamine prescriptions except for a few special conditions—thus profiting from the Swedish experience.

The actual Swedish amphetamine experience, investigated there for this Consumers Union Report, suggests a very different perspective.

Amphetamine was first placed on sale in Sweden in 1938, three years after its introduction into the practice of medicine in the United States.[1] The Swedes, however, were much more prompt in recognizing the potential hazards of the drug; in 1939, though sales were still very small, they placed amphetamines on the list of drugs available only on prescription—a step that the United States did not take until 1954.

Swedish physicians apparently found the drug useful, for by 1942 they were prescribing it to about 3 percent of the population.[2]

Some 6,000,000 doses were prescribed during the year. A survey[3] indicated that most Swedish users were using amphetamine sensibly and in moderation:

- 140,000 were occasional users, taking four amphetamine tablets or fewer per year. No doubt, like Americans at the same time, they used amphetamine on rare days when they had to work longer than usual, or faced some extraordinary challenge, or woke up depressed and out of sorts and needed something to "pull themselves together."
- 60,000 others were also occasional users, but with somewhat greater frequency; their usage ranged from five times a year to twice a month.
- 4,000 users took amphetamine only once a week or so, but often took two or three tablets at a time—perhaps for a Saturday-night "high."
- 3,000 users might be described as "borderline." Their frequency of use varied from several times a week to daily—and they sometimes took from five to ten tablets in a single day.
- 200 users—less than a tenth of one percent—could properly be la-

beled "abusers." They took from ten to a hundred or more amphetamine tablets a day, more or less regularly.

This spectrum of use suggests that amphetamines prescribed by physicians are drugs with only a modest potential for misuse. The figures may be contrasted with the estimated 10 to 12 percent of alcohol users who become problem drinkers or alcoholics, and the estimated one percent who become skid-row alcoholics.

The Swedish authorities, however, were not comforted by such statistical comparisons. Warnings against the amphetamines were circulated to all practicing physicians—and in 1944 the prescribing of amphetamines was placed under much more rigid legal restrictions.

The new restrictive measures, of course,.engendered nationwide publicity and once more alerted Swedes of all ages to the remarkable effects of the amphetamines. Thus at a time when these drugs were still known to only a minority in the United States, in Sweden they had achieved the status of near-universal familiarity, as a result of repressive measures.

The first effects of the tighter restrictions appeared to be favorable. "Sales dropped for a few years by one-half," [4] Professor Gunnar Inghe of the world-renowned Karolinska Institute in Stockholm reports. But, as in the United States and other countries where the authorities rely on drug repression, undesirable side effects of the repressive measures made their appearance: increased use, a black market in amphetamines, the rise of an amphetamine-centered subculture, and the appearance of the "speed freak."

In the middle of the 1940s, [Professor Inghe continues,] it became obvious that misuse of central stimulants was now taking shape in gangs on [a] collective basis, at first especially among Bohemians, writers, actors, musicians and other artists and their sycophants and admirers. At first there was only oral administration. Among the misusers there were however a few morphinists, and probably in the early fifties subcutaneous and later intravenous injection of central stimulants started. These forms of administration have gradually become the most common among large-dose addicts. Misuse had now very obviously started spreading among asocial and criminal groups, among whom it can be said to have become endemic. In the middle of the fifties instances of breaking into chemists' shops, forging of prescriptions, etc. became common, the number of narcotic gangs increased and the seizing of smuggled tablets started.[5]

Each of these incidents, of course, was accompanied by widespread publicity; indeed, the antiamphetamine publicity in effect took the place of paid advertising in maintaining a booming sale of black-market amphetamines year after year.

The drive against smuggled amphetamine tablets no doubt helped raise prices and attract more smugglers, as in the United States. High prices also encouraged the switch from oral use to mainlining. In addition, however—as in the United States—repression and high prices led to the popularization of amphetamine substitutes: cocaine in the United States, phenmetrazine (sold under the trade name Preludin) in Sweden.

Preludin was introduced into Sweden in 1955.* "It was observed at once," Professor Inghe reports, "that this drug produced euphoria. It became rapidly popular in addict circles in preference to other central stimulants which it replaced." [6] The parallel between Swedish and American policies and results is thus complete. The only difference is that the Swedes were far ahead of the Americans. The Swedes instituted anti-amphetamine measures somewhat earlier—and thus popularized both the amphetamines and amphetamine substitutes somewhat earlier.

In 1959 the Swedes took the next obvious step. They subjected Preludin to the same strict legal controls as amphetamine, morphine, and heroin. A special prosecuting attorney was also appointed to concentrate on drug-law enforcement. "Since then, however," Professor Inghe reports sadly, "illegal import of Preludin has increased steadily." Originally "it came from the Boehringer factories in Germany." When the Swedes put economic and diplomatic pressure on the German government—much as the United States has been pressuring the Turks and the French to cut off opium and heroin trafficking—the smugglers switched their source of supply from Germany to Spain. Pressure on Spain was also effective. "Next came the smuggling of Preludin tablets from Belgium and various other countries, notably Italy," [7] Professor Inghe states. Other amphetamine substitutes also became popular. "Phenmetrazine [Preludin] is still the most in demand," Professor Inghe reported in November 1968, "but amphetamine, methamphetamine, dexamphetamine, methylphenidate, and other drugs are used as well. Recent reports tell of an increasing abuse of weight-reducing preparations, which include diethylpropion [Tenuate, Tepanil]. . . . The misusers themselves have an incredible capacity for rapidly progressing to new euphoria-inducing preparations, which apparently without exception can prove both habit-forming and dependence-forming." [8]

By November 1968, as smuggling controls over amphetamines and amphetamine substitutes became somewhat more effective, the Swedish black market, like the American black market a few years earlier, took the next obvious counterstep. As noted above, the raw materials out of which the amphetamines are made are common industrial chemicals, used in great quantity in ordinary manufacturing processes. Sweden imports these raw materials. A slight increase in such imports is very hard to detect—yet sufficient to produce vast amounts of amphetamines. This, Professor Inghe told an international amphetamine conference in Novem-

---

* It is used in the United States as a "diet drug."

ber 1968, was beginning to occur in Sweden.* "This means that some part of the market now, as far as one can judge, is covered by illegal factories, at least partly situated in Sweden." [10] The Swedes had belatedly discovered the "speed labs" which had begun flourishing in the United States six years earlier.

The Swedish response to this 1968 development was to ban altogether —except for a few uncommon conditions—the prescribing of amphetamines and related drugs. Special permission was required from the National Board of Health and Welfare for each patient receiving amphetamines; during the second half of 1968, only 343 such permissions were granted for the entire country.

The sensible and occasional use of amphetamines under medical supervision was thus effectively curbed—but a visit paid Stockholm in November 1970, in the course of research for this Consumers Union Report, indicated that the black market still flourished. Amphetamines and other stimulants were freely on sale in the city's large black market behind the Central Station—a region of impressive new skyscrapers roughly comparable to New York City's Park Avenue in the fifties. The Swedes are convinced that they have today the worst amphetamine problem of any country on earth—and they are almost certainly right.

The outcome of Swedish efforts to suppress amphetamine misuse between 1942 and 1970 can now be objectively evaluated. Prior to the repression, 240,000 Swedes received amphetamines legally on prescription from their physicians and used them occasionally and sensibly to help meet the minor crises of life—chiefly overtime work and feeling out of sorts or depressed. This occasional legal use of amphetamines has now ended. Yet the "abusers"—200 in 1944—had by 1970 become an army estimated at more than 10,000—and many had become mainlining speed freaks. The question inevitably arises whether Sweden might not have been wiser in 1944 to try, quietly and without publicity or publicized warnings, to reduce the number of its "serious" misusers from 200 to 150 or perhaps even 100, rather than trying to "stamp out amphetamine abuse."

One more parallel between the Swedish and American experience— and between heroin and the amphetamines—deserves mention. Because the United States has by far the largest heroin problem on earth, Americans also have the greatest number of heroin experts; at meetings of the United Nations, the World Health Organization, and other international agencies, the United States urges other countries to follow its lead in repressing the traffic in heroin. Other countries, looking at the results in the United States, are naturally loath to comply. The same is true of Sweden and the amphetamines. Through the years Swedish delegates to international conferences have urged that other countries

---

* According to another Swedish source, however, clandestine speed labs had operated in Sweden for some time; they simply escaped official attention until 1968. [9]

also launch nationwide drives against the amphetamines, place them under the same controls as heroin and morphine, and curb international smuggling. Since the Swedish experts have had the longest and most extensive experience with amphetamine abuse, they consider themselves the best-informed experts. Other countries, however, have proved understandably reluctant to set off down the path that, beginning as early as 1944, led Sweden to its current amphetamine situation.

But if the facts are as here presented, what of the story, circulated in the United States for several years, that the Swedes have been tolerant of the amphetamines, have given them away free to addicts, and are suffering an amphetamine disaster as a direct result of this toleration?

The facts are quite simple and uncontroversial. In 1965, after Sweden had exhausted all repressive approaches to the amphetamines and amphetamine substitutes, a group of physicians applied for permission to supply modest numbers of amphetamine users with amphetamines as a research project. Permission was granted, subject to the condition that no physician supply more than 10 users. Two physicians exceeded the limit, so that as many as 250 or 300 users may have been supplied with amphetamines in the course of the project—250 or 300 out of an estimated 10,000 amphetamine abusers at the time the project was launched. The project gave added reason to conclude that an amphetamine maintenance program has little or nothing to recommend it, and it was abandoned after two years.

Thus, Sweden's amphetamine problem has been blamed in the United States on the experimental prescription of amphetamines to a few hundred users in a dispensing project that *followed* rather than preceded Sweden's amphetamine explosion.

Japan, like Sweden, experienced an epidemic of excessive amphetamine use after World War II. According to reports by Japanese and American observers,[11] Japan successfully curbed this epidemic by law-enforcement methods—sweeping arrests, stiff prison sentences and curtailing supplies. If true, this marks one of the few victories of law enforcement over drugs in the history of drug use. No on-site review of the Japanese experience was made, however, in the course of research for this Consumers Union Report; and no objective evaluation of the Japanese experience was found in the medical literature available in English. Nor have we found any cogent explanation of why law-enforcement methods that proved counterproductive in the United States, in Sweden, and in other countries— against other drugs as well as the amphetamines—proved so successful in Japan. Whether, on closer scrutiny, the Japanese amphetamine stories circulating in the United States might prove as misleading as the stories emanating from Sweden, is an issue of considerable importance which warrants further inquiry.

40.

Should the amphetamines be prohibited?

Why shouldn't the amphetamines be banned altogether, as in Sweden—except, perhaps, for a few essential medical purposes?

Like all such prohibition proposals, this one is highly rational. It is the ideal solution to the speed problem and to the amphetamine problem in general. The only possible objection that can be raised against banning amphetamines is that, like alcohol prohibition and heroin prohibition, it won't work. To evaluate the likelihood that amphetamine prohibition will work, let us examine in more detail the ways in which amphetamines are manufactured and marketed in the United States today.

Before the Federal Drug Abuse Control Amendments of 1965, illicit speed labs had to compete with diverted legal tablets priced at wholesale as low as thirteen or fourteen tablets for a penny—75 cents per thousand. When enforcement of the Drug Abuse Control Amendments at least partially dried up those low-priced legal supplies, the door was opened for profitable illicit manufacture on a far larger scale. Dr. Roger C. Smith's unpublished 1969 report, "The Marketplace of Speed," supplies some of the details for the San Francisco Bay area.

"A speed laboratory," the Smith report notes, "may range from a well-organized, highly efficient operation, capable of producing five to twenty-five pounds [from about 225,000 to about 1,125,000 ten-milligram doses] of speed per week consistently, to a kitchen or bathroom in a small apartment, producing less than an ounce per week, to a college chemistry laboratory where a student produces speed only occasionally, when he needs money or feels that the chances of detection are slight. . . . They usually operate in secluded areas well removed from neighborhoods of high use. This pattern has also been described as typical of operations in the Midwest and East Coast." [1]

The very large labs, the report continued, have skilled chemists and a reliable source of the chemical precursors required to manufacture speed; these precursors are standard chemicals that have a wide variety of industrial uses, and have until recently been readily available from wholesale chemical supply companies and from other suppliers. During the past few years, narcotics officers have checked the records of these companies for clues that might lead to the speed labs, and some labs have been "busted" as a result. The surviving labs have therefore developed subtle indirect ways of securing their raw materials.

[299]

One informant described how he secured precursor chemicals for a friend who was setting up a lab:

I just walked into this store . . . it's a funny kind of store. Two old people work there who are about 50 years old, and they look at you and smile and say "what would you like?", and you would say that we want P-2-P [phenyl-2-proponol] and so on, and you would just run down the list and they would say "fine, come back in two days," and you would have to leave half the money as a deposit, and you could come back in two days and there they were, along with 20 other orders lined up on the floor, right in the middle of the store. These two people knew what was going on, because one time we went in there and the people asked how the crank [speed] was coming . . . completely blew my mind, seeing this sweet old lady asking how the crank was coming. . . . This world is getting pretty heavy.[2]

"The cost of production," the Smith report continues, "is directly related to the source of chemicals. In a large laboratory, producing from 10 to 25 pounds per week with a steady source of supply, the basic cost may be $50 a pound."[3] This is slightly less than the wholesale price of legally manufactured amphetamines—75 cents per thousand for five-milligram tablets, or about $70 per pound. "In a small operation, making a pound or less per week, buying chemicals from street sources, the cost per pound will exceed $200."[4] This raises the raw-materials cost per dose to almost a third of a cent. In the speed black market, as elsewhere, volume counts.

After a while, knowledge of how to manufacture speed spread from chemists to the laymen who worked with them and watched their techniques closely. By 1969 Dr. Roger C. Smith was able to report: "The low-level chemist is often a speed user, often without any formal training in chemistry, who learns the process . . . by working with a more experienced chemist or by following a 'recipe' which can easily be obtained in the speed community."[5] As an example, he cited a fifteen-year-old girl "who had operated her own speed lab in the Haight-Ashbury." Asked how she learned the technique, she replied:

I moved into this house with a friend of mine in Seattle and this guy was making it in the bathroom, and I'm very interested. I like to learn things, so I just stayed up with him on three different nights and he would go through all the steps and I would write down how to do it. And he taught me and the next time I helped him do it. We did this around five times and I learned a lot. I can do it now, and I know most of the chemicals. I have all of it written down and I have to go by it, the temperature and everything. I couldn't remember it all, it's too complicated. *And people think it's easy to do, but it's not.*[6] [Italics in original]

The way in which black-market speed is clandestinely manufactured is relevant to the problem of illicit drugs in general. LSD can be similarly manufactured in "bathtub labs," at low cost and in enormous quantities. The possibility that THC—an active ingredient in marijuana—might be clandestinely manufactured is reviewed in Part VIII. That synthetic heroin, or a wide range of synthetic heroin substitutes, might also be turned out clandestinely is an ever-present possibility. Nor should one ignore the possibility that new psychoactive drugs, more potent and more hazardous than any now known, may sooner or later emerge from bathtub labs. The two essential preconditions for the success of the clandestine laboratories are the banning of legally manufactured drugs and intensive policing of the ban.

But even if all the amphetamines on earth, clandestine as well as legal, were eradicated forever, not very much would be accomplished—for many users would turn (indeed, some already are turning) to cocaine again.

41.

Back to cocaine again

By the mid-1960s, as we have shown, the market for amphetamines and related stimulants was being supplied in at least four ways: (1) physicians were prescribing these drugs for patients; (2) domestic supplies of legal stimulants were being diverted to the black market; (3) legal stimulants were being exported from the United States to Mexico and smuggled back into the United States; (4) speed labs were manufacturing illicit stimulants.

As the 1960s drew to a close, however, all four of these sources of supply were under increasing pressure. The medical journals carried papers warning physicians not to overprescribe stimulants. The United States Bureau of Customs was on guard against stimulant smuggling. The Bureau of Narcotics and Dangerous Drugs, the Food and Drug Administration, and state and local police agencies battled against both the diversion of legal stimulants and the illicit speed labs. Securing the precursor chemicals for speed manufacture became increasingly risky. The net effect was a notable expansion of a fifth source of supply of stimulants—a boom in *cocaine* smuggling.

"More and more cocaine, worth millions of dollars," correspondent George Volsky reported from Miami in the New York *Times* for February 1, 1970, "is being smuggled into the United States from Latin America, much of it through this area, according to Federal law enforcement officials and narcotics agents." [1]

Volsky then went on to quote Dennis Dayle, supervisory agent of the Federal Bureau of Narcotics and Dangerous Drugs in Miami, as saying: "The traffic of cocaine is growing by leaps and bounds. It was insignificant only a few years ago, but now it has become a significant problem." [2]

Agent Dayle failed to link the revival of cocaine smuggling with the efforts his bureau was making to curtail the availability of speed. But John J. Bellizzi, director of the New York State Bureau of Narcotics in Albany, explained to Volsky why cocaine smuggling was on the increase —"because younger drug users are finding out about it. The kids are beginning to learn that it's pretty much like speed." [3]

Nationally, Volsky reported, Bureau of Customs cocaine seizures rose from 22 kilograms in 1967 to 90 kilograms in 1969.* And he quoted a

* Seizures increased markedly in 1970; indeed, 200 kilograms were seized in New York and Miami during the last three months of 1970. The New York *Times,* however, commented: ". . . few of the men involved in this dangerous work have any illusions

rule-of-thumb estimate that for every kilogram seized, ten kilograms get through—or an estimated 900 kilograms successfully imported during 1969. (Nine hundred kilograms is enough to provide from 18,000,000 to 27,000,000 cocaine doses of the size Sigmund Freud took during the 1880s.)

Volsky added details concerning the economics of cocaine smuggling—details reminiscent of the heroin smuggling market described in Part I. Pure cocaine, he was informed by Wilbur Underwood of the Bureau of Customs, can be purchased in Latin America for $3,000 to $5,000 per kilogram (2.2 pounds). After importation, it is diluted or "cut" so that one gram of pure cocaine produces 16 grams of "street" cocaine. The street cocaine, Underwood told Volsky, is sold at $50 a gram. Thus the 900 kilograms of pure cocaine supposed to have been smuggled into the United States in 1969 represented 14,400 kilograms of street cocaine worth $50,000 per kilogram, or—if those Bureau of Customs figures are to be believed *—$720,000,000.

With so vast a total markup, it is easy to see why smugglers who lost $495,000 worth of cocaine (at South American prices) to the Bureau of Customs in 1969 continued to smuggle cocaine in 1970 and 1971. Even if the Bureau of Customs retail price estimates are divided by ten, the loss due to interception of smuggled consignments remains trivial in comparison to the total markup.

On the basis of data supplied by Bureau of Narcotics supervisory agent Dayle, Volsky described a typical smuggling operation in these terms:

There are two principal partners, one controlling operations in South and Central America and the other in Miami.

The syndicate boss abroad, through a number of subordinates, buys coca leaves, sets up laboratories, maintains contact with local officials, arranges for payoffs, and recruits and dispatches local couriers with cocaine to the United States, mostly by plane.

The Miami boss, like a head of a large commercial corporation, has deputies in charge of travel, transportation, personnel, security, accounting, and quality control—"cutting" pure cocaine for wholesale and retail trade.

Several years ago, modest Latin-American women were usually employed as "body carriers," smuggling into Miami from two to four kilograms of pure cocaine. . . . Some women carriers posed as being pregnant. . . . After passing through Customs at the Miami International Airport, these couriers—who were given precise but simple instructions and who had little information about the syndicate—usually proceeded to a downtown hotel where cocaine and cash transportation payment changed hands.[6]

---

about reducing the flow."[4] As in the case of heroin, the arrest of a courier does not close off a conduit.

* One observer has suggested that the law-enforcement practice of "attributing 'retail' value to bulk merchandise [such as cocaine] is similar to attributing the value of 100 Christian Dior dresses to a bale of cotton."[5]

Once federal agents learned of these procedures, of course, it was easy to keep an eye open for modest Latin American women—especially the ones who looked pregnant. After a few of them had been arrested, however, the syndicates simply changed the style of their couriers. Subsequent reports indicated that couriers looked like businessmen or college students.

As noted in Part I, the United States law-enforcement system tends to catch price-cutting newcomers to the black market rather than established syndicates; law enforcement thus tends to perpetuate these syndicates and to keep prices high. A United States narcotics agent stationed in South America explained to a New York *Times* reporter in some detail just how this happens in the case of cocaine.

The narcotics agent, "who cannot be named," told of a small-time procurer of prostitutes in New York City who became interested in the high prices paid by his girls for cocaine, and decided to get in on the racket. "When he learned that the stuff came from Chile, he bought a $550 roundtrip airline ticket and came down," [7] the *Times* reported on January 25, 1971. Cocaine is readily available in kilo lots in Chile and other Latin American countries. The New York procurer bought a kilo for $1,800. "An experienced buyer could have gotten the cocaine for about $900," the United States narcotics agent commented.

The procurer safely returned to New York with his kilo, adulterated it to make two kilos, and sold them for $15,000 each to the dealer who had been supplying cocaine to his girls. This was price-cutting, and horning in on the trade of the established importer who had previously supplied the same dealer. Following a second trip to South America, the procurer cut prices even lower—selling 75 percent pure cocaine for $18,000 to $20,000 a kilo.

Retribution swiftly followed. "A member of an organized drug-peddling group informed on the independent operator and he was seized [by the authorities] upon returning from his third trip to Chile." [8] It would be hard to find a clearer example of how vigorous United States law enforcement buttresses the monopoly of the established distributors of illicit drugs—and thus keeps both consumer prices and the profits of established traffickers exorbitantly high.

The flooding of the market with cocaine after 1968 represented a threat to the established black-market amphetamine interests. But the United States Bureau of Narcotics and Dangerous Drugs, which in 1968 had from four to seven agents in its Miami office, increased its Miami staff to over thirty agents early in 1970—and more were being trained. [9] To the extent that such increased cocaine policing is effective, of course, it will protect the illicit speed market from too much cocaine competition.

The developments of the 1960s can now be summed up. The decade began with almost all stimulants being supplied by reputable manufacturers; their low-cost amphetamines had almost driven cocaine off the market. The withdrawal of intravenous amphetamines from the legal market opened the door for the illicit speed labs. The Drug Abuse Control Amendments of 1965 curbed the direct diversion of legal amphetamines to the black market; this opened the door for the smuggling of exported amphetamines back into the United States. By 1969, law-enforcement efforts had raised black-market amphetamine prices and curbed amphetamine supplies sufficiently to open the door for renewed cocaine smuggling. All of these modes of supplying the black market shared the benefits of vigorous law enforcement, for it was law enforcement that prevented the flooding of the market with excess supplies of both cocaine and amphetamines that might threaten the price structure. If the various black-market suppliers had conspired among themselves to limit production and imports, they would have been in violation of the antitrust laws. But no conspiracy was necessary; law enforcement limited supplies, thus playing the role that is ordinarily played by conspiracies in restraint of trade.

Viewed from this perspective, the proposals current in 1971 to ban (with certain minor exceptions) the legal use of amphetamines, even on a doctor's prescription, seem less persuasive. Such a measure, it is true, would promptly curb the use of these drugs by patients *under medical supervision*; but there is not the slightest reason to expect that it would significantly curtail the overall consumption of amphetamines, cocaine, and other stimulants. On the contrary, it would deliver over to the cocaine smugglers, illicit speed labs, and other black-market suppliers at least some of the millions of users who now secure their euphoriants and central nervous system stimulants on a doctor's prescription—and it would thus protect the black market from the last remaining vestiges of low-priced legal competition. This, of course, was precisely what the Harrison Narcotic Act had accomplished for the morphine and heroin black market back in 1914 (see Part I).

42.

A slightly hopeful postscript

While law enforcement serves mainly to raise prices and thus attract additional black-market entrepreneurs rather than to curb consumption, and while antidrug propaganda campaigns have helped to popularize drugs like the amphetamines more than to discourage their use, the current outlook is not altogether hopeless. Progress is actually being made against the "speed freak" phenomenon in its original home and major citadel, California—and no doubt elsewhere as well.

California observers of the "youth drug scene" (see Part IX) report that *fewer young people are being attracted to speed.* There is nothing mysterious about this. New arrivals on the youth drug scene look at the speed freaks, the acid (LSD) droppers, the grass (marijuana) smokers, and decide to stick with acid and grass. They don't want to become like the speed freaks. The speed-freak phenomenon is in this respect self-limiting.

Young drug users need not rely solely on their own observations, moreover, for throughout the youth drug scene today there are "indigenous institutions," such as free clinics and "hot lines," devoted to helping them. These institutions, which will be discussed at length in Part IX, are not trying to stamp out illicit drug use. Instead, most of them are trying to *minimize the damage done by drugs,* both licit and illicit. Thus, instead of railing against marijuana, they are pointing out to drug novices just what happens to the speed freak.

Unlike other warnings against drugs, the comments of these indigenous institutions ring true to young people. One reason is that they *are* true; youthful recruits to the drug scene can confirm what they are told merely by looking around them at the drug scene's speed freaks. Another reason is that the indigenous institutions do not destroy their own credibility with dire warnings against marijuana—warnings that are *not* confirmed when young people look around them. Finally, the indigenous institutions are dedicated, and are *seen* to be dedicated, to helping young drug users rather than to repressing them. What they say need not be discounted by the young. As a result of the efforts of these indigenous institutions, and of young drug users' own observations, the number of new users recruited to speed—the mainlining of amphetamines in large doses— appears to be dropping. The drug scene itself, in short, is beginning to curb speed mainlining after the United States Bureau of Customs, the United States Bureau of Narcotics and Dangerous Drugs, the Food and Drug Administration, and nationwide propaganda efforts have failed.

A second factor in curbing the "speed freak" phenomenon is reminiscent of Dr. W. S. Halsted, who cured himself of his cocaine addiction—a close parallel of speed addiction—by going on morphine and thus salvaging his surgical career (see Chapter 5). California speed freaks in large number are similarly deserting speed for heroin. This reduction in the number of speed freaks spreading the speed gospel also tends to curb the recruitment of new speed freaks. If these trends continue, the speed freak may in the not too distant future be merely a historical oddity—unless, of course, a new wave of antispeed propaganda alerts a new generation of young people who have never seen a speed freak, and a new wave of speed mainlining is triggered.

The future of the ex-speed freaks who convert to heroin depends on the future of heroin addicts generally. If we leave them at the mercy of the American black market, the high prices and adulterants will ruin and perhaps kill them. But this, as we saw in Part I, is an avoidable outcome if society decides to avoid it.

Part VI

Inhalants and Solvents — and Glue-Sniffing

The first two anesthetic gases, *nitrous oxide* (N_2O, "laughing gas") and *ether,* were used recreationally prior to their adoption for surgical anesthesia. Nitrous oxide can produce a relatively shallow anesthesia, useful in dentistry and during childbirth, and, together with other anesthetics, in surgery. Ether has been widely used as a general anesthetic, but its flammability and other disadvantages have seen it largely replaced by newer anesthetics. *Chloroform* is still sometimes administered in obstetrics, but its use otherwise is greatly limited because of possible undesirable side effects from moderate doses and possible death or liver damage from overdose.

Organic solvents, such as gasoline, benzene, and related chemical substances, are toxic when inhaled for lengthy periods in unventilated areas, such as some industrial settings. Brief inhalation of these and similar substances can also produce many of the effects of alcohol intoxication and, sometimes, a hallucinogen-like "trip." The best-known example is *glue-sniffing,* which involves inhaling the organic solvents found in "hobby glue," mainly toluene.

43.

The historical antecedents of glue-sniffing

That drugs of many kinds reach the brain more rapidly and efficiently when they are sniffed rather than swallowed is a commonplace of physiology. The lung, after all, is designed to admit oxygen promptly and effortlessly into the bloodstream; and such drugs as heroin, nicotine, and cocaine readily follow the same short route when they are inhaled, reaching the brain in seconds. Nicotine and marijuana are customarily taken via the lung route. Inhalation is also commonly used to produce anesthesia with ether, chloroform, nitrous oxide (laughing gas), and a wide range of newer anesthetic agents. In this chapter we shall review the nonmedical use of these anesthetic inhalants, and of a number of other mind-affecting substances—most of them organic solvents extracted from petroleum— that are commonly inhaled.

"The voluntary inhalation of vapors for the purpose of altering psychological states has a long history," Edward A. Preble and Gabriel V. Laury noted in the Fall 1967 issue of the *International Journal of the Addictions*. "At Delphi, in the ancient Greek world, the Pythia sat on a tripod above a cleft in the rocks and inhaled cold vapors emanating from inside the earth, which induced in her an ecstatic alteration of mind. In this altered state she uttered mystical observations in the presence of the Delphi Prophet, who translated them into oracular pronouncements.

"In the ancient Judaic world, the vapors from burnt spices and aromatic gums were considered part of a pleasurable act of worship. In *Proverbs* (27:9), it is said that 'ointment and perfume rejoice the heart.' Perfumes were widely used in Egyptian worship. Stone altars have been unearthed in Babylon and Palestine which have been used for burning incense made of aromatic wood and spices."[1] While casual readers today may interpret such practices as mere satisfaction of the desire for pleasant odors, this is almost certainly an error; in many or most cases, a psychoactive drug was being inhaled. In the islands of the Mediterranean 2,500 years ago and in Africa hundreds of years ago, for example, leaves and flowers of a particular plant were often thrown upon bonfires and the smoke was inhaled; the plant was marijuana (see Chapter 53). The inhalation of LSD-like snuffs by North and South American Indians is similarly well-documented. Thus drug inhaling as it is known today has a long tradition.

With the dawn of modern chemistry, new substances were discovered that had mood-altering effects—effects usually resembling those of alcohol, but in some cases producing in addition the equivalent of a short, mild hallucinogenic "trip." The late Dr. David R. Nagle, assistant professor of pharmacology at the University of Kentucky, made a historical study of these newer substances; following his death, his findings were published in the Spring 1968 issue of the *International Journal of the Addictions.*

Nitrous oxide (N₂O). This gas was discovered in 1776 by Sir Joseph Priestley, and was first synthesized in the same year by an English chemist, Humphrey (later Sir Humphrey) Davy. Davy exposed nitrous peroxide (N_2O_4) to iron and thus removed three of the four oxygen atoms. When inhaled, Davy learned, the gas N_2O produces initially a state of excitement often accompanied by loud laughter; hence nitrous oxide came to be called "laughing gas." Davy soon gathered around him for nitrous-oxide parties, Dr. Nagle reports, "a group of gay spirits who were perhaps more interested in seeking 'pleasurable effects'—getting drunk— than in scientific research." [2] Among those who inhaled nitrous oxide with Davy were the poets Coleridge and Southey, the potter Josiah (later Sir Josiah) Wedgwood, and Roget of *Roget's Thesaurus.* The experience was pleasant and a little like getting drunk—but it had several major advantages over alcohol drunkenness. The N_2O effect sets in within thirty seconds after inhaling the gas, and the peak effect lasts only two or three minutes. Unlike alcohol, moreover, there is no tendency to increase the dose at each inhalation. On the contrary, experienced N_2O inhalers report an increase in effects *without* increasing the dose, as is also the case with marijuana. Davy apparently thought of marketing the new gas, for he calculated that he could supply it in bags at a lower price than was then being charged for alcoholic beverages—and alcohol at the end of the eighteenth century was notoriously cheap. Southey commented after one of Davy's N_2O parties that the atmosphere of the highest of all possible heavens was no doubt composed of nitrous oxide.

Noting that pains vanished under the influence of nitrous oxide, Davy proposed in 1799 that it be used in surgical operations; but no one bothered to test this possibility for another forty-five years.

Dr. Nagle cites several references to nitrous-oxide intoxication in American medical publications of the early 1800s. There are also nineteenth-century American references to the use of nitrous oxide by students, indicating that N_2O sniffing—for its "exhilarating" effects[3]—was endemic among American students. One young American medical student, Gardner Quincy Colton, decided—like Sir Humphrey Davy—that nitrous oxide might be profitably marketed in competition with alcohol as a recreational drug; when his first public demonstration of the gas netted him $535, he quit medical school and went into the nitrous-oxide business. An advertisement for his nitrous-oxide demonstration in Hartford, Connecticut, in 1844 read as follows:

A Grand Exhibition of the effects produced by inhaling Nitrous Oxid, Exhilarating or Laughing Gas! will be given at Union Hall this (Tuesday) Evening, Dec. 10th, 1844.

Forty gallons of Gas will be prepared and administered to all in the audience who desire to inhale it.

Twelve Young Men have volunteered to inhale the Gas, to commence the entertainment.

Eight Strong Men are engaged to occupy the front seats to protect those under the influence of the Gas from injuring themselves or others. This course is adopted that no apprehension of danger may be entertained. Probably no one will attempt to fight.

The effect of the Gas is to make those who inhale it either Laugh, Sing, Dance, Speak or Fight, and so forth, according to the leading trait of their character. They seem to retain consciousness enough not to say or do that which they would have occasion to regret.

N.B.—The Gas will be administered only to gentlemen of the first respectability. The object is to make the entertainment in every respect a genteel affair.* [4]

Among those who attended Colton's Hartford demonstration was a young dentist, Horace Wells, who was particularly impressed when one of the nitrous-oxide sniffers tripped and fell to the ground, gashing his leg in the process. To the victim's own astonishment, the wound was unaccompanied by pain. Wells questioned the young man closely about this—and was so impressed by the absence of pain that the next day he had Colton pull one of his teeth under nitrous-oxide anesthesia. Feeling no pain, Wells exclaimed, "A new era in tooth-pulling!" Thereafter he used nitrous oxide on several patients in his Hartford dental practice —and a few weeks later, on January 10, 1845, he demonstrated the use of nitrous oxide during surgery at the Massachusetts General Hospital in Boston. Unfortunately, the patient came out of the anesthesia too soon and screamed in pain; Wells was laughed out of the hospital.[5] Despite this unfortunate inaugural, the use of N_2O as an anesthetic spread, and the gas is in common use today for the reduction of pain during tooth extractions and other dental procedures, during childbirth, and (in association with other more potent and longer-acting anesthetics) during surgery.[6]

That nitrous-oxide inhalation for recreational purposes has continued on a small scale, with few interruptions, to the present time, seems well

* The twenty-five-cent admission charge included a dose of N_2O.

established. Use among young people was reported from Maryland in 1971,[7] and was observed in Vancouver, British Columbia, in the course of research for this Consumers Union Report. In 1970, Dr. Edward J. Lynn and his associates at Michigan State University, in cooperation with the staff of the East Lansing Drug Information Center, made a survey of the nonmedical use of N_2O in mid-Michigan.

It was not uncommon [they reported] to hear from individuals who had been to parties where a professional (doctor, nurse, scientist, inhalation therapist, researcher) had provided nitrous oxide. There also were those who work in restaurants who used the N_2O stored in tanks for the preparation of whip cream. Reports were received from individuals who used the gas contained in aerosol cans both of food and non-food products. At a recent rock festival nitrous oxide was widely sold for 25 cents a balloon. Contact was made with a "mystical-religious" group that used the gas to accelerate arriving at their transcendental-meditative state of choice. Although a few, more sophisticated users employed nitrous oxide–oxygen mixes with elaborate equipment, most users employed balloons or plastic bags. They either held a breath of N_2O or rebreathed the gas. There were no adverse effects reported in the more than one hundred individuals surveyed.[8]

The Michigan group also supplied nitrous oxide to 34 volunteers who breathed it under laboratory conditions. "Subjective findings generally indicated pleasurable effects," which set in within fifteen to thirty seconds. Tests were administered shortly after inhaling; "cognitive defects were noted during the peak high but returned to normal within five minutes." Adverse effects in general were described as "minimal." The Lynn group reported their findings at the May 1971 meeting of the American Psychiatric Association.

Ether. Though ether is available as a liquid, it vaporizes very easily at room temperature; it can therefore be either swallowed or inhaled. The effects are quicker when it is inhaled but are otherwise much the same. This drug is manufactured by distilling alcohol and sulphuric acid together—a discovery said to date from the thirteenth century. "A dose of a little more than [a teaspoonful]," *Encyclopaedia Britannica* reported back in 1911, "will produce a condition of inebriation lasting from one-half to one hour, but the dose must soon be greatly increased. The after-effects are, if anything, rather pleasant, and the habit of ether-drinking is certainly not so injurious as alcoholism."* [9]

Ether was introduced into medicine under the trade name Anodyne by Friedrich Hoffmann (1660–1742). Hoffmann recommended his Anodyne

* This comparison is quoted here as a common opinion in England at the time rather than as an established medical fact.

for pains due to kidney stones, gallstones, intestinal cramps, earache, toothache, and painful menstruation. Ether labeled as Anodyne, Dr. Nagle notes, is "still available over the counter in some countries. Genteel ladies who would never think of touching sinful whiskey have been known to treat their ills with the drops." [10] A 1761 textbook on pharmacology recommended ether as "one of the most perfect tonics, friendly to the nerves, cordial, and anodyne," directing that three to twelve drops be taken on a lump of sugar, swallowed with water.[11]

Ether was also used for recreational purposes at least as early as the 1790s, when James Graham (1745-1794), described by Dr. Nagle as "a famous London quack, proprietor of the Temple of Hymen and owner of the Celestial Bed," [12] was accustomed to inhale an ounce or two several times a day, in public, "with manifest placidity and enjoyment." [13] There are accounts of ether drinking and ether sniffing at universities in both England and the United States during the nineteenth century. But the major nineteenth-century outbreak occurred in Ireland, under circumstances that carry a lesson. Dr. Nagle reports: "About 1840 a Catholic priest, Father Matthew, led a great temperance crusade through England, Scotland, and Ireland. It was one of the most successful that ever occurred; thousands took the pledge." One of them was an alcoholic physician named Kelly who practiced in Draperstown, Northern Ireland. "Aghast at the pleasure he had given up, but not wishing to break his pledge, [Dr. Kelly] cast about for a substitute. He had prescribed ether by mouth on occasion and knew of its pleasant effects. After a few personal experiments he imparted the knowledge to his friends and patients who had also taken the pledge ." [14] Ether sniffing became endemic in Draperstown.

Fifteen years later, when the British government placed a stiff tax on alcoholic beverages and when the constabulary clamped down on home-distilled Irish whiskey, Kelly's discovery was recalled and exploited to the hilt. Ether, which was not subject to the tax, was distilled in London and shipped to Draperstown and other places in Northern Ireland by the ton. Ether "was preferred in some ways, and especially among the poor, to the now-expensive whiskey. The drunk was quick and cheap, and could be achieved several times a day without hangover. If arrested for drunkenness, the offender would be sober by the time the police station was reached." [15]

A surgeon visiting Draperstown in 1878 remarked that the main street smelled like his surgery, where ether was used as an anesthetic. Old ether topers, he added, could finish off a three-ounce wineglassful at a single swig, without even water for a chaser. "Everyone who discussed this particular phenomenon," Dr. Nagle notes, "admitted that there appeared to be less chronic damage than with alcohol." But hazards were also noted: chronic gastritis, deaths from overdosage, and fatal burns from smoking while drinking—for ether is extremely flammable.

"By 1890," Dr. Nagle continues, "the pressure of temperance societies, aided by an article by the editor of the *British Medical Journal*,[16] and loss of tax revenue, caused a Parliamentary committee to investigate.[17] Subsequently, regulations limiting the sale of this ether were imposed." As in the case of heroin prohibition, alcohol prohibition, marijuana prohibition, and other forms of prohibition, however, ether prohibition failed. In 1910, ether drinking was still prevalent in Draperstown. It died out in the 1920s, "replaced by [alcoholic] beverages that were cheaper and more easily available."

Ether turned up again in the United States during the alcohol Prohibition era (1920-1933), when nonalcoholic "near beer" and other "soft" drinks were frequently "spiked" with ether as well as with alcohol; and ether was drunk in Germany during World War II, when alcoholic beverages were rationed, expensive, and of poor quality.[18]

Ether *inhalation* has a similarly long and fascinating history. It was inhaled at Harvard by students during the nineteenth century, for example —and by at least one professor, Dr. Oliver Wendell Holmes of the Harvard Medical School.* No doubt this college use was one of the factors that led William T. G. Morton, a dentist studying medicine at the Harvard Medical School, to ask permission to use ether as an anesthetic at the Massachusetts General Hospital on October 16, 1846 [20]— one of the several occasions sometimes cited as the birth of modern inhalational anesthesia.

Thereafter, Dr. Nagle adds, ether continued in recreational use in many countries, and was sniffed as well as drunk. "For example, ether inhalation as a substitute for ingestion of alcohol was felt to be widespread among the upper classes in England during the late 19th century.[21] Yvonne, mistress of Guy de Maupassant and a ballet dancer, said that

---

* Dr. Holmes inhaled ether at a time when it was popularly supposed to produce mystical or "mind-expanding" experiences, much as LSD is supposed to produce such experiences today. Here is his account of what happened: "I once inhaled a pretty full dose of ether, with the determination to put on record, at the earliest moment of regaining consciousness, the thought I should find uppermost in my mind. The mighty music of the triumphal march into nothingness reverberated through my brain, and filled me with a sense of infinite possibilities, which made me an archangel for a moment. The veil of eternity was lifted. The one great truth which underlies all human experience and is the key to all the mysteries that philosophy has sought in vain to solve, flashed upon me in a sudden revelation. Henceforth all was clear: a few words had lifted my intelligence to the level of the knowledge of the cherubim. As my natural condition returned, I remembered my resolution; and, staggering to my desk, I wrote, in ill-shaped, straggling characters, the all-embracing truth still glimmering in my consciousness. The words were these (children may smile; the wise will ponder): 'A strong smell of turpentine prevails throughout.'"[19]

she and her fellow dancers, and even the director of the *corps de ballet*, took ether for a pick-me-up when they were dancing." [22] France, Russia, Norway, and Michigan were also reputed to have ether users; and there were reports of the simultaneous sniffing and swallowing of ether.

Is ether sniffed and drunk in the United States today? Though reports are few, it seems highly likely. Ether sniffing by a child was reported in Salt Lake City in 1962.[23] Dr. Nagle states that "there are anesthetists in this country who have become addicted to anesthetic agents. Anecdotal accounts are not uncommon in professional circles. All the major agents, including ether, nitrous oxide, cyclopropane, ethyl chloride, ethylene, thiopental and halothane have been indicted." [24]

Chloroform. This is a liquid at room temperatures but it gives off vapors which are highly potent when inhaled. It was discovered independently and simultaneously in Germany, France, and the United States in 1831; and its recreational use in the United States began concurrently with its discovery. "During the last six months," Samuel Guthrie, the American discoverer, reported in his paper announcing the discovery, "a great number of persons have drunk of the solution . . . in my laboratory, not only very freely, but frequently to the point of intoxication, and so far as I have observed, it has appeared to be singularly grateful, both to the palate and stomach, producing a lively flow of animal spirits, and consequent loquacity; and leaving, after its operation, little of that depression consequent upon the use of ardent spirits [alcohol]." [25] In other words, no hangover.

Sixteen years later chloroform was introduced into Scotland by Dr. James Y. Simpson for anesthesia during surgery and childbirth. Strong opposition to its obstetrical use immediately came from some clergymen who argued that obstetrical anesthesia violated God's word in Genesis 3:16: "In pain you shall bring forth children." Dr. Simpson responded by quoting Genesis 2:21 to show that God used anesthesia before extracting Adam's rib to fashion Eve: "So the Lord God caused a deep sleep to fall upon the man, and while he slept took one of his ribs. . . ." The controversy was calmed, and chloroform popularized, when Dr. Simpson gave Queen Victoria chloroform during the birth of her eighth child.* [26]

Chloroform gradually fell into medical disrepute, however, due in part to the hazard of sudden death from overdose and in part to the rise in popularity of other anesthetics. Its occasional recreational use continued, sometimes with fatal outcomes. Dr. Nagle reports: "Although chloroform never achieved ether's spectacular success in replacing liquor for whole areas, individual case reports have been published in most countries. Indeed, the total number of such reports is greater than with ether, since a dead patient is more likely to be written up than a chronic drunk. . . .

* The Queen knighted Dr. Simpson for his pioneering work.

The use of chloroform for addiction is now considered rare, but it is not totally extinct" [27]—and as evidence, Dr. Nagle cites cases published in the *Bulletin of the Menninger Clinic* (1945) and the *Journal of the American Medical Association* (1963).

Other organic solvents. These include a broad range of chemicals, many of them secured through the distillation of petroleum. When their vapors are inhaled, these can produce intoxication resembling alcoholic drunkenness—and in some cases effects resembling those of a short hallucinogenic trip. Many, such as gasoline, are highly flammable and even explosive.

A wide variety of common household products contain these organic solvents, whose rapid evaporation speeds drying—for example, paint thinners, lacquers, enamels, varnishes, varnish removers, glues and cements, cigarette lighter fluids, charcoal lighter fluids, fingernail polishes and polish removers, spot removers, and other dry-cleaning products.

The effects of inhaling gasoline fumes, Dr. Ewart A. Swinyard of the University of Utah College of Medicine points out in Goodman and Gilman's textbook (1970), can be similar to those of drinking an alcoholic beverage. "The signs and symptoms include incoordination, restlessness, excitement, confusion, disorientation, ataxia, delirium, and, finally, coma that may last for a few hours to several days." Most gasoline sniffers stop long before the severer symptoms set in, of course, just as most alcohol drinkers stop before they pass out cold. *Repeated* inhalation of gasoline fumes, Dr. Swinyard adds, "induces dizziness, giddiness, a 'butterfly feeling,' and hallucinations. If the desired end point is exceeded, unconsciousness results." Dr. Swinyard adds that "prodromal symptoms such as headache, blurred vision, vertigo, ataxia, tinnitus, nausea, anorexia, and weakness are not uncommon" with low concentrations of gasoline fumes; and that *chronic* exposure to gasoline fumes may produce "muscular weakness, listlessness, fatigue, nausea, vomiting, abdominal pain, and weight loss" along with "neurological effects such as confusion, ataxia, tremor, paresthesias [itching], neuritis, and paralysis of peripheral and cranial nerves." [28]

If Dr. Swinyard is correct—and there is no reason to doubt his long lists of signs and symptoms—why does anyone sniff gasoline vapors? The answer becomes clear when we move from the confines of the pharmacological textbooks to the world of real children and young people. There it appears that gasoline sniffing, like numerous other common activities, *makes you feel good* (or better). One of the best descriptions of gasoline sniffing as it actually occurs was published in 1955 by the late A.E. ("Tajar") Hamilton of the Hamilton School in Sheffield, Mass., in his classic account of children at work and play, *Psychology and the Great God Fun*. One day when the other children had gone on an expedition, Tajar Hamilton reports, he found a boy nicknamed Bullet with a can of gasoline and a gasoline-soaked rag. After a few preliminary questions, Tajar (with Bullet's consent) turned on a recorder and preserved the dialogue for posterity.

Tajar: Bullet, you said you would come up to the attic and tell me about the gasoline and the bicycles. Will you talk your story into the mike, just as you remember it?

Bullet: Well, I was awful mad when they said I couldn't go on the trip. Sure I picked up the axe when Martha told me not to, but I put it back again. Then she said I couldn't go, and Donnie was going, and when they all went I didn't have anything to do to have fun and I began to get madder and madder all the time. It made me feel kind of sick to be so mad, so I went where they keep the gasoline can and I started to smell it.

Tajar: What made you want to smell gas, Bullet?

Bullet: Well, when you feel bad, you smell it and it makes you feel kind of hot and kind of drowsy, like you was floating through the air. It makes you feel sort of hot inside and different from the way you were before.

Tajar: And after you smelled the gas and felt better, what did you do?

Bullet: Then I began to feel mad again and had to do something, so I found a nail. It was an old rusty one, and I got a piece of board to push it with so it wouldn't hurt my hand, and I made holes in all the tires except Donnie's.

Tajar: Why not in Donnie's?

Bullet: Because they're solid and you can't. . . .

Tajar: And after you had punched all those holes what did you do?

Bullet: Mary hollered to come to dinner, so I went and we had hot dogs at the Council ring and then we had some games and then I didn't feel so good, so I went and smelled the gas again.

Tajar: How long have you liked to smell gas, Bullet?

Bullet: Well, here at camp, ever since about two weeks after I came to the farm. I showed Donnie how to smell it. It makes you feel like you was in fairyland or somewhere else than where you are. . . .

Tajar: Bullet, how come so much gas was spilled on the cellar floor?

Bullet: Oh, I just wanted to get more on my rag. If you have a lot it makes you sort of dream. It gets all dark and you see shooting stars in it, and this time I saw big flies flying in it. They were big and green and had white wings.

Tajar: And you feel better about yourself and about people after you have one of those dreams?

Bullet: Yep, until I begin to feel bad again, or get mad.

Tajar: Okay, Bullet, that's all for now. Thank you for being truthful with me.[29]

The solvents found in the other common household products listed above have effects on the whole quite similar to those Bullet described for gasoline. Whether these substances are addicting, or, indeed, what permanent effects if any result from recreational use, remains undetermined. In two bulletins of the National Clearinghouse for Poison Control Centers (a unit of the United States Public Health Service), one dated

February-March 1962 and the other July-August 1964, Mr. Henry L. Verhulst and Dr. John J. Crotty reviewed both the older toxicological literature on organic solvents and recent laboratory studies on glue-sniffing in particular. The older literature was based on exposure among industrial workers who breathed solvent fumes eight hours a day, five days a week for months or years. The workers suffered adverse effects like those listed by Dr. Swinyard, as well as serious damage to the brain, liver, and kidneys. Solvent sniffing for recreational purposes, however, involves only a transient rather than a prolonged exposure. Hence, Verhulst and Crotty concluded, the older toxicological data on industrial exposure could not be extrapolated to cover occasional recreational sniffing.[30]

Solvent sniffing in general was not particularly widespread in the 1950s, and there is no reason to believe that it is any more widespread today. But there is one startling exception. *Glue*-sniffing, almost unknown before 1959, became a source of nationwide concern and a major form of drug use shortly thereafter. The factors that led to the almost overnight popularization of glue-sniffing deserve close scrutiny; they are therefore reviewed in detail in the following chapter.

44.

How to launch a
nationwide drug menace

During the 1960s, Dr. Ralph M. Susman of the United States Department of Health, Education, and Welfare, and his associate Lenore R. Kupperstein, prepared a "Bibliography on the Inhalation of Glue Fumes and Other Toxic Vapors," which they published in the Spring 1968 issue of the *International Journal of the Addictions*. Despite diligent search, the earliest references to glue-sniffing in either the medical or the popular literature that they were able to find dated from 1959.[1] A similarly thorough search in the course of preparing this Consumers Union Report has turned up no earlier mention of glue-sniffing. Other documented studies of glue-sniffing are similarly void of references earlier than 1959. Thus, while it is likely that children (and adults as well) sniffed glue on occasion before 1959, the practice either went unobserved or, more probably, was not deemed worthy of recording.

The first known mentions of glue-sniffing in print date from 1959 and concern the arrest for sniffing glue of children in Tucson, Arizona, Pueblo, Colorado, and perhaps other Western cities. Laws against sniffing glue or sniffing anything else, of course, did not yet exist. Accounts of these remarkable arrests reached Denver, where two reporters investigated. Their account of glue-sniffing—the first full description in the mass media that has yet turned up—appeared in *Empire*, the Sunday magazine supplement of the Denver *Post*, on August 2, 1959. The article reported: "Police in Pueblo, Colo. and several other cities in the West and Midwest report that juveniles seeking a quick bang and a mild jag spread liquid glue on the palms of their hands, then cup their hands over their mouth and nose and inhale deeply."[2]

Alerted by these police actions in other cities, the two reporters interviewed Denver police officers concerned with juvenile problems, and other authorities, to learn about glue-sniffing in Denver. Apparently Denver had no cases to report, for the story led off with an account of a child *accidentally* affected by glue fumes in a poorly-ventilated basement room; and an expert the two reporters interviewed—Dr. Samuel Johnson, director of Denver's Poison Control Center—similarly warned against using quick-drying glue in a room with the windows closed, lest intoxication *accidentally* result.

Dr. Johnson was on the whole reassuring about the glue "menace." If a person is affected by the fumes, he said, he need only go out and breathe fresh air to recover. Permanent injury is possible only if the exposure is prolonged and heavy—as when a worker in a glue factory breathes the stuff all day long every day. Yet the pioneer Denver story, setting a pattern soon to be followed by newspapers and magazines throughout the country, carried a scare headline:

SOME GLUES ARE DANGEROUS
Heavy Inhalation Can Cause Anemia or Brain Damage

This and subsequent warnings in the mass media were all based on the results of earlier industrial studies that, as noted above, could not be justifiably applied to the glue-sniffing fad.

The newspaper story also explained that one way to inhale glue is to "soak a handkerchief with glue and hold it over the mouth and nose." A photograph accompanying the article showed a young man demonstrating how the glue-soaked handkerchief should be held. Interesting results were promised if the glue were sniffed as directed: "The first effect of breathing the undiluted fumes is dizziness, followed by drowsiness. There is a feeling of suspension of reality. Later there is lack of coordination of muscle and mind." In a word, it was like getting drunk.

The effects of this newspaper article, published August 2, 1959—and no doubt of other similar articles and broadcasts in other Denver mass media thereafter—were visible by June 1960, when Denver police reported that during the past six or eight months they had investigated some 50 cases of glue-sniffing. In addition to these 50 cases, of course, there were no doubt many hundreds of others which had not come to the attention of the police. Denver was thus experiencing what—so far as the available literature reveals—was the earliest of many similar local glue-sniffing epidemics throughout the country.

Denver police met the new peril in the usual way—by escalating the warnings. In August 1959, Denver glue-sniffers had been threatened merely with anemia and brain damage. In June 1960 a spokesman for Denver's Juvenile Police Bureau was quoted as saying: "This practice is extremely dangerous, and a kid can die from it if he gets too much." A second police spokesman added that "inhaling large quantities of the cement fumes can lead to permanent injury of the respiratory system and could cause death." And the head of the Police Crime Laboratory warned: "I'm afraid some kid will get hold of too much of the stuff and we'll have a fatal case on our hands." [3] In October 1961 a Denver police lieutenant was quoted as explaining that glue fumes "diminish the oxygen supply to the blood" and "cause severe brain damage and death." [4] A representative in the state legislature warned that glue-sniffing "can result in permanent damage to the brain." [5] In April 1962 Denver youngsters were warned that glue-sniffing causes "stimulation of the central nervous system, followed by depression and often convulsions," and that "it can affect the respiratory tract, mucous membranes, skin, liver, kidneys, heart and blood—depending on what type of glue is used." [6]

The headline over the June 1960 story presented the two central themes which were later to characterize anti-glue-sniffing propaganda in other cities as well:

COULD BE FATAL

Plane Glue Gives Kids a Kick

Far from ending Denver's glue-sniffing epidemic, however, these warnings were followed by a further spread of the epidemic. The warnings seemed to function as lures. By October 23, 1961, the chief probation officer of the Denver Juvenile Court was able to announce: "We are averaging about 30 boys a month now on this glue-sniffing problem." Worse yet, he added, the custom was spreading from the high schools into the junior highs and "even into the grade schools." [7] A police spokesman similarly announced that glue-sniffing, unknown 26 months earlier, was now "a major problem among juveniles in Denver." He noted that 278 arrests were made for glue-sniffing in 1961, as compared with only 95 in 1960. [8]

Nor was the problem limited to Denver. Tom Adams, director of the state reform school in Golden, Colorado, was quoted in October 1961: "Right now I have about 50 boys here because of this glue-sniffing." [9]

Since no city or state law against glue-sniffing had yet been passed, the reporter who covered the story felt called upon to explain how 278 arrests could be made in 1961 for glue-sniffing and how 50 children could be incarcerated in a reform school for the same offense. His explanation, however, did not entirely clarify the mystery. All he could say was that "the youths are charged under juvenile delinquency procedures when they are found sniffing glue." A police spokesman added a detail: the 278 Denver arrests for glue-sniffing were classed for statistical purposes as "drunkenness arrests."*

Throughout 1960 and 1961, Denver police made further headlines by periodic raids on glue-sniffers. A typical 1961 example was headed:

---

* Readers should not be surprised at this development, for a substantial proportion of arrests and incarcerations of juveniles throughout the country are for actions which are not prohibited by any law and which would not be crimes if indulged in by adults. (See Ruth and Edward Brecher, *The Delinquent and the Law*, Public Affairs Pamphlet No. 337 [New York: Public Affairs Pamphlets, 1962]; also, *The Challenge of Crime in a Free Society*, A Report by the President's Commission on Law Enforcement and Administration of Justice [New York: Avon Books, 1968], pp. 227–228.)

7 DENVER YOUTHS ARRESTED
FOR DEADLY "GLUE-SNIFFING"

The story began:

Seven Denver teen-agers were arrested over the weekend for "glue-sniffing," a new thrill-seeking activity that juvenile authorities label "extremely dangerous."

Five of the boys, four of them 16 and the other 17, are in City Jail. Two others, 13 and 14, were lodged in Juvenile Hall.

All seven were arrested Sunday near the Curtis Park Recreation Center, 50th and Curtis Sts., by Patrolmen Dale Nelson and Donald Smith.[10]

Thus the broad pattern was established—the dramatic police raids and the imprisonment of children and teen-agers, accompanied by dire warnings of physical and psychological damage. The next element in the pattern was soon added: proposals for specific antiglue legislation.

On December 8, 1961, just six weeks after the sensational Curtis Park police raid, the Denver papers reported that State Representative Ben Klein, a former probation officer, would "propose to the January [1962] session of the Colorado Legislature three new laws to deter youngsters from sniffing airplane glue. . . ."[11] Denver youngsters no doubt noted the order of events: arrests and jailings first, legislation later—a sequence unlikely to encourage respect for law.

In support of his three new laws, Representative Klein quoted Denver's Juvenile Court Judge Philip Gilliam as saying that he considered glue-sniffing to be now "the Number 1 juvenile problem in the metropolitan area." Glue-sniffing had achieved this preeminence within two and a half years after the two writers in *Empire* had found no evidence of glue-sniffing in Denver.

Representative Klein's three laws would make it an offense (1) to sell glue to minors without parental consent, (2) to drive a car while under the influence of glue, or (3) to *sniff* glue. This last proposed offense was remarkable—for, as noted in Part I, it is not an offense to *use* even such drugs as heroin, in Denver or elsewhere in the United States. Representative Klein said his legislation would also require retailers "to keep a registry of sales . . . similar to the registry of sales of narcotics drugs." Thus glue-sniffing was more or less subtly linked with heroin.

Just as arrests for glue-sniffing were followed by laws against glue-sniffing, so medical warnings were followed by medical studies designed to justify the warnings. A study undertaken by Dr. Oliver Massengale, director of the Adolescent Clinic at the University of Colorado Medical Center, and Dr. Helen Glaser, assistant professor of pediatrics at the university, was no doubt the first scientific research on the recreational aspects of glue-sniffing in the history of the medical sciences.

[324]

Dr. Massengale explained that he became interested in glue-sniffing way back in 1960, when early newspaper reports of glue-sniffing hazards had appeared. A mother almost in tears, he recalled, had brought her son to his office.

"He's sniffing glue," the mother declared. "You've got to stop him before he dies."

A reporter for a Denver paper, in an interview with Drs. Massengale and Glaser published April 29, 1962, cited these researchers as authority for the statement that some types of plastic cement "may cause damage to the liver, kidneys and brain." [12] When the full text of the Glaser-Massengale study was published in the *Journal of the American Medical Association* for July 28, 1962, however, certain details were added that the newspaper interview had neglected. Cases of damage from glue all involved either the *swallowing* of substantial amounts or else the continuous day-after-day exposure to high concentrations among workers in industrial plants.

"Although a great deal of concern about the ill effects of this practice is expressed by parents, school personnel, juvenile authorities, and the children themselves," the medical experts noted in the medical publication, "very little is actually known about possible damage to organ systems resulting from deliberate inhalation of cement vapors. Many children share the so far unsubstantiated belief that glue-sniffing produces insanity and death, and we know of one case in which glue was first used by an adolescent boy in an attempt to commit suicide." [13]

Drs. Glaser and Massengale then presented six cases of juvenile Denver glue-sniffers. In none of them was any physical damage attributable to glue-sniffing; and in none of them was glue-sniffing the source of the child's psychological problems. Case Number 1, for example, concerned an eleven-year-old boy; "his mother worked at night; his parents were separated; and he had not seen his father for six years." The mother of Case Number 2 "was an alcoholic and was possibly also psychotic. The parents were separated, and the patient lived in a foster home, where he was unhappy. . . . He was . . . depressed, anxious, and fearful, and longing for affectional security. Seeing the world as hostile and pain-inflicting, he tended to withdraw into passive, immature forms of behavior." Patient Number 3 was a fourteen-year-old whose father had died when he was five, "and he had been taken out of the custody of his alcoholic mother but subsequently had been returned to her. A few months before being seen in the clinic the boy had spent eight months in a reformatory because of stealing." Case Number 5 was the boy who tried to commit suicide by sniffing glue. "This boy's father, possibly acting out of a cultural pattern of insecurity and fear, was very strict and rigid and was looked upon by the patient as a tyrant. His mother was a weak, inadequate person who sided with her son but was unable to rebel against her husband in his behalf." Case Number 6 was a fifteen-year-old; "the patient's father, who had been very strict and punitive, had died about six months before, and the mother was finding her son increasingly unmanageable and destructive. This boy had been in trouble even before his father's death because of writing obscenities in school books, running away, and joy-riding." [14]

In all cases, the child's problems and disturbances had antedated the glue-sniffing. Just what good was accomplished by arresting and incarcerating these troubled youngsters for sniffing glue did not appear in the study.

It should be noted, moreover, that these were not *typical* glue-sniffers. Rather they were typical of the small subsample of glue-sniffers who were *caught at it*—arrested by the police and referred to the university's adolescent clinic.

The Glaser-Massengale paper in the *Journal of the American Medical Association* confirmed the incredible speed with which glue-sniffing had spread following the first accounts in the mass media: "Glue sniffing, almost unheard of two years ago, has become a serious threat in some communities. In the Denver area it is considered by responsible juvenile authorities to be the most serious problem they face currently in working with known delinquents and other youngsters brought to the attention of the court because of violations of the law."* The 130 Denver children arrested in the two-year period for glue-sniffing "ranged in age from 7 through 17, with a mean age of 13 years, and all but 6 were boys." [15] Eighty percent had Spanish surnames; this high incidence was perhaps due as much to the arresting practices of the police as to the frequency of glue-sniffing among those children. Glue-sniffing children in middle-class white neighborhoods are customarily seen by pediatricians in private practice.

The remainder of the Denver story need here be only briefly summarized through selected newspaper items:

- January 18, 1965: Legislation introduced to ban glue-sniffing.[16]
- March 21, 1965: Juvenile court lays plans for preventive approach to glue-sniffing.[17]
- April 22, 1965: Adams County sheriff announces breakup of juvenile glue-sniffing activities with arrest of nineteen-year-old girl.[18]
- April 29, 1965: Thirteen-year-old leader of glue-sniffing gang admits burglaries.[19]
- June 25, 1965: Glue-sniffing charges against boy will be dismissed if he enlists in armed services before September 13.[20]

* As noted above, however, there was as yet no law to be violated.

• July 2, 1965: United States Department of Health, Education, and Welfare makes $85,500 grant to finance study of glue-sniffing in Denver.[21]

• January 11, 1966: Thirteen-year-old resident of county receiving home hangs himself after being scolded for sniffing glue.[22]

• May 18, 1966: Twenty-one-year-old jailed after admitting he burglarized drugstore to get glue to sniff.[23]

• June 10, 1966: Three with Spanish surnames sentenced to 30 days each in County Jail after pleading guilty to sniffing glue.[24]

• October 30, 1966: An additional $44,923 HEW grant is made to study glue-sniffing in Denver. . . .[25]

While Denver was in all probability the first city in the world to suffer a major glue-sniffing epidemic, other cities soon followed Denver's example. In New York City, for example, the New York *Times* ran a story about glue-sniffing on October 6, 1961: "L.I. Youths Inhale Glue in Model Kits For Narcotic Effect." [26] Other New York area newspapers— and no doubt radio and television stations as well—ran similar stories.

As in Denver, the New York stories stressed the hazards of glue-sniffing. The initial New York *Times* story, after stating that youngsters sniff glue to "obtain a feeling of elation similar to that of narcotics," and that youngsters who sniff glue are "found in seemingly drunken stupors," went on to cite the Nassau County Health Department as authority for the warning that toluene, the organic solvent most commonly used in model airplane glue, "dulls the brain when it is inhaled and could kill a person. It can cause damage to the liver and bone marrow if it is taken in small repeated doses. The chemical has an irritating effect on the lungs and can cause pain, vomiting, headaches, confusion, and ultimately coma. It can also cause the heart to beat irregularly and can result in transient euphoria. The lethal dose is unknown. No fatalities have been recorded." These warnings, like the earlier Denver warnings, seemed to be highly effective lures. Within fifteen months, New York City police had made 778 arrests for glue-sniffing [27]—and the city authorities were seriously considering proposals to make glue-sniffing illegal. In 1963, New York City arrests totaled 2,003.[28] Many tens of thousands of others, of course, were no doubt sniffing glue by then without coming to the attention of the police.

Salt Lake City was another city where local news media publicized glue-sniffing early, and where the glue-sniffing epidemic had an early start. Twelve boys, aged fourteen to eighteen, were apprehended there for glue-sniffing and interviewed in 1962; the interviews were of particular significance in revealing the way in which glue-sniffing, which a few years earlier was only one of a number of forms of sniffing, had become the prime form of sniffing. "Seven of the boys had previously inhaled the fumes of other substances, notably the fumes of gasoline (6 boys), ether, and nasal inhalers (one each), and one of these boys had been smoking marijuana." Glue-sniffing had recently, however, far outstripped the other sniffings, "to the extent that in one small town the practice was considered virtually universal among boys. Girls, as yet, have not been widely involved." [29] Marijuana smoking did not catch up with glue-sniffing among children until a major antimarijuana campaign was launched a little later.

The glue interests contributed notably to expanding the anti-glue-sniffing campaign from a local to a nationwide phenomenon. As early as 1962 the Hobby Industry Association of America, representing 1,100 industry members, announced that it was spending $250,000 a year to combat glue-sniffing.

"To help inform communities about the sniffing problem," the *Wall Street Journal* announced on its front page on December 7, 1962, "the Hobby Industry Association has produced a 15-minute color film 'The Scent of Danger,' which it soon will release to local civic groups. The film describes the harm done by glue sniffing and mentions other products, such as cleaning fluid and nail polish, which also contain solvents that can cause intoxication. It recommends that communities make it illegal to sniff any substance with an intoxicating effect." [30] For this the hobby industry won rewards of two kinds—public approval for its dedication to the anti-glue-sniffing campaign, and a marked rise in glue sales during the subsequent years.

The early anti-glue-sniffing laws were remarkable in several respects. One of the first of them—perhaps the very first—was Ordinance Number 1722, passed by the City of Anaheim, California, on June 6, 1962. This ordinance made it illegal for any person to "inhale, breathe, or drink any compound, liquid, chemical, or any substance known as glue, adhesive cement, mucilage, dope, or other material or substance or combination thereof, with the intention of becoming intoxicated, elated, dazed, paralyzed, irrational or in any manner changing, distorting or disturbing the eyesight, thinking process, balance, or coordination of such person." [31] Whiskey drinking was no doubt illegal under this ordinance.

A Maryland law enacted a little later was not quite so broad; this statute made it "unlawful for any person under twenty-one years of age to deliberately smell or inhale such excessive quantities of any narcotics, drugs, or any other noxious substances or chemicals containing any ketones, aldehydes, organic acetates, ether, chlorinated hydrocarbons or any other substances containing solvents releasing toxic vapors, as cause conditions of intoxication, inebriation, excitement, stupefaction, or dulling of the brain and nervous system. . . . Any person violating this section will be guilty of a misdemeanor and upon conviction thereof shall be fined. . . ." [32] Why glue-sniffing by adults aged twenty-one or older was exempted from the Maryland law is not apparent.

[328]

Other cities and states passed laws restricting the *sale* of glue in various ways—though this approach was opposed by the Hobby Industry Association. At the beginning of 1968 the Kupperstein-Susman bibliography listed 13 states and 29 counties and municipalities that had already passed glue-sniffing laws; additional states, counties, and municipalities had such laws under consideration.

The national news media contributed notably to the glue-sniffing campaign. In its issue of February 16, 1962, for example, the weekly news magazine *Time* carried an item headed "The New Kick," which declared: "The newest kick is glue-sniffing. A 14-year-old sniffer explains: 'You take a tube of plastic glue, the kind squares use to make model airplanes, and you squeeze it all out in a handkerchief, see. Then you roll up the handkerchief into a sort of tube, put the end in your mouth and breathe through it. It's simple and it's cheap. It's quick, too. Man!' " [33]

As is customary, the information about how to get high on glue was accompanied in *Time* by ritual warnings—much as crime movies of the era, after glorifying the heroic criminals, ended with their tragic deaths. *Time* quoted Dr. Alan K. Done, director of Salt Lake City's Poison Control Center, as saying: "I have found definite evidence of effects on the kidneys from glue sniffing. It is too soon to know whether this effect is temporary or permanent damage." [34] Neither *Time* nor the other media, however, publicized the findings of Dr. Massengale and his Denver associates indicating that glue-sniffing did *not* produce kidney damage in Denver.

Newsweek followed on August 13, 1962, with a story entitled "The New Addicts." It began:

You're in outer space. You're Superman. You're floating in air, seeing double, riding next to God. It's Kicksville. Are these the fantasies of narcotics addicts on a pop? No. More disturbingly, these hopped-up reactions are those of teenagers hooked on goofballs, model airplane glue, and cough medicine. Across the nation, police last week reported case after case of this alarming trend. [35]

In Miami, *Newsweek* noted, "a 12-year-old boy, discovered sniffing airplane glue by his father, snatched up a knife and threatened to kill him." A police officer with the Miami Juvenile Bureau was then quoted as commenting: "It's common for the boys who sniff glue to become belligerent. They are willing to take on a policeman twice their size." And *Newsweek* added: "Glue sniffers—while not physiologically addicted—can do equal damage to their systems. Some of the long-term effects [include] burned-out nose membranes, liver damage, perforations of the gall bladder, destruction of bone marrow, blindness, and possible death. But," *Newsweek* cogently went on, "this threat doesn't deter youngsters from squeezing up to five tubes of glue daily into a paper bag and breathing the fumes." [36]

Consumer Reports, the magazine of Consumers Union, also ran a warning against glue-sniffing—a bit more restrained than the others—in January 1963. "Although there is as yet no documented evidence . . . ," the *Consumer Reports* article cautiously noted, "CU's medical consultants are convinced that the inhalation of sufficient solvent vapors to produce the mental effects the sniffers seek probably will also produce damage to the liver, kidneys, respiratory organs, and possibly other organs as well." [37]

Even the Federal Bureau of Investigation took a hand in the anti-glue-sniffing campaign. Its *FBI Law Enforcement Bulletin* for October 1965 carried an article by Dr. Jacob Sokol, chief physician for the Los Angeles County Probation Department, entitled "A Sniff of Death." The tenor of the article was summarized in the subhead: "Glue-sniffing—in all its horrifying and alarming ramifications, mentally, physically, and medically—is discussed by Dr. Sokol in plain, lay language. His report should be of the utmost interest to law enforcement officers, parents, teachers, civic leaders, and all persons concerned with the welfare and health of young people." [38] The *FBI Bulletin* article, moreover, cited a new argument by Dr. Sokol against glue-sniffing:

Glue sniffers have described to me how a number of children, boys and girls, meet in unoccupied houses where they sniff glue together and later have sexual relations—both homosexual and heterosexual. To my knowledge this practice has not, however, come to the attention of law enforcement agencies.

Recently, while conversing with deputy probation officers, I have been informed that several episodes of homosexual relations have occurred between adults and children under the influence of glue. Some of these sexual perverts are encouraging the children to sniff glue with the intensions of having homosexual relations with them.[39]

Just where the "sexual perverts" got this idea of giving children glue was not discussed; perhaps it was from reading the anti-glue-sniffing campaigns in the mass media.

To end the glue menace, the *FBI Bulletin* article recommended seven measures, including the following: "1. We should arouse public opinion as to the dangers of this practice. . . .

"7. Legislation should be passed which would prohibit the sale of glue containing certain toxic chemicals to persons under 21 years of age." [40]

One side effect of the anti-glue-sniffing campaign, which continued throughout the 1960s, calls for special mention. The campaign produced subtle changes in the relations of parents and teachers to children. A child was now a suspect to be spied upon lest he secretly be sniffing glue. Health departments and other authoritative agencies encouraged this espionage, and listed the symptoms adults should be on the alert for: "Parents suspecting or told that their children have deliberately sniffed glue should take them to a doctor without delay.

"Schoolteachers should note irritability, inattentiveness, sleeping or loss of consciousness as symptoms of glue sniffing." [41]

The one voice of reason and common sense amid the near-hysterical concern with glue-sniffing was found in the Verhulst-Crotty bulletin issued by the National Clearinghouse for Poison Control Centers, cited earlier. Summing up the evidence from the studies of glue-sniffers reviewed by the authors, the bulletin noted:

By speculation, projection, and imagination, one can . . . build up quite a case for the potential hazards of the repeated inhalation of organic solvents such as those used in plastic cements. It behooves us, however, to ascertain facts in this regard. [One expert] inferred from his contact with a number of boys who practice glue-sniffing that the boys could and would give up the practice readily if they were convinced it was dangerous. At the same time, however, it became evident that the transparent misinformation or contradictory statements by authorities concerning the dangers of these practices would be completely disregarded by these boys and taken as evidence that none of the information was true. It also became apparent that, if the boys gave up glue-sniffing, they would take up other habits which would provide a comparable effect. [One expert] points out that, in our present state of knowledge, toluene (one of the more commonly used solvents in plastic cements) is considerably safer than many other organic solvents. [42]

The mass media of the early 1960s were filled with reports of deaths due to glue-sniffing. The Verhulst-Crotty bulletin tracked down these reports and found a total of nine alleged glue-sniffing deaths—each one reported many times. Six of the nine were not due to glue fumes but to asphyxiation, which occurred when the victim's head was covered by an airtight plastic bag. A seventh death was probably also a plastic-bag case. In an eighth case there was no evidence whatever that the victim had been sniffing glue before his death, and no toluene was found at autopsy. The last case was probably not due to glue-sniffing; the victim had been ill and had sniffed gasoline. Thus among tens of thousands of glue-sniffers prior to 1964, no death due unequivocally to glue vapor had as yet been reported. The lifesaving advice children needed was not to sniff glue with their heads in plastic bags.

The Verhulst-Crotty bulletin also reviewed behavioral effects of glue-sniffing; children unquestionably did all sorts of silly and potentially dangerous things when high on glue—much the same things they would have done if drunk on alcohol.

Those bulletins, unfortunately, were distributed in mimeographed form to only a short list of recipients. They had no visible effect on the nation-wide anti-glue-sniffing campaign.

The toxicology of recreational solvent-sniffing at this writing remains very much where it was at the time of the 1964 Verhulst-Crotty summary. No one is prepared to say that occasional solvent sniffing is safe, and some studies suggest that frequent sniffing may be moderately harmful.

Later in the decade, it was widely observed that young people paid little or no attention to dire warnings against the hazards of marijuana smoking, LSD-using, and other forms of drug use. It seems highly likely, in retrospect, that the exaggerated warnings against glue-sniffing were among the factors desensitizing some young people to drug warnings in general. Most teenagers knew of others in their own neighborhoods who had sniffed glue repeatedly, and who did not drop dead or go to the hospital with brain damage, kidney damage, or liver damage. Children may be ignorant, but they are not stupid. When the evidence of their own experience contradicts adult propaganda, they (like sensible adults) rely on their own experience—and tend to distrust in the future a source of information which they had found unreliable in the past.

The nationwide anti-glue-sniffing campaign, it should be noted, *preceded* the anti-LSD campaign, to be described later, and in part set the model for it. The anti-LSD campaign, like the antiglue campaign, featured solemn warnings of dire damage, laws against LSD, sensational police raids, scientific studies demonstrating hazards—and an endless bombardment of publicity concerning all of these other factors. Both campaigns were followed by increased use of the drugs attacked.

There was also one difference. In the case of LSD (see Chapter 50), the drug was popularized through the simultaneous efforts of LSD enthusiasts and LSD enemies. But glue-sniffing had no Timothy Leary to advertise and praise it. The enemies of glue-sniffing popularized the custom all by themselves.

At the beginning of the decade, gasoline sniffing was the most common form of organic solvent inhalation. Paint-thinner sniffing, varnish-remover sniffing, cigarette-lighter-fluid sniffing, glue-sniffing, and the others were not-very-common phenomena to which no one paid much attention. So far as can be determined, gasoline sniffing at the end of the 1960s was neither more nor less popular than at the beginning. The same was true of the sniffing of other readily available organic solvents. Only *glue*-sniffing was the target of a nationwide campaign—and only *glue*-sniffing became a popular youth pastime. It seems clear that the damage done by the arrests and imprisonments of children for glue-sniffing during the 1960s far exceeded the damage done by glue-sniffing during that sorry decade—and served to popularize rather than to discourage the practice.

Just how popular it became, many recent surveys reveal.

In 1969, 1,348 high-school seniors in Montgomery County, Maryland, filled out a drug-use questionnaire. Of these, 7.4 percent stated that they had sniffed glue, and 1.0 percent described themselves as current glue-sniffers. Similarly, among 1,429 Montgomery County junior-high-school students, 6.6 percent reported that they had sniffed glue.[43]

Among 781 sophomores, juniors, and seniors in five high schools in Madison, Wisconsin, filling out a questionnaire in 1969, 5.1 percent stated that they had sniffed glue. The replies indicated that 0.8 percent sniffed glue frequently, 1.0 percent sniffed glue infrequently, and the remaining 3.3 percent had sniffed glue only once or twice.[44]

Among 47,182 students in Utah high schools and junior highs answering a questionnaire in 1969, 7.1 percent reported that they had at some time sniffed glue; 9.5 percent of the boys and 4.8 percent of the girls had sniffed. Among the boys, 3.5 percent had sniffed only once, 3.8 percent had sniffed several times, and 2.2 percent had sniffed more than 10 times. The returns indicated that 1.8 percent of the boys and 0.9 percent of the girls had sniffed glue within the past few weeks.[45]

Among 1,379 high-school seniors in 11 selected Michigan high schools in 1968, 8.1 percent in one school reported glue-sniffing, as compared with 7.0 percent in another, 4.7 percent in a third, and none at all in two small high schools.[46]

Among 1,225 students at Mamaroneck (New York) Senior High School answering a questionnaire in 1967, 6.1 percent reported having sniffed glue and 2.0 percent had sniffed glue more than once. Among 1,294 Mamaroneck Junior High School students, 8.3 percent reported having sniffed glue, and 1.4 percent had sniffed glue more than once.[47]

These and other similar surveys suggest that at a rough estimate, at least 5 percent of all young Americans graduating from high school—perhaps 150,000 in each annual cohort—have sniffed glue at least once. This level of use can be contrasted with the level before 1959, when glue-sniffing was essentially unknown and unpublicized.

On July 20, 1971, the New York *Times* heralded yet another nationwide campaign against yet another inhalant menace with a front-page headline:

AEROSOL SNIFFING: NEW AND DEADLY CRAZE

The story, by Grace Lichtenstein, echoed closely the kickoff of the anti-glue-sniffing campaign a decade earlier: "Physicians, government officials, drug experts and chemical manufacturers are growing increasingly worried about a deadly and relatively new drug-abuse problem among the nation's children: the inhalation of aerosol sprays."

As in the earlier stories about glue-sniffing, precise details were supplied on how to get high on aerosols: "The aerosol product—hair spray, deodorant, household cleaners or some other—is sprayed into a paper bag or balloon and then inhaled because the propellant produces a strange, floating kind of high."

There followed the usual warnings of disastrous effects:

According to the Food and Drug Administration, more than 100 youths have died from deliberate aerosol sniffing since 1967, with an average of four deaths a month currently being recorded. . . . It appears that death occurs after a youngster deeply inhales an aerosol spray for a prolonged period, either on a single occasion or on several occasions. The fluorocarbon propellant Freon, the best-known brand of fluorocarbon, can make the heart beat irregularly and then stop.

An expert was quoted as adding: "Once the final event begins, it's quick, sudden, and irreversible." [48]

An earlier round of aerosol inhaling by children, the story noted, had centered around a spray-on product used to chill cocktail glasses. This product had therefore been removed from the market. Little was accomplished, however, for "experts stress that any of the 300 kinds of aerosol products now on the market can be equally abused because all use similar propellants."

Like the glue industry in the earlier glue-sniffing campaign, the aerosol industry entered the aerosol-sniffing campaign through an "Inter-Industry Committee on Aerosol Use." "The campaign includes a filmstrip, 'Rap On,' that has been distributed to 3,000 school districts. The industry has also put out a booklet, 'Will Death Come Without Warning?' which declares that aerosol products are safe when used as directed."

"They're really trying awfully hard," said B. J. Burkett, spokesman for the Inter-Industry Committee and public relations manager of the Freon Products Division of E. I. du Pont de Nemours & Co.

There was as yet no suggestion that aerosol sniffing be made a criminal offense; but laws were being proposed to require a warning—perhaps even a skull-and-crossbones—on the label of all aerosol products. Such measures, however, had been decided against as of this writing.

But, one might wonder: Here we go again?*

---

* The first effort to repress the recreational use of nitrous oxide (laughing gas) was also instituted in 1971. *Psychiatric News* reported: "Strict regulations have been placed on the distribution and sale of nitrous oxide in Maryland by Dr. Neil Solomon, state secretary of health and mental hygiene, following reports that the gas is being used by some young people as an inhalant to produce an exhilarating effect. This is the first regulatory action taken in the nation concerning improper use of nitrous oxide, according to information from the Food and Drug Administration. . . ." [49]

Part VII

LSD and LSD-Like Drugs

Scores of substances with widely varying chemical compositions are known to have effects similar (not identical) to that of *LSD* on the human mind. In general there are three major sources for these drugs. Some are natural plant substances—for example, *peyote,* a cactus plant. Some are extracted from such substances; thus *mescaline* is derived from peyote. Some—LSD, mescaline, psilocybin, and others—can be manufactured synthetically.

To an even greater extent than for other psychoactive drugs, the effects of these drugs vary with the expectations of the user, the setting in which they are used, and other nonpharmacological factors. Three drugs in the group—LSD, mescaline, and psilocybin—have been used in psychotherapy, and LSD is still used as an adjunct to psychotherapy in countries other than the United States.

These drugs are commonly taken orally. They are not addicting. Tolerance for LSD builds up very rapidly, but no withdrawal syndrome has been reported. LSD is longer-acting (usually seven hours or more) and is effective in smaller doses (as little as 25 micrograms) than most other drugs in the group. Effects, both undesirable and favorable, are primarily psychological. The lethal dose of LSD is not known; no human fatalities have been recorded.

Part VII

LSD, and LSD-like Drugs

45.

Early use of LSD-like drugs

LSD was not discovered until 1938, and its effects on the human mind remained unknown until 1943; but numerous other drugs producing LSD-like effects have been known since time immemorial, and have been used by peoples throughout the world, especially by North and South American Indians. The plants that produce these drugs grow almost anywhere —in temperate as well as tropical climates; in deserts as well as forests. Almost everywhere, the effect of such drugs was considered a mystical and religious phenomenon, an experience that brings man closer to the gods and to nature.

Peyote. Peyote (in Aztec, *peyotl*) is a spineless cactus with a small crown or "button" and a long carrot-like root. The crown is sliced off and dried to form a hard brownish disk known as a mescal button. The dried button is generally held in the mouth until soft and then swallowed unchewed; several buttons may be required to achieve a peyote "trip." "Native to the deserts of central and northern Mexico," Professor Richard Evans Schultes reports, "peyote claims centuries of use . . . and was basic to pre-Columbian religious practices of the Aztec and other Mexican Indians." [1] Much of the account that follows is based on a 1969 survey by Professor Schultes, director of the Botanical Museum of Harvard University and one of the nation's foremost authorities on ethnobotany.*

The peyote effect is highly complex and variable, Dr. Schultes notes. "Its most spectacular phase . . . comprises the kaleidoscopic play of visual hallucinations in indescribably rich colors, yet auditory and tactile hallucinations and a variety of synesthesias are among the effects." [2] A typical synesthesia is the "seeing" of music in colors or the "hearing" of a painting as music. In addition to these sensory experiences, there is often a mystical experience of insight into a reality deeper than mere everyday appearances, or of communion with the gods; hence peyote was revered as a sacred medicine and used in healing rites and ceremonies.

The Spanish warriors and priests who conquered and ruled Mexico viewed peyote, and other LSD-like drugs in common use among the Aztecs, as diabolical. Neither the civil authorities nor the Spanish Inquisition, however, was able to stamp out peyotism altogether; "primitive peyote religious dances still survive among the Cora, Huichol, and Tara-

---

* Readers interested in further details should consult Professor Schultes's paper in *Science,* January 17, 1969, or his "Botanical and Chemical Distribution of Hallucinogens," in the *Annual Review of Plant Physiology,* 21 (1970): 571–598.

humare of northern Mexico," [3] Professor Schultes reported in 1969.* Indians on the United States side of the Mexican–United States border—notably the Mescalero † Apaches—adopted the custom from the Mexican Indians.

Farther north, early white traders introduced the Indians to alcohol; and as the post–Civil War tide of white settlers and United States Army expeditions drove the Indians from their lands and onto the newly established reservations, alcoholism became a major problem among them. The peyote cult, with its mystical setting and religious rites, then spread northward in competition with alcohol. The Comanches and the Kiowas adopted peyotism in the 1870s; the Shawnees, Pawnees, Delawares, Cheyennes, Arapahoes, and numerous other tribes followed.[5] Great Indian prophets like Quanah Parker (a Comanche), and John Wilson (part Caddo, part Delaware) carried both the drug and its meaningful ritual from tribe to tribe.[6] By 1954, it was estimated that one-half of all American Indians had experienced the peyote "trip." [7]

Before discovering peyote, we are told, Quanah Parker "was dedicated to destroying every white man he came in contact with. He had more scalps in his tepee than all the other chiefs combined." [8] As the white man continued to come west in ever larger numbers, however, Parker saw he was fighting a losing battle. He accordingly went alone into the wilderness "where he could think and pray to the Great Spirit Within." After many moons, we are told, the Great Spirit Within appeared and spoke to him:

Lay down your arms, Quanah Parker. Your solution, as is the solution of all creatures, is personal. Turn your energies toward conquering the self. . . . Only through this will you and your people have a freedom that exceeds the white man's.

I have planted my flesh in the cactus pioniyo [peyote]. Partake of it, as it is the food of your soul. Through it you will continue to communicate with Me. When all of those with the skin of red-earth clay are united by pioniyo, then and only then will they once again reign supreme. The white civilizations will destroy themselves and the Indian will return to nature, master over himself and at peace with all.[9]

When Quanah Parker returned to his people, we are further told, he called together his council and they adopted the peyote ritual, "which still prevails to this day. They broke the bow and arrow, signifying the ending of killings and wars. Quanah Parker was never to kill another man after that day." [10]

* For a detailed account of how peyotism survives in a rigorous framework of ritual and shamanism in Mexico, readers are referred to *The Teachings of Don Juan* (1968), by Carlos Casteneda, an anthropologist at the University of California at Los Angeles.
† Whence the name of the drug mescaline.[4]

Anthropologists are quite generally agreed that the migration of peyote and its associated religion northward to the beleaguered Indians of the United States brought many advantages. The peyote cult required total abstinence from alcohol—and there is abundant evidence that Indians who accepted peyotism did in fact abandon alcohol in substantial numbers.[11] In some tribes, where some members have adopted peyotism while others continue on alcohol, the contrast is quite striking. In addition the peyote cult eased the Indians' acceptance of their subjugation by the white man, and brought a sense of solidarity and brotherhood within that subjection. Finally, peyote was shared by many tribes and was thus a step toward pan-Indianism, the awareness of common interests that is a dominant theme of American Indian culture today.

Land speculators, who coveted the tribal lands where the peyote rites were practiced, and Christian missionaries sought to have peyote outlawed.[12] They scored modest successes in a few state legislatures. They were less successful, however, in getting antipeyote legislation through Congress;[13] anthropologists and friends of the Indians joined with the Indians themselves to defeat such legislation year after year. Even some of the state legislatures that had passed antipeyote laws later repealed them.

Oklahoma, the first state to outlaw peyote (1899), repealed its law in 1908 after Comanche Chief Quanah Parker himself testified before a legislative committee. Efforts to reenact the Oklahoma law in 1909 and 1927 were defeated. New Mexico outlawed peyote in 1929, but the law was not enforced—and in 1959 it was amended to permit ritual use. Montana also has legalized the use of peyote in worship.[14]

A major factor in maintaining the legal status of peyote has been the Native American Church of North America, an organization that claims some 250,000 Indian members from tribes throughout the United States and Canada. In addition to successfully opposing Congressional action against peyote and securing the repeal of state laws, the Native American Church has succeeded in several states in having such laws declared unconstitutional as a violation of freedom of religion.

To supply peyote to Indian tribes throughout the United States, mail-order companies sprang up that sold the dried buttons at very low prices. Interest in the drug widened, stimulated by books and by magazine articles such as Alice Marriot's sensitive account in the *New Yorker* (1954) of her experience with peyote among the Indians of South Dakota. The mail-order companies began advertising in college newspapers and other publications during the late 1950s and early 1960s.* Although peyote was

* During the 1950s, the cost per trip was as low as 32 cents. When *Life* magazine published an article by R. Gordon Wasson on psychoactive mushrooms, a woman reader wrote the editors: "Sirs: I've been having hallucinatory visions accompanied by space suspension and time destruction in my New York apartment for the past

not illegal, there were periodic raids on those in possession of it. In 1960, 311 peyote buttons were confiscated from a New York City coffeehouse.[16] Still, peyote remained generally available and openly used until LSD took over its market in the 1960s.

A recent study [17] of peyote use among American Indians today was presented at the 1971 meeting of the American Psychiatric Association (and later published in the *American Journal of Psychiatry*) by Dr. Robert L. Bergman, chief of the United States Public Health Service's mental health program serving 125,000 Navajo Indians in the Southwest.

Dr. Bergman had attended many peyote ceremonials and had interviewed some 200 peyote users, members of the Native American Church. Its religious services, he reported,

are highly serious and arduous. They follow a prescribed form which is derived largely from the ceremonial symbolism and practices of many tribes. A considerable difference from other Christian religions is the fact that until relatively recently all meetings were held for the purpose of praying for the cure of a sick person. This is still frequently the case, and all meetings must still have a specific purpose such as praying for the well being of children about to leave home for boarding school, or giving thanks for the safe return of a soldier from Vietnam. . . . The service is directed by a road chief assisted by several other officers, but is participated in almost equally by all present. Road chiefs learn their work through an apprenticeship usually lasting several years, but all have other occupations. There is no professional clergy.

The formal portion of a meeting begins at sunset and ends at sunrise. . . .

The group sits in a circle around a central altar and fireplace. The time is organized by a set order of service, and after a certain point in the service, Peyote is passed around the circle of worshippers and each is free to take whatever amount he wishes. This process is repeated during the night, and later each person is free to use a personal supply of medicine, which most bring with them. Amounts used vary greatly even within the same meeting. . . .

Much of the night is spent in the singing of religious songs: mostly Christian ideas expressed in various Indian languages and set to traditional Indian melodies. The songs are led by each person in turn and accompanied by a drum and by gourd rattles. There are also group and individual prayers, which are spontaneous, as well as many opportunities for the members of the group to address one another. Though there is some variation, portions of many meetings resemble group therapy. For example, I was present at a meeting held for a woman suffering from a mild menopausal depression. Older women present described their feelings about aging and the end of child-bearing and towards

---

three years . . . produced by eating American-grown peyote cactus plants. . . . I got my peyote from a company in Texas which makes C.O.D. shipments all over the country for $8 per 100 'buttons.' It usually takes about four 'buttons' for one person to have visions." [15] An interesting sign of the times was the fact that the writer signed her name.

morning, the patient's husband said that he had realized that he was partly to blame for his wife's difficulties.

"I have been so busy with church work," he said, "that I don't think I've been paying much attention to my companion. It came to me during the night that the reason I've been working hard is that I've prayed for a lot of people and sometimes they get better, but sometimes they don't, and sometimes they're grateful for what I did, but a lot of times they're not, and so I guess I began to have my doubts about religion, and the more I had doubts the harder I made myself work so I would forget about them."

The meeting ends with the consumption of symbolic foods and water, and then everyone goes outside into the early light, shakes hands and wishes everyone else good morning. It is a moment much like that at the end of a Jewish High Holy Day service when everyone exchanges wishes for a happy new year. . . .

As hostility toward LSD spread through the United States during the 1960s (see below), hostility toward the peyote religion also increased. "There have been attempts lately to limit the freedom of the members of the Native American Church to practice their religion," Dr. Bergman noted. "There have been a few journalistic reports depicting them as drug abusers." Peyote ceremonials were attracting "popular, official, and scientific interest because of the growing concern over the use of hallucinogens by students and others in the population at large. The main source of this new attention is fear that the ceremonial consumption of Peyote may be dangerous."

To determine the extent of this danger, Dr. Bergman and his associates launched their study. "For a period of four years, we have followed up every report of psychotic or other psychiatric episodes said to arise from Peyote use. There have been forty or fifty such reports. The vast majority have been hearsay that could never be traced to a particular case. Some have been based on a physician's belief that Navajo people use Peyote and if a particular person became disturbed it must be for this reason." In the end, the study found "one relatively clearcut case of acute psychosis and four cases that are difficult to interpret."

The clear-cut case involved a Navajo who attended a peyote meeting after having taken alcohol—several drinks. "Ordinarily, no one is allowed to participate if he has been drinking, but the road man did not realize that this person had been." The Navajo became panicky and disoriented, then violent—but recovered within twenty-four hours and remained well on follow-up six months later. "It is noteworthy," Dr. Bergman added, "that members of the church warn that the combination of alcohol and Peyote is very dangerous." Reactions in the other four cases were minor, and their relationship with peyote was doubtful.

Dr. Bergman then went on to calculate that even if all five of these incidents were to be classified as adverse reactions, "the resulting, probably overestimated, rate [over the four-year period] would be one bad reaction per 70,000 ingestions."

Dr. Bergman continued:

In describing some of the ways in which the Native American Church avoids harming its members, I have implied some ways in which I feel that it helps them. That is a subject for another and longer paper, but this one would be incomplete without saying that we have seen many patients come through difficult crises with the help of this religion and it appears to me that for many Indian people threatened with identity-diffusion it provides real help in seeing themselves not as people whose place and way in the world is gone, but as people whose way can be strong enough to change and meet new challenges. The Peyotists themselves are proud in particular of the help the church has been to Indian people who have drinking problems. In fact, Levy and Kunitz report a greater success rate for the Peyotists than for any other agency working with alcoholics in one part of the Navajo Reservation.

Dr. Bergman also describes in fascinating detail the precise ways in which the potential hazards of peyote are minimized and its potential for good enhanced by the peyote ritual. "Some of the crucial factors," he explains,

are a positive expectation held by Peyotists, an emphasis on the real interpersonal world rather than the world within the individual, an emphasis on communion rather than withdrawal during the drug experience, an emphasis on adherence to the standards of society rather than on the freeing of impulses, and certain practices during the meetings. . . .

The whole spirit of the religion seems best characterized as communion—with God and with other men. Meetings are experienced as a time of being close and growing closer to one another. . . . Distortions of time sense are counteracted by the various events of the service which take place at precisely defined times of the night. . . .

Road men are trained to look after people who become excessively withdrawn. If a participant begins to stare into the fire fixedly and seems unaware of the others in the meeting, the road man will speak to him, and if necessary go to him to pray with him. In the process of praying with such a person, he may fan him with an eagle feather fan, splash drops of water on him and fan cedar incense over him. All of these processes are regarded as sacred and helpful, and it appears to me they provide stimulation in several sense modalities to draw one back to the interpersonal world. Another safeguard is the custom that no one is to leave the meeting. Considerable efforts are made if necessary to prevent someone who has been eating Peyote from going off into the night alone. This factor is probably important too, in the customary activities of the morning after the meeting. Everyone stays together and socializes until well after the time the drug effect is over.

[342]

These safeguards, as we shall see below, are strikingly similar to the safeguards necessary for minimizing the hazards of LSD.

Dr. Bergman concluded his paper with a plea for further study of peyotism among the Indians—"not only to avoid injustice but also to learn from these people who use a potentially dangerous drug well and who, after all, have much longer experience in these matters than we have."

At the conclusion of Dr. Bergman's paper, the audience stood and applauded—a rare event at meetings of the American Psychiatric Association.

Fly agaric. Concerning this mushroom, Dr. Schultes reports,

The hallucinogenic use of the fly agaric *(Amanita muscaria)* by primitive tribesmen in Siberia came to the attention of Europeans in the 18th century. This fungus—widespread in north-temperate parts of both hemispheres—has long been recognized as toxic; its name refers to the European custom of employing it to poison flies. In recent times, its use as an inebriant has been known in only two centers: extreme western . . . and extreme northeastern Siberia. . . . Tradition established the use of fly agaric by witch doctors of the Lapps of Inari in Europe and of the Yakagir of northernmost Siberia. Formerly, the narcotic employment of *Amanita muscaria* was apparently more widespread, and it has even been suggested that the ancient giant berserkers of Norway induced their occasional fits of savage madness by ingesting this mushroom. . . .

Effects . . . vary appreciably with individuals and at different times. An hour after the ingestion of the mushrooms, twitching and trembling of the limbs is noticeable with the onset of a period of good humor and light euphoria, characterized by macroscopia, visions of the supernatural and illusions of grandeur. Religious overtones—such as an urge to confess sins—frequently occur. Occasionally, the partaker becomes violent, dashing madly about until, exhausted, he drops into a deep sleep.[18]

No use of fly agaric has been reported in the United States.

Other mushrooms. According to Dr. Schultes,

Archeological "mushroom stones" indicate that a sophisticated mushroom cult existed in Guatemala 3500 years ago. Early Spanish chroniclers wrote in detailed opposition to the diabolic mushrooms of the Aztec, *teonanacatl* ("food of the gods"),* eaten ceremonially for divination, prophecy, and worship; but since four centuries failed to produce evidence of such use of mushrooms, the suggestion that the chroniclers had confused the dried mushrooms with the dried crowns of the hallucinogenic peyote cactus was accepted. Only during the past two decades have ethnobotanical studies elucidated the extent of modern use in southern Mexico of at least 20 species of mushrooms in four genera among nine

---

* This also has been translated to mean "god's flesh." [19]

tribes. . . . Many, if not all, contain psilocybin . . . and an unstable derivative psilocin.

Psilocybe yungesis has been suggested as the identification of a "tree fungus" reported by early missionaries as the source of an intoxicating beverage of the Yurimagua of Amazonian Peru. No evidence, however, points to the present use of an hallucinogenic mushroom in that area.[20]

Reports are occasionally made of the use of such mushrooms by Americans today. The active principles in several of them—psilocybin and psilocin—have been isolated and synthesized,[21] and are occasionally marketed. They have been placed under legal control.

Nutmeg. "It is interesting," Dr. Schultes continues, "that primitive American cultures have discovered [hallucinogenic] properties in *Virola*, since the related Asiatic *Myristica fragrans*—the common nutmeg—is hallucinogenic and is thought to have been employed narcotically in southeastern Asia. It is occasionally so employed in . . . Europe and in the United States. . . ."

DMT. "*Yurema*," Dr. Schultes states, "an hallucinogen of the Kariri, Pankararu and other Indians of eastern Brazil, prepared from *Mimosa hostilis*, forms the center of a cult using an infusion of the root to bring on glorious visions of the spirit world. The active principle has been identified as *N, N-dimethyltryptamine*. . . ." [22]

N,N-dimethyltryptamine, or DMT, is outlawed by Congress and some state legislatures. It has been called "the businessman's LSD" because it produces an LSD-like trip lasting only an hour or two—and can therefore be taken during the lunch hour.[23]

Morning glory. During the 1960s, the seeds of two varieties of morning glory were reported to produce LSD-like effects. With respect to hallucinogenic morning-glory seeds, Dr. Schultes has this to say:

The early Spanish chroniclers of Mexico reported on numerous occasions the religious use of the lentil-like seeds of the Aztec *ololiuqui*, a sacred, hallucinogenic vine with cordate leaves. Several illustrations of the plant—the best in a voluminous study of the medicinal plants, animals, and stones of "New Spain" by Hernández, personal physician to the King of Spain who worked in Mexico from 1570 to 1575—leave no doubt that ololiuqui represented a morning glory. Most of the chroniclers were ecclesiastical authorities who railed against this "diabolic seed," and Christian persecution drove the native cults into hiding.

Corroboration of the identity of ololiuqui waited for 400 years, since no morning glory was found employed in pagan religious rites. The apparent absence of hallucinogenic use of a . . . plant [resembling the morning glory], together with the fact that no intoxicating constituent was known to exist in the family, led ethnobotanists to assume that ololiuqui must have been one of the several narcotic species of *Datura*—despite the insistence of reliable Mexican botanists that the plant was a morning glory. . . . Only in the late 1930's was actual voucher botanical material of a morning glory employed as an hallucinogen collected in Mazatec country in Oaxaca, and the accuracy of the ancient reports seemed to be vindicated by modern fieldwork. Later, another psychotomimetic morning glory—*badoh negro* of the Zapotec of Oaxaca—was found.

Among the natives of Aztec Mexico, ololiuqui was used for divination perhaps even more than peyote and teonanacatl. Hernández wrote that: ". . . when the priests wanted to commune with their gods . . . ," they ate ololiuqui seeds, and ". . . a thousand visions and satanic hallucinations appeared to them. . . ." Believed to possess a deity of its own, this plant was an ingredient also of magical ointments and enjoyed an exalted place in Aztec medicine. Modern Indians grind the seeds on a stone, soak them in water or alcoholic drinks, and filter them; ingest the filtrate, since the hard impervious testa may otherwise allow the seeds to pass intact through the digestive tract.[24]

For many years chemists sought to isolate the active principle in these morning-glory seeds, without success. Since 1960, the mystery has been solved. The hallucinogenic seeds contain a chemical very closely related to LSD. Most of the morning-glory seeds available in the United States, however, are believed to lack both this drug and the LSD-like effect.

Numerous other Old World and New World plants with LSD-like effects have been used through the centuries. It is the ready availability of low-cost black-market LSD itself (see below) that makes the cultivation or even harvesting of such plants uneconomic for clandestine users. Since LSD weighs much less per dose, is much less bulky, and keeps better than the natural substances, it is better adapted to black-market distribution. In the event that the supply of LSD should be cut off or that prices should rise unduly, however, an increase in the growing and harvesting of plant materials would no doubt follow.

46.

LSD is discovered

On the afternoon of April 16, 1943, Dr. Albert Hofmann, a chemist working at Sandoz Laboratories—a pharmaceutical firm in Basel, Switzerland—fell ill; and a few days later he recorded the curious nature of his illness in his notebook:

Last Friday . . . I had to interrupt my laboratory work in the middle of the afternoon and go home, because I was seized with a feeling of great restlessness and mild dizziness. At home, I lay down and sank into a not unpleasant delirium, which was characterized by extremely excited fantasies. In a semiconscious state, with my eyes closed (I felt the daylight to be unpleasantly dazzling), fantastic visions of extraordinary realness and with an intense kaleidoscopic play of colors assaulted me. After about two hours this condition disappeared.[1]

At the time of this curious experience, Dr. Hofmann had been working with two chemicals, both derivatives of ergot, whose effects were well-known; they could not have produced his symptoms. In addition, however, he had manufactured that morning a few milligrams of a third ergot derivative, d-lysergic acid diethylamide, which he and a Sandoz associate, Dr. W. A. Stoll, had discovered five years before. Since this was the twenty-fifth compound in the lysergic acid series synthesized at Sandoz, it had been nicknamed LSD-25. When preliminary tests on animals revealed nothing of interest in LSD-25, it had been put aside without human testing.

To find out if this relatively untested drug, unwittingly ingested, could have caused his strange symptoms, Dr. Hofmann administered to himself the following week what he thought would be a trifling amount—one-quarter of a milligram—of LSD-25. Then he sat down with his notebook to await developments. After forty minutes he noted "mild dizziness, restlessness, inability to concentrate, visual disturbance and uncontrollable laughter."[2] There the notebook entry abruptly came to an end. A quarter of a milligram of LSD, we now know, is a very substantial dose. Dr. Hofmann had embarked on his second LSD "trip," and was in for a rough six hours.

"The last words were written only with great difficulty," Dr. Hofmann noted after he had recovered.

I asked my laboratory assistant to accompany me home as I believed that I should have a repetition of the disturbance of the previous Friday. While we were cycling home (a four-mile trip by bicycle, no other vehicle being available because of the war), however, it became clear that the symptoms were much stronger than the first time. I had great difficulty in speaking coherently and my field of vision swayed before me and was distorted like the reflections in an amusement park mirror. I had the impression of being unable to move from the spot, although my assistant later told me that we had cycled at a good pace. . . .

By the time the doctor arrived, the peak of the crisis had already passed. As far as I can remember, the following were the most outstanding symptoms: vertigo, visual disturbances, the faces of those around me appeared as grotesque, colored masks; marked motoric unrest, alternating with paralysis; an intermittent feeling in the head, limbs, and the entire body, as if they were filled with lead; dry, constricted sensation in the throat; feeling of choking; clear recognition of my condition, in which state I sometimes observed, in the manner of an independent, neutral observer, that I shouted half insanely or babbled incoherent words. Occasionally I felt as if I were out of my body.

The doctor found a rather weak pulse, but an otherwise normal circulation. . . . Six hours after the ingestion of the LSD, my condition had already improved considerably.

Only the visual disturbances were still pronounced. Everything seemed to sway and the proportions were distorted like the reflections in the surface of moving water. Moreover, all objects appeared in unpleasant, constantly changing colours, the predominant shades being sickly green and blue. With closed eyes multihued, metamorphizing fantastic images overwhelmed me. Especially noteworthy was the fact that sounds were transposed into visual sensations so that from each tone or noise a comparable colored picture was evoked, changing in form and color kaleidoscopically.

The next day, Dr. Hofmann added, he felt "completely well, but tired." [3]

During the years since April 16, 1943, hundreds of psychiatrists, psychologists, and other professionals have taken LSD themselves, and have observed the effects in others. Dr. Hofmann's accounts of his trips have been repeatedly confirmed and in many respects expanded. His initial accounts are of particular interest, however; for it is now known that the nature of an LSD trip is profoundly affected by the *expectations* of the person taking the LSD, and of the persons administering the LSD and observing the effects. Dr. Hofmann's LSD experiences were not only the first; they were also among the few not contaminated by expectations on the part of the experimenter, the observer, or the subject.

Psychiatrists at the University of Zurich and elsewhere to whom Sandoz initially supplied experimental quantities of LSD soon established that very small doses have profound effects. Most drug doses are measured in milligrams, or thousandths of a gram; LSD doses are measured in micrograms—millionths of a gram. As little as twenty-five micrograms, it was learned, produces noticeable psychological effects in some people; 100 micrograms produces a full-scale LSD trip in most people.[4] An amount of LSD weighing as little as the aspirin in a five-grain tablet is enough to produce effects in 3,000 people.

The early experiments promptly established the fact that LSD is not addicting; and experience since then has uniformly confirmed this finding. The LSD experience is so massive that very few people want to experience it oftener than once a week—and longer intervals between trips are the common pattern.[5]

Because it was thought to produce hallucinations, LSD was soon classified (along with mescaline) as a *hallucinogen*. This label, however, has been questioned. A true hallucination is something you see and think is there but that really isn't—like the snakes and green elephants seen by an alcoholic during delirium tremens. The LSD user for the most part sees what *is* there, but he sees it in distorted, wavering, or kaleidoscopically changing forms—and he misinterprets what he sees. He may also see patterns, geometrical figures, or in rare cases even panoramas that aren't there; but unlike the true victim of hallucinations, he does not ordinarily accept them as real. He remains aware that what he is experiencing is a drug-induced phenomenon, and so experiences for the most part what Dr. Jerome Levine has labeled *pseudo-hallucinations*.[6] Exceptions to this rule are discussed below.

Still later, when LSD came into use as an adjunct to psychotherapy, it was dubbed a *psycholytic* drug because it was thought to dissolve or lyse a patient's resistance to therapy. The term *psychedelic* also came into common use; it was coined by Dr. Humphrey Osmond [7] to indicate that LSD is "mind-manifesting" or "mind-expanding." And the term *psychotomimetic* was introduced because LSD was thought to induce symptoms mimicking those of psychosis.[8] All of these terms, of course, indicate a point of view. In this Report we shall for the most part use a more neutral terminology: "LSD and LSD-like drugs."

47.

LSD and psychotherapy

For a time after 1943, LSD was a drug in search of a use. The United States Army tested its usefulness for brainwashing, and for inducing prisoners to talk more freely. Later, LSD was stockpiled in very large amounts by the American armed forces for possible use in disabling an enemy force.* [2] Military interest in LSD waned, however, when psychoactive chemicals such as BZ, capable of producing even more bizarre effects, were developed.†

Psychiatrists were naturally interested from the beginning in LSD effects. Many of them took the drug themselves, and gave it to staff members of mental hospitals, in the belief that its effects approximate a psychotic state and might thus lead to better understanding of their patients. Some of those who tried LSD reported that it did enable them to achieve greater empathy with their psychotic patients. It was as an adjunct to psychotherapy, however, that LSD came into widespread use.

Drs. Anthony K. Busch and Warren C. Johnson secured a supply of LSD from Sandoz in 1949, and published the first report on its psychotherapeutic use in twenty-one hospitalized psychotic patients in 1950. They concluded that "LSD-25 may offer a means for more readily gaining access to the chronically withdrawn patients. It may also serve as a new tool for shortening psychotherapy. We hope further investigation justifies our present impression." [5] Other reports soon followed. In 1950, Rosta-

---

* Brigadier General J. H. Rothschild, commanding general of the United States Army Chemical Corps Research and Development Command, in a book that he wrote following his retirement, *Tomorrow's Weapons* (1964), noted: "It is easy to foresee that a military commander under the effects of LSD–25 would lose his ability to make logical, rational decisions and issue coherent orders. Group cooperation would fall apart. . . . Think of the effect of using this type of material covertly on a higher headquarters of a military unit, or overtly on a large organization. Some military leaders feel that we should not consider using these materials because we do not know exactly what will happen and no clearcut results can be predicted. But imagine where science would be today if the reaction to trying anything new had been, 'let's not try it until we know what the results will be.'" [1]

† While most information about BZ is a military secret, the chemical is said to produce not only hallucinations, disorientation, giddiness, headache, drowsiness, and sometimes maniacal behavior, but also retention of urine and constipation. Field dispensers and bombs for delivering BZ to the enemy have been developed. [3] A major feature of LSD, BZ, and other psychochemicals is that even very small nations can develop and stockpile them. "The psychochemicals will be the most difficult of all weaponry to control and supervise if disarmament ever comes," Dr. Sidney Cohen notes. [4] The demobilization of United States biological warfare facilities in 1970 and 1971 did not include chemical agents.

finski in Poland told of giving LSD to eight patients with epilepsy.[6] In 1952 Dr. Charles Savage, who had first received LSD for use in a United States Navy project, reported lack of success in fifteen patients suffering from depression.[7] In 1953, Liddell and Weil-Malherbe in England reported favorable effects in patients suffering from a number of mental disorders.[8] By 1954 LSD was being used therapeutically in Baghdad.[9] Also in 1954, Federking in Germany reported the comparative effects of 60 LSD trips and 40 mescaline trips among neurotic patients refractory to psychotherapy; he thought LSD more effective than mescaline.[10] By 1965, it was estimated that between 30,000 and 40,000 psychiatric patients around the world had received LSD therapeutically; and additional thousands of normal volunteers had received it experimentally.[11] Countless experiments had been run on animal species ranging from the spider and the snail to the chimpanzee. It was estimated in 1965 that some 2,000 papers on LSD effects had been published.[12] Few drugs known to man have been so thoroughly studied so promptly.

At a 1965 LSD conference Dr. Sidney Cohen, an American authority on LSD, summed up the claims made for LSD and LSD-like drugs by psychiatrists:

1. They reduce the patient's defensiveness and allow repressed memories and conflictual material to come forth. The recall of these events is improved and the abreaction is intense.

2. The emerging material is better understood because the patient sees the conflict as a visual image or in vivid visual symbols. It is accepted without being overwhelming because the detached state of awareness makes the emerging guilt feelings less devastating.

3. The patient feels closer to the therapist and it is easier for him to express his irrational feelings.

4. Alertness is not impaired and insights are retained after the drug has worn off.

Under skilled treatment procedures, the hallucinogens do seem to produce these effects and one more which is not often mentioned. That is a marked heightening of the patient's suggestibility. Put in another way, the judgmental attitude of the patient toward the experience itself is diminished. This can be helpful, for insights are accepted without reservations and seem much more valid than under nondrug conditions.[13]

"It is curious," Dr. Cohen added,

how under LSD the fondest theories of the therapist are confirmed by his patient. Freudian symbols come out of the mouths of patients with Freudian analysts. Those who have Jungian therapists deal with the collective unconscious and with archetypal images [two key Jungian concepts]. The patient senses the frame of reference to be employed, and his associations and dreams are molded to it.[14]

Dr. Cohen did not conclude, however, that this curious LSD phenomenon invalidates LSD results. Instead, he called attention to an explanation first offered by a California psychoanalyst, Dr. Judd Marmor, who pointed out that while the technical terms used by different therapists may vary,

each interpretation has a definite relationship to the life pattern of the patient. A Freudian may express it in terms of unresolved Oedipal complexes, a Jungian will speak of archetypes, a Rankian of separation anxiety, and a Sullivanian of oral dynamisms. Marmor's point is that they are all structuring the data in their own terminology, but that a common core of reality underlies each of the explanations.[15]

Dr. Daniel X. Freedman, chairman of the department of psychiatry at the University of Chicago–Pritzker School of Medicine, has pointed out yet another feature of the LSD experience, one which he calls "portentousness": [16] the sense that something—even a trivial platitude—is fraught with a cosmic significance too profound to be adequately communicated.* Whether or not LSD does in fact enable users on occasion to grasp significant new insights into themselves or the world about them—a much-debated issue—the drug certainly gives many users a *feeling* that they have achieved profound new insights.

LSD was tried for the treatment of alcoholism at several research centers after 1952. The early reports suggested that a single large dose of LSD, given under appropriate circumstances, might profoundly affect drinking patterns and even produce total abstinence—reports curiously paralleling nineteenth-century and recent accounts of abstinence from alcohol among Indians entering the peyote cult. One LSD report of this kind from the Mendocino State Hospital in Talmadge, California, in 1967 concerned the effects of large doses (400 to 800 micrograms) of LSD on 71 women alcoholics with an average of 7.8 years of uncontrolled drinking:

Most of the women enjoyed the music though some wanted it turned off later in the day. Most lay quietly on the lounge and showed some feelings. Some thought of issues as large as the meaning of life and their place in it, while many considered tearfully their relationship to husband, children or boyfriends. . . . They often lay peacefully from 8 to 1 o'clock with a little leisurely moving about from 1 to 3 or 4 p.m. . . . Only three sessions [out of 82] were terminated early

* Ether was once thought to have a similar effect. Dr. Oliver Wendell Holmes, it will be recalled (see Chapter 43), took ether in the hope of achieving a mystical insight into the nature of the universe and felt that he had in fact achieved one. The insight, laden with a sense of portentousness, he recorded verbatim: "A strong smell of turpentine prevails throughout." [17]

because of the subject's reaction. . . . Most indicated no physical discomfort or fear of dying and found the experience intensely memorable and real. Almost none felt suspicious of others or unduly influenced by the others present. They felt a high level of of trust and affection . . . 75 percent felt a spiritual bond with others, 72 percent felt a unity of all things and that they were part of this unity, which 60 percent were willing to call God; 80 percent felt they gained a more complete acceptance of others; 84 percent felt their own understanding was enhanced.[18]

Bad trips occasionally occurred when LSD was used in psychotherapy —but these, too, were sometimes therapeutic. At a Wesleyan University LSD conference in 1967, Dr. Albert A. Kurland of the Maryland Psychiatric Research Center cited a remarkable example from among the 177 patients whom he and his associates—Drs. Charles Savage, John W. Schaffer, and Sanford Unger—had treated up to that time. This patient was a forty-year-old male alcoholic, black, brought to the hospital from jail after ten days of uncontrolled drinking. He had dropped out of the fourth grade at the age of twelve and had an I.Q. of 70. "He had been draining whiskey barrels at his place of work, a distillery. He gave a history of excessive alcohol consumption over the past four years. . . . The only limit on his drinking was his low income and the need to support five children. During these years his marriage had deteriorated." [19]

Given a week of preparation and a single large dose of LSD, this patient felt (among other things) that he was being chased, struck with a sword, run over by a horse, and frightened by a hippopotamus—a quite typical "bad trip." His own verbatim report of his trip then continued:

I was afraid. I started to run, but something said "Stop!" When I stopped, everything broke into many pieces. Then I felt as if ten tons had fallen from my shoulders. I prayed to the Lord. Everything looked better all around me. The rose was beautiful. My children's faces cleared up. I thought of alcohol and the rose died. I changed my mind from alcohol toward Christ and the rose came back to life. I pray that this rose will remain in my heart and my family forever. As I sat up and looked in the mirror, I could feel myself growing stronger. I feel now that my family and I are closer than ever before, and I hope that our faith will grow forever and ever.[20]

This patient was given psychological tests both before and after his LSD experience. His score on the Eysenck neuroticism scale before LSD had been in the eighty-eighth percentile—highly neurotic. One week after LSD his score had swung to the normal portion of the scale. His pre-LSD depression, as measured by the Minnesota Multiphasic Personality Inventory (MMPI), had lifted and his score was greatly improved. Tested a third time, six months after LSD, his depression score on the MMPI was

still within normal limits. More important—"He had been totally abstinent, and his wife reported that there was a peace and harmony in the
home that had never existed before and that he had never been better." [21]

A full year after the single LSD treatment, "the family picture remains
the same. He is still sober, although there has been one brief break in
abstinence following the loss of his job." [22]

The credit for this and similar one-shot successes with alcoholics, Dr.
Kurland believes, is traceable only in part to the LSD experience itself.
"This particular patient was fortunate in having a family that reinforced
his new-found feeling of love and affection for them. A patient who goes
back to a rejecting family is very likely to return to drink." [23] Observations
such as this have led some therapists to offer the LSD experience to the
spouses of patients as well as to the patients themselves.

"What seems striking about this particular case," Dr. Kurland concluded, "is not only that an alcoholic's drinking has been arrested, but
that an illiterate, culturally deprived man of low intelligence could apparently be reached through a psychotherapeutic procedure. . . ." [24]

Another field in which LSD has been used at a number of medical
centers is the palliation of terminal cancer. Beginning in 1964, a Chicago
anesthesiologist, Dr. Eric C. Kast of Cook County Hospital, published a
series of reports on LSD given to 128 terminal cancer patients in great
pain.[25] LSD proved about as effective as the usual opiates in relieving this
pain—and the effect was much longer-lasting. Indeed, the pain relief
continued even after the LSD trip terminated. More remarkable still,
many patients retained their equanimity for several weeks after the pain
returned; they no longer considered the pain *important*.

Dr. Kast's findings were confirmed by Dr. Sidney Cohen in his work with
terminal cancer patients,[26] and by Dr. Kurland and his associates in
Maryland. The Maryland research was launched under dramatic circumstances.

"A professional member of our own research department, a woman in
her early forties, developed a progressive neoplastic disease [cancer],"
Dr. Kurland explained at the 1967 Wesleyan University conference. "She
had undergone radical mastectomy [breast removal], and subsequent surgery had revealed inoperable metastases to the liver. Although still ambulatory, she was in considerable physical distress—unable even to breathe
deeply without severe pain. She was fully aware of the gravity of her
condition, and her depressed and distraught psychological state was
steadily worsening." In these desperate straits, the patient requested LSD
therapy. "After discussion with her husband and her surgeon, and with
the approval of all concerned, a course of psychedelic therapy was
initiated." [27]

A week was devoted to preparation. Then LSD was administered. Two days later the patient went on a two-week vacation with her husband and children. Upon her return she wrote the following report:

The day prior to LSD, I was fearful and anxious. I would, at that point, have gratefully withdrawn. By the end of the preparatory session, practically all anxiety was gone, the instructions were understood, the procedure clear. . . .

The morning was lovely—cool and with a freshness in the air. I arrived at the LSD building with the therapist. Members of the department were around to wish me well. It was a good and warming feeling.

In the treatment room was a beautiful happiness rosebud, deep red and dewy, but disappointingly not as fragrant as other varieties. A bowl of fruit, moist, succulent, also reposed on the table. I was immediately given the first dose and sat looking at pictures from my family album. Gradually my movements became fuzzy and I felt awkward. I was made to recline with earphones and eyeshades. At some point the second LSD dose was given me. This phase was generally associated with impatience. I had been given instructions lest there be pain, fear or other difficulties. I was ready to try out my ability to face the unknown ahead of me, and to triumph over any obstacles. I was ready, but except for the physical sensations of awkwardness, and some drowsiness, nothing was happening.

At about this time, it seems, I fused with the music and was transported on it. So completely was I one with the sound that when the particular melody or record stopped, however momentarily, I was alive to the pause, eagerly awaiting the next lap in the journey. A delightful game was being played. What was coming next? Would it be powerful, tender, dancing, or somber? I felt at these times as though I were being teased, but so nicely, so gently. I wanted to laugh in sheer appreciation. . . . And as soon as the music began I was off again. Nor do I remember all the explorations.

Mainly I remember two experiences. I was alone in a timeless world with no boundaries. There was no atmosphere; there was no color, no imagery, but there may have been light. Suddenly, I recognized that I was a moment in time, created by those before me and in turn the creator of others. This was my moment, and my major function had been completed. By being born, I had given meaning to my parents' existence.

Again in the void, alone without the time-space boundaries. Life reduced itself over and over again to the least common denominator. I cannot remember the logic of the experience, but I became poignantly aware that the core of life is love. At this moment I felt that I was reaching out to the world—to all people—but especially to those closest to me. I wept long for the wasted years, the search for identity in false places, the neglected opportunities, the emotional energy lost in basically meaningless pursuits.

Many times, after respites, I went back, but always to variations on the same themes. The music carried me, and sustained me.

Occasionally, during rests, I was aware of the smell of peaches. The rose was nothing to the fruit. The fruit was nectar and ambrosia (life), the rose a beautiful flower only. When I finally was given a nectarine, it was the epitome of subtle, succulent flavor.

[354]

As I began to emerge, I was taken outdoors to a fresh, rain-swept world. Members of the department welcomed me and I felt not only joy for myself but for having been able to use the experience these people who cared wanted me to have. I felt very close to a large group of people.

Later, as members of my family came, there was a closeness that seemed new. That night, at home, my parents came, too. All noticed a change in me. I was radiant, they said. I seemed at peace, they said. I felt that way too. What has changed for me? I am living now, and being. I can take it as it comes. Some of my physical symptoms are gone. The excessive fatigue, some of the pains. I still get irritated occasionally and yell. I am still me, but more at peace. My family senses this and we are closer. All who know me well say that this has been a good experience.[28]

Psychological tests were administered to this patient both before and after LSD therapy. "The retesting indicated a significant reduction on the depression scale and a general lessening of pathological signs." The patient "returned to work and appeared in relatively good spirits" for five weeks. Then she was hospitalized for accumulation of fluid caused by the cancer, and died three days later.

"Investigation of the utility of psychedelic therapy with terminal patients is continuing," Dr. Kurland concluded his 1967 report, "with the collaboration of staff at the Sinai Hospital in Baltimore. . . ."[29]

Through the years of LSD psychotherapy from 1949 to the mid-1960s, psychiatrists and others relearned the lesson American Indian users of LSD-like drugs had learned long before: that the setting in which the drug is given, the expectations aroused in the patient prior to the experience, the people and objects present during the experience, the reassurance given the patient as the trip progresses, and countless similar ancillary factors are as significant in molding the experience as the drug itself—and are essential safeguards against adverse effects.

Ultimate pharmacological proof of the effectiveness of LSD in psychotherapy has not been established. Ideally, candidates for therapy should be divided at random into two groups, one of which is given the medication while the other is treated in exactly the same way except that it is given a placebo instead. To guard against bias, moreover, the procedure must be "double-blind"; neither doctor nor patient must know whether the patient is receiving the active drug or a placebo. The effects of LSD are so obvious, however, that the "double-blind" requirement is utterly impractical; any physician will recognize within a very short time whether a patient has in fact received LSD.

Despite lack of a control group, both patient and psychiatrist may conclude that the patient's life pattern has improved under treatment. The patient is in this respect his own control: a comparison of his condition before and after therapy takes the place of a comparison between treated and untreated patients. So it was with the use of LSD in psycho-therapy. It survived and spread in the United States from 1949 into the mid-1960s, and continues in use in other countries, because psychiatrists and patients alike have been impressed by the changes experienced. As Dr. Sidney Cohen points out, "No method of using LSD therapeutically has as yet met rigid scientific requirements, which include long-term follow-up and comparison of patients receiving LSD with a control group who receive identical treatment except for the LSD. But, in truth, no other type of psychotherapy has been fully tested by these exacting methods." [30]

48.

Hazards of LSD psychotherapy

From the very beginning, psychiatrists were aware that LSD, like most other medicaments, poses hazards. The hazards visible during the early years were summed up in a classic 1960 paper, "Lysergic Acid Diethylamide: Side Effects and Complications," by Dr. Sidney Cohen.[1]

Dr. Cohen sent a questionnaire to 66 researchers who were known to have administered LSD or mescaline to humans, either therapeutically or experimentally. Forty-four of them replied; they had administered LSD on more than 25,000 occasions to nearly 5,000 men and women. Dr. Cohen also searched the medical literature for published reports of adverse effects.

From the *physical* point of view, LSD was found to have a remarkable record. "No instance of serious, prolonged physical side effects was found either in the literature or in the answers to the questionnaires. When major untoward reactions occurred they were almost always due to psychological factors."[2] No physical complications were observed even when LSD was given to skid-row alcoholics with impaired liver function and generally deteriorated health.

As for adverse *psychological* reactions, Dr. Cohen noted that the published LSD literature "directly records only one suicide and that in a schizophrenic patient, and a small number of short, self-limited psychotic reactions and other lesser side effects."[3]

Dr. Cohen's survey of LSD therapists, however, turned up several kinds of adverse psychological reactions. These he divided into immediate and subsequent.

The most common, but still infrequent, immediate problem [Dr. Cohen reported] was one of unmanageability. This apparently occurs when insight into the situation is lost and the individual acts upon delusory, usually paranoidal ideas. Instances of running away from the tester, disrobing, or accidental self injury were described. . . .

Panic episodes were likewise mentioned. When these develop early they seem to represent the terror involved with the loss of ego controls. At the height of the reaction panic may be precipitated. . . . Finally, after many hours of frightening dissociation the subject could develop an intense fear that he will not be able to get back to his ordinary state.* [4]

* Others have similarly commented that the *duration* of the LSD trip—more than six hours in most cases—is a disadvantage. Few trials have as yet been made of psychotherapy with short-acting LSD-like drugs such as DMT.

Certain kinds of people, the Cohen survey revealed, are particularly likely to have bad trips of these kinds. "Those with excessive initial apprehension" are the prime example; fear of a bad trip increases the likelihood of a bad trip. Dr. Cohen also mentioned people with "rigid but brittle defensive structures, or considerable subsurface guilt and conflict." [5]

People hostile to LSD were also noted as likely to have bad trips. "Invariably, those who take hallucinogenic agents to demonstrate that they have no value in psychiatric exploration have an unhappy time of it. In a small series of four psychoanalysts who took 100 [micrograms] of LSD, all had dysphoric [unpleasant] responses. Two Zen Buddhists were given LSD in order to compare the drug state with the transcendent state achieved through meditation. Both Zen teachers became so uncomfortable that termination [of the trip] became necessary." [6]

The Cohen survey also noted two kinds of hazard during the day or two after LSD. "The first is a simple prolongation of the LSD state. Ordinarily, after a night's rest it is to be expected that complete cessation of the drug effect will have occurred. However, the persistence of anxiety or the visual aberrations for another day or two in wavelike undulations has been described." [7] More frequent were short-lived depressions following LSD. These, Dr. Cohen noted, might be due to simple "letdown" on returning to humdrum everyday life, or to other factors.

While bad trips were infrequent, Dr. Cohen offered a number of suggestions for reducing the frequency still further. One was adequate screening of patients through a preliminary psychiatric interview and history-taking—especially to exclude schizophrenics and schizoids. The briefing of the patient in advance is also "a matter of some importance, with the value of the drug interview sometimes depending on the preliminary instructions. Something of the nature of the experience and the expectations for the session are communicated at this time. Misconceptions are corrected and necessary reassurances are given." [8]

Precautions *during* the LSD trip are also essential. "That the person under the influence of LSD should not be left alone is universally agreed. Human contact is comforting and serves as a pivot between every day reality and the strange world of LSD. Without it the patient can readily lose all orientation. Personnel in contact with the subject should be experienced and sympathetic. . . . The [LSD] state is a highly suggestive one with the patient responding strongly to environmental cues. He can sense the therapist's unspoken feelings with phenomenal accuracy. Impersonality, coldness and disinterest is the equivalent of being left alone." [9]

Finally, Dr. Cohen noted that although they are rarely needed, LSD antagonists should be on hand. Several drugs are capable of terminating an LSD trip quite promptly. Psychological measures such as reassurance rather than drugs, however, are commonly used today to abort an LSD bad trip.

A much feared aftermath of LSD during the 1950s was suicide—in part because of widespread rumors of a European suicide following LSD use, and in part because one actual LSD suicide had been reported in the medical literature. In this respect, the 1960 Cohen survey was reassuring.

The patients given LSD included many who were seriously depressed or suffering from other severe forms of mental illness. In such a population, the incidence of suicide is relatively high. Among the patients covered in the Cohen survey, the suicide rate was one per 2,500 patients. Among healthy experimental subjects given LSD, the suicide rate was zero. The rate of suicide attempts among psychiatric patients given LSD was 1 in 800; the rate among experimental subjects given LSD was zero.

During a four-year period ending in 1964, among 150 patients given from one to eighty LSD doses by Dr. E. F. W. Baker of the University of Toronto and Toronto General Hospital, one patient committed suicide a few weeks after an LSD trip and one died of "unknown causes." "This experience is not out of line with ordinary suicide risk in a comparable group of patients not subjected to this form of treatment," Dr. Baker noted. "We know of at least nine serious suicidal attempts made by patients in this particular group before LSD therapy was instituted." [10]

Finally, and perhaps most important, psychiatrists in 1960 were concerned that LSD might trigger not just a brief "bad trip" but a prolonged psychotic reaction lasting more than forty-eight hours. The Cohen survey confirmed that such cases do occur. They are most likely to occur, the questionnaire returns indicated, among schizophrenic or schizoid patients; hence such patients should not receive LSD. The frequency of prolonged reactions was low, however. Only one such case was reported among 1,300 experimental subjects who received LSD—and he recovered within a few days. There were seven prolonged reactions among the psychiatric patients—a rate of one per 550 patients. "These breakdowns happened to individuals who were already emotionally ill," Dr. Cohen commented; "some had sustained schizophrenic breaks in the past. In certain instances the unskillful management of the patient contributed to the undesirable outcome." [11]

Dr. Cohen concluded:

This inquiry into the adverse effects of the hallucinogenic drugs indicates that with proper precautions they are safe when given to a selected healthy group. Their use in [psychiatric] patients has been associated with an occasional complication. An analysis of these incidents suggests that with the application of certain safeguards many of these side effects might have been avoided.[12]

Drs. Jerome Levine and Arnold M. Ludwig, then psychiatrists at the United States Public Health Service Hospital in Lexington, Kentucky, commented on the Cohen survey findings that they "better support a statement that the drug is *exceptionally safe* rather than dangerous. [Italics in original.] Although no statistics have been compiled for the dangers of psychological therapies, we would not be surprised if the incidence of adverse reactions, such as psychotic or depressive episodes and suicide attempts, were at least as high or higher in any comparable group of psychiatric patients exposed to any active form of therapy." [13]

Another questionnaire survey on the use of LSD in psychotherapy was undertaken in Britain in 1969 by Dr. Nicolas Malleson, psychiatrist, Fellow of the Royal College of Physicians, and member of the Advisory Committee on Drug Dependence of the United Kingdom Home Office. Dr. Malleson's survey [14] differed from Dr. Cohen's in only a few respects. He received replies from substantially all of the therapists who had ever administered LSD to patients in the United Kingdom over a span of nearly twenty years—66 therapists in all. The replies covered 4,303 patients, given a total of more than 50,000 sessions (almost all of them LSD, the remainder psilocybin), plus 169 experimental subjects given a total of 448 sessions. The handful of therapists not included in the survey consisted of a few who had given LSD only to animals, plus a few who had treated only a very small number of cases. Thus for practical purposes the survey covered substantially all patients receiving LSD therapeutically in Britain down to 1969.

Two suicides were reported among the 4,303 patients:

1. "Female, late 20's, married, an atypical manic-depressive. Admitted [to mental hospital] depressed. Anti-depressant drugs and 'other therapies' having failed, LSD therapy attempted. Some symptomatic improvement. Went on leave from hospital one week after an LSD session and was found dead from barbiturate and carbon monoxide poisoning three days after."
2. Male, early 20's, psychopath, given one very small dose of LSD [25 micrograms, the minimum likely to secure even a slight effect]. Showed no significant response. Left hospital against medical advice a few days later and hanged himself. "I think it is difficult to say," the psychiatrist reporting the case noted, "whether the patient's suicide was connected with his medication or not."

Twenty attempted suicides were reported; but "four of these were quite possibly only gestures and for seven no precise details were available." Several had made repeated suicide attempts before taking LSD.

Thirty-seven patients developed psychoses of more than forty-eight hours' duration. Of these, 9 patients recovered completely within two weeks, and 10 remained chronically psychotic; in some of these chronic cases, the reporting therapists expressed the opinion that these were potential chronic psychotics before LSD.

There were also two natural deaths during the 50,000 LSD sessions or shortly thereafter. One asthmatic patient died of acute asthma twelve hours after his third session; another dropped dead for reasons unknown during his seventh session. There was one proved coronary attack and two suspected attacks during sessions, as well as an epileptic attack in one patient without a prior history of epilepsy. One patient in a panic jumped out of the window, with superficial injuries; another pushed her hand through a windowpane and suffered cuts.

The bulk of the adverse reactions were among the patients receiving LSD from therapists with little LSD experience. Hospitals with the greatest experience reported relatively few adverse reactions; at Marlborough Day Hospital, for example, 6,522 LSD sessions and 50 psilocybin sessions were given to 507 patients with no suicides, no serious suicide attempts, no accidents, and only four psychotic reactions. "Treatment with LSD is not without acute adverse reactions, but given adequate psychiatric supervision and proper conditions for its administration, the incidence of such reactions is not great," Dr. Malleson concluded. Whether a like number of equally ill patients given psychotherapy *without* LSD would have had more or fewer adverse effects could not be determined.

A substantial majority of the British therapists who answered Dr. Malleson's questionnaire in 1969 were apparently of the opinion that LSD therapy is well worth the risk in cases where it is indicated. Asked whether they were still using LSD, and if not, why not, the 63 therapists who answered this question replied:

Still using LSD in 1969	37
Stopped for reasons not associated with LSD	
(e.g., retired from practice, change of field, etc.)	11
LSD not effective	7
LSD too dangerous	4
Fear of genetic damage	2
Reasons for stopping not given	2
Total	63

49.

Early nontherapeutic use of LSD

Long before LSD was discovered, some investigators interested in the working of the human mind had from time to time taken LSD-like drugs, especially peyote, and reported on their experiences; Havelock Ellis was an early example. Philosophers, theologians, and clergymen interested in the mystical religious experience had similarly experimented. Such informal use continued after the discovery of LSD; Aldous Huxley, for example, reported favorably on his experiences with mescaline in *The Doors of Perception* (1954). As LSD became available in the 1950s, this personal use of such drugs, and especially of LSD itself, for nontherapeutic or quasitherapeutic purposes became much more common. Developments of this kind in California during the 1950s and early 1960s have been described by Dr. Richard H. Blum and his Stanford University associates in *Utopiates* (1964), a review of the early LSD experiences of 92 men and women.[1]

Among the first to use LSD privately for nontherapeutic purposes, the Blum group reported, were physicians, psychiatrists, and other mental-health professionals, plus laymen who took LSD in their company.[2] The Blum group studied 24 LSD users in this category, some of whom had begun LSD use as early as 1956.

Most of the group were initiated to LSD use by psychiatrist friends, others by friends, teachers, or husbands. "In every case the initiator had himself taken the drug before offering it to a novice. . . . Only two persons initiated themselves; for the rest, LSD was a social event in which someone else gave them the drug and was with them during the experience. Most took LSD in a private home, either their own or that of an 'experienced' LSD user."[3] Having used LSD themselves, moreover, a majority of this group went on either to initiate or to encourage at least one other person to use LSD. (This desire of LSD users to enlist others runs as a common theme throughout the Blum report.) One reason for this proselytizing enthusiasm was that a majority of the sample "felt that LSD had improved their lives or persons,"[4] and wanted their friends to experience similar benefits.

Volunteers who had received LSD as part of an experiment in a university, hospital, or other bona fide research setting formed another category of early LSD users; the Blum group studied 15 examples, mostly male students or former students aged twenty-one to thirty. The majority in this group reported "some beneficial psychological changes as the result of having taken LSD, although they have not reoriented their goals or interests. The amount of change most report in response to LSD is not great. . . ." [5] About half stated that they had influenced others to use LSD following their own favorable experience.

From these very early user groups, LSD spread to others who took LSD "without benefit of either institutional setting or the presence of any medical or mental-health professional." [6] The Blum group studied 12 men and women in this category, all of whom knew one another and formed part of an active social circle. LSD among members of this circle "was usually taken in a party setting. It was just one of a number of hallucinogenic or intoxicating drugs which were used. Everyone reported pleasant reactions or 'kicks'—being 'high' or having 'freedom from troubles,' for example. The majority also discussed aesthetic experiences; some were passive ones in which music or a painting was more appreciated; others were active in that users would paint, make montages or mobiles, or write. Some of the sample also spoke of their mystical religious experiences and most described unusual feelings of closeness and special appreciation of others. Upon occasion, we were told, these interpersonal delights became quite specific as the partying people took off their clothes and played romantic roulette." [7]

Members spent "much of their social life with like-minded drug-taking persons," [8] and actively recruited additional LSD users—"there was pride when a father or an aunt could be persuaded to join the inner circle." [9] They saw nothing wrong with a fourteen-year-old taking "acid"—but they did hesitate to initiate "unstable" people. "I feel I have a responsibility when I 'turn someone on' to LSD; you want to be sure they won't go sour"; and again, "You want them to have enough sense to know how to act; I mean to be discreet and not get themselves or anybody else in trouble." [10] Thus there was at least a casual "screening" process among nontherapeutic users, with few seriously disturbed individuals given LSD.

Most of the members of the circle were in their twenties, some in their teens—but the ages ran up into the forties and fifties as the users "turned on" their parents and other older people. "They were well educated, socially respectable, and ambitious as far as career goals were concerned. All but two appeared to make excellent work adjustments. None appeared to have serious personality pathology." [11] The high ambitions and good work adjustments during this early LSD period stand in marked contrast to later reports that many or most LSD users were "dropouts" from school or society.

This circle, the Blum group concluded, was generally happy; members were motivated to use LSD by a "desire to enhance an already pleasurable state rather than a desperate need to escape misery. . . ." [12] Many other such LSD circles arose in other parts of the country.

[363]

The Blum group also studied 8 patients given LSD therapeutically in a free public clinic, 13 private patients who took LSD therapeutically in the home or private office of their psychiatrist, and 20 who paid as much as $500 for LSD sessions at a "center," opened in 1960, which promised both therapeutic and religious-mystical benefits. Most of the "center" users were in their thirties.

"Nearly all center sample members report self-improvement as a consequence of LSD use," the Blum group noted; "often personal changes, spiritual benefits, and reduction in competitive or material concerns are cited. Although practically none of the sample had originally had any interest in having a religious experience through LSD, nearly half reported a religiously significant experience." [13]

The majority in this sample "described both pleasant and unpleasant reactions to the drug. For most, the unpleasantness was recalled as initial and transient. Frequently the unpleasant features were said to have been valuable, 'part of the price of self-knowledge.' Quite clearly, several people felt it was necessary to suffer to gain from LSD. The belief that suffering is a necessary requirement for salvation is extensive in our culture. It is found in psychoanalysis, in the Christian doctrine of salvation from sin, and in the Protestant work ethic which holds that good things do not come easily. One suspects that the welcome accorded to the painful facets of the center LSD experience is not unrelated to these larger themes." [14] One may also have here an explanation of the strange fact that some people who have personally experienced a bad trip nevertheless take LSD again—and recommend it to their friends. Others, of course, abandon the drug.

Reviewing the 92 LSD users in their sample, the Blum group found that many of them reported various benefits—"as a therapeutic tool, a means for enhancing values or expanding the self, a road to love and better relationships, a device for art appreciation or a spur to creative endeavors, a means to insight, and a door to religious experience." [15] Also mentioned were *pleasurable* effects—"release from anxiety or troubles, euphoria, heightened sensations, fantastic images or hallucinations, orgiastic excitement, and the like." [16] In recruiting new users and talking about "what LSD has done for me," the Blum group noted, the emphasis was generally on the ethical and aesthetic "changes for the good" rather than on these transient pleasures of the LSD experience.

A notable finding of the Blum study was the extent to which both the benefits and the unpleasantnesses of LSD varied among the groups studied. Thus more than 90 percent of the "informal professional" and "religious-medical-center" groups claimed that they benefited in their personal adjustments; the proportion was lower among those receiving LSD therapeutically from private psychiatrists, still lower from those receiving LSD at a public clinic, and lowest of all among healthy volunteers who received LSD as part of an experiment.[17] Among the informal professionals the chief unpleasant reactions were "physical distress [and] feelings of helplessness or loss of control." The clinic patients said that they "felt self-conscious or were embarrassed by what they did or felt during the experience." The patients of psychiatrists in private practice "suffered raw fear—of madness, of loss of control, of the unknown lying ahead." In the social circle using LSD for pleasure, "the one bad effect was disappointment at the failure of LSD to meet their expectations—to produce the desired aesthetic, euphoric, or self-expanding sensations." [18]

These and other differences among the groups—plus data from countless other studies—serve to underline the fact that "the LSD experience," to an even greater extent than experiences with most other drugs, varies with the setting, the expectations, the motivations of both giver and receiver, the companionship, and a variety of similar ancillary factors. In this study, interestingly enough, the group receiving LSD from psychiatrists in psychotherapy reported neither experiencing as much benefit as the nontherapeutic users, nor enjoying as much freedom from undesirable effects. The Blum sample of 92 was much too small, of course, to supply reliable data on such occurrences, rare at that time, as suicide, attempted suicide, accidents, or prolonged psychotic reactions following LSD.

50.

How LSD was popularized, 1962-1969

The creation of an LSD black market. Prior to 1962, LSD was a little-known drug, available only on a small scale, and used by relatively few people. Substantially all of the LSD and psilocybin available in the United States and Canada was produced by Sandoz Laboratories and legally distributed by them to psychiatrists, psychologists, and others who certified their qualifications to use it. Each LSD container was labeled, as required by FDA regulations: "Caution: New drug—limited by Federal law to investigational use." Throughout the 1950s and early 1960s, the supply of LSD for informal use had been uncertain. Sometimes Sandoz LSD was available; sometimes it was not. When it wasn't, users turned to psilocybin, mescaline, peyote, and other LSD-like substances.

In 1962, a new tranquilizing drug, thalidomide, was also distributed for testing under the FDA's IND (investigational new drug) regulations to 1,267 American physicians, and reached hundreds of pregnant women. In other countries it was distributed on a far larger scale. A worldwide epidemic of deformed babies followed. During the next few years, the FDA tightened up its IND regulations, many states outlawed LSD, and Congress passed a new law further restricting the use of investigational drugs—including LSD. Sandoz responded by sharply limiting LSD distribution.

The new laws, the new FDA regulations, and the Sandoz restrictions were followed by a marked *increase* in the availability of LSD. The drug is only moderately difficult to synthesize in a modest chemistry laboratory. The formula can be secured from the United States Patent Office for fifty cents, and the precursor chemicals are not hard to acquire. The quantities producible are very great; million-dose batches of clandestine LSD were in fact produced.* (A million 250-microgram doses weigh about nine ounces.) The clandestine supply soon exceeded the domestic demand, and the American black market thereupon became a large-scale exporter of clandestinely manufactured LSD to Canada and Europe.

In 1970, the Advisory Committee on Drug Dependence of the United

---

* In fiscal 1967, government agents seized clandestine laboratories said to have a production capacity of more than 25,000,000 doses of LSD and LSD-like drugs per year. In fiscal 1968, the production capacity of the clandestine laboratories seized was reported to be more than 40,000,000 doses per year.[1] Consumption, of course, fell far short of this production capacity. No estimate is available of the production capacity of the clandestine LSD labs that *escaped* seizure.

Kingdom Home Office reported: "Probably the bulk of [British LSD] is smuggled in from the USA. We are told that users preferred .the American [black-market] LSD and regarded the English product as inferior." The LSD smuggled into Britain from the United States was originally "impregnated into innocent objects such as sugar cubes, sweets and blotting paper. More recently it has been coming in in tablet or capsule form under such exotic names as 'cherry top,' 'purple haze,' and 'blue cheer.' " [2] Canada's Le Dain Commission similarly reported in 1970 that Canadian black-market LSD was coming "mainly from clandestine factories in the United States." [3] Since LSD is odorless, tasteless, and colorless, weighs only a trifle and occupies a negligible volume, few shipments are intercepted.

Thus, by shutting off the relative trickle of Sandoz LSD into informal channels, Congress and the Food and Drug Administration had unwittingly opened the sluices to a veritable LSD flood. By 1970 it was estimated that between 1,000,000 and 2,000,000 Americans had taken an LSD trip.[4]

In 1964, Drs. Arnold M. Ludwig and Jerome Levine, then at the United States Public Health Service Hospital in Lexington, Kentucky, investigated the beginnings of the LSD black market by talking with drug users from all over the country. They reported their findings in the *Journal of the American Medical Association* in 1965:

The drug, as obtained through illicit channels, is usually deposited on sugar cubes. It has also been obtained in liquid form in small ampules, in crystalline form (in capsules or by the spoonful), or as a small white pill. The drug was also distributed on animal crackers when certain enforcement agencies declared sugar cubes to be contraband.

In the Boston, Mass. area the drug was purchased for $1 per cugar cube, whereas in New York, N.Y. and Miami, Fla., a cube might cost from $2 to $7. In Harlem, gelatin capsules containing powdered LSD were bought for $2 to $10 depending on the size of the capsule. One quarter of a teaspoon of [diluted] LSD (equivalent to seven to ten capsules) sold for $35. . . .

The drug is usually referred to as LSD but has also been called "25" (apparently from LSD-25). In the Boston area the designation "crackers" (from animal crackers) was used, and when people considered obtaining the drug they often stated, "Let's get some coffee," because the drug was frequently acquired in coffee houses.[5]

The first clandestinely synthesized LSD, according to knowledgeable sources, was of excellent purity and quality. Excellent black-market LSD is also available today. But in addition, the market since 1963 has been flooded with adulterated LSD, contaminated LSD, improperly synthesized LSD containing a variety of related substances whose effects are little known, and LSD of unknown dosage. It is impossible to determine how many of the adverse reactions noted after 1962 were traceable to these factors.

LSD publicity. Glue-sniffing, it will be recalled (Chapter 44), was popularized by antiglue warnings emanating from medical and law-enforcement authorities and widely publicized in the mass media. LSD was similarly publicized by anti-LSD warnings; but, in addition, praise of LSD by its proponents was also widely publicized. It is impossible to determine which contributed more to the growth of the demand for black-market LSD between 1962 and 1969: the warnings or the praise. The combination of warnings and praise triggered a publicity barrage that grew far out of rational proportion. The net effect was to make LSD familiar to everyone in the land, and to arouse nationwide curiosity. From curiosity to experimentation is only one short step.

There were many propagandists for LSD before 1962, but no one paid much attention to them, and they had little effect. This was still true when Timothy Leary, an instructor at Harvard University's Center for Research in Human Personality, first started work with LSD. Leary had been much impressed by the effects of some Mexican psilocybin mushrooms that he had tried in the summer of 1960. "It was the classic visionary voyage and I came back a changed man," he wrote in 1967. "You are never the same after you've had that one flash glimpse down the cellular time tunnel. You are never the same after you've had the veil drawn." [6]

At Harvard that fall, Dr. Leary and an associate, Dr. Richard Alpert, secured a supply of psilocybin from Sandoz for use in an experiment with prisoners at the Massachusetts Correctional Institution in Concord. The first results seemed promising: prisoners released from the institution following a psilocybin trip seemed less likely to be rearrested and returned for parole violation than other parolees. Critics of the experiment noted, however, that it might have been association with the two charismatic young instructors, Drs. Leary and Alpert, rather than the drug that produced the favorable results. In addition, Leary continued to take trips himself, to confer with other psychedelic enthusiasts such as Aldous Huxley and Allen Ginsberg, and to gather around him a clique of Harvard young people dedicated to the LSD-like drugs. He remained little-known outside his small Cambridge circle.

In 1962, however, Leary's activities attracted the attention of the FDA and Massachusetts law-enforcement officials, who made inquiries. Harvard and the Harvard *Crimson* responded by warning students against taking LSD. The warnings were picked up by the mass media—and were among the first nationally circulated publicity for LSD. As the FDA and state officials continued their investigation, a scandal broke. Leary, the focus of the scandal, became a national figure overnight. He used his new eminence to propagandize for LSD on a national scale.

Leary and Alpert left Harvard under fire in the spring of 1963—to the accompaniment of more nationwide publicity. Leary was thereafter harassed by both local and federal law-enforcement authorities, imprisoned for violation of the Marijuana Tax Act, released when the United States Supreme Court found portions of that Act unconstitutional,[7] arrested again, reindicted, retried, and reimprisoned for the same marijuana offense. He escaped to Europe, avoided United States attempts to extradite him, and at this writing is living in Switzerland. Each stage in his strange odyssey, and each crackdown by law-enforcement authorities, added to his status as a martyr and culture hero—and served to publicize LSD even more widely.

Medical authorities also contributed to the inflation of publicity with exaggerated and unsubstantiated reports of LSD effects, such as that it rotted the mind and destroyed motivation. The chairman of the New Jersey Narcotic Drug Study Commission in 1966 called LSD "the greatest threat facing the country today . . . more dangerous than the Vietnam war." [8]

Confusing marijuana with LSD. The use of LSD was further encouraged and advertised by the antimarijuana publicity of the 1960s. Marijuana and LSD were constantly (and mistakenly) bracketed together in government and medical statements. Official pronouncements repeatedly labeled marijuana, like LSD, a "hallucinogen," leading people to conclude that the effects were similar. The fact that many of the warnings against marijuana were patently false (see Part VIII) helped destroy the credibility of LSD warnings from the same sources.

In addition, the shortage of marijuana around September 1969, when Mexican border crossings were closely screened for drugs in "Operation Intercept," caused many marijuana users who had no particular interest in LSD to turn to that drug in place of marijuana (see Page 442). This occurred in Canada as well as the United States; Canada's Le Dain Commission commented in 1970: "We have been told repeatedly that LSD use increased rapidly during periods when cannabis [marijuana] was in short supply. Drug users and non-users alike have suggested that the effectiveness of Operation Intercept in the United States in reducing the supply of marijuana available in Canada was a major cause of the increase in the demand for 'acid.' " [9]

The period following Operation Intercept also brought stories of LSD use among "square" young people who hardly could have been attracted to the drug a few years earlier—such as military personnel manning American missile defenses. United Press International reported one such instance in October 1969:

10 ARMY MISSILE MEN HELD IN MIAMI ON DRUG CHARGES

MIAMI, Oct. 3 (UPI)—At least 10 Army missile men manning Nike-Hercules batteries near Miami have been arrested on drug abuse charges in a joint crackdown by Army and civilian authorities.

Details came to light today when two enlisted men appeared in court on charges of possession or sale of LSD, a hallucinatory drug.

An Army spokesman at the 47th Artillery Brigade said the arrests took place over a four-month period with the Army's Criminal Intelligence Division working closely with civilian authorities. There were reports that other arrests were expected.

The information officer said elaborate security measures would prevent a "turned-on" GI from triggering a missile.

"No one man can work alone near the weapons which are capable of carrying nuclear warheads," the spokesman said. "And it takes roughly 15 men working in unison to accomplish a launch." [10]

LSD legislation. The barrage of publicity that popularized LSD was intensified by a wave of prohibitive legislation. New York's 1965 penalties for the "possession, sale, exchange, or giving away" of LSD or LSD-like drugs without a special license provided for a maximum of two years' imprisonment. Sponsors of a bill to increase the penalties cited two newspaper stories as illustrations of the LSD menace: one reported that a five-year-old Brooklyn girl had swallowed an LSD-impregnated sugar cube left in the refrigerator by her young uncle.[11] Her stomach was pumped— a useless measure which, several physicians noted, was probably more traumatic than the drug effect—but she recovered. The other newspaper story reported that a thirty-two-year-old ex–mental patient charged with the brutal murder of his mother-in-law claimed to have been "flying" on LSD, and to remember nothing about the homicide.[12] Law-enforcement officers promptly labeled this case an "LSD murder." (At the man's trial, psychiatrists testified that he suffered from chronic paranoid schizophrenia. He was found not guilty by reason of insanity; the issue of insanity due to LSD was not raised.) [13] These two incidents—the accidental poisoning and the homicide—were interpreted as reasons to increase LSD criminal penalties in 1966 to a maximum of twenty years' imprisonment. The Speaker of the New York State Assembly, A. J. Travia, announced that the LSD problem was so urgent, he would defer hearings on the law increasing penalties until *after* the law was passed.[14]

The same year, Donald Grunsky introduced a bill in the California State Senate prohibiting the possession as well as the manufacture, sale, or importation of LSD and DMT. The same New York "LSD murder" case was referred to, and lurid color photographs of a psychotic reaction to LSD were circulated by the state attorney general's office.[15] Four witnesses testified against the bill in the California House of Representatives: a Jesuit priest, a psychologist, and two physicians. "They agreed that controls on LSD manufacture and distribution were needed," an observer later noted, "but argued that outlawing use and possession would result in the prosecution of young persons whose intentions were not antisocial; that its use was often nothing more than youthful adventure; and that some of the most creative students were among those experimenting with the drug. They further argued that fear of arrest would discourage users from seeking psychiatric aid should they need it." [16] Convinced by these arguments, the House committee voted not to report out the bill. This action was promptly labeled "irresponsible" by some state senators; the state attorney general added that LSD and LSD-like drugs "present the most crucial drug problem which the U.S. has faced." Governor Pat Brown, gubernatorial candidate Ronald Reagan, and other candidates for office announced that they favored the bill; and a Los Angeles *Times* editorial expressed amazement that the House committee was unaware of the LSD menace. The committee stood firm for a time, but as political pressure mounted, it compromised and ultimately yielded. The Grunsky bill became law in 1966.

Three years later, Maryland's legislature, considering anti-LSD legislation, heard an hour of testimony by Dr. Charles Savage, director of medical research at Spring Grove State Hospital and professor of psychiatry at Johns Hopkins, whose experience with LSD in psychotherapy covered nineteen years. Dr. Savage stressed, as had other witnesses, that the nonmedical use of LSD constituted a serious problem, but he pointed out numerous reasons for concluding that making possession a criminal offense would exacerbate the problem. LSD distribution in Maryland, he testified, was still on a small-scale, amateur basis with low prices. When the California legislature outlawed LSD, the immediate effect was a trebling of the cost (from $3 to $10 per trip); this price increase had attracted additional LSD distributors. The same would no doubt happen in Maryland. "When you make it illegal, you make it more lucrative for sellers," Dr. Savage said. Nor would the law significantly interfere with LSD distribution. "It's . . . easily concealed. The law would be very difficult to enforce. Prohibition did not stop drinking and the marijuana laws have not stopped kids from smoking marijuana." Finally, Dr. Savage testified that the people likely to be imprisoned under such a law "are largely normal adolescents that are attracted to LSD . . . essentially good kids, the future leaders of our society. If they are picked up and charged, they become criminals. . . . The passage of more and more legislation creates more and more criminals. [The LSD user] gets the idea that the law is just one more silly game he has to play and he loses respect for it." [17]

Nevertheless, the law was passed.

The passage of federal and state anti-LSD laws was followed (a) by an increase in the availability of LSD, and (b) by an increase in the demand. The increased availability can be explained in part by the higher prices which law enforcement engendered, and which attracted more distributors. The increased demand can similarly be explained in part by the LSD publicity that legislative action engendered. As in the case of the opiates, the barbiturates, the amphetamines, glue, and other drugs, the warnings functioned as lures.

Curtailment of LSD research. From 1962 on, Sandoz distributed LSD with caution to qualified investigators. In 1965, as anti-LSD sentiment rose to new peaks and as laws against LSD were pending both in Congress and in the state legislatures, Sandoz decided to stop distributing the drug altogether. It recalled the supplies outstanding and turned them over to the National Institute of Mental Health, which doled out small quantities to a few researchers—many of whom were experimenting only on animals. Dr. Harold A. Abramson, director of research in a large New York State mental hospital, cited the result at a 1965 LSD conference:

It's virtually prohibited now for a private physician to use LSD unless his patient buys it on the black market and comes in with the drug. That is, unfortunately, the situation in the United States today. I must say that I have had patients who tell me, "If you won't give me LSD, I'll get it and then come in." Naturally, I disapprove of this. . . . I must say that some of these people had had LSD under suitable medical auspices. They are very intelligent, capable people, and it has helped them so much to find themselves. It has given them a sense of being somebody.[18]

Dr. Abramson summed up: "Everybody seems to be able to get LSD and similar drugs except physicians."[19]

In Britain, when the Sandoz LSD supply was cut off, the medical profession took effective measures to secure an alternative supply; LSD of pharmaceutical quality was legally secured from Czechoslovakia,[20] and it is still in legal use, as the Malleson survey noted, by 37 British therapists. When the Advisory Committee on Drug Dependence of the United Kingdom Home Office investigated this use in 1970, it concluded that LSD psychotherapy should continue: "There is no proof that LSD is an effective agent in psychiatry. Equally there is no proof that it is an exceptionally hazardous or prohibitively dangerous treatment, in clinical use, in the hands of responsible experts and subject to appropriate safeguards. We see no reason to recommend arrangements which would prohibit the continued careful clinical and experimental use of LSD by approved and responsible practitioners."[21]

The Advisory Committee further concluded: "The supply of LSD for use in clinical practice should not be withheld from any doctor, whether in

National Health Service or private practice, who can establish a claim to its legitimate use, and can show he has the proper facilities available for the care of a patient who is undergoing treatment, and for the storage of the drug." [22]

The LSD chromosome scare, 1967. A wide variety of agents—including X rays, virus infections, fever, caffeine, and in some studies aspirin—have been shown to damage white-blood-cell chromosomes either in animals, in humans, or in test tubes. In March 1967, Dr. Maimon Cohen of the State University of New York at Buffalo reported that LSD damaged white-blood-cell chromosomes in test tubes.[23] Unlike earlier chromosome studies of other agents, the LSD finding made front-page headlines from coast to coast. Reporters (and physicians as well) speculated in print and on television and radio that LSD, like thalidomide, might cause a vast epidemic of tragically malformed babies.*

Subsequent chromosome studies produced mixed results; some seemed to exonerate LSD, while others seemed to confirm Dr. Cohen's findings. Only the confirmatory studies received wide attention in the mass media. The stories based on these studies usually failed to mention that damage to white-blood-cell chromosomes is far from a reliable index of *genetic* damage.

In response to the fear of deformed babies, many young people temporarily stopped taking the drug. Others continued on the theory presented in the mass media that the damage had already been done—that a single dose of LSD is all that is needed to damage chromosomes. Some pregnant young women secured abortions, legal or illegal; some couples refrained from having babies they wanted; and some LSD users switched from LSD to mescaline, psilocybin, or other LSD-like drugs. (Since drugs sold under these names were often in fact LSD, little was accomplished by the switch.)

The facts soon overtook the warnings. All over the country, obviously healthy babies were born to LSD users. A thorough California study of 120 "LSD babies" (to be reviewed in detail in Chapter 52) showed birth defects no more common than in babies of non–LSD users. Thus the credibility of official and medical pronouncements was once again severely shaken—and LSD use increased again.

Much the same sequence of events was experienced in Britain. A United Kingdom Home Office report stated in 1970:

The possibility of genetic damage from LSD has received a great deal of publicity both here and in the United States, but the presentation has been

---

* A relatively restrained and qualified warning entitled "LSD: Danger to Unborn Babies," which appeared in *McCall's* magazine for September 1967, was written by the senior author (E. M. B.) of this Consumers Union Report.

one-sided. Those findings that suggest danger have had extensive coverage whilst those that did not suggest a hazard have not been noticed. We have little doubt that this has had a major effect in dissuading young people from experimenting with the drug. Witnesses made it clear to us, however, that among young people, particularly among the more sophisticated of those who might be tempted to experiment, any evidence of potential damage is coming to be discounted. It seems probable, therefore, that this risk is ceasing to be a major deterrent.[24]

51.

How the hazards of LSD
were augmented, 1962-1969

As LSD use became more widespread the drug also became far more hazardous. Many reports appeared of large numbers of LSD users hospitalized—some of them for considerable periods—following LSD trips. Reports of LSD accidents also increased—falls or jumps from windows, death when someone on LSD threw himself in front of a passing car, and so on.

There is adequate reason to believe that such hospitalizations and accidents did in fact occur with markedly increased frequency from 1962 until about 1969. The increase in adverse effects, moreover, did not result simply from an increase in the number of users; the *proportion* of adverse effects per 1,000 users also increased. At least twelve reasons for this increase warrant discussion.

1. Increased expectations of adverse effects. The American Indians who used LSD-like drugs learned long ago that the *expectations* present in the mind of a user before he takes the drug are among the major factors determining the nature of his reaction to the drug; they took the drug within a framework that dictated favorable expectations. Scientists subsequently confirmed this phenomenon for LSD itself. Dr. Sidney Cohen, for example, had noted in 1960 that "those with excessive initial apprehension" are particularly likely to experience bad trips.[1]

One effect of the nationwide warnings against LSD from 1962 on was to arouse "excessive initial apprehension" in the minds of countless LSD users. The result was what might have been anticipated. Bizarre behavior increased markedly from 1962 to 1969. Some users, warned that LSD might cause them to jump out of the window, did in fact jump out of the window. Many who were warned that LSD would drive them crazy did in fact suffer severe panic reactions, fearing that LSD had driven them crazy. Thus the warnings proved self-fulfilling prophecies, and enhanced the hazards of the drug.

2. Unknown dosages. Patients and others who took LSD before 1962 received precisely measured doses. When the curtailment of the Sandoz supply triggered the clandestine manufacture of black-market LSD, no such precision was possible. An LSD sugar cube or capsule might contain too little LSD to engender a trip—or many times the recommended amount. The classic example was the Haight-Ashbury's "Pink Wedge incident" on November 11, 1967, when a batch of LSD shaped like pink wedges, and adulterated with another LSD-like drug, STP, hit the San Francisco market. "We treated 18 cases of acute toxic psychosis generated by the 'Pink Wedge' in a five-hour period," Dr. David E. Smith of the Haight-Ashbury Medical Clinic later recalled. "Most of the people seen were having acute panic reactions due to the strength of the dose, which was more than most of the young persons had been used to." [2]

3. Contamination. Some of the black-market LSD available after 1962, as noted earlier, was of excellent quality. But other batches, synthesized by amateurs, were contaminated. As we have shown, true LSD-25— d-lysergic acid diethylamide—was one of twenty-five closely related ergot derivatives synthesized by Sandoz before 1938, and many more were to follow. The effects of many of these LSD congeners are poorly understood. Even a slight error in the process of synthesizing LSD-25 may result in an end product containing not only the desired chemical but also admixtures of these potentially hazardous congeners. Many analyses of black-market LSD have shown the presence of substances that are not in fact LSD but apparently some unknown congener. It is impossible to determine how much of the difference between pre-1962 and post-1962 LSD effects resulted from this kind of contamination.

4. Adulteration. In addition to contaminants accidentally introduced into black-market LSD through errors of synthesis, some black-market suppliers deliberately adulterated their LSD with a variety of substances, including amphetamines * and even strychnine. It was necessary, of course, to mix LSD with a bulking agent of some kind; the amount of LSD needed for one trip is so small as to be barely visible and it cannot be safely or conveniently handled. One reason for using potent substances as bulking agents may have been to provide an *immediate* effect; half an hour or more is likely to elapse before the first effects of true LSD-25 are felt. Or potent drugs may have been used as adulterants merely because the distributors of clandestine LSD happened to have them conveniently available.

Some of the adulterants also complicated the *therapy* for adverse reactions. "The admixture of chemicals with atropine-like properties to LSD changes the response to the usual antidotes to LSD which may, under these circumstances, instead of lessening the effects of a 'bad trip,' actually increase the toxic reaction." [4]

* Dr. David E. Smith said (1967): "Methamphetamine crystals or 'speed' . . . have appeared in great abundance in the Haight-Ashbury. Because of its small cost and ease of synthesis, it is often mixed with small quantities of LSD, and sold as 'pure acid.' This mixture increases the likelihood of a 'bad trip', primarily due to the intense sympathomimetic effects of the amphetamines. The tachycardia, muscle tremor, and anxiety produced by 'speed' is often magnified by the LSD-sensitized mind into a panic reaction." [3]

5. Mistaken attribution. A substantial proportion of LSD users experiencing adverse reactions also used other drugs—either at the same time or at other times. There was a widespread tendency to attribute adverse effects to the LSD rather than to the other drugs—especially in statements designed to warn against LSD.

6. Side effects of law enforcement. The imprisonment of young people while they were on "trips" unquestionably contributed to adverse effects. One well-known example occurred on June 21, 1967, when 5,000 tablets of the LSD-like drug STP were distributed without charge at a celebration in San Francisco's Golden Gate Park. Scores of young people suffered bad trips; 60 of the 5,000 users came to professional attention. Of the 60, 32 were treated at the Haight-Ashbury Medical Clinic. "All but one of these 32 patients were returned to their homes or to the care of their friends within a few hours, following explanation and very mild sedation," [5] Dr. David E. Smith subsequently reported. Seven other users, however, were arrested and imprisoned—and then, as their symptoms grew worse, were taken to the San Francisco General Hospital. They suffered much more severe and prolonged illnesses. "Our hypothesis is," Dr. Smith explained, "that these patients differed from those seen at the Clinic, not so much in the intensity of their reaction as in its management. In the supportive atmosphere of the room of a friend or the Clinic, the patient recognized the drug-induced nature of his experience. If he was incarcerated, his paranoid, hallucinatory behavior was intensified and prolonged." [6]

7. Lack of supervision. "That the person under the influence of LSD should not be left alone is universally agreed," Dr. Sidney Cohen had noted in 1960. As LSD became freely available on the black market, this safeguard was occasionally ignored. More commonly, the others present were also "tripping" on LSD, and were concerned primarily with their own trips. Or unskilled young people panicked when one of their number panicked, and thus compounded his reactions. No one took the simple measures which can favorably alter the course of an LSD trip—assuring the user, for example, that this is just a drug experience and that it will in due course fade away, or distracting his attention from whatever unpleasant is preoccupying him to something else: a rose, a tune, a photograph. In the absence of such simple supervisory techniques, the proportion and severity of bad trips increased.

8. Mishandling of panic reactions. When an LSD user and the people around him panicked, the user was sometimes rushed to the emergency room of a nearby hospital; indeed, most of the accounts of adverse LSD effects during the 1960s came from these emergency rooms, where personnel in those days were usually quite inexperienced. They sometimes did not diagnose an LSD trip correctly. Whether or not they diagnosed it

[377]

correctly, they sometimes used wholly inappropriate treatment such as washing out the patient's stomach (a traumatic experience in any event, and far more so in the middle of an LSD trip); or they initiated other procedures that frightened the patient and complicated his bad trip. Even in the absence of such procedures, the impersonal hostility to drug users in some emergency rooms was a complicating factor. As better ways of treating bad trips were introduced (see Part IX), their severity declined.

9. *Misinterpretation of reactions.* Before 1962, when LSD bad trips occurred, they were accepted as an inherent part of the total LSD experience; sometimes they were even perceived as therapeutic in themselves, and therefore welcomed. After 1962, however, these bad trips were labeled *psychotic.* From a review of the medical literature of the 1960s it is evident that some of the "psychotic reactions" of that decade were actually bad trips similar to what therapists and patients alike had taken in their stride during the 1950s. Indeed, the label "psychotic" itself affected the reactions of both physicians and patients and thus contributed its share to making bad trips worse.

10. *Flashbacks.* One widely publicized adverse effect of the LSD trip is the "flashback"—a sudden and unexpected reexperiencing of some portion of an earlier trip, weeks or even months afterward.

Dr. Sidney Cohen, interestingly enough, did not receive a single report of flashbacks during his 1960 study of adverse LSD reactions.[7] No doubt some earlier users experienced flashbacks—but they were not perceived in those days as adverse reactions. As late as 1967, only 11 cases of flashbacks were reported in the medical literature, though no doubt more were occurring. Then the flashback hazard was widely publicized—and a flood of reports promptly followed. By 1969, according to Dr. M. J. Horowitz, about one out of every 20 "hippies" who used LSD suffered flashbacks of some kind. Characteristically, Dr. Horowitz reported, such flashbacks occur without apparent stimulus, and are not subject to the volitional control of the individual. Those who used LSD repeatedly seemed to encounter the most severe forms of flashback. Dr. Horowitz noted that out of 22 cases of "massive drug use, defined as a history of more than 15 LSD 'trips' and considerable use of other agents," 7 cases reported flashbacks.[8]

A simple explanation of LSD flashbacks, and of their changed character after 1967, is available. According to this theory, almost everybody suffers flashbacks with or without LSD. Any intense emotional experience—the death of a loved one, the moment of discovery that one is in love, the moment of an automobile smashup or of a narrow escape from smashup—may subsequently and unexpectedly return vividly to consciousness weeks or months later. Since the LSD trip is often an intense emotional experience, it is hardly surprising that it may similarly "flash back." Once flashbacks were labeled as "psychotic episodes" and warned against, they could no longer be taken in stride. They produced anxiety, even panic, in some LSD users.

It should be added, however, that some LSD users who have experienced flashbacks report the LSD flashback to be altogether different from the recurrence of emotionally laden nondrug experiences. We shall return to this issue.

11. Preexisting pathology. A major cause of the increase in adverse LSD effects after 1962 was almost certainly the drug's availability to everyone, including schizophrenics and schizoid personalities, who are most likely to experience adverse effects. Indeed, there is some reason to believe that the youth drug scene in general, and LSD in particular, had a special attraction to these troubled people. Among 47 users of LSD and LSD-like drugs admitted to Bellevue Hospital, New York, during the first half of 1967, "almost 50 percent . . . showed signs of schizophrenia or were treated for that condition before ever taking LSD." An additional 20 percent "showed schizoid features prior to the hallucinogen intake." [9]

This does not mean, of course, that *only* schizophrenics or schizoid personalities suffer severe or prolonged effects following LSD. In a 1970 *Archives of General Psychiatry* paper entitled "Chronic Psychosis Associated with Long-Term Psychotomimetic Drug Abuse," Drs. George S. Glass and Malcolm B. Bowers of the Connecticut Mental Health Center in New Haven reported 4 cases of psychosis requiring prolonged hospitalization in young male LSD users. "Their personalities had allegedly been very different prior to their beginning of heavy drug ingestion," Drs. Glass and Bowers noted. After repeated LSD trips, "these individuals were withdrawn and isolated on the ward. Their affect was shallow, and thought processes, while not loose, were bizarre and centered on eastern religious mysticism. Primarily these patients utilized mechanisms of denial and projection, even to the extent of paranoid delusion formation. . . . The overwhelming passivity, evasive style of interaction, and peculiar manner of thinking seemed not to be a part of an acute process, but rather an integral part of each patient's personality." [10] No doubt other cases might be cited of apparently psychotic reactions following LSD in persons who revealed no visible foreshadowings of psychosis before LSD. The incidence of such cases, however, remains in doubt. One might also question whether lengthy hospitalization is the treatment of choice in such cases, or whether it might prolong and exacerbate the symptoms.

12. Unwitting use. A number of adverse reactions during the 1960s resulted from the administering of LSD covertly to people who did not know they were receiving it. Sometimes the LSD was given as a prank; sometimes it was a well-meant but misguided effort to provide the benefits of the LSD experience to a reluctant nonuser. In either case, a person experiencing a 'trip" without knowing he has taken a drug naturally concludes that he has suddenly "gone crazy"—a highly traumatic experience.

Some observers have suggested that adolescents may be more vulnerable than adults to the adverse effects of LSD, and that the increase in adverse effects after 1962 may be due in part to increased LSD use by adolescents. Other observers, however, believe that adolescents are better able than adults to take LSD effects in their stride. No comparative studies exist on this issue.

The twelve factors cited above—increased expectation of adverse effects engendered by anti-LSD warnings, unknown and in some cases excessive dosages of black-market LSD, contaminated black-market LSD, adulterated black-market LSD, the popular attribution to LSD of the adverse effects of other drugs, the arrest and incarceration of LSD users while they were on "bad trips," trips taken without skilled supervision, the mishandling of panic reactions, the labeling of "bad trips" and of "flashbacks" as "psychotic," the failure to screen out schizophrenics and schizoid personalities, and the unwitting consumption of LSD—serve to explain at least in considerable part why a drug that produced relatively few adverse effects during the 1950s became the "horror drug" of the 1960s. By altering those factors, a notable reduction in the damage done by LSD could no doubt be achieved, even though its use were to continue. There would no doubt remain some adverse effects, which might prove serious in isolated cases—but the scale of the damage might be markedly reduced.

Since the adverse effects of LSD from 1962 to 1969 were in considerable part traceable to the anti-LSD publicity and to other nonpharmacological factors, there was reason to hope that once the excitement died down, the acute adverse effects would become fewer and less severe—and this is what has now happened. The re-emergence of LSD as a less hazardous drug is discussed more fully in Parts IX and X.

52.

LSD today: the search for a rational perspective

The use of LSD by 1970 had become endemic in the United States among some segments of the youthful white society, much as peyote became endemic in the American Indian society a century earlier. But the great majority of LSD users, having learned how to use the drug, no longer engage in behavior of the type which engenders headlines or necessitates hospitalization.

But what of the *long-range* effects of LSD on its users, as distinct from the acute immediate effects? By far the best data on long-range LSD effects have been assembled by two psychologists at the University of California at Los Angeles, Drs. William H. McGlothlin and David O. Arnold.[1] In 1967, they secured from three Los Angeles psychiatrists the names of men and women who had received LSD during the period 1956–1961. Some were patients who had received the drug as part of their psychotherapy; others were healthy volunteers who had participated in LSD experiments. The long-term effects on these two different classes of users were determined separately, and compared.

Some of these early LSD users, moreover, had discontinued the drug at the end of the therapy or experiment; others had gone on to use black-market LSD. The long-term effects on these disparate groups were also compared.

The psychiatrists who used LSD in psychotherapy had also, of course, provided psychotherapy *without* LSD to other patients. In ingenious ways a control group was drawn from these non-LSD patients receiving psychotherapy—matched in as many ways as possible to the group that received LSD. And a second control group was also set up to match the patients who had subsequently taken LSD nonmedically. Thus a variety of intergroup comparisons and contrasts was possible.

In all, 247 patients and volunteers who had taken LSD before 1962 were included in the study. They were intensively interviewed, subjected to a battery of psychological tests, and asked to fill out a lengthy questionnaire. Their automobile driving records were checked, and the birth certificates of their babies. In many cases the wives or husbands of the LSD users were also questioned. It is quite possible, of course, that some long-term effects of LSD, favorable or adverse, may have escaped the numerous McGlothlin-Arnold checks; but if so, they were almost certainly rare, or mild, or both.

The researchers found that only 58 of the 247 patients and volunteers continued to use LSD nonmedically after their therapy or the experiment was discontinued. Only 22 of these 58 took more than ten subsequent LSD trips. Only one of the 22 used LSD oftener than once a week; this exception took it twice a week. Only one or two others took LSD even once a week. None of the users showed a pattern of *increasing* use. Finally, all but three users either discontinued LSD use altogether after a few years or else took only one, two, or three trips a year thereafter. Only 9 of the original 247 took LSD in 1967. The pattern of use among the 22 (out of 247) who took more than ten nonmedical trips is shown in Table 4.

As shown in the column at the far right of Table 4, 9 of the 22 users indicated that they might take LSD in the future, while 8 thought they would not and 5 were undecided.

Of the 58 who used LSD nonmedically, only one said he discontinued LSD because it was unavailable. Thus, law-enforcement efforts to curb availability of LSD did not account for the decline in use. Despite the fact that the McGlothlin-Arnold study was conducted mostly in 1967 and 1968, at the height of the anti-LSD publicity, only 9 of the 58 said they stopped for fear of bad trips or physical harm. The reasons given for either continuing or discontinuing LSD use are shown in the following table.[2]

Reasons for continuing	
Self-exploration	16
Mystical experiences	4
Euphoria, pleasure	3
Total	23
Reasons for discontinuing	
Concern about bad trips; physical or mental harm	9
No need; had enough	10
Prefers nondrug methods	5
Illegality; current bad reputation	4
Doesn't like effect	3
Need to integrate with therapy	2
Prefers peyote	1
LSD unavailable	1
Total	35
TOTAL	58

"Compulsive patterns of LSD use," Drs. McGlothlin and Arnold concluded, "rarely develop; the nature of the drug effect is such that it becomes less attractive with continued use and in the long term, is almost always self-limiting."[3] They give this explanation:

Table 4. Patterns of Nonmedical LSD Use: Yearly Exposures [5]

Age at Time of Interview	Sex	Year												Future Use
		1956	1957	1958	1959	1960	1961	1962	1963	1964	1965	1966	1967	
44	M	—	—	—	20	100	110	150	100	100	100	100	100[a]	Yes
46	M	—	—	—	—	—	19	50	50	50	50	50	50	Yes
28	F	—	—	—	—	—	15	20	20	—	65	65	3	P.
45	M	3	12	12	0	0	0	2	0	22	3	2	0	No
35	F	—	—	—	0	—	—	—	—	0	0	0	0	No
43	M	—	—	—	—	—	—	—	15	10	3	0	0	No
36	M	—	—	—	—	—	—	—	3	3	3	3	3	Yes
31	M	—	—	—	—	—	—	—	—	3	3	3	3	Yes
39	M	15	20	10	9	8	2	2	5	2	2	0	0	No
44	M	—	—	—	—	—	—	10	5	2	2	0	0	P.
37	F	—	—	—	—	—	—	—	—	—	45	45	3	No
31	M	—	—	—	—	—	5	5	2	2	2	2	2	P.
53	M	6	6	6	6	6	6	6	6	6	6	2	5	Yes
31	M	—	3	4	5	6	6	6	6	6	6	6	0	No
57	M	—	—	—	2	5	5	0	0	0	0	0	0	No
46	M	—	—	—	—	2	2	5	0	0	0	0	1	P.
42	F	—	—	—	—	8	8	2	1	1	1	0	0	Yes
38	F	—	—	—	—	7	12	0	0	0	0	0	0	Yes
44	M	—	—	—	—	—	8	2	1	1	0	0	0	Yes
42	M	—	—	—	—	—	—	—	—	0	0	0	0	Yes
34	M	—	—	—	—	—	—	—	6	3	3	3	2	P.
52	F	—	2	1	1	3	1	2	3	3	3	3	0	No

[a] Of this LSD user, McGlothlin and Arnold noted that his twice-a-week use of LSD "appeared to be motivated as much by his role as an LSD proselytizer as by the effects of the drug." [4]

There are several reasons why hallucinogens would not be expected to give rise to long-term chronic abuse of the type frequently encountered with most other mind-altering drugs. First, of course, there is no development of physiological dependence. Second, at least for those hallucinogens for which reliable data are available, daily use leads to rapid build-up of tolerance, such that for practical purposes these drugs cannot be used more than twice a week without losing much of their impact. Equally relevant is the fact that the intense emotional effects of hallucinogens produce a type of psychological satiation which, for most persons, results in much longer intervals between use than is necessary to avoid tolerance effect. A third reason why the hallucinogens appear not suitable for long-term use is their lack of dependable effects. Habitual drug users seek to satisfy particular needs—escape, euphoria, anxiety relief, feeling of inadequacy, etc. To qualify for long-term use, a drug must *consistently* produce the type of mood alteration desired. Hallucinogens are quite inconsistent in terms of mood alteration, and in addition, often produce a feeling of increased awareness which is incompatible with the need for escape and withdrawal. The fourth and probably most important reason to expect individuals to decrease rather than increase their hallucinogen use over time is to be found in the characteristics of the drug effect. As described earlier, the major effect of the hallucinogens is to temporarily suspend the normal mode of perception and thinking. The utility of the experience lies in the uniqueness of the new modes of perception and thought which become available under these conditions. However, as one repeats the experience many times, what was initially unique becomes more commonplace and there is a process of diminishing returns. The effect of hallucinogens is indeed "a trip," and trips tend to lose their appeal when repeated too often.[6]

This pattern of declining use, and of stopping LSD altogether, does not, however, mean that LSD use is dying out. On the contrary, new users are continuously being recruited. Indeed, LSD use among high-school and college students is believed to have reached a new high in 1970.* What the evidence indicates is that LSD is, for almost all users, a phase to be lived through rather than a continuing way of life.

The great majority of the 247 LSD users in the McGlothlin-Arnold sample reported, years later, that their experience with the drug had benefited them. "These reports of change show a fairly consistent pattern," Drs. McGlothlin and Arnold note—"more understanding of self; more tolerance of others; less egocentricity; a less materialistic and aggressive orientation; and more appreciation of music, art, and nature."[8] The proportions reporting such favorable effects were very high; among 97 patients who received LSD only in therapy, for example, 94 percent reported "more understanding of self and others." Among 58 patients who

* A December 1970 Gallup poll of 1,063 students on 61 college campuses indicated that 14 percent had tried LSD—as compared with 4 percent reporting LSD use in a comparable poll one year earlier. Six percent in the 1970 poll reported having taken LSD during the previous month.[7]

in addition used black-market LSD, 95 percent reported this effect. Sixty-one percent of the former group and 63 percent of the latter reported "less anxiety." [9]

But here the importance of *controlled* studies leaps into view. When the patients who had received psychotherapy without LSD, and the non-LSD users who were matched to the black-market users, were asked the same questions, they also reported that through the years they had become "more understanding of self and others," suffered less anxiety, were more tolerant of the viewpoints of others, and so on.[10] In only two respects did the favorable reports of LSD users differ significantly from the favorable reports of nonusers; the patients who had used black-market as well as psychotherapeutic LSD reported "more appreciation of music" and "more appreciation of art" much oftener than their matched control group. (This was not true of the patients who received LSD only in psychotherapy and *their* control group.) [11]

In sum, the McGlothlin-Arnold study found most LSD users still convinced, from seven to twelve years after their first use of LSD, that the drug experience had significantly benefited them—but matched non-LSD users reported similar self-improvement.

LSD had a long-term effect in reducing alcohol consumption in only a modest proportion of cases.[12] But the subjects in this study were not alcoholics.

When the records of the California Department of Motor Vehicles were checked for accidents and traffic violations, no significant differences were found between the LSD users and the control groups.[13]

All of these findings are subject to qualification. The LSD users in the sample, all of whom had used LSD before 1961, were not typical of the later generation of "hippie" users. Many in the sample had received LSD only a few times. They were in general older and better established in life. The findings are nevertheless of great importance—for they demonstrate the modest effects *of the LSD itself,* as distinct from the effects of the other aspects of the LSD-using hippie subculture in the 1960s.

It is commonly believed that LSD affects the beliefs and values of the LSD subculture, changes attitudes, alienates users from society, reduces political and organizational activity, and so on. Drs. McGlothlin and Arnold explored all of these possibilities in their sample of 247 LSD users by means of tests and rating scales. Minor differences were found between the LSD users and the control groups—but the overall conclusion was negative: "There is little evidence that a few administrations of LSD will produce measurable lasting personality, belief, value, attitude, or behavior changes in a relatively unselected population of adults. . . ." [14] To the extent that such changes appear in LSD subcultures, they are quite probably traceable to nonpharmacological aspects of the subculture.

Twenty-six of the 247 LSD users in all categories felt that LSD had harmed them in various ways. Many of the same 26 also felt that it had helped them. The same effect that some users considered beneficial others considered harmful. Thus, while two-thirds of the LSD users listed "more tolerant of opposing viewpoints" as a benefit of LSD, the comment was also made: "When you see both sides it is more difficult to decide, and therefore less efficient in the Western sense." Another negative comment: "I was unprepared to have my world and moral structure broken down and it has taken time and much effort to rebuild." Several of the comments were ambivalent: "It loosened me up in a way that is both positive and negative—like an artist that previously could draw precise work. Afterward he could draw freely, but not precisely." "I have lost some of my goals. I don't know if this is harm—my boss would say so." [15]

"Seven respondents [out of 247] felt their LSD experiences had contributed to increased anxiety and/or depression," Drs. McGlothlin and Arnold noted. "Three thought they had suffered some physical harm, e.g., numbness and tingling in legs and impaired eyesight. One individual felt his LSD use had resulted in memory loss and another stated it had caused serious marital conflict. Three regarded it as a painful memory of a horrible experience, and two others thought they 'would be better off without knowledge of the means to escape to another world.'" [16] The striking fact, however, is the rarity of such negative comments. At a time when the country was being warned that LSD was the greatest threat to the nation —worse even than the Vietnam war—221 out of 247 people with LSD experience had no negative comments whatever to make about the drug's long-range effects on themselves.

Subjective reports, of course, do not tell the whole story. In addition to asking respondents whether they thought they had been harmed, Drs. McGlothlin and Arnold diligently searched for objective evidence of harm. They found very little.

Suicides. Among approximately 140 users who first took LSD as part of a scientific experiment, there were no suicides. Among approximately 140 users who received LSD as part of their psychotherapy, one committed suicide within two years of his last LSD use and 6 committed suicide from two to ten years after the last use. [17] No comparable figures are available on the suicide rate among psychotherapy patients who do not receive LSD.

Psychosis. One LSD-linked psychotic reaction occurred among the 247 LSD users in this sample. This patient "received three LSD treatments in psychotherapy, was hospitalized for one week following the third exposure, and was unable to work for an additional three months." [18] Another patient had been hospitalized for psychiatric illness before taking LSD. Thereafter, she suffered a "nervous breakdown" of two years' duration, which she herself attributed to LSD. The "breakdown" did not require hospitalization however—and it did not occur until four years after her last LSD experience.[19]

Flashbacks. In reporting on the flashback phenomenon, Drs. McGlothlin and Arnold emphasized that while "a spontaneous experience subjectively described as LSD-like" may follow LSD use, there is no certainty that such an experience was *caused* by the use of the drug.[20] The investigators asked the 247 LSD users three related questions:

Subsequent to your use, have you experienced any uncontrolled LSD-like experiences without using drugs?

What were they like?

Did you find them frightening or disturbing?

Thirty-six of the LSD users did experience something that might be considered a flashback.

Eight of them reported "mild, pleasant phenomena related to environment or self-suggestion." One recalled, for example, that "music [that had been] played during LSD session brings back some of the feelings." Another described his "flashback" as a feeling of oneness with the world."

Seven reexperienced "minor perceptual changes"—for instance, seeing a flash in the periphery of the visual field. Whether such "minor perceptual changes" are more or less common among people who have not taken LSD was not discussed.

Six LSD users out of the 247 reported experiencing "vague anxiety"—for example, fear of driving a car—which they described as similar to the initial part of the LSD trip.

Seven reported unusual phenomena related to sleep, sex, or alcohol intoxication. For example, one reported an intense fear of death experienced while drunk on alcohol. Why this was attributed to the LSD rather than to the alcohol was not indicated.

This left *eight* reports of what might properly be considered brief "psychotic" flashbacks among the 247 LSD users. Five of these were perceptual changes: recurring undulation of visual field, seeing objects as weird animals, repeats or "playbacks" of frightening scenes experienced on an LSD trip, auditory hallucinations. The other three were depersonalization experiences—as if the mind had left the body. One of these experiences occurred while the subject was driving a car, and an accident followed.

"In summary," Drs. McGlothlin and Arnold concluded, "the majority of the descriptions cited relatively minor, isolated events. Only one case fits Horowitz's definition of 'repeated intrusions of frightening images in spite of volitional efforts to avoid them.' In very few instances does there appear to be substantial evidence of a causal relationship between the LSD experiences and the incidents described. In the large majority of cases, there seems to be nothing more than the association of two events bearing certain similarities." [21]

Drs. McGlothlin and Arnold did not discuss the possible relationship between LSD flashbacks and nondrug recurrences of emotion-laden experiences. They did suggest, however, that reports of flashbacks among youthful "hippie" LSD users "may be related to their relative instability and a tendency to use the hallucinogens frequently * in high doses," or to the fact that these users "are exceptionally suggestible, prone to believe in all kinds of magical and fanciful phenomena." [22]

Effects on thinking. Drs. McGlothlin and Arnold suggest rather tentatively one possible long-term effect of repeated LSD use—an effect that, they point out, is often viewed as favorable rather than unfavorable. They call this a "structure-loosening" effect.[23] LSD proponents call it a "mind-expanding" effect. The effect is a subtle one, and no cogent description of it has been found. More research is clearly called for on this point—as well as more serious consideration of whether the effect (if it in fact exists) should be welcomed or worried about. Meanwhile, it would seem evident that the "mind-expanding" or "mind-loosening" effect here referred to differs appreciably from the "mind-rotting" effect widely publicized in the 1960s.

Brain damage. Drs. McGlothlin and Arnold selected from their sample 16 "heavy" LSD users who had taken at least 20 and as many as 1,100 LSD trips, nonmedical as well as medical; most of the 16 had also used other LSD-like drugs (peyote, mescaline, psilocybin, mushrooms, DMT, etc.). A control group, matched with the heavy LSD users in as many ways as possible but with no use of LSD or LSD-like drugs, was also selected.[24]

The 16 heavy users were interviewed by Dr. Daniel X. Freedman. Each interview lasted from one to two hours, and was specifically directed "toward detecting any clinical evidence of organic impairment.[25] . . . The psychiatric interviews did not reveal clinically significant signs of organic impairment in behavior or life situations. For some, there were characterological and psychological features which were somewhat eccentric; but, over-all, the ability to judge, to acquire competence and new learning, to focus attention and concentrate, to recall and retrieve relevant information, appeared intact. Where unusual personality traits were encountered, they seemed to have been present in the pre-LSD life history, style, and subculture of the subjects." [26]

The Freedman interviews established that LSD, at least in this sample of heavy users, had produced no evidence of brain damage of a kind that could be identified by a skilled psychiatric interviewer. But what of subtler forms of brain damage—impairments that can be diagnosed only

---

* That is, once or twice a week.

through precise psychological tests? To check for these subtler forms of injury, Drs. McGlothlin and Arnold gave both the heavy LSD users and the nonuser controls thirteen psychological tests of the kinds most likely to reveal brain damage.

With respect to twelve of these thirteen tests, the LSD users did a little better on some and a little worse on others than the controls; the differences were not significant in either direction.[27] In this respect, the McGlothlin-Arnold study confirmed a parallel study by Drs. Sidney Cohen and A. E. Edwards, who gave a battery of fifteen such tests to 30 young people who had taken 50 or more LSD trips. Drs. Cohen and Edwards found no significant difference on thirteen out of the fifteen tests between the heavy LSD users and a control group.[28]

When Drs. McGlothlin and Arnold compared their test results with those of Drs. Cohen and Edwards, a curious inconsistency emerged. The two tests on which LSD users in the Cohen-Edwards sample had done significantly less well than their controls were a test for visual perception, known as "Trail-Making A," and a test for spatial orientation. In the McGlothlin-Arnold study, heavy LSD users also showed somewhat poorer scores on those two tests, but the differences were not significant. Moreover, the heavy users did somewhat *better* than their controls in a quite similar test, "Trail-Making B." [29] On even closer analysis, some features of the McGlothlin-Arnold results tended to confirm the Cohen-Edwards findings on the "Trail-Making A" and spatial-orientation tests, while others tended to cast further doubt on them.

The one test in the McGlothlin-Arnold battery on which the heavy LSD users did significantly less well than the controls was the Halstead category test—a nonverbal measure of the ability to discern abstract principles. But when Drs. Cohen and Edwards had given the same test to *their* sample they "found no difference between LSD and comparison groups...." [30]

The whole issue might be summarized succinctly: Who knows? Maybe heavy LSD users do significantly less well on these three tests and maybe they don't. And even if it were proved that they do less well, the question whether this is due to brain damage or some other factor—less interest in passing tests, for example—would remain unanswered.

Taken together, the Cohen-Edwards and McGlothlin-Arnold studies would appear to rule out the possibility of major brain damage from LSD, even after scores or hundreds of trips. Further studies on larger populations, of course, might reveal some form of brain damage that is subtle, or rare, or both—but the same could be said of further studies of virtually any other substance.

Babies born to LSD users. Drs. McGlothlin and Arnold have also provided by far the best available evidence concerning possible damage to babies born to LSD users. In cooperation with a pediatrician, Dr. Robert S. Sparkes, they traced the outcome of 120 live births occurring among their sample of 247 LSD users.[31] These births fell into four categories.

• One hundred and six of the 120 babies were born in good health and with no identifiable birth defects whatever.

• Seven babies showed minor defects which "ran in the family" before LSD was discovered. For example, 3 babies in one family were born pigeon-toed; their father and the father's mother both had the same condition.

• Two babies who were born prematurely showed conditions associated with premature birth rather than LSD—hyaline membrane disease and acute pulmonary edema. The baby with acute pulmonary edema was the only baby among the 120 who died. The proportion of premature births in the sample was about what would be expected among babies born to parents who had never used LSD.

• Four other babies showed miscellaneous birth defects—about the number that would be expected in a population this size, even in the absence of LSD. One had a turned-in left foot (corrected with shoes). A second had pyloric stenosis (corrected with surgery). A third was pigeon-toed, and a fourth had cystic fibrosis.

The McGlothlin group concluded that "there is no evidence of a relation between parental LSD exposure and major congenital defects in their offspring." [32]

The group noted two limitations on their study. First, like LSD users generally, few of the parents had used LSD in high dosages over long periods of time. Second, the study did not rule out the possibility that LSD on rare occasions *might* cause a birth defect. The same might be true, of course, of virtually any other substance. Subject to these qualifications, there was no evidence that LSD, taken either by the mother or the father, "increased the risk of having a child with a congenital defect." [33]

The McGlothlin-Sparkes-Arnold study casts little light, it should be stressed, on the effects of LSD taken by the mother *during* pregnancy; in only twelve of the pregnancies was LSD taken. Nor is there any other reliable study on this point, either for LSD or for many other drugs. Hence the advice given by Consumers Union to readers of *Consumer Reports* [34] concerning medicines in general during pregnancy applies equally to LSD:

• No chemical known to science has been proved to be entirely harmless for all pregnant women and their babies during all stages of pregnancy. Hence, do not take any drug during pregnancy unless there is a specific medical need for it.

• If there *is* a medical need, however, and if your physician prescribes a drug to meet that need, take it scrupulously, in the amounts and at the times specified. Don't increase or lower the dose; don't discontinue sooner or continue longer than directed. Remember that your unborn baby's health can be adversely affected by your failure to take a needed drug as well as by your indulgence in unprescribed medication.

• If you are pregnant or potentially pregnant,* be sure to tell your doctor so whenever he is prescribing a drug for you. If your regular doctor refers you to someone else while you are pregnant or potentially pregnant, be sure to tell the second doctor, too.

• During pregnancy and potential pregnancy, curtail the use of over-the-counter "home remedies" as well as drugs available only on a doctor's prescription. Even common self-prescribed medicines like aspirin, for example, should be taken sparingly—except on your doctor's advice. The same goes for vitamin preparations.

• Interpret the term "drugs" broadly to include many things besides oral preparations and injections—for example, lotions and ointments containing hormones or other drugs that may be absorbed through the skin; vaginal douches, suppositories and jellies; rectal suppositories; medicated nose drops; and so on.

• A number of drugs exert their adverse effects during the first weeks following a missed menstrual period—the weeks when you are likely to be wondering whether you are pregnant. Hence discontinue all self-prescribed remedies within a few days after an expected menstrual period fails to occur, and recheck with your doctor concerning drugs prescribed for you previously.

• Mothers who breast-feed their babies should continue to exercise prudence until weaning time. Numerous drugs taken by the mother are secreted in her milk and reach the nursing baby.

These precautions apply equally to LSD and to medicaments in general. When presented in this general framework, young women are far more likely to respect the recommended precautions than when they are presented as if they applied to LSD alone, in an anti-LSD campaign that many young people discount.

Spontaneous abortion. In addition to the search for birth defects, the McGlothlin-Sparkes-Arnold study also inquired into the incidence of spontaneous abortions (miscarriages). They reported three findings:

* A woman of childbearing age should assume that she is potentially pregnant during any month when she engages in sexual intercourse without adequate contraceptive measures.

The spontaneous abortion rate was somewhat high—15 percent—among those who took LSD only medicinally, but this was still "within the usual range."

The spontaneous abortion rate was lower when only the father took LSD.

Among women who took LSD nonmedicinally (usually black-market LSD), the spontaneous abortion rate was shockingly high: 50 percent. Of the ten spontaneous abortions in this group, however, five were accounted for by one woman—and she had had one abortion *before* taking LSD. "Habitual aborters," who lose one baby after another, are well-known in the medical literature among women who do *not* take LSD; it was hardly significant that one habitual aborter should be found in this LSD-using group.

The somewhat higher spontaneous abortion rate among the mothers who took LSD, however, did appear to be significant even when the one habitual aborter was excluded. Drs. McGlothlin, Sparkes, and Arnold therefore cautiously concluded: "There is some indication that the use of LSD prior to conception by women may increase the incidence of spontaneous abortions, although the data do not permit the establishment of a clear-cut causal relationship." [35]

The findings of the McGlothlin group were published as the lead article in the *Journal of the American Medical Association* for June 1, 1970. With a few exceptions, the mass media found little newsworthy in the reassuring aspects of the study; but they heralded in headlines the cautious statement that there was *some* evidence that LSD *might* increase the incidence of spontaneous abortions.*

The question of subtle chromosome damage which does not affect the children of LSD users but which may affect subsequent generations is

---

* Thus the Los Angeles *Times*–Washington *Post* Service syndicated to newspapers an account of the McGlothlin-Sparkes-Arnold study which began: "A woman who takes LSD may have more chance of having a miscarriage than a woman who does not, though she takes the drug before she gets pregnant, a University of California at Los Angeles study . . . shows." [36] The Detroit *News* ran this syndicated dispatch on June 4, 1970, under the headline: "LSD May Foster Miscarriages." The twelve-paragraph dispatch noted in a single sentence in the third paragraph the McGlothlin-Sparkes-Arnold finding that "LSD has no discernible effect on a couple's chances of having a deformed or premature baby." A press release sent to science writers by *Medical World News* went even farther in this direction. The release was headed: "NEW STUDIES ON LSD LINK MENTAL ILLNESS, ABORTIONS TO ITS USE." [37] Six paragraphs were devoted to the McGlothlin-Sparkes-Arnold study. There was no mention whatever of the finding—the first such finding on a large scale in the history of LSD research—that 106 of the 120 babies were born in good health without birth defects, and that the other 14 cases were about what would be expected if the parents had *not* taken LSD. Yet to a country that had been warned to expect an epidemic of malformed "LSD babies," this was surely a sensational finding, which the public was entitled to know.

too complex to be reviewed in detail here. The essential point is that LSD is *at most* a trivial factor in the problem. Yale University investigators, for example, studied 4,500 consecutive births in New Haven. Twenty-two of the 4,500 babies showed visible chromosome abnormalities. None of the parents of the 22 affected babies reported having taken LSD. The study concluded that about 20,000 babies with visible chromosome abnormalities are born in the United States each year to parents who do *not* take LSD. All 14 of the babies in the sample whose parents did report taking LSD had normal chromosomes.[38]

Consumers Union's conclusions and recommendations concerning LSD appear in Part X.

Part VIII

Marijuana and Hashish

Marijuana is the popular name for a plant, *Cannabis sativa,* also known as hemp. *Marijuana* is also the common name of the drug prepared by drying the leaves and flowering tops of the plant. The leaves and tops contain several members of a group of chemicals known as the cannabinols. *Hashish* is the drug produced by drying the resin exuded by the marijuana plant. The resin is richer in cannabinols than the leaves and tops—one gram of hashish is said to have the effectiveness of five to eight grams of marijuana—but the potency of both marijuana and hashish varies widely from sample to sample. One of the cannabinols, delta-9-tetrahydrocannabinol or THC, was for a time believed to be the major active ingredient; the role of THC in the marijuana experience, however, is now in question.

Under the name Extract of Cannabis, marijuana was once widely used medically in the United States, and it still has minor medicinal uses in other countries. Though sometimes classed as a hallucinogen (LSD-like drug), marijuana is in fact unique, both chemically and in psychological effects produced. Hallucinations are not a common effect of the drug, but (like alcohol hallucinations) a symptom of overdose.

Marijuana and hashish are commonly smoked in the United States; they can also be taken orally in foods or beverages. They are not addicting. Neither tolerance nor withdrawal symptoms have been reliably reported. The lethal dose is not known; no human fatalities have been documented.

53.

Marijuana in the Old World

The "weed" that in the United States and Mexico is commonly called marijuana, hemp, or cannabis is in fact a highly useful plant cultivated throughout recorded history and perhaps much earlier as well. There is only one species—its scientific name is *Cannabis sativa*—which yields both a potent drug and a strong fiber long used in the manufacture of fine linen as well as canvas and rope. The seeds are valued as birdseed and the oil, which resembles linseed oil, is valuable because paints made with it dry quickly.

Since cannabis is the only plant that yields both a drug or intoxicant and a useful fiber, its early history can be readily traced through references to a plant that yields both.

A Chinese treatise on pharmacology attributed to the Emperor Shen Nung and alleged to date from 2737 B.C. contains what is usually cited as the earliest reference to marijuana. According to one tradition, it was Shen Nung who first taught his people to value cannabis as a medicine.[1] Shen Nung, however, was a mythical figure, and the treatise was compiled much later than 2737 B.C.

The first known reference to marijuana in India is to be found in the Atharva Veda, which may date as far back as the second millennium B.C.[2] Another quite early reference appears on certain cuneiform tablets unearthed in the Royal Library of Ashurbanipal, an Assyrian king. Ashurbanipal lived about 650 B.C.; but the cuneiform descriptions of marijuana in his library "are generally regarded as obvious copies of much older texts,"[3] says Dr. Robert P. Walton, an American physician and authority on marijuana who assembled much of the historical data here reviewed. This evidence "serves to project the origin of hashish back to the earliest beginnings of history." References to marijuana can also be found, Dr. Walton adds, in the *Rh-Ya* [sic], a Chinese compendium dating from the period 1200-500 B.C.; in the *Susruta,* an Indian treatise originating before 400 A.D.; and in the Persian Zend-Avesta, originating several centuries before Christ.[4]

The ancient Greeks used alcohol rather than marijuana as an intoxicant; but they traded with marijuana-eating and marijuana-inhaling peoples. Hence some of the references to drugs in Homer may be to marijuana—including Homer's reference to the drug which Helen brought to Troy from Egyptian Thebes.[5] Certainly Herodotus was referring to marijuana when he wrote in the fifth century B.C. that the Scythians cultivated a plant that was much like flax but grew thicker and taller; this hemp they deposited upon red-hot stones in a closed room—producing a vapor, Herodotus noted, "that no Grecian vapor-bath can surpass. The Scythians, transported with the vapor, shout aloud." [6]

Herodotus also described people living on islands in the Araxes River, who "meet together in companies," throw marijuana on a fire, then "sit around in a circle; and by inhaling the fruit that has been thrown on, they become intoxicated by the odor, just as the Greeks do by wine; and the more fruit is thrown on, the more intoxicated they become, until they rise up and dance and betake themselves to singing." * [7] Other passages assembled by Dr. Walton—from Pliny, Dioscorides, Paulus Aegineta, Abu Mansur Muwaffaq, *The Arabian Nights*, Marco Polo, and others— leave little room for doubt that marijuana was cultivated both for its fiber and for its psychoactive properties throughout Asia and the Near East from the earliest known times to the present.

Like the ancient Greeks, the Old Testament Israelites were surrounded by marijuana-using peoples. A British physician, Dr. C. Creighton, concluded in 1903 that several references to marijuana can be found in the Old Testament.[9] Examples are the "honeycomb" referred to in the Song of Solomon, 5:1, and the "honeywood" in I Samuel 14: 25-45. (Others have suggested that the "calamus" in the Song of Solomon was in fact cannabis.)[10]

The date on which marijuana was introduced into western Europe is not known; but it must have been very early. An urn containing marijuana leaves and seeds, unearthed near Berlin, Germany, is believed to date from 500 B.C.[11]

Cloth made from hemp (cannabis), we are told, "became common in central and southern Europe in the thirteenth century" and remained popular through the succeeding generations; fine Italian linen, for example, was made from hemp as well as flax—"and in many cases the two fibers are mixed in the same material." [12] Nor were Europeans ignorant of the *intoxicating* properties of the plant; François Rabelais (1490-1553) gave a full account of what he called "the herb Pantagruelion." [13]

The use of marijuana as an intoxicant also spread quite early to Africa. In South Africa, Dr. Frances Ames of the University of Cape Town reports, marijuana "was in use for many years before Europeans settled in the country and was smoked by all the non-European races, i.e. Bushmen, Hottentots and Africans. It was probably brought to the Mozambique coast from India by Arab traders and the habit, once established, spread inland. . . .

* The use of marijuana on a campfire has also been reported from Africa; [8] the high price no doubt inhibits similar use in the United States today.

"The plant has been used for many purposes in South Africa. Suto women smoke it to stupefy themselves during childbirth;* they also grind up the seeds with bread or mealie pap and give it to children when they are being weaned." [15] A 1916 report noted that marijuana smoking was not only permitted but actually encouraged among South African mine workers because "after a smoke the natives work hard and show very little fatigue." The usual mine practice, the report continued, was to allow three smokes—resembling "coffee breaks"—a day.[16] Farther north, "the lives of some tribes in the Congo center on hemp, which is cultivated, smoked regularly and venerated. Whenever the tribe travels it takes the Riamba [a huge calabash pipe more than a yard in diameter] with it. The man who commits a misdeed is condemned to smoke until he loses consciousness." [17]

Most Americans today think of marijuana as a substance to be smoked; but countless other ways of using it have also been developed—even its use as a flavoring or seasoning for common foodstuffs. Nowhere have the modes of use multiplied more lavishly through the centuries than in India; Colonel Sir R. N. Chopra, Director of the Drug Research Laboratory, Jammu and Kashmir, and his son, Dr. I. C. Chopra, a pharmacologist, have described some Indian modes of use in the United Nations *Bulletin on Narcotics* (1957).

Three separate grades of marijuana product have traditionally been recognized in India, the Chopras point out:[18]

Bhang, a weak preparation of the leaves and flowering tops of the plant —roughly comparable to marijuana grown and harvested in the United States.

Ganja, a significantly stronger preparation, which includes some of the potent resin as well as the leaves and flowering tops—roughly comparable to potent marijuana imported into the United States from Mexico or Vietnam.

---

* The use of marijuana to ease the pangs of childbirth has been discussed in the United States as well. In 1930 a Pennsylvania physician sent this query to the *Journal of the American Medical Association:*

"If cannabis is taken to a point of intoxication during labor, what effect will it have on labor and on the newborn child?"

The AMA's consultants replied:

". . . Its chief effects are on the central nervous system. There is a mixture of depression and stimulation similar to that occasionally seen under morphine. Soon after its administration the patient passes into a semiconscious state in which judgment is lost and vivid dreams occur. The sensation of pain is distinctly lessened or entirely absent and the sense of touch is less acute than normally. Hence a woman in labor may have a more or less painless labor. If a sufficient amount of the drug is taken, the patient may fall into a tranquil sleep from which she will awaken refreshed. Some degree of tolerance for this drug is rapidly acquired and death from acute poisoning is rare. As far as is known, a baby born of a mother intoxicated with cannabis will not be abnormal in any way." [14] This opinion, of course, is subject to qualification today. The effect is not similar to morphine, and tolerance is not acquired.

Charas, the highly potent resin in pure or almost pure form—the product known in the United States and elsewhere as hashish (or "hash"). The effects of charas are roughly comparable to those of the weaker forms—but it is said to take from five to eight grams of bhang (or of American-grown marijuana) to equal the effect of one gram of charas or hashish. (These estimates were made before reliable methods of measuring potency were developed, and may be subject to revision.)

Bhang and ganja are used primarily by the lower classes in India—those that cannot afford alcohol. "The low cost and easy availability of these drugs," the Chopras report, "are important factors in their use by the working classes, whose economic condition is low in this country. Cannabis drugs are perhaps the only narcotic drugs which fall comfortably within their meagre means, and they make use of them as occasion arises. A dose worth an anna or two (one or two U.S. cents) is often sufficient for producing the desired effect"—not only for the purchaser but for one or two of his friends as well.

The two stronger forms, ganja and charas, are smoked much as marijuana is smoked in the United States: "The smoke is retained in the lungs for as long as possible and is then allowed to escape slowly through the nostrils, the mouth being kept shut. The longer the smoke is retained, the more potent are the effects obtained. Experienced smokers are able to retain the smoke for quite a long while." [19]

The weakest marijuana, bhang, is in India customarily eaten or drunk in a variety of forms. The Chopras explain that it is "always taken by mouth either in the form of a beverage or a confection. . . . The simplest bhang beverage consists of a drink made by pounding bhang leaves with a little black pepper and sugar, and diluting with water to the desired strength. Various kinds of special beverages are prepared by the middle and well-to-do classes by the addition of almonds, sugar, iced milk, curds, etc. . . .

"Bhang leaves are sometimes chewed for their sedative effects. This is done particularly at times when it is inconvenient for the *habitué* to prepare the beverage, as, for example, when travelling. During cold weather, when the system does not require large quantities of fluid or in the case of mendicants (sadhus and fakirs) who cannot afford the expense of preparing the beverage, the chewing of leaves may be substituted for the beverage. On festive occasions bhang may be incorporated in a variety of sweetmeats. Ice-cream containing bhang is also sometimes available in large towns during the hot weather." [20]

Like marijuana smoking in the United States today, the eating and drinking of bhang in India is almost always a social occasion, indulged in primarily among friends. "Even up to the present day," the Chopras wrote in 1957, "at the occasion of some festivals, a large iron vessel full of a bhang drink is sometimes kept for public consumption. It is rare to find *habitués* indulging in these drugs without company, except in the form of pills or sweets or at other occasions when company is not available. Our experience is that even those who have bought their own supplies always enjoy them in company if possible." [21]

Marijuana is also commonly used in the Hindu (Ayurvedic) and Mohammedan (Tibbi) systems of medicine in India; and it has ceremonial significance. "In Bengal, for instance," the Chopras report, "the custom still persists among certain classes of offering a beverage prepared from the leaves of the cannabis plant to the various family members and to guests on the last day of Durga Puja . . . which is the biggest Hindu festival in that state. . . . It is also taken by certain classes on the occasion of the Holi and Dewali festivals, marriage ceremonies, and other family festivities. . . . Assam is the only state where bhang is practically not used at all at present, probably because of the prevalance there of the use of opium." [22]

The Chopras in addition report a use of bhang resembling the chewing of coca leaves among the mountain people of South America (see Part V):

Cannabis drugs are reputed to alleviate fatigue and also to increase staying power in severe physical stress. In India, fishermen, boatmen, laundrymen and farmers, who daily have to spend long hours in rivers, tanks and waterlogged fields, often resort to cannabis in some form, in the belief that it will give them a certain amount of protection against catching cold. Mendicants who roam about aimlessly in different parts of India and pilgrims who have to do long marches often use cannabis either occasionally or habitually. Sadhus and fakirs visiting religious shrines usually carry some bhang or ganja with them and often take it. It is not an uncommon sight to see them sitting in a circle and enjoying a smoke of ganja in the vicinity of a temple or a mosque. Labourers who have to do hard physical work use cannabis in small quantities to alleviate the sense of fatigue, depression and sometimes hunger. A common practice amongst labourers engaged on building or excavation work is to have a few pulls at a ganja pipe or to drink a glass of bhang towards the evening. This produces a sense of well-being, relieves fatigue, stimulates the appetite, and induces a feeling of mild stimulation, which enables the worker to bear more cheerfully the strain and perhaps the monotony of the daily routine of life. [23]

In addition to these common uses of bhang in moderate doses, resembling American uses of caffeine and nicotine, marijuana products are sometimes taken in larger doses, the Chopras note, "to induce a state of intoxication which will excite emotion and give a sense of bravado so that daring acts will be committed." They add that "indulgence in cannabis drugs, unlike alcohol, rarely brings the *habitué* into a state of extreme intoxication where he loses entire control over himself. As a rule, the intoxication produced is of a mild nature, and those who indulge in it habitually can carry on their ordinary vocations for long periods and do not become a burden to society or even a social nuisance." [24]

Finally, the Chopras report that cannabis, presumably in the form of charas, can be "employed to produce a state of intoxication so intense that the individual may lose all control of himself." This use, they add, is rare; "these drugs are not often indulged in to such an extent as to constitute a definite abuse and menace." [25]

Marijuana appears to occupy fourth place in worldwide popularity among the mind-affecting drugs—preceded only by caffeine, nicotine, and alcohol. As in the cases of caffeine, nicotine, and alcohol, attempts have occasionally been made to suppress the traffic in marijuana and to eradicate its use, sometimes by means of extreme penalties. Thus the Emir Soudoun Sheikhouni of Joneima in Arabia is said to have ordered in the year 1378 that all hemp plants in his territory be destroyed and that all marijuana eaters be imprisoned. He further decreed that anyone convicted of eating the plant should have his teeth pulled out. Many were in fact punished in this way. But fifteen years after the Emir's decree, Dr. Louis Lewin reports in *Phantastica*, "the use of this substance in Arabian territory had increased." [26]

No successful effort to suppress marijuana use has been found in a review of the historical literature for this Report. In the early 1950s, a report to the United Nations estimated that there were then 200,000,000 marijuana users in the world.[27] In 1969, Dr. Stanley Yolles of the National Institute of Mental Health estimated the number at between 200,-000,000 and 250,000,000.[28] Thus, if there have in fact been any successful antimarijuana drives through the centuries, they have almost certainly been successful only on a small scale or for a limited period of time.

54.

Marijuana in the New World

The first definite record of the marijuana plant in the New World dates from 1545 A.D., when the Spaniards introduced it into Chile.[1] It has been suggested, however, that African slaves familiar with marijuana as an intoxicant and medicine brought the seeds with them to Brazil even earlier in the sixteenth century.[2]

There is no record that the Pilgrims brought marijuana with them to Plymouth—but the Jamestown settlers did bring the plant to Virginia in 1611, and cultivated it for its fiber.[3] Marijuana was introduced into New England in 1629.[4] From then until after the Civil War, the marijuana plant was a major crop in North America, and played an important role in both colonial and national economic policy. In 1762, "Virginia awarded bounties for hempculture and manufacture, and imposed penalties upon those who did not produce it."[5]

George Washington was growing hemp at Mount Vernon three years later—presumably for its fiber, though it has been argued that Washington was also concerned to increase the medicinal or intoxicating potency of his marijuana plants.*

British mercantile policy hampered American hemp culture for a time during and after the colonial period by offering heavy bounties on hemp exported from Ireland; but the American plantings continued despite this subsidized competition. At various times in the nineteenth century large hemp plantations flourished in Mississippi, Georgia, California, South Carolina, Nebraska, and other states, as well as on Staten Island, New York.[8] The center of nineteenth-century production, however, was in Kentucky, where hemp was introduced in 1775. One Kentuckian, James

---

* The argument depends on a curious tradition, which may or may not be sound, that the quality or quantity of marijuana resin (hashish) is enhanced if the male and female plants are separated *before* the females are pollinated. There can be no doubt that Washington separated the males from the females. Two entries in his diary supply the evidence:

May 12–13, 1765: "Sowed Hemp at Muddy hole by Swamp."

August 7, 1765: "—began to seperate [sic] the Male from the Female Hemp at Do— rather too late."[6]

George Andrews has argued, in *The Book of Grass: An Anthology of Indian Hemp* (1967), that Washington's August 7 diary entry "clearly indicates that he was cultivating the plant for medicinal purposes as well as for its fiber."[7] He might have separated the males from the females to get better fiber, Andrews concedes—but his phrase "rather too late" suggests that he wanted to complete the separation *before the female plants were fertilized*—and this was a practice related to drug potency rather than to fiber culture.

L. Allen, wrote in 1900: "The Anglo-Saxon farmers had scarce conquered foothold in the Western wilderness before they became sowers of hemp. The roads of Kentucky . . . were early made necessary by the hauling of hemp. For the sake of it slaves were perpetually being trained, hired, bartered; lands perpetually rented and sold; fortunes made and lost. . . . With the Civil War began the decline, lasting still." [9] The invention of the cotton gin and of other cotton and wool machinery, and competition from cheap imported hemp, were major factors in this decline in United States hemp cultivation.

The decline in commercial production did not, however, mean that marijuana became scarce. As late as 1937, the American commercial crop was still estimated at 10,000 acres, much of it in Wisconsin, Illinois, and Kentucky. [10] Four million pounds of marijuana seed a year were being used in bird feed. During World War II commercial cultivation was greatly expanded, at the behest of the United States Department of Agriculture, to meet the shortage of imported hemp for rope. Even decades after commercial cultivation has been discontinued, hemp can often be found growing luxuriantly as a weed in abandoned fields and along roadsides. Indeed, the plant readily spreads to additional territory. The area of Nebraska land infested with "weed" marijuana was estimated in 1969 at 156,000 acres.* [11]

The medicinal use of marijuana in the United States. It has often been alleged that American marijuana, cultivated primarily as a fiber, has little or no psychoactive effect. Nineteenth-century observers knew better. Dr. Walton sums up:

> Hemp grown for fiber in Kentucky has been shown to contain a substantial degree of . . . potency. H. C. Wood, in 1869, prepared an alcoholic extract of hemp grown near Lexington and proceeded to test the product himself. A large [oral] dose (20 to 30 grains) produced marked effects and, on subsequent occasions, milder but definite effects were obtained with doses as low as ¼ grain. This latter dose is lower than the usual dose of the Indian extract and was probably the result of a more than usually selective extraction. Houghton and Hamilton in 1908 concluded from animal experiments that the Kentucky hemp was fully as active as the best imported Indian product. In any event, it is clear that the potentiality of hashish abuse has always existed with this type of hemp production. [12]

Comparative studies made by the National Institute of Mental Health on marijuana experimentally grown at the University of Mississippi in 1969 and 1970 indicate that the relative low potency of American-grown marijuana is determined primarily by the seed planted. [13] Marijuana grown in Mississippi from high-quality Mexican seed proved to contain much

---

* One acre of good land yields about one thousand pounds of marijuana, enough for almost one million marijuana cigarettes.

more of the psychoactive substance (THC) than marijuana from domestic seed grown on the same plot and harvested and processed in the same way.[14]

The NIMH studies also refute the widespread belief that the female marijuana plant yields a more potent leaf. Flowers and leaves of male plants from Mexican seeds yielded 1.47 percent THC as compared with 1.31 percent for female plants.[15] The female plant does, however, yield more resin or hashish.

Laboratory tests of United States "weed" marijuana indicate that its THC content is very low. A 1971 study published in *Science,* however, suggests that the THC determinations as currently made are a poor index of the effectiveness of marijuana when smoked; the smoke may be considerably more potent than the THC determinations indicate.[16]

Between 1850 and 1937, marijuana was quite widely used in American medical practice for a wide range of conditions. The *United States Pharmacopeia,* which through the generations has maintained a highly selective listing of the country's most widely accepted drugs, admitted marijuana as a recognized medicine in 1850 under the name *Extractum Cannabis* or Extract of Hemp,[17] and listed it until 1942.[18] The *National Formulary* and United States *Dispensatory,* less selective, also included monographs on marijuana and cited recommendations for its use for numerous illnesses. In 1851 the United States *Dispensatory* reported:

Extract of hemp is a powerful narcotic [here meaning sleep-producing drug], causing exhilaration, intoxication, delirious hallucinations, and, in its subsequent action, drowsiness and stupor, with little effect upon the circulation. It is asserted also to act as a decided aphrodisiac, to increase the appetite, and occasionally to induce the cataleptic state. In morbid states of the system, it has been found to cause sleep, to allay spasm, to compose nervous disquietude, and to relieve pain. In these respects it resembles opium; but it differs from that narcotic in not diminishing the appetite, checking the secretions, or constipating the bowels. It is much less certain in its effects, but may sometimes be preferably employed, when opium is contraindicated by its nauseating or constipating effects, or its disposition to produce headache, and to check the bronchial secretion. The complaints in which it has been specially recommended are neuralgia, gout, rheumatism, tetanus, hydrophobia, epidemic cholera, convulsions, chorea, hysteria, mental depression, delirium tremens, insanity, and uterine hemorrhage.[19]

Many eminent British and American physicians recommended marijuana as an effective therapeutic agent. Dr. J. Russell Reynolds, Fellow of the Royal Society and Physician in Ordinary to Her Majesty's (Queen Victoria's) Household, reported in *Lancet* in 1890, for example, that he had been prescribing cannabis for thirty years and that he considered it "one of the most valuable medicines we possess."[20] Sir William Osler, professor of medicine at the Johns Hopkins and later Regius Professor of Medicine at the University of Oxford, stated in his 1898 discussion of migraine headaches that marijuana "is probably the most satisfactory remedy" for that distressing condition.* [28]

To meet the substantial nineteenth- and early twentieth-century medical demand for marijuana, fluid extracts were marketed by Parke Davis, Squibb, Lilly, Burroughs Wellcome, and other leading firms,[29] and were sold over the counter by drugstores at modest prices. Grimault and Sons actually marketed ready-made marijuana cigarettes for use as an asthma remedy.[30] As medicine progressed after 1903, marijuana's use declined, but its therapeutic value remained unchallenged, and doctors continued to prescribe it.

Early recreational use of marijuana in the United States. A number of colorful references to the recreational use of marijuana and hashish in the nineteenth century are available. Lush descriptions of their personal experiences were published by Baudelaire, Gautier, Dumas *père,* and other members of a Parisian institution, the Club des Hachichins,[31] where strong forms of marijuana were eaten. In December 1856 a young American, Fitz Hugh Ludlow, of Poughkeepsie, New York, published an account of his own marijuana-eating experiences in *Putnam's Magazine,* which he then expanded to 371 pages in *The Hasheesh Eater,* a book published by Harper and Brothers the following year.

Young Ludlow had read De Quincey's *Confessions of an English Opium-Eater,* and was probably influenced as well by the French accounts of hashish eating published in the 1840s. His interest in drugs thus kindled, he made friends with a Poughkeepsie apothecary named Anderson and soon Anderson's drugstore was his favorite "lounging place."

Here, many an hour have I sat . . . , [he later wrote,] and here especially, with a disregard to my own safety which would have done credit to Quintus Curtius, have I made upon myself the trial of the effects of every strange drug and chemical which the laboratory could produce. Now with the chloroform bottle beneath my nose have I set myself careering upon the wings of a thrilling and accelerating life, until I had just enough power remaining to restore the liquid to its place upon the shelf, and sink back into the enjoyment of the delicious apathy which lasted through the few succeeding moments. Now ether was substituted for chloroform, and the difference of their phenomena noted,

* Others who recommended marijuana for migraine headaches included the Committee on Cannabis Indica of the Ohio State Medical Society (1860); [21] Dr. G. S. D. Anderson in the *Boston Medical and Surgical Journal* (now the *New England Journal of Medicine*) (1863); [22] Dr. Edward John Waring in his textbook, *Practical Therapeutics* (1874); [23] Dr. C. W. Suckling in the *British Medical Journal* (1881); [24] Dr. J. B. Mattison in the *St. Louis Medical and Surgical Journal* (1891); [25] and Dr. A. A. Stevens in his textbook, *Modern Materia Medica* (1903).[26] (We are indebted to Dr. Tod H. Mikuriya [27] for a number of these and other historical references to the medical history of marijuana.)

and now some other exhilarant, in the form of an opiate or stimulant, was the instrument of my experiments, until I had run through the whole gamut of queer agents within my reach. . . .[32] When the circuit of all the accessible tests was completed, I ceased experimenting, and sat down like a pharmaceutical Alexander, with no more drug worlds to conquer.[33]

He was sixteen years old at this time.

One spring morning in the early 1850s, however, apothecary Anderson greeted young Ludlow with a question: "Have you seen my new acquisitions?"

Ludlow "looked toward the shelves in the direction of which he pointed, and saw, added since my last visit, a row of comely pasteboard cylinders inclosing vials of the various extracts prepared by Tilden & Co. . . . I approached the shelves, that I might take them in review." [34] One of the Tilden products was a marijuana extract. After consulting the United States *Dispensatory* (quoted above) and Johnson's *Chemistry of Common Life,* Ludlow took ten grains of it. Nothing happened. A few days later he took fifteen grains. Again nothing happened.

Gradually, by five grains at a time, I increased the dose to thirty grains, which I took one evening half an hour after tea. I had now almost come to the conclusion that I was absolutely unsusceptible of the hasheesh influence. Without any expectation that this last experiment would be more successful than the former ones, and indeed with no realization of the manner in which the drug affected those who did make the experiment successfully, I went to pass the evening at the house of an intimate friend. In music and conversation the time passed pleasantly. The clock struck ten, reminding me that three hours had elapsed since the dose was taken, and as yet not an unusual symptom had appeared. I was provoked to think that this trial was as fruitless as its predecessors.

Ha! what means this sudden thrill? A shock, as of some unimagined vital force, shoots without warning through my entire frame, leaping to my fingers' ends, piercing my brain, startling me till I almost spring from my chair.

I could not doubt it. I was in the power of the hasheesh influence.[35]

Ludlow went on eating marijuana extract on occasion for the next four years, from the age of sixteen to the age of twenty. Then he stopped, and reported his experiences at inordinate length.

Marijuana continued in use after the Civil War as a rare and exotic drug claiming relatively few devotees by twentieth-century standards. The *Scientific American* reported in 1869: "The drug hashish, the cannabis indica of the U.S. Pharmacopeia, the resinous product of hemp, grown in the East Indies and other parts of Asia, is used in those countries to a large extent for its intoxicating properties and is doubtless used in this country for the same purpose to a limited extent." [36]

The December 2, 1876, issue of the *Illustrated Police News* confirmed that conjecture with a drawing showing five attractive young women in exotic clothing, reclining on divans—several of them visibly intoxicated. The drawing was captioned, "Secret Dissipation of New York Belles: Interior of a Hasheesh Hell on Fifth Avenue." Water pipes (hookahs) similar to those used for smoking hashish were conspicuously displayed.[37]

The most impressive evidence of hashish smoking in nineteenth-century America appears in an anonymous * article published in *Harper's New Monthly Magazine* for November 1883, entitled "A Hashish-House in New York." It opened with a dialogue:

"And so you think that opium-smoking as seen in the foul cellars of Mott Street and elsewhere is the only form of narcotic indulgence of any consequence in this city, and that hashish, if used at all, is only smoked occasionally and experimentally by a few scattered individuals?"

"That certainly is my opinion, and I consider myself fairly well informed."

"Well, you are far from right, as I can prove to you. . . . There is a large community of hashish smokers in this city [New York], who are daily forced to indulge their morbid appetites, and I can take you to a house up-town where hemp is used in every conceivable form, and where the lights, sounds, odors, and surroundings are all arranged so as to intensify and enhance the effects. . . ."[38]

The next night the author with his friend visited a "hasheesh house" on or near Forty-second Street west of Broadway. The hashish smokers there, the author was informed, "are about evenly divided between Americans and foreigners; indeed, the place is kept by a Greek, who has invested a great deal of money in it. All the visitors, both male and female, are of the better classes, and absolute secrecy is the rule. The house has been opened about two years, I believe, and the number of regular habitués is daily on the increase."[39] Dr. Kane was also told: "Smokers from different cities, Boston, Philadelphia, Chicago, and especially New Orleans, tell me that each city has its hemp retreat, but none so elegant as this."[40]

The maintenance of secrecy, the date of opening (presumably 1881), and other aspects of the New York City account suggest that when police pressure was put on opium-smoking dens in New York City and elsewhere after 1875 (see Chapter 6), their place was taken by "hasheesh hells" modeled after them.

* The *Oxford English Dictionary* attributes the article to Dr. H. H. Kane, author of a standard 1880 textbook on the medical uses of morphine (see Chapter 2) and an 1882 study of opium smoking. The article was recently discovered by lexicographer David Rattray, who sent a copy to the poet Allen Ginsberg, who passed it on to Dr. Michael Aldrich of the Marijuana Research Association, who in turn made it available for this Report.

Liquid cannabis plus ergot—the drug from which LSD was later derived—were taken by Frank Dudley Beane, M.D., and reported by him in the *Buffalo Medical Journal* in 1884. Dr. Beane's "trip," after a period of "hilarious exhilation and constant volubility," ended in deep sleep.[41]

The ready availability of hashish in candy form in Baltimore was reported in 1894 by Dr. George Wheelock Grover in his book, *Shadows Lifted or Sunshine Restored in the Horizon of Human Lives: A Treatise on the Morphine, Opium, Cocaine, Chloral and Hashish Habits:* "Once while passing down the leading business street in Baltimore, I saw upon a sign above my head, 'Gungawalla Candy, Hashish Candy.' I purchased a box of the candy and, while waiting with two or three medical friends at the Eutaw House in Baltimore, determined that I would experiment upon myself [and] test the power of this drug. I took a full dose at 11 o'clock in the forenoon." Hashish taken orally is much slower-acting than smoked hashish, and Dr. Grover felt nothing for about three hours. Then the drug "manifested its peculiar witchery with scarcely prelude or warning." Dr. Grover remarked to his friends, sitting at the dining room table with him:

It is undoubtedly here a day of jubilation or of something in the way of celebration. You perceive that the tables are set with golden plate, that the waiters all seem to be dressed in velvet costumes, and that hundreds of canary birds are singing in gilded cages. It must be a celebration of a good deal of magnitude, as the many bands of martial and orchestral music seem all to be playing at once.[42]

The occasional use of cannabis for recreational purposes continued into the twentieth century. One New York City physician, Dr. Victor Robinson, reported in 1910 that he personally had taken fluid extract of cannabis (U.S.P.) and had on several occasions supplied it to his friends —in part out of scientific curiosity but also just for fun.[43] General John J. Pershing's troops were said to have brought marijuana back with them from Mexico where they were chasing Pancho Villa in 1915.[44]

"Old persons in Kentucky report seeing colored field hands break up and load their pipes with dried flowering tops of the plants and smoke them," Dr. J. D. Reichard of Lexington, Kentucky, told a scientific meeting in 1943.[45]

In short, marijuana was readily available in the United States through much of the nineteenth and early twentieth centuries, its effects were known, and it was occasionally used for recreational purposes. But use was at best limited, local, and temporary. Not until after 1920 did marijuana come into general use—and not until the 1960s did it become a popular drug.

55.

Marijuana and alcohol prohibition

It was a change in the laws rather than a change in the drug or in human nature that stimulated the large-scale marketing of marijuana for recreational use in the United States. Not until the Eighteenth Amendment and the Volstead Act of 1920 raised the price of alcoholic beverages and made them less convenient to secure and inferior in quality did a substantial commercial trade in marijuana for recreational use spring up.

Evidence for such a trade comes from New York City, where marijuana "tea pads" were established about 1920. They resembled opium dens or speakeasies except that prices were very low; a man could get high for a quarter on marijuana smoked in the pad, or for even less if he bought the marijuana at the door and took it away to smoke. Most of the marijuana, it was said, was harvested from supplies growing wild on Staten Island or in New Jersey and other nearby states; marijuana and hashish imported from North Africa were more potent and cost more. These tea pads were tolerated by the city, much as alcohol speakeasies were tolerated. By the 1930s there were said to be 500 of them in New York City alone.[1]

In 1926 the New Orleans *Item* and *Morning Tribune*, two newspapers under common ownership, published highly sensational exposés of the "menace" of marijuana.[2] They reported that it was coming into New Orleans from Havana, Tampico, and Vera Cruz in large quantities, plus smaller amounts from Texas. "In one day, ten sailors were followed from the time they left their ships until they delivered their respective packages of the drug to a particular block in the Vieux Carré."[3] The sailors, it was said, bought marijuana in the Mexican ports for $10 or $12 per kilogram (2.2 pounds) and sold it in the Vieux Carré for $35 to $50.[4] This was far more profitable than smuggling a comparable weight of whiskey.

Much of the smuggled marijuana was smoked in New Orleans; but some, it was said, was shipped up the Mississippi and "found its way as far north as Cleveland, Ohio, where a well-known physician said it was smoked in one of the exclusive men's clubs."[5]

In New Orleans, the reporters in 1926 laid particular stress on the smoking of marijuana by children. "It was definitely ascertained that school children of 44 schools (only a few of these were high schools) were smoking 'mootas.' Verifications came in by the hundreds from harassed parents, teachers, neighborhood pastors, priests, welfare workers and club women. . . . The Waif's Home, at this time, was reputedly full of children, both white and colored, who had been brought in under the influence of the drug. Marijuana cigarettes could be bought almost as readily as sandwiches. Their cost was two for a quarter. The children solved the problem of cost by pooling pennies among the members of a group and then passing the cigarettes from one to another, all the puffs being carefully counted." [6]

A Louisiana law passed in 1927, after the newspaper exposé, provided a maximum penalty of a $500 fine or six months' imprisonment for possession or sale of marijuana.* [7] There followed "a wholesale arrest of more than 150 persons. Approximately one hundred underworld dives, soft-drink establishments, night clubs, grocery stores, and private homes were searched in the police raids. Addicts, hardened criminals, gangsters, women of the streets, sailors of all nationalities, bootleggers, boys and girls—many flashily dressed in silks and furs, others in working clothes— all were rounded up in the net which Captain Smith and his squad had set." [8]

The newspaper investigation, the new law, and the heavily publicized police roundups did not, however, accomplish their purpose. On the contrary, according to Commissioner of Public Safety Frank Gomila, during the next few years New Orleans "experienced a crime wave which unquestionably was greatly aggravated by the influence of this drug habit. Payroll and bank guards were doubled, but this did not prevent some of the most spectacular hold-ups in the history of the city. Youngsters known to be 'muggle-heads' fortified themselves with the narcotic and proceeded to shoot down police, bank clerks and casual by-standers. Mr. Eugene Stanley, at that time District Attorney, declared that many of the crimes in New Orleans and the South were thus committed by criminals who relied on the drug to give them a false courage and freedom from restraint. Dr. George Roeling, Coroner, reported that of 450 prisoners investigated, 125 were confirmed users of marihuana. Mr. W. B. Graham, State Narcotic Officer, declared in 1936 that 60 percent of the crimes committed in New Orleans were by marihuana users." [9]

Intensive patrolling of the New Orleans harbor tended to curb imports; but Louisianans were little inconvenienced by the smuggling curbs; they simply began to grow their own marijuana. "The first large growing crop in the city was found in 1930 and its value estimated at $35,000 to $50,000. . . . In 1936 about 1,200 pounds of bulk weed were seized along with considerable quantities of cigarettes. On one farm, 5½ tons were destroyed and other farms yielded cultivated areas of about 10 acres. . . .

* The penalties were later escalated to include thirty years at hard labor or the death sentence for sale of marijuana to anyone under twenty-one years of age (first offense). We have found no record, however, of the actual imposition of the death sentence in a United States marijuana case.

One resident of the city was found growing 100 large plants in his back-yard." [10] The net effect of eleven years of vigorous law enforcement was summed up by Commissioner Gomila in 1938: "Cigarettes are hard to get and are selling at 30 to 40 cents apiece, which is a relatively high price and a particularly good indication of the effectiveness of the present control." [11] Marijuana smoking, in short, had become endemic in New Orleans—and remains endemic today. What years of law enforcement had accomplished was to raise the price from two for 25 cents to 30 cents or 40 cents apiece—and even this increase might be attributable in part to inflation.

In Colorado, the Denver *News* launched a similar series of sensational marijuana exposés following the pattern set in New Orleans.[12] Mexican laborers imported to till the Colorado beet-sugar fields, it seems, had found Prohibition alcohol very expensive and so had resorted instead to marijuana, bringing their supplies north with them. A Colorado law against marijuana was duly passed in 1929.[13]

These sensational newspaper accounts and early efforts to outlaw marijuana should not, however, be taken as evidence that marijuana smoking was in fact widespread. In 1931 the United States Treasury Department, then responsible for enforcing both the federal antinarcotics and the federal antialcohol laws, indicated that the marijuana exposés in the newspapers were quite possibly exaggerated:

A great deal of public interest has been aroused by newspaper articles appearing from time to time on the evils of the abuse of marihuana, or Indian hemp, and more attention has been focused on specific cases reported of the abuse of the drug than would otherwise have been the case. This publicity tends to magnify the extent of the evil and lends color to an inference that there is an alarming spread of the improper use of the drug, whereas the actual increase in such use may not have been inordinately large.[14]

56.

Marijuana is outlawed

Following the legalization of weak beer in 1933 and the return of hard liquor the following year, the modest, localized popularity of marijuana during the Prohibition years might have declined further. But additional legal developments intervened.

On January 1, 1932, the newly established Federal Bureau of Narcotics, a unit in the Treasury Department, took over from the Alcohol Unit of the department the enforcement of the federal antiopiate and anticocaine laws; and former Assistant Prohibition Commissioner Harry J. Anslinger took over as commissioner of narcotics. Commissioner Anslinger had no legal jurisdiction over marijuana, but his interest in it was intense. The Bureau's first *Annual Report* under his aegis warned that marijuana, dismissed as a minor problem by the Treasury one year earlier, had now "come into wide and increasing abuse in many states, and the Bureau of Narcotics has therefore been endeavoring to impress on the various States the urgent need for vigorous enforcement of the local cannabis laws." [1]

During his first year as commissioner of narcotics, Mr. Anslinger secured from the National Conference of Commissioners on Uniform Drug Laws the draft of a "Uniform Anti-Narcotics Act," designed for adoption by state legislatures. The conference failed to include a ban on marijuana in the main text of this model law; but it did supply to the states an "optional text applying to the restriction of traffic in Indian hemp." [2] Commissioner Anslinger and his bureau urged on the states the adoption of this "optional text" as well as the basic act; and state after state complied.

Commissioner Anslinger's report for 1935 noted: "In the absence of Federal legislation on the subject, the States and cities should rightfully assume the responsibility for providing vigorous measures for the extinction of this lethal weed, and it is therefore hoped that all public-spirited citizens will earnestly enlist in the movement urged by the Treasury Department to adjure intensified enforcement of marijuana laws." [3]

By 1937, forty-six of the forty-eight states as well as the District of Columbia had laws against marijuana. [4] Under most of these state laws, marijuana was subject to the same rigorous penalties applicable to morphine, heroin, and cocaine, [5] and was often erroneously designated a narcotic.

Commissioner Anslinger's next campaign was for a federal marijuana law. Professor Howard S. Becker, a sociologist now at Northwestern University, has documented in detail the magazine phase of this campaign. The *Readers' Guide to Periodical Literature,* Professor Becker notes, failed to list a single article on marijuana from January 1925 through June 1935.[6] Four such national magazine articles, however, were indexed for the period July 1935 through June 1937, and seventeen more were indexed between July 1937 and June 1939. The production of antimarijuana articles then tapered off again to four between July 1939 and June 1941, with one lone article indexed in the period July 1941 to June 1943.

Of the seventeen articles during the peak of the drive, Professor Becker continues, "ten either explicitly acknowledged the help of the Bureau in furnishing facts and figures or gave implicit evidence of having received help by using facts and figures that had appeared earlier, either in Bureau publications or in testimony before the Congress. . . ."[7]

Typical of the articles in this magazine campaign was one signed by Commissioner Anslinger himself, in collaboration with Courtney Ryley Cooper, which appeared in the *American Magazine* for July 1937. It contained such atrocity stories as the following:

An entire family was murdered by a youthful [marihuana] addict in Florida. When officers arrived at the home they found the youth staggering about in a human slaughterhouse. With an ax he had killed his father, mother, two brothers, and a sister. He seemed to be in a daze. . . . He had no recollection of having committed the multiple crime. The officers knew him ordinarily as a sane, rather quiet young man; now he was pitifully crazed. They sought the reason. The boy said he had been in the habit of smoking something which youthful friends called "muggles," a childish name for marihuana.[8]

Four of the sixteen other articles indexed in *Readers' Guide* for the peak period contained this same story.

Many readers in the 1970s, familiar with the mild, often calming effect of marijuana on young people in their own neighborhoods, will dismiss these accounts of wild crimes of violence committed under the influence of the drug as sheer nonsense or malicious propaganda—but this is far from certain. LSD, it will be recalled, was converted as a result of anti-LSD publicity from a relatively bland drug before 1962 to a drug that evoked the most bizarre behavior after that date. It is quite possible that marijuana effects were similarly altered during the 1920s and 1930s— that some children solemnly warned in advance that marijuana would madden them and cause them to commit the most awful crimes, including crimes of violence, really did lose self-control and commit such crimes thereafter when they smoked marijuana. Whether or not there was some truth in the antimarijuana stories, however, they were certainly exaggerated—as one of the cases reported in a 1937 bulletin of the Foreign Policy Association demonstrates.

The cases presented in the bulletin were described as "culled at random from the files of the U.S. Bureau of Narcotics." [9] One such story concerned a young man identified as "J. O.," who was said to have confessed that he murdered a friend and put his body in a trunk "while under the influence of marijuana." [10]

The story turned out to be partly true. Dr. Walter Bromberg, psychiatrist-in-charge at the Psychiatric Clinic, New York County Court of General Sessions, described the case of J. O. in greater detail in a 1939 issue of the *Journal of the American Medical Association.* No doubt J. O. really had murdered a friend and stuffed his body into a trunk. But the remaining details differed notably from the bureau's version. "J. O. was examined in this clinic," Dr. Bromberg reported; "although he was a psychopathic liar and possibly homosexual, there was no indication in the examination or history of the use of any drug. The investigation by the probation department failed to indicate use of the drug marijuana." [11] The only known relationship of the crime to drugs was that the *victim* was a *heroin* addict.

Dr. Bromberg's debunking of the story of J. O., however, did not retire that story from circulation. It bobbed up again, with additional verisimilitudinous details, in the United Nations *Bulletin on Narcotics* for April-June 1966, in an article by Dr. James C. Munch, identified as "Member, Advisory Committee, U.S. Bureau of Narcotics." In this version J. O. was quoted as saying: "I was fearless after smoking marijuana cigarettes but would not have done this without marijuana." [12]

The news media frequently may omit mentioning that a criminal was drunk on alcohol when he committed his crime, but when marijuana (or LSD) is supposedly involved in a case, that fact is often given prominence. Dr. Lawrence Kolb has supplied a striking example: "Two young men had some drinks of whiskey in a hotel room where they were celebrating. They then smoked a marijuana cigarette, after which they had some more whiskey and left the hotel room. Shortly thereafter, one of the men shot another man for some trifling reason. This story was played up in the press as a vicious, marijuana-induced murder." [13]

Commissioner Anslinger's drive for federal as well as state antimarijuana legislation shifted into high gear in 1937, when his superiors in the Treasury Department sent to Congress the draft of a bill that became the Marijuana Tax Act of 1937. This bill, modeled on the Harrison Narcotic Act of 1914, did not on its face actually ban marijuana. It fully recognized the medicinal usefulness of the substance, specifying that physicians, dentists, veterinarians, and others could continue to prescribe cannabis if they paid a license fee of $1 per year, that druggists who dispensed the drug should pay a license fee of $15 a year, that growers of marijuana should pay $25 a year, and that importers, manufacturers, and compounders should pay $50 a year. Only the *nonmedicinal, untaxed* possession or sale of marijuana was outlawed.[14]

At hearings on this bill before Senate and House committees, Commissioner Anslinger appeared as the chief witness, buttressed by members of his staff. He told horror stories similar to the ones in his *American Magazine* article quoted above. Another witness was the prosecuting attorney from New Orleans, who told of how criminals used marijuana in that city. In addition to stressing the relationship between marijuana and crime, witnesses testified that marijuana "addicts" went crazy.[15]

Curiously, Commissioner Anslinger himself refuted one charge against marijuana now commonly made. In the course of the House hearings, Representative John Dingell of Michigan remarked, "I am just wondering whether the marijuana addict graduates into a heroin, an opium, or a cocaine user."

Commissioner Anslinger replied, "No, sir; I have not heard of a case of that kind. The marijuana addict does not go in that direction." [16]

By 1955, however, Commissioner Anslinger was testifying before a Senate committee that "eventually if used over a long period, [marijuana] does lead to heroin addiction." [17]

No *medical* testimony in favor of the proposed federal antimarijuana law was presented at the 1937 Congressional hearings. Indeed, the only physician to testify was a representative of the American Medical Association—and he *opposed* the bill.[18] Marijuana, he pointed out, was a recognized medicine in good standing, distributed by leading pharmaceutical firms, and on sale at many pharmacies. At least twenty-eight medicinal products containing marijuana were on the market in 1937.

Although the proposed federal law preserved the right of physicians to prescribe marijuana and of pharmacists to dispense it,[19] an editorial in the *Journal of the American Medical Association* for May 1, 1937, vigorously opposed the legislation.

The medical profession today seldom dispenses the drug [the *JAMA* editorial conceded]. Many physicians will, however, probably feel it necessary to preserve their right to use it if and when circumstances make it advisable to do so and accordingly will feel compelled to pay the tax. Pharmacists presumably seldom have calls for cannabis, but they must nevertheless be prepared to dispense it when a call does come, so they will have to pay the tax. . . . The million dollars to be collected annually by the federal government will no doubt be charged as a part of the cost of practising medicine, dentistry, and pharmacy. So also will the expense of record keeping and reporting, called for under the bill. All this will in the end be paid for by the patient and thus will go to swell the cost of sickness. Thus the sick and injured must contribute toward federal efforts to suppress a habit that has little or no relation to the use of cannabis for medicinal purposes and that is already within the jurisdiction of the several states.[20]

The *JAMA* editorial also took a dim view of the likelihood that the new law would succeed in its purpose of discouraging the *nonmedicinal* use of marijuana. Its words have a prophetic ring:

After more than twenty years of federal effort and the expenditure of millions of dollars, the opium and cocaine habits are still widespread. The best efforts of an efficient bureau of narcotics, supplemented by the efforts of an equally efficient bureau of customs, have failed to stop the unlawful flow of opium and coca leaves and their compounds and derivatives, on which the continuance and spread of narcotic addiction depends. The best efforts of the Public Health Service to find means for the prevention and cure of narcotic addiction have not yet accomplished that end. Two federal narcotic farms, operating under the supervision and control of the U.S. Public Health Service, cannot yet guarantee the cure of narcotic addiction. What reason is there, then, for believing that any better results can be obtained by direct federal efforts to suppress a habit arising out of the misuse of such a drug as cannabis? Certainly it is almost as easy to smuggle into the country and to distribute as are opium and coca leaves. Moreover it can be cultivated in many parts of the United States and grows wild in field and forest and along the highways in many places.[21]

The proposed federal antimarijuana law was also considered at the June 1937 convention of the American Medical Association in Atlantic City. The "Report of the AMA Committee on Legislative Activities" at that convention noted:

There is positively no evidence to indicate the abuse of cannabis as a medicinal agent or to show that its medicinal use is leading to the development of cannabis addiction. Cannabis at the present time is slightly used for medicinal purposes, but it would seem worth while to maintain its status as a medicinal agent for such purposes as it now has. There is a possibility that a restudy of the drug by modern means may show other advantages to be derived from its medicinal use.*

* This "restudy of the drug by modern means" has now begun. At the University of Vermont College of Medicine, for example, researchers announced in August 1970 that they were testing THC for the alleviation of pain in cancer patients. The project was approved by local medical and legal officials, the United States Food and Drug Administration, and the National Institute of Mental Health. The THC was offered for voluntary oral use to patients at the Medical Center Hospital of Vermont. "The background for this study," the hospital's newsletter explained, "is the fact that cancer patients frequently require large doses of sedatives, antidepressants and pain killers toward the terminal part of the illness. Search is therefore being made for a

Your committee also recognizes that in the border states the extensive use of the marijuana weed by a certain type of people would be hard to control.[24]

Dr. William Woodward, a specialist in legal medicine and a lawyer as well as a physician, testified as a representative of the board of trustees of the American Medical Association in opposition to the proposed marijuana legislation at the 1937 Congressional hearings. He pointed out that the case against marijuana rested merely on newspaper stories and was not proven, and he opposed the law as likely to be a nuisance to the medical profession.[25]

Also testifying against the law were the distributors of birdseed, who complained that canaries would not sing as well, or might stop singing altogether, if marijuana seeds were eliminated from their diet.[26]

Congress recognized the legitimacy of the opposition from the birdseed manufacturers, and the bill was amended before enactment to exclude *sterilized* marijuana seed.[27] But the AMA's opposition was ignored, and the law was passed without other amendment.

Having secured both state and federal antimarijuana legislation, Commissioner Anslinger's next goal was to drive marijuana out of legitimate medical practice, despite the promarijuana stand of the American Medical Association. One step in this direction was his successful effort to persuade Dr. Ernest Fullerton Cook, chairman of the Committee on Revision of the *United States Pharmacopeia (U.S.P.)*, to have marijuana deleted from that official compendium.* Commissioner Anslinger made use of Dr. Cook's well-known opposition to "shotgun remedies" containing two or more active ingredients. "I recollect very well my conversation with . . . Dr. Fullerton Cook in relation to removing marijuana from the *Pharma-*

---

drug which could produce mood elevation in cancer patients without undesirable side effects." [22] This study was never completed.

In Britain, too, the reevaluation of cannabis as a medicine is under way, with government approval. The Baroness Wootton Subcommittee of the United Kingdom Home Office's Advisory Committee on Drug Dependence commented on this trend in 1968:

"At present cannabis can be prescribed by doctors in the form of extract of cannabis and alcoholic tincture of cannabis. Until very recently the demand for these preparations has been virtually negligible. In recent months however, there has been a striking increase in the amounts prescribed. Our enquiries, supported by what we were told by our witnesses, indicate that there are a number of doctors who are beginning to experiment with the use of cannabis in the treatment of disturbed adolescents, heroin and amphetamine dependence and even alcoholism. Whilst we do not expect cannabis prescription will ever become standard medication in the treatment of these conditions, it is quite likely that the amount dispensed on medical prescriptions will continue to increase and that this process may be accelerated when synthetic cannabis derivatives, properly standardised, become available. We see no objection to this and believe that any new legislation should be such as to permit its continuance. We think, however, that when cannabis or its derivatives are prescribed, records of the kind that can be inspected by H.M. Inspectors of Drugs should be available. This will enable the prescribing trend over the next few years to be kept under methodical review." [23]

* Cannabis is still an accepted drug in the *British Pharmacopoeia.*

copeia," the former commissioner wrote in 1970. "He made the decision to remove it after I pointed out that it was being used purely in shotgun prescriptions. In one case, a woman had her prescription refilled 300 times and wound up in Bellevue Hospital as a mental case." [28]

Commissioner Anslinger's campaign against medicinal use of marijuana was almost wholly successful. During the year ending December 31, 1970, only 38 American physicians paid their tax under the Marijuana Tax Act of 1937 and received licenses to prescribe marijuana.[29]

Since 1937, restrictive legislation on marijuana has increased in quantity and severity. Most state marijuana laws specified that marijuana penalties should be the same as heroin penalties. Thus, as heroin penalties were escalated through the decades, marijuana penalties rose automatically. Nineteen states, moreover, made no distinction between mere possession of one marijuana cigarette and the sale of large quantities of heroin. Under both federal law and the laws of many states, as noted earlier, the giving or furnishing of a narcotic drug or of marijuana was included in the definition of "sale."

Here are some of the penalties in force as of January 1, 1970: [30]

• In Alabama, a judge was required to sentence the possessor of one marijuana cigarette to not less than five years; he could hand down a ten-year sentence, and as much as forty years for a second-possession offense. Suspended sentences and probation were prohibited in all cases.

• In Colorado, the mandatory minimum for a first-possession offense was two years and for a first-sale offense ten years; no parole was permitted until these minimum sentences had been served.

• In Georgia, sale of marijuana to a minor was punishable by life imprisonment, even if it was a first offense—though the jury could recommend ten-to-twenty years instead. A second such offense was punishable by death—but the jury could recommend life imprisonment or ten-to-twenty years instead. No mitigation of sentence (suspension, probation, or parole) was permitted; the constitutionality of this clause was in question.

• In Illinois, the penalty for a first-sale offense was not less than ten years and as much as life. A mandatory life sentence was in effect for a second-sale offense. These penalties remained in effect after a 1968 amendment to the law reduced the penalties for possession of small amounts.

• In Louisiana, anyone over twenty-one years of age possessing marijuana was subject to a mandatory minimum sentence of five years at hard labor for a first offense; the judge could impose a fifteen-year sentence. Possessors under twenty-one could be sentenced to not more than ten years, with or without hard labor. An adult selling marijuana to another adult was subject to a minimum mandatory sentence of ten years at hard labor and a maximum sentence of fifty years at hard labor for a first offense. If the seller were under twenty-one, sentences ranged from five to fifteen years. If the buyer were under twenty-one, however, a first-sale offense required a mandatory minimum sentence of thirty years at hard labor and could draw a death sentence. No suspended sentences or probation was permitted for any sale offenses or for second-possession offenses.

• In Massachusetts, it was a felony punishable by not more than five years in prison to be in a place where marijuana was kept or deposited, or to be in the company of anyone known to be in illegal possession of marijuana.

• In Missouri, the judge could hand down a life sentence for a second-possession offense or a first-sale offense, without possibility of suspended sentence, probation, or parole. If the buyer were a minor, a death sentence was possible for a first-sale offense.

• In Rhode Island, a mandatory minimum sentence of ten years was decreed for a first offense of possession with intent to sell. The mandatory minimum for the first actual sale was twenty years, and a forty-year first-offense sentence could be imposed.

• In Texas, the penalty for a first-possession offense was not less than two years, but the judge could impose a life sentence for a first-possession offense. A second-possession offense carried a mandatory minimum ten-year sentence or a possible life sentence.

• In Utah a life sentence was possible for a first marijuana sale offense or for a second possession-with-intent-to-sell offense.

Congress also from time to time escalated federal marijuana penalties along with federal heroin penalties. In 1951, mandatory minimum sentences were fixed for all marijuana offenses, and all but first-time offenders were rendered ineligible for suspended sentence or probation. In 1956, the mandatory minimum for first-offense possession was fixed at two years (with a ten-year term possible). The mandatory minimum for a second-possession offense was fixed at five years (with a twenty-year term possible), with parole as well as probation and suspended sentence prohibited. For sale offenses, the mandatory minimum was set at five years for a first offense and ten years for a second; terms of twenty years for a first offense and forty for a second were possible—and parole as well as suspended sentence and probation were banned for all sale offenses.[31]

The Comprehensive Drug Abuse Prevention and Control Act of 1970 subsequently reduced federal penalties for marijuana possession.

As in the case of similar penalties for the possession or sale of heroin, these "mandatory" penalties were in fact rarely invoked; the offender was usually allowed to plead guilty to a lesser offense. When extreme penalties were handed down, there usually appeared to be some other reason—

some conduct or advocacy—aside from involvement with marijuana. Ordinary people, it is commonly agreed, rarely draw such sentences. "In California," one youth leader explains, "it is illegal to smoke marijuana unless you have your hair cut at least once a month." [32] The children of governors, senators, and others in the public eye, when arrested for marijuana offenses, rarely receive even short prison terms. Inequities of sentencing are no doubt among the factors bringing the marijuana laws, and drug law enforcement generally, into disrepute.

Continuing antimarijuana propaganda kept pace with the continuing antimarijuana legislation after 1937. And people generally believed the propaganda. In a National Institute of Public Opinion (Gallup) poll of a cross-section of 1,539 adults in 300 localities, made in October 1969, only 12 percent of the respondents thought that use of marijuana should be legalized; 84 percent were opposed, and 4 percent had no opinion. Among grade-school children, opposition to marijuana was even more prevalent; 6 percent thought it should be legalized, while 91 percent were opposed, and 3 percent had no opinion. [33] When adult respondents were asked to describe the effects of smoking marijuana, they gave the following replies. [34]

	Percent of Respondents
Harms mind and nervous system	17
Leads to use of stronger drugs	12
Dulls the senses	9
Harmful to the health	9
Makes user "high"	8
Addictive, habit-forming	7
Makes user lose control of his actions	7
Leads to irresponsibility, affects judgment	3
Neither habit-forming nor harmful	3
Leads to crime	1
Harmful to unborn children	1
Generally unfavorable comments	6
Miscellaneous	1
Unable to give answer	35
	119

"The total adds up to more than 100 percent since some persons gave more than one response," the Gallup organization explained. That only 3 percent of respondents considered marijuana "neither habit-forming nor harmful" is worthy of particular note. From the point of view of antimarijuana laws and antimarijuana publicity alike, the United States in the 1960s was superbly protected against this hated drug.

57.

America discovers marijuana

Here are some of the results of a third of a century of antimarijuana laws, escalated penalties, and intensive antimarijuana propaganda.

On September 17, 1969, a spokesman for the United States Department of Health, Education and Welfare—Dr. Stanley F. Yolles, then Director of the National Institute of Mental Health—informed a Senate Judiciary Subcommittee that somewhere between 8,000,000 and 12,000,000 Americans had smoked marijuana at least once.[1] This estimate was based on a wide range of surveys made among high-school students, college students, and the public at large.

Of those 8,000,000 to 12,000,000 marijuana smokers, Dr. Yolles continued, about 65 percent (5,000,000 to 8,000,000) were "experimenting, trying the drug from one to ten times, and then discontinuing its use." (Many of those who discontinued marijuana no doubt concluded that they preferred alcohol.) Another 25 percent (2,000,000 to 3,000,000 smokers) were "social users, smoking marijuana on occasion when it is available, usually in a group context." The remaining 10 percent or less (800,000 to 1,200,000 marijuana smokers) "can be considered chronic users who devote significant portions of their time to obtaining and using the drug."[2]

This burgeoning of marijuana smoking can hardly be blamed on lax law enforcement. In California, where marijuana smoking was most prevalent, marijuana arrests had increased enormously between 1954 and 1968:

Year	Number of marijuana arrests, California
1954	1,156 [3]
1960	5,155
1962	3,793
1964	7,560
1966	18,243
1968	50,327 [4]

Marijuana arrests accounted for 27 percent of all California drug arrests in 1960; by 1968 this figure had increased to 58 percent. Comparable figures are not available for other states or for the country as a whole.*

---

* This is a shocking gap, indeed, in the nation's statistical resources. Although both Congress and the state legislatures have been passing antimarijuana laws through

By the spring of 1970, as additional survey data flowed in, the official United States estimates of 8,000,000 to 12,000,000 users were raised. The number of individuals who had "ever smoked" marijuana, it was reported, "may be closer to 20 million." [5]

Here are some of the surveys on which these estimates were based.

In May 1969, the Gallup Poll reported results of a survey of college students. "Interviews were conducted for the poll with students across the nation—in private institutions such as Harvard University, in state-supported institutions such as Ohio State University, and in denominational or church-related institutions such as Notre Dame University." Twenty-two percent of the respondents stated that they had smoked marijuana.[6] (By December 1970, the comparable Gallup Poll figure was 42 percent.[7]) In contrast, only 10 percent said that they had taken a barbiturate and only 4 percent that they had tried LSD.

"Less stigma seems to be attached to the use of marijuana now than a year ago," the 1969 Gallup college report noted; "many students admit to taking marijuana as readily as they do to drinking beer." [8]

In October 1969, the Gallup Poll estimated that 10,000,000 Americans —half of them under twenty-one—had smoked marijuana. Based on the same sample of 1,539 adults in 300 localities described above, the poll concluded that 4 percent of all adults over twenty-one (6 percent of men and 2 percent of women) had smoked marijuana. Smokers ranged from 2 percent of the adults sampled in the Midwest and South to 5 percent in the East and 9 percent in the West. Twelve percent of men and women twenty-one to twenty-nine years of age had smoked marijuana, 3 percent of those thirty to forty-nine, and one percent of those fifty and over.[9] The nonusers, moreover, included many who said they *would* smoke marijuana if it were offered them.

At the University of Maryland, Dr. James D. McKenzie, a psychologist, has for several years been polling students enrolled in psychology and business courses. In 1967, 15 percent of responding students stated that they had smoked marijuana at least once; by 1969 this figure had increased to 35.6 percent.[10] The most dramatic increase occurred among women students.

Among the 600 students polled by Dr. McKenzie in 1969, 25.4 percent stated that they had smoked marijuana in the past and intended to continue smoking it or were currently smoking it at least once every two weeks. Among students living off campus, nearly half had smoked marijuana. Forty-eight percent of all students polled, including many who

---

the years, the number of people arrested under those laws, the number found guilty, the number serving prison terms, the length of terms served, and other data essential to wise legislative decisions have never been determined.

did not smoke marijuana themselves, believed that marijuana should be legalized.

"All kinds of students are using it—even the fraternity types," Dr. McKenzie was quoted as saying. "You can't talk about a drug-using type of student when you are talking about marijuana. Most of the use is very casual, like beer drinking on Saturday night." [11]

In September 1966, a drug-use questionnaire was distributed to medical students enrolled at the Albert Einstein College of Medicine in New York. Fourteen percent of the freshman (Class of 1970) medical students reported that they had smoked marijuana.[12] One year later, the same questionnaire was distributed again to the same Class of 1970 medical students. This time 31 percent reported that they had smoked marijuana —indicating that 17 percent had smoked it for the first time during their first year at medical school. Among freshman (Class of 1971) medical students included in the second survey, 22 percent reported smoking marijuana, as compared with the 14 percent for the Class of 1970 at the comparable point in its medical-school career. The Albert Einstein surveys also noted a modest decrease in alcohol use among medical-school students as marijuana use increased. The proportion of Class of 1970 students who stopped using alcohol between the 1966 and 1967 questionnaires was the same as the proportion who started smoking marijuana: 17 percent.[13]

In the spring of 1970, a poll was taken among 1,057 seniors at four medical schools—two in the East, one in the Middle West, and one on the West Coast. The medical schools were not named; but the psychiatrists who undertook the study were from the Harvard Medical School, the State University of New York Medical School at Buffalo, the University of Nebraska College of Medicine, and the Stanford University Medical School.

When asked whether they had ever used marijuana, only 16 percent of the seniors at one medical school said yes. At the other three medical schools, the replies were 46 percent, 68 percent, and 70 percent affirmative.[14]

Dr. Samuel G. Benson, the Stanford University psychiatrist who reported these figures at the 1971 meeting of the American Psychiatric Association, added this comment: "The large numbers of respondents indicating experience with marijuana (over two-thirds at Schools A and C) place medical students among the greatest users of cannabis yet reported. Only University of California law students and Vietnam combat soldiers were reported to have equivalent usage. No other survey published in medical literature reports comparable figures." [15] Of 466 medical students in the four-school study who had smoked marijuana, more than 275 reported that they were current marijuana smokers, and 114 reported that they had smoked marijuana more than a hundred times.[16]

Among 491 prospective lawyers enrolled in the Columbia University Law School who filled out a 1969 questionnaire, 69 percent said that they had smoked marijuana at least once. Fewer than 7 percent had smoked it only once. Among the marijuana smokers, 40 percent said that they smoked it "infrequently"; 53 percent said that they smoked it once or twice a month; and 7 percent said that they smoked it daily.*[17]

It is commonly supposed that marijuana smoking is particularly prevalent among students; but a study of 1,104 San Francisco residents aged eighteen and over, conducted in 1967–1968 by Dean I. Manheimer, Glen D. Mellinger, and Mitchell B. Balter, casts doubt on that supposition. One-half of the men and one-third of the women aged eighteen to twenty-four in the sample had smoked marijuana at least once; but "the proportion of students who report using marijuana does not differ markedly from the corresponding proportion among non-students" in the same age brackets. For all ages, 13 percent reported using marijuana—18 percent of the men and 9 percent of the women; no doubt these percentages have increased since the years 1967–1968. One-fifth of the marijuana smokers in the San Francisco sample were over thirty-five.[18]

The Manheimer-Mellinger-Balter survey also showed interesting correlations between marijuana smoking and cigarette smoking. Among those aged eighteen to thirty-four who smoked a pack or more of cigarettes daily, 51 percent of the men and 42 percent of the women had smoked marijuana; among those in the same age bracket who did not smoke cigarettes, only 17 percent of the men and 8 percent of the women had smoked marijuana.

Polls taken among American servicemen in Vietnam indicated high levels of marijuana smoking there.

A study made in February 1970 by Major John J. Treanor, chief medical officer of the 173rd Airborne Brigade, for example, showed that of 1,064 soldiers questioned, 32 percent stated that they had *not* smoked marijuana; 37 percent said that they had tried it once or twice, 15 percent said they used it one or more times a week, and 16 percent said that they used it "about every day" or "more often than once a day." [19]

"Contrary to a widely held opinion that most marijuana smoking is done among soldiers in large rear-base camps," the New York *Times* reported, "the [Treanor] study found that nearly two-thirds of the soldiers who had admitted smoking marijuana were stationed at forward base camps and had spent most of their time on 'field duty' or combat and pacification operations in the countryside." [20]

The Associated Press reported corroborative details from Detroit under a June 22, 1971, dateline:

---

* When it is recalled that the possession of marijuana was a felony in most states, the willingness of so many students and adults alike—including doctors-to-be and lawyers-to-be—to admit to marijuana smoking is particularly impressive.

A Congressional Medal of Honor winner says he was "stoned" on marijuana the night he fought off two waves of Vietcong soldiers and won America's highest military honor. . . .

It was April 1, 1970, when Mr. [Peter] Lemon, an Army Specialist 4, used his rifle, machine gun and hand grenades to smash a large attack on his position.

He fought the enemy single-handed and dragged a wounded comrade to the rear before collapsing from exhaustion and three wounds. At a medical center, he refused treatment until more seriously injured men had been cared for.

The dispatch quoted the injured hero as explaining: "It was the only time I ever went into combat stoned.

"You get really alert when you're stoned because you have to be. We were all partying the night before. We weren't expecting any action because we were in a support group."

Mr. Lemon continued: "All the guys were heads [confirmed marijuana smokers]. We'd sit around smoking grass and getting stoned and talking about when we'd get to go home." [21]

New York *Times* correspondent B. Drummond Ayres reported in March 1970, after a year in Vietnam:

The first American combat unit had not been in Vietnam very long before it was noted locally that the big, fair-skinned soldiers had an affinity not only for chewing gum but also for a weed that grew wild. Quickly, the entrepreneur that lurks in every Vietnamese took over, and almost overnight there were places in the fertile Mekong delta where peasants were row-cropping marijuana.

When the United States command learned of this agricultural brazenry, it immediately imported Federal narcotics agents to direct a crackdown. They came on very strong, with pot-sniffing police dogs, a series of surprise barracks inspections, television and radio commercials and a program for training Vietnamese law officers in narcotics suppression. Even helicopters were enlisted in the struggle.[22]

The explosive increase in marijuana smoking in Vietnam, as in the United States, followed rather than preceded such intensive law-enforcement and public-relations efforts.

The military campaign against marijuana eased in 1971, when it was discovered that an estimated 15 or 20 percent of United States military personnel in Vietnam had at least sampled heroin, and that many thousands were smoking or sniffing heroin daily. Thereafter, primary military emphasis shifted to a campaign against heroin, and marijuana again became regularly available. The drive against marijuana in Vietnam, as noted in Chapter 20, was an important factor in the sudden rise in heroin use.

One of the most significant yet rarely cited marijuana surveys was that made in 1967 for the Special House Committee on Narcotics of the Michigan House of Representatives, with Representative Dale Warner of Lansing as chairman. The Committee's fact-finding task force decided for several reasons to concentrate on drug use among high-school seniors; and in December 1968, its findings were reported to the committee by Richard A. Bogg of the University of Michigan School of Public Health, Dr. Roy G. Smith, a physician representing the Michigan State Department of Public Health, and Susan D. Russell, research assistant.[23]

The task force had great difficulty in finding schools that would permit their students to be surveyed on drugs; but eleven schools eventually agreed. These included a distinguished private coeducational preparatory school sending its graduates to the country's leading colleges and universities, two urban slum schools, three suburban schools, and several schools in remote rural areas. Data were collected from most schools in May 1968.

Marijuana use varied widely from school to school. No marijuana smoking whatever was reported from two rural high schools, while 33.7 percent of the 89 respondents in the private preparatory school reported that they had smoked marijuana at least once.

Unlike most drug-use studies, the Bogg-Smith-Russell Michigan survey then went on to ask about *alcohol* use. Alcohol, it should be noted, was also illegal for those under twenty-one years of age. Here the figures were much higher, varying from 49 percent to 81 percent. The marijuana-*vs.*-alcohol comparisons, school by school, are shown in Table 5.

As in other surveys, a higher proportion of male than of female respondents reported smoking marijuana—except at the private preparatory school, where 18 of the 30 marijuana smokers were female.

Much more detailed questions about drug use were asked at six of the eleven schools. The relation between marijuana smoking and alcohol drinking, for example, was explored in some detail. It turned out that among the 535 respondents who drank alcoholic beverages, 107 (20 percent) had also smoked marijuana at least once. Among the 322 who did not drink alcohol, only 5 (1.6 percent) had ever smoked marijuana. These figures suggest a close relationship between alcohol drinking and marijuana: there was a negligible likelihood that a Michigan high-school senior who did not drink alcohol would smoke marijuana.

Many of the high-school drinkers, moreover, didn't just try a beer occasionally. Among the 525 respondents who reported drinking alcoholic

Type of High School	Percentage Who Have Smoked Marijuana One or More Times	Percentage Who Consume Alcoholic Beverages
Private N = 89	33.7	81
Suburban N = 319	10.3	60
Central City A N = 148	12.2	69
Central City B N = 89	12.4	70
Urban Community A N = 113	8.0	50
Urban Community B N = 99	11.1	49
Small Town Upper Peninsula N = 104	5.0	74
Small Town Lower Peninsula N = 132	7.6	64
Rural Community A Lower Peninsula N = 64	0.0	57
Rural Community B Lower Peninsula N = 66	0.0	56
Rural Community Upper Peninsula N = 156	5.7	79

Table 5. Marijuana and Alcohol Usage in High Schools [24]

beverages, nearly half (258) reported that on at least one occasion they had drunk enough to cause vomiting. Thirty-seven percent reported that they had drunk enough to produce "blackout" (inability to remember the next day what had happened during the drinking). One-fifth said that they had drunk enough to lose consciousness (pass out).[25] These data suggest that, even in schools where marijuana use is widespread, alcohol remains the major drug *problem* among high-school seniors.

[428]

In general, the marijuana smokers in the sample were somewhat more likely than the nonsmokers to have experienced vomiting, blackout, or unconsciousness following excessive alcohol consumption. Whether their unpleasant experiences with alcohol were among their motives for trying marijuana was not determined, but is an obvious possibility.

An association was found between tobacco smoking and marijuana smoking; among 351 respondents who smoked tobacco, 24 percent also smoked marijuana; among 507 respondents who did not smoke tobacco, only 5 percent smoked marijuana. The associations among alcohol drinking, cigarette smoking, and marijuana smoking were the strongest statistical associations found in the entire study.

The use of marijuana among adults in business and the professions is, of course, more difficult to document. In the New York *Times* Magazine for August 23, 1970, however, Sam Blum did supply some anecdotal evidence of increasing use among such groups.[26] "Undoubtedly, the most important reason for the sudden outbreak of marijuana use in the adult working world is that young people have grown older," Mr. Blum explains. "The pot-smoking art student of 1965 is the pot-smoking art director of 1970. The pot-smoking coed of last year is today's pot-smoking 'assistant buyer of better dresses.'"

Mr. Blum then goes on to quote one of these assistant buyers: "You go into a [garment district] showroom, and there's a straight set of salesmen for the old ladies, and they offer the old ladies a drink, but there are also hip salesmen, guys with real long hair and groovy clothes; and they just take you in the back and turn you on [with marijuana]. In some of the houses the designer, the models, everybody is spaced out of his mind [high on marijuana]. . . ."

Then Mr. Blum continued: "Statistics don't exist on this matter, but it is this observer's impression that in New York marijuana is being used most widely by adults in the arts and the commercial arts, in the teaching profession (where it is argued that one could not conceivably understand the students if one did not grasp their highs), and in the 'helping' professions such as social work and psychiatry."

Mr. Blum interviewed four psychoanalysts—all members of the New York Psychoanalytic Society. All four "agreed on the estimate that 95 percent of their colleagues in their own age group (between 35 and 45) had experimented with marijuana and that many continued to use it from time to time. Moreover, to the best of their knowledge, all of the psychiatrists under the age of 35 whom they personally knew, and certainly all of their own psychiatric residents, smoked pot regularly, many of them daily. Knowledgeable Bostonians suggest that their psychoanalytic community is equally turned on."

Society in the New York area, Mr. Blum went on to report, is becoming stratified into marijuana-*vs.*-alcohol subgroups. "Recently, for example, a New York editor found that he was excluded from a grass-smoking dinner party because he had let slip that he had never learned to inhale. To make up for the slight, his hostess invited him to a second dinner party with a bunch of drinkers. . . ." [27]

The United States, in short, had at long last discovered marijuana.

58.

Can marijuana replace alcohol?

Optimists sometimes argue that the increased popularity of marijuana should be welcomed and encouraged, since increased marijuana use means a decline in alcohol consumption and of the evils associated with alcohol drunkenness and alcoholism (see Part IV). Pessimists maintain that far from supplanting the evils of alcohol, the evils of marijuana are simply being added on.

Most of the data currently available on this point indicate that marijuana smoking tends to replace alcohol drinking, but some contrary indictions have recently appeared. Let us first review the optimistic evidence.

There are no doubt some individuals and some small social groups who give up alcohol altogether after discovering marijuana. Sam Blum supplied details, in the same New York *Times* Magazine article[1] cited in Chapter 57. The middle-aged marijuana smoker in the New York area, he notes, is likely to "use marijuana precisely the way he previously used alcohol, and there are now middle-aged circles in which the drinking of liquor has almost disappeared." A forty-year-old financier told Blum over a glass of nonalcoholic mineral water: "Well, I can hardly remember the last time I saw a drink at a dinner party. In fact, I can't remember the last time I had a drink.

"You know, the homes to which I get invited aren't that remarkable. I'd say they're upper-middle-class, typical East Side Manhattan, South Shore folks . . . but it is a rarity in their homes that I'm not offered pot in beautifully rolled joints."

A housewife in her mid-thirties told Blum: "I'd go to parties and hold one drink all night. I hated the taste of alcohol. And it made me dizzy, and it left me with a hangover. Marijuana was a godsend. It's much milder than liquor and much pleasanter, so I carry my own. When everyone else drinks, I open my cigarette case, pull out a joint; and everyone is very impressed. . . . But I just smoke enough to get a slight high. I don't really like the super-boo that takes the top of your head off. I just want to feel more relaxed, more in the mood for a party. I love it."[2]

In 1968, Professor Alfred R. Lindesmith, Indiana University sociologist, commented: "It is of incidental interest that some pot smokers, both old and young, have developed an aversion to alcohol, regarding it as a debasing and degrading drug, a view which is standard among the Hindus of India where alcohol is strongly taboo for religious reasons. Some of these people were heavy users of alcohol before they tried marijuana and feel that the latter saved them from becoming alcoholics." [3]

Professor John Kaplan of the Stanford University Law School has assembled further evidence on this point in his 1970 study, *Marijuana— The New Prohibition.*

"There is already data," Professor Kaplan points out, "showing that a sizeable percentage of marijuana users . . . cut down their alcohol consumption on taking up their new drug. Thus, Richard Blum's data shows that 54 percent of the regular (weekly) marijuana-users decreased their alcohol consumption after taking up marijuana, while only two percent increased their alcohol use. With respect to the daily marijuana-users, the difference was even more striking. Here eighty-nine percent of the users had decreased their alcohol consumption.

This type of data is confirmed from several other sources. Another study at a California college showed that while in the sample marijuana use had climbed from nineteen to forty-three percent between 1967 and 1968, use of alcohol in the "more than once a month" category had fallen from twenty-nine to fourteen percent, while use in the "more than several times a month" category had fallen from seventeen to twelve percent. And one of the most recent surveys, at Stanford University, showed that, at a time in their lives when students typically increase their alcohol consumption significantly, only three percent of the marijuana-users had increased the frequency or quantity of their hard-liquor consumption while thirty-two percent reported a decrease.[4]

Anecdotal evidence tends to confirm these findings. In the New York *Times* for August 9, 1970, for example, correspondent Frank J. Prial wrote:

In some parts of the country, marijuana appears to be making inroads on the sale of liquor. While most tavern owners and liquor salesmen deny that the [marijuana] joint has replaced the [alcohol] jigger, or ever will, there are signs of at least a partial trend around the country toward drugs at the expense of drinks.

A beer distributor in Denver said that 1969 sales at one college tavern were down 27 percent from a 1967 base. They were also down 53 percent at a second place near a campus and 71 percent at a third.

Then the Denver beer distributor added: "Our retailers say they can tell when a big shipment of marijuana hits town. The [beer] sales go down."

The assistant manager of an alcohol-dispensing discotheque called Evil People, in Miami, Florida, was quoted as saying: "Marijuana spells disaster to the liquor trade. If they ever legalize it, the liquor business is dead." He contended that if his young patrons could buy marijuana legally, they "wouldn't touch liquor." [5]

Professor Kaplan also cites Dr. Seymour Halleck, professor of psychiatry at the University of Wisconsin, as the authority for the view that the evils of marijuana are not simply being added to the prior evils of alcohol. Dr. Halleck, after noting in 1968 the rapid increase in marijuana smoking on the Wisconsin and other campuses, made this comment:

Perhaps the one major positive effect of the drug [marijuana] is to cut down on the use of alcohol. In the last few years it is rare for our student infirmary to encounter a student who has become aggressive, disoriented, or physically ill because of excessive use of alcohol. Alcoholism has almost ceased to [be] a problem on our campuses.[6]

While those reports may have quite accurately described the situation in 1968, 1969, and perhaps even 1970, there is also growing evidence that points in the opposite direction. Just as youthful drug users during the 1960s periodically discovered marijuana, LSD, the amphetamines, the barbiturates, and other "new" drugs, so, it seems, they are now discovering yet another strange intoxicant: alcohol—liquor, beer, and wine. (Wine manufacturers responded swiftly, and a burgeoning number of low-cost, exotically labeled wines have become available.) Moreover, marijuana users were said to be drinking the alcoholic beverages *along with* smoking the marijuana joints. One survey even suggested that the heaviest marijuana smokers were also the heaviest alcohol drinkers.[7]

The moral here is clear. Marijuana can be smoked alone, or it can be smoked along with the drinking of alcohol. The patterns of use—one drug or a mixture of two—is not inherent in their chemical molecules but is determined by a host of legal, social, psychological, and economic factors. A knowledgeable society, noting a few years ago that some of its members were switching from alcohol to a less harmful intoxicant, marijuana, might have encouraged that trend. At the very least, society could have stressed the advantages of cutting down alcohol consumption if you smoke marijuana. But no such effort was made here. It may yet not be too late to present that simple public-health message.

59.

The 1969 marijuana shortage and "Operation Intercept"

The extent of marijuana use and distribution in the United States was brought to nationwide attention in the spectacular failure of "Operation Intercept," an elaborate and determined effort by the government to shut off the flow of smuggled marijuana from Mexico. The program was based on the belief that Mexico was and would remain the primary source of marijuana for Americans.

Operation Intercept was launched at 2:30 P.M. Pacific Daylight Time on Sunday, September 21, 1969, and abandoned on October 11—just 20 days later. Felix Belair, Jr., broke the story two weeks in advance, in the New York *Times* under a September 8 dateline from Washington: "At the direction of President Nixon Federal enforcement agencies are preparing an all-out drive on the smuggling of drugs into the United States from Mexico. Details of the drive . . . are being kept a closely guarded secret pending a joint statement later this week by the Secretary of the Treasury and the Attorney General. In personnel and equipment it will be the nation's largest peacetime search and seizure operation by civil authorities." [1] So important was the drive that President Nixon had discussed it at his September 8 meeting with President Gustavo Diaz Ordaz of Mexico. "On this side of the border pursuit planes and some motor torpedo boats will be employed for the first time. Additional observation planes will be placed at the disposal of a strengthened border patrol." Operation Intercept was to be concerned partly with heroin and other drugs—but primary emphasis was to be placed on marijuana, the bulkiest of the drugs commonly smuggled and therefore the easiest to intercept.

The drive to close the American border was strategically timed for the September 1969 marijuana harvest. The American marijuana supply was already far short of the demand, and the closure was intended to intensify the shortage.

"Pot began to be scarce in June [1969]," Peggy J. Murrell explained in the *Wall Street Journal* for September 11, 1969, "when Mexico started cracking down on shipments of the weed smuggled into the U.S." [2] A college sophomore named Frank, vacationing in New York City's East Village, was quoted as saying: "Nobody can get any grass. After all this damned LSD, speed, and mescaline that's going around, it sure would be great to get back to some nice, soft pot." Miss Murrell then explained:

"Frank had intended to stock up on marijuana in New York and take it to his friends at college, but the 'pot drought' has left him empty-handed. 'It's really awful,' he complains. 'What will I tell the kids?' "

A *Wall Street Journal* reporter had interviewed Larry Katz, head of the Justice Department's Bureau of Narcotics and Dangerous Drugs in San Diego, who explained that the summer marijuana shortage started in Mexico "because of a drought and a killing. Lack of summer rains thinned the grass [marijuana] crop. Then a Mexican official who had ordered the burning of 50 acres of what was left, was shot and killed. . . . As a result of the killing, martial law has been declared. They have moved in troops for a house-to-house search throughout the state (of Sinaloa) and every road leading out of Mexico is heavily guarded. The Mexican government now maintains squads that constantly destroy marijuana wherever they find it." [3]

Though the *Wall Street Journal* failed to mention it, the burgeoning demand for marijuana on the part of a rapidly growing mass of users was also no doubt a major factor in the midsummer 1969 "pot shortage." Supplies were lagging far behind demand—at least temporarily.

"Far from rejoicing at the marijuana shortage," Miss Murrell's *Wall Street Journal* dispatch continued, "some narcotics officials are now afraid that pot smokers may switch to other, more dangerous routes to euphoria." [4] One of these officials was William Durkin, head of the New York Bureau of Narcotics and Dangerous Drugs, who was quoted as saying: "Youthful drug experimenters, if they can't get one kind of drug, will look for something else."

A twenty-one-year-old Radcliffe College senior interviewed by Miss Murrell emphatically confirmed this official view. "I really didn't want to try acid (LSD) before," she was quoted as saying. "But there's no grass around, so when somebody offered me some (LSD), I figured, 'What the hell.' I didn't freak out or anything, so I've been tripping [taking LSD] ever since."

"The objective of the [Operation Intercept] program," Secretary of the Treasury David M. Kennedy and Attorney General John N. Mitchell declared in a joint statement released at precisely 2:30 P.M. on Sunday, September 21, 1969, "is to reduce the volume of narcotics, marijuana, and dangerous drugs which are smuggled into the United States from Mexico." [5] The statement added that "more than 80 percent of the marijuana smoked in the United States" entered the country illegally from Mexico. If this 80 percent could be cut off, all would be well. That, at least, was the official hope.

Traffic at the border "was backed up for more than two and a half miles within an hour after Operation Intercept began," Felix Belair, Jr., of the New York *Times* reported from San Ysidro, California, on September 21. "And as the usual Sunday exodus from the Tijuana bullfight and racetrack approached the border station in late afternoon, traffic was backed up for six miles"⁶ in the border dust and heat. No doubt the officials who planned Operation Intercept had had this peak traffic flow in mind when they set 2:30 P.M. on Sunday afternoon as H-hour. By then a maximum number of Americans would have entered Mexico for the afternoon, and would be caught in the operation en route home.

Halted motorists "expressed their feeling in the classical manner" by blowing their horns. "They're playing our song," a customs agent remarked.

Similar scenes, the *Times* dispatch continued, were "being enacted at the 30 other border-crossing stations along the 2,500-mile-long border between the two countries. In between, special radar installations have been set up by the Federal Aviation Administration to enable waiting customs agents to detect any attempt to cross the border unobserved.

Military pursuit planes borrowed from the Air Force were poised to chase any aircraft that failed to file a pre-flight plan before heading across the border.

The surveillance network was spread out to sea, with Navy boats plying the Gulf of Mexico and a variety of patrol craft in coastal waters. The "intensified inspection of vehicles and persons crossing the border" was in effect also at the 27 airports at which international flights are authorized to land.⁷

"Despite complaints about zealous inspectors peeking into the purses and lunchboxes of school children and forcing travelers to strip for personal searches, the United States said today that it has been successful in its Mexican-border crackdown on drug smuggling,"⁸ said the lead on an Associated Press dispatch from Los Angeles on the eighth day of the operation. Although only small quantities of drugs had been seized during the week, a federal spokesman was quoted as saying: "We're measuring our success not by the quantity of seizures made but by the price of marijuana, heroin, and other drugs on the market. It is raising their cost beyond the means of most young people in America.

"We're positive we're stopping narcotics and dangerous drugs from coming into this country. No large seizures have been made since Intercept was launched last Sunday, because obviously the big smugglers have gotten the word." Obviously the small smugglers had also gotten the word. "We know we're succeeding," the federal spokesman continued, "therefore we feel that most Americans will agree it is worth our effort, the manpower and expense involved." The New York *Daily News* ran the dispatch under the headline "GRASS CURTAIN A SUCCESS."

As might be expected, however, Operation Intercept engendered a number of protests. The earliest of these came from along both sides of the border.

"In the 30 twin cities that straddle the United States–Mexican border from here to the Gulf," Mr. Belair of the New York *Times* again reported from San Ysidro on the third day of the operation, "the government's drive on marijuana smuggling has become one of the hottest issues since Pancho Villa raided frontier towns.

Commerce and tourism are grinding slowly to a halt. Retail business on the American side has dropped more than 50 percent. And with no relief in sight, the merchants are up in arms because Mexican customers won't waste two to four hours waiting to go through customs inspection.

It's the same in the cities and towns on the Mexican side that depend on weekend tourists and commuter shoppers. . . .

Absenteeism is rampant among Mexican . . . workers with permits that allow them to live in Mexico and work in the United States. Mexican school children attending public and private schools in the United States have been showing up two to three hours late or don't show up at all. . . .

The impact of the operation hit like a windstorm at Chula Vista, the nearest shopping center to this major gateway. . . . Chula Vista business establishments count on Mexican customers for about 70 percent of their trade. Yesterday, they catered to a handful of local customers.[9]

On the second day of Operation Intercept, the dispatch continued, "the United States–Mexican Border Cities Association decided to do something about it. It began organizing a protest, urging its 30 twin city members to get in touch with their Congressmen, governors, and mayors and demand a modification. . . ." The head of the association also sent telegrams to all affiliated chambers of commerce on the United States side, warning that "time is short, and the need for action immediate." In a telephone interview he added: "The economic life's blood of these communities is based on a free flow of vehicular and pedestrian traffic in both directions. Disrupt that flow, and the economy dies, people are thrown out of work and the communities will become ghost towns. . . ."

On the seventh day of the operation, the New York *Times* reported from Mexico City:

Indignation mounted here yesterday in the press and business and government circles against the measures adopted by the United States in an anti-narcotics drive on the Mexican border.

"Humiliating Mexicans" was the banner headline published by *La Prensa*, one of the largest newspapers in the country. It emphasized a theme that was echoed in many other dailies.

In the Chamber of Deputies, representatives of all parties protested vigorously against Operation Intercept on the border as a program that "damages the dignity of Mexicans and constitutes an unfriendly act. . . ."

[437]

The National Confederation of Chambers of Commerce here termed the operation "an absurd and exaggerated program" for the meager results it has produced.[10]

President Diaz of Mexico, who in early September had paid a courtesy visit to Washington during which his relations with President Nixon had been cordial, in early October personally denounced Operation Intercept as "a bureaucratic error" that had "raised a wall of suspicion between Mexico and the United States."[11]

The protest spread from Mexico to other Latin American countries. An ambassador from one such country, stationed in Mexico City, told a reporter: "It is the old story of United States policy decisions that affect a Latin-American country profoundly being taken for domestic political reasons without consultation or consideration."[12] Another ambassador likened Operation Intercept to the United States military intervention in the Dominican Republic in 1965.

Prior to Operation Intercept, border inspectors worked on a schedule that allowed them on the average one minute per vehicle crossing the border. During Operation Intercept, this quota was increased to an average of two or three minutes per vehicle—hardly enough for a really thorough search. Further extending the duration of searches, of course, would have further extended the delays and the lines of cars.

Some persons desiring to enter the United States were required to strip to the skin for a personal inspection. Official reports revealed that during the first week of Operation Intercept 1,824 border crossers were stripped and searched. This left some 1,978,000 persons who had crossed the border with only a superficial search or none at all. Most of the 1,824 "skin searches," incidentally, proved fruitless; there were only 33 arrests along the border during the week.[13]

"Ten days of relentless warfare on the smuggling of marijuana and dangerous drugs across the Mexican border has convinced United States enforcement officials of the futility of trying to dry up the illicit traffic with currently available money, manpower, and equipment,"[14] Mr. Belair reported from San Ysidro on October 1. At that time nearly 2,000 agents and inspectors, including many transferred to the border from other posts, were at work in the operation.

"Attempts to get the drugs across border highway crossings concealed in motor vehicles have almost ceased. But enforcement officials say that illegal air traffic continues to move through the Mohawk Valley in Arizona, Laredo, Texas, and the rugged approaches to El Centro and San Diego, Calif. . . .

"Meanwhile, with supplies of marijuana and dangerous drugs piling up south of the border as a result of the drive on land, Mexican distributors are changing smuggling methods. Checked at the normal crossing points, they have started to probe the fences along remote mountain trails and in the desolate flatlands where Mexican roads parallel the border by fewer than 100 yards." An undetermined amount of marijuana and other drugs was also being smuggled in by plane despite newly installed FAA radar equipment and Air Force intercept planes lent for the operation. "Recently positioned radar installations . . . showed the blips of intruding aircraft from the south but the blips faded from scanning screens as the planes dropped between mountain ranges and canyon corridors or passed beyond range of the truck-mounted sensors." * 16

On October 8, 1969, a delegation of Mexican officials headed by Mexican Attorney General David Rodriguez conferred in Washington with a delegation of American officials headed by United States Attorney General Mitchell. As late as the afternoon of October 9, after two full days of these talks, Mr. Belair reported from Washington to the New York *Times* that "the United States has rejected a Mexican government appeal for a prompt termination of Operation Intercept. . . . A source close to the con-

---

* This discovery by drug smugglers of the vulnerability of the United States–Mexican border to aerial intrusion was to have disastrous aftereffects. Long after Operation Intercept itself was discontinued, aerial smugglers continued to use the techniques pioneered in September 1969.

"They fly low and slow, by the light of the moon, and make $50,000 a night," Robert Lindsey reported in the New York *Times* in November 1971.[15]

"They use some private planes and old military transports and land on deserted airstrips or sagebrush-covered desert. Their cargo is marijuana, cocaine and heroin.

"Along the sparsely settled frontier that divides the United States and Mexico, airborne drug-runners are doing a booming business, and Federal agents say they do not know how to stop them.

"On most nights, the agents estimate, at least 10 planes cross the border with marijuana and other drugs. On rare occasions, the smugglers are caught by United States agents flying their own planes. But usually they land unnoticed. . . ."

"Anybody who knows how to fly can get into the business and make a lot of money . . . ," one customs agent was quoted as saying; and an official of the Bureau of Narcotics and Dangerous Drugs added: "They're developing their own air force, and it's getting bigger and bigger."

Most of the planes used were small, but a Department of Justice official noted that recently (November 1971), "a lot of them are starting to use bigger planes—DC–3's, surplus military transports, turbo-prop executive planes, and we have our eye on one group that has a Constellation."

A Constellation can carry twenty tons of cargo—enough to supply the entire United States heroin market for three or four years with the fruits of a single flight.

Despite the fact that marijuana weighs far more than heroin per dose and sells for far less, it, too, can be profitably smuggled by air. The Department of Justice official told reporter Lindsey how "in the interior of Mexico, you can buy weed [marijuana] for as low as $2 a brick [2.2 pounds], but if you don't know your way around, you will probably have to pay closer to $30. It doesn't take a very big plane to fly 500 bricks if you take out the seats and strip it down. . . .

"Say [a smuggler] buys it for $30 and sells it in the states for $130; that's a profit on 500 bricks of $50,000 for a night's work." At $130 per brick or kilogram, moreover, the cost per half-gram marijuana cigarette works out at 6.5 cents—hardly an exorbitant price, even at wholesale.

ferees said the United States had no intention of calling off the drive or of substantially modifying border inspections. . . ." [17]

But the next day, Operation Intercept was called off.

"In a dramatic overnight reversal of position," Mr. Belair announced under an October 10 dateline, "the United States bowed today to Mexican demands and ordered a strategic retreat in its war on the smuggling of marijuana and dangerous drugs into this country.

"A joint statement by representatives of both Governments after three days of conferences on Operation Intercept said it had been superseded by Operation Cooperation. It added that the United States would 'adjust' its border inspection procedures 'to eliminate unnecessary inconvenience, delay and irritation.'

"Precisely what happened to cause the about-face by United States delegates was not immediately clear and the Federal enforcement officials who are most concerned with the problem said they were 'too sick to talk about it.'" Mr. Belair added, however, that State Department officials had first proposed the retreat, that Justice Department officials had agreed; "this left the Treasury Department contingent under Assistant Secretary Eugene T. Rossides standing alone without White House support. . . . As the showdown approached today, the White House was advised of the pending decision but decided against any direct involvement." [18] Traffic across the border began flowing freely again on the next day—Saturday, October 11.

"An immediate problem for enforcement officials," Mr. Belair added, "was how to soften the impact of today's retreat on the morale of customs agents and inspectors and members of the Border Patrol who have been working 12 and 14 hours a day to make Operation Intercept a success."

While primary responsibility for ending Operation Intercept was commonly attributed to the protest from Mexico, from the rest of Latin America, and from American border businessmen and their Congressmen, the statistics of drugs seized may also have played a role. During the year ending June 30, 1969, United States customs officials had seized 57,164 pounds of marijuana—about 150 pounds per day. During the three weeks of Operation Intercept, they had seized 3,202 pounds of marijuana—about the same amount per day.[19] Operation Intercept had enormously inflated marijuana publicity, but had not increased marijuana seizures. How much smuggling increased elsewhere as a result of the transfer of customs officials and narcotics agents to the Mexican border is not known.

A statement by then Deputy Attorney General Richard G. Kleindienst and Assistant Secretary of the Treasury Eugene T. Rossides, released by the United States Department of Justice twelve days after the termination of Operation Intercept, claimed a modest success. It described marijuana as "unavailable in Miami and almost unavailable in New York," as well as "almost unavailable at Yale, Harvard and the University of California [Berkeley and Los Angeles]. A similar or even more tight supply condition exists at the University of Chicago, Rice Institute, Oklahoma University, Southern Methodist University and Northwestern University." [20]

This announcement from Washington evoked a bitter retort from Professor Charles R. Beye, chairman of the classics department at Boston University, who declared in a letter to the editor of the New York *Times*:

In their elation at having made marijuana scarcer on our college campuses, could the Federal narcotics agents ponder for a moment the ugly repercussions of their campaign?

Many dealers responding to this scarcity are blending in all kinds of other ingredients to provide strange psychic effects neither sought nor planned. The high price of marijuana is moving the high school crowd into some really weird trip-causing agents, of which glue is only the mildest.

The intensive police pressure reinforces the sense of being criminal and thus antisocial. Then, too, instead of your friendly student dealers, older men suspiciously criminal-looking, are beginning to push the pot; obviously the student amateurs are being closed out of the increasingly profitable marijuana business and organized crime is being given another avenue of exploitation.

As someone who spends a great deal of time with the young I must say that marijuana is here to stay. As a father I can only hope that these hypocritical, viciously unnatural laws and the people who enforce them are removed before an entire generation is perverted morally and corrupted physically.[21]

Professor Beye's concern that marijuana users deprived of marijuana might shift to other substances was confirmed in some detail in a study of what actually happened among Los Angeles marijuana smokers during Operation Intercept. The study was undertaken by two graduate students in psychology at the University of California at Los Angeles, Kay Jamison and Steven Rosenblatt, in collaboration with Dr. William H. McGlothlin of the UCLA psychology department.[22] Questionnaire returns were secured in this project from 478 UCLA undergraduate and graduate students, and from 116 patients attending the Los Angeles Free Clinic. The great majority of both the students and clinic patients were marijuana smokers who had smoked marijuana ten or more times.

One question which the study sought to answer was whether there had actually been a marijuana shortage before and during Operation Intercept —a shortage sufficient to curtail marijuana use. Deputy Attorney General Kleindienst and Assistant Secretary of the Treasury Rossides, it will be recalled, had announced on October 23 that marijuana was "almost unavailable" at UCLA. The study did not bear this out. "Of those using marijuana ten or more times," the Los Angeles group reported, "44 percent of the students and 51 percent of patients reported that their frequency of marijuana use was below normal at some time between May and October 1969, as a consequence of the unavailability of marijuana." [23] The other half of the respondents were able to go right on smoking marijuana at their customary frequency despite the shortage that preceded Operation Intercept and despite Operation Intercept itself.

The respondents were also asked how much they had been paying for marijuana in May 1969, and how much in October 1969. The responses, when averaged, worked out to $10.13 per ounce in May and to $11.87 per ounce in October. About 60 half-gram marijuana cigarettes can be made from one ounce of marijuana. Thus the price as reported by Los Angeles smokers rose from about 16.9 cents per marijuana cigarette in May to about 19.8 cents in October. [24]

Finally, the Los Angeles study sought to determine how the marijuana shortage affected the consumption of *other* drugs. "Of those reporting a shortage of marijuana," the UCLA researchers noted, "76 percent of students and 84 percent of patients reported that they increased their consumption of one or more other drugs (including alcohol) because of the unavailability of marijuana." [25] Here are the drugs to which these respondents turned as a result of the marijuana shortage. [26]

Drug	Students (Percentage)		Free Clinic (Percentage)	
	Male	Female	Male	Female
	(N = 56)	(N = 30)	(N = 24)	(N = 25)
Hashish	52	37	54	44
Alcohol	55	23	50	48
Sedatives	9	10	29	24
Stimulants	11	7	21	16
LSD	16	7	50	48
Other strong hallucinogens	23	13	37	28
Opiates or cocaine	2	3	25	24

The temporary shortage of Mexican marijuana led to a marked increase in the importation into the United States of highly potent marijuana from Vietnam. Some of it was mailed home through GI channels; far larger amounts were brought home by military personnel returning from the war. San Francisco observers reported a flood of Vietnamese marijuana on the market immediately following the docking of each homebound troopship. There were few prosecutions, however—perhaps because officials did not welcome the political repercussions which might follow the large-scale criminal prosecution of veterans freshly returned from war.

Another effect of Operation Intercept was to open the United States for the first time to the large-scale importation of North African and Near Eastern *hashish*. There is a delicate balance between marijuana prices and hashish prices. Hashish is more costly to produce because it takes much more labor during the brief harvest period—but it is easier to smuggle because a comparable dose weighs only one-fifth to one-eighth as much. Trivial amounts of hashish had long been available in the United States. The tight marijuana supply before and during Operation Intercept triggered a large-scale increase in hashish smuggling.

Numerous instances were cited in newspaper dispatches before, during, and after Operation Intercept: For example, the New York *Times* reported from Washington, D.C., on August 17, 1969, that "the smuggling of hashish, a concentrated form of marijuana, has sharply increased," according to Myles J. Ambrose, then Bureau of Customs Commissioner. Seizures for the year ending June 30, 1969, totaled 623 pounds—"up from 311 pounds the previous year. Only about 70 pounds had been seized in 1966 and 1967." Marijuana seizures did not increase. An assistant commissioner of customs cited three reasons for the rise in hashish smuggling: it is far less bulky than marijuana, it is highly potent, and it appeals to the "hippie type" of tourist.[27]

On October 6, 1969, Sydney H. Schanberg reported in the New York *Times* from Srinagar, Kashmir, that Kashmiri hashish formerly went mostly to the Middle East. "But now," he quoted the local chief of police as saying, "there is a new market—Europe and America. And therefore the price has gone very high." [28]

On October 10, 1969, Dana Adams Schmidt reported in the New York *Times* from Beirut, Lebanon, that "eleven Americans are in prison in Lebanon on charges of using or trafficking in hashish." He went on to explain: "Two pounds of hashish selling here for $40 to $80 can be resold in the United States for that amount an ounce." [29]

The Burlington, Vermont, *Free Press* reported on March 17, 1970, that hashish purchased for $3,000 in Ibiza, Spain, and alleged to be worth $350,000 in the United States market had been seized in Vermont after it had been shipped by freight from Ibiza to Casablanca, to Marseilles, to St. Thomas, Ontario, to Tonawanda, New York, and then to Rutland and Plainfield, Vermont.[30]

Finally, the marijuana shortage induced many industrious people to spend more time harvesting domestic "weed" marijuana, growing throughout the United States.

Under ordinary circumstances, with high-quality Mexican marijuana available at moderate prices, there is relatively little incentive to harvest the domestic weed supply. The hourly wage rate is much higher in the United States than in Mexico, and harvesting marijuana takes time. When

[443]

prices rise and supplies become scarce, however, people take to the harvest fields in large numbers. Edward B. Zuckerman described the marijuana-harvesting process in a dispatch from North Judson, Indiana, published in the *Wall Street Journal* of August 20, 1969:

The elderly farmer escorts a visitor around his prosperous-looking farm near this quiet northern Indiana town. There's the corn field, he says, and there's the potatoes. And over there is the marijuana.

The farmer hastens to point out that he doesn't cultivate the marijuana—it just grows wild. Indeed, he considers it a headache. "It gets so thick around my storage lot that I have to pay good money to spray it so I can find my machinery," he says. "Then, I'm always shooing away people who come on my land to pick the stuff."

The farm is a typical one in this lush farming area not far from Chicago. The hardy marijuana plant . . . grows in weedlike abundance along roads and drainage ditches here. It's difficult and expensive to kill, and it has made the region something of a mecca for enterprising devotees . . . who drive to the farmlands to help themselves rather than pay the $15 to $20 an ounce that processed marijuana brings on the clandestine market.

"We've arrested every type of individual—white, colored, male, female, young and old—a real cross-section of the population," says Sgt. Harry Young of the Indiana State Police, whose members regularly inspect cars parked along the roads near here. . . .

Marijuana came to North Judson, as well as to other areas of the Midwest where it grows in abundance, as the upright and respectable hemp plant. . . . Mills that converted the tough fibers of the plant's stalk into rope used to dot the Midwest. . . . Hemp cultivation has all but ceased in the U.S. but the plant hangs on. "It's extremely hardy and adaptable—we've seen it growing in sandy soil and in the most swampy areas," says University of Illinois botanist Alan W. Haney. "It's also very hard to get rid of. It takes a high concentration of poison to do the job. I've seen plants that wilted after being sprayed, but sprang back within two weeks." [31]

By early November 1969, the marijuana famine was over—in considerable part as a result of increased harvest of the domestic American "weed" supply. Reporter John Kifner supplied the details in a dispatch from Lawrence, Kansas, which appeared in the New York *Times* for November 7, 1969, less than a month after the abandonment of Operation Intercept:

Only a few of the plants—8 to 10 feet tall with clusters of seven sharply serrated leaves—are still green. Most of the stalks are brown and withering after the first frosts.

Some harvesters, who contend that a field-dried crop yields the best product, are still gathering tops and leaves.

But much of the work—the hurried chopping under the hot sun, the heaving of armsful of plants into automobile trunks and the stumbling around in the dark with flashlights and pillowcases to be filled—has been done.

The last crop is hanging, upside down so the precious sap can flow into the leaves, in garages, backyards and dormitories waiting to be dried and processed. The harvesters are settling back and lighting up to enjoy the fruits of their labors.

The crop is marijuana, and this has been a good growing year, particularly here in the flat Middle Western plains, where the Cannabis sativa plant grows wild along the edges of fields, river banks and railroad tracks, and sometimes in cultivated plots.

"The marijuana has been like a super benefit to this community," a student at the University of Kansas said with a grin. "A lot of people have got new motorcycles and things because of it."

The director of the Kansas Department of Agriculture's Noxious Weeds Division reported that there were 52,050 acres of marijuana in the state in 1968—the figure is probably higher this year. The plant is also growing in wild profusion throughout Nebraska, Iowa and Illinois.

It is a strong and hardy plant that resists efforts at eradication by fire or chemicals, to the delight of the young and the distress of the law enforcement officials and politicians. . . .

In Indiana, farmers complain of the difficulty of clearing the plant from the edges of their fields. According to underground sources, an elderly farmer in the Champaign-Urbana area, near the University of Illinois, has simply let a field go to marijuana.

He sits in his farmhouse with field glasses, these sources say, waiting for youths to come and pick the crop. Then he calls the police and collects an informer's fee.

While the Middle West is the main center for wild marijuana, the plant is being harvested more and more secretly in small cultivated patches throughout the country.

In Vermont, the state police say there are vast quantities of marijuana growing wild in the Champlain Valley and being regularly harvested at night.

Policemen destroyed tons of marijuana over the summer months, but the crop was too big for the available manpower and equipment. . . .

Detective Cpl. William Chilton said he believed the quality of Vermont marijuana was almost as good as that of most of the Mexican varieties.

There are scattered fields throughout Georgia, including a patch in the Okefenokee Swamp, and Joseph Weldy, the state's chief drug inspector, said he expected to find "a lot of marijuana fields in the spring."

In Austin, Tex., marijuana has been found growing on the State Capitol grounds and at the municipal golf course. Crafty planters frequently sow their crop on public ground, where it will be well-tended by unsuspecting gardeners.

In Oregon, state agents had 3,000 plants under surveillance in the Cornelius Pass west of Portland last August. They were thwarted when an industrious Washington County lawman destroyed the plants with chemicals. There was a lack of communication, officials said.

Law enforcement and underground sources agree that the domestic marijuana harvest this summer and fall was probably the biggest yet. It was centered largely in the Middle West and particularly in Kansas.

The reasons for this, they agreed, are the shortage of Mexican marijuana, caused by Operation Intercept and other American pressures on the Mexican Government, and the rapidly increasing numbers of marijuana smokers.

The harvesting season runs generally from July to late October, with September the prime time. Throughout these months, hundreds of young people have been busily working in isolated fields, and rural sheriffs have been just as busily responding to calls from farmers reporting "a bunch of hippies in the fields" acting strangely.

Melwyn Purdy, an agent of the campus Bureau of Investigation here who is assigned to narcotics problems said there were 175 arrests for marijuana harvesting in this state since July 4. Last year, there had been about 40 arrests.

He described those arrested as "mostly young subjects, of college age with no criminal background."

Some of those arrested, Mr. Purdy said, had road maps or hand-sketched charts showing where patches of marijuana might be found. Some of the areas of heaviest growth, he added, are along the Republican River in north central Kansas and in the eastern part of the state.

Gov. Robert Docking has expressed alarm at the situation, particularly at the possibility that organized crime might be moving into Kansas. . . . Farmers, however, are not enthusiastic about the Governor's plan to put marijuana under the weed control program since they would have to undergo the trouble of eradicating it from their own lands. Some conservationists and ecologists have expressed alarm at the potential destruction of ground cover.

A more powerful lobby—hunters and sportsmen—is also worried about the program. Quail feed on marijuana seeds, and organized hunters fear that a favorite quarry will be reduced in number. . . .

The increase in the marijuana market has led to shady business practices. Kansas marijuana is being wrapped in Mexican newspapers and sent to California masquerading as the imported variety.

Most smokers seem to feel that Kansas marijuana is better than none at all, so the young people in and around Lawrence seem particularly happy about this year's crop.[32]

Another report, perhaps apocryphal, says that there was *too much* marijuana growing in Kansas in 1969; hence "the professional pot harvesters there have formed an association in violation of the Sherman Anti-Trust Act to maintain price levels by destroying part of the crop."[33]

The United States House of Representatives' Select Committee on Crime in the fall of 1969 took an interest in this harvesting of domestic weed marijuana to supplement and perhaps replace imported Mexican marijuana. One witness it called was Lieutenant Wayne F. Rowe of the Nebraska State Highway Patrol; Lieutenant Rowe was questioned by Larry Reida, the Select Committee's associate chief counsel, and by Con-

gressmen Claude Pepper of Florida, the committee chairman, and Robert
V. Denney of Nebraska.

Mr. Reida. Mr. Rowe, could you make an estimate, based on your information
and experience in the field of marijuana control for the last couple of years,
as to the number of acres of marijuana in Nebraska?
Mr. Rowe. No, sir, I couldn't make this estimate. We had a discussion group
yesterday. The experts said it was considerable.
Mr. Reida. We are talking about thousands of acres, right?
Mr. Rowe. Right.
Mr. Denney. We heard one estimate of 156,000 acres in Nebraska, right?
Mr. Pepper. Yes, we did.
Mr. Reida. As a matter of fact, it grows in clumps; you don't have a 100-acre
field of marijuana.
Mr. Rowe. No, sir. You may find one plant on an acre and in other fields the
entire field would be infested.

This "weed" marijuana, Lieutenant Rowe continued, was attracting
"hempleggers" from all over the country:

Now, last year was the first year that we had a great deal of experience
with marijuana harvesters coming in from out of State. In the year of 1968
we documented 40 arrests for marijuana harvesting. These were all people
from out of State.
To date in 1969 we have documented 81 arrests of people from outside
of Nebraska who have come in to harvest the marijuana that is growing here.
This represents over a 100-percent increase over last year.
Mr. Pepper. How many arrests have you made?
Mr. Rowe. I have a breakdown in States: 32 arrests of California residents,
six arrests of New York residents, six arrests of Massachusetts residents, five
New Mexico, five from Washington, four from Virginia, three from Pennsylvania, three from Wyoming, three from Colorado, two from Michigan,
two from Kansas, two from Utah, one from Ohio, one from Wisconsin, one
from Arizona, one from Iowa, one from Oregon, one from Idaho, one from
Montana, and one from Oklahoma. . . .
Mr. Pepper. Did you notice that those arrests increased as the supply of marijuana coming into this country was diminished?
Mr. Rowe. Yes, sir. The spring crop of marijuana in Mexico,* as I understand it,
was bad because of the weather. They were unable to dry it out. We also
understand from the people whom we have apprehended that Mexican
marijuana is not available in supply as is demanded by the present market.
Mr. Pepper. From that experience, would you anticipate that if we are successful in our effort to diminish the available quantity of marijuana in other
parts of the country, there will be greater effort to get it from Nebraska and
Iowa than there is today?

* In Mexico, the same field may yield three or even four crops of marijuana per year.

Mr. Rowe. Yes, sir, this will be what will happen. By coming to Nebraska they eliminate the dangers of crossing an international border.[34]

The way in which Nebraskan and other Midwestern marijuana is subsequently distributed throughout the United States was indicated in an Associated Press dispatch from Freeport, Long Island, New York, dated October 4, 1970:

Five men were arrested here today in a raid in which police confiscated 300 pounds of marijuana said to be worth $600,000 at retail.

According to Nassau County and Freeport police, three of the men had driven from California in a panel truck, stopping on the way in Frank, Neb., to harvest a crop of marijuana they knew was growing in an open field there. Using machetes, the men cut enough marijuana to fill 15 duffle bags, the police said.[35]

The three were identified as a twenty-four-year-old unemployed high-school teacher, a twenty-four-year-old professor at an unaccredited California college, and a twenty-eight-year-old student at a state university.

The suggestion that 300 pounds of weed marijuana, requiring only a machete for harvesting and a panel truck for transportation, would yield $600,000 for a few days' work was obviously grossly exaggerated—but the influence of such police estimates in attracting additional entrepreneurs to marijuana harvesting and distribution should not be underestimated.

Clandestine marijuana plantations have also made their appearance on a modest scale.

Not only is clandestine pot farming being carried on all over the country, [columnist Nicholas von Hoffman reported in the Washington *Post*] but many people are at work developing higher yields, more potent strains so that good quality grass should be increasingly available at moderate prices. In addition to the thousands who're in this new industry for profit, there appears to be tens of thousands who grow pot at home for their own use. It's an indomitably hardy vegetable that grows anywhere, even in closets or basement. People plant it [indoors] in flower pots, train an electric light on it and wait for the high harvest.[36]

Mr. Zuckerman's August 1969 dispatch to the *Wall Street Journal*, quoted earlier, similarly reported that "some intrepid users have taken to growing the stuff on their own." He cited as an example a twenty-year-old college student who lived with his family in a Detroit suburb and who had cultivated a small crop in his family's garden each summer since he was seventeen.

"Every year I tell my mother I'm growing gourds, and every year when there aren't any gourds I tell her that I planted them late or something," the student was quoted as saying. He worried a bit when he saw his father in the marijuana patch—"but it was all right. He'd very considerately put stakes on my plants and tied them for support." [37]

Once the plants are grown and harvested, the *Wall Street Journal* dispatch continued, this student "speeds the drying process by tying his leaves in a pillowcase and running them through the clothes dryer." The student was quoted as explaining: "At the end of the summer, you'll usually find two or three of my friends waiting for their pillowcases" at a nearby launderette. This home-grown marijuana development resembles in several respects the home fermenting of grapes, the home brewing of beer, and the manufacture of gin in home bathtubs during Prohibition (1920–1933).

"Other amateurs," the *Wall Street Journal* added, "go in for marijuana cultivation in a bigger way. A hip young farmer in upstate New York, where wild marijuana is scarce and local police are less vigilant, is raising 500 plants for his friends in New York City. 'Why should they pay for the stuff, when I can grow it so easily?' he says."

An observer living in one New England township, formerly an agricultural center, says that marijuana is beginning there to take the place of other cash crops no longer profitable. "The only farms yielding a profit in our entire township are the three marijuana plantations." [38]

The chief problem in growing marijuana secretly, either outdoors or indoors, is the excessive height of the plant—often eight to ten feet at harvest time, and sometimes even higher. This height, of course, is the result of the fact that for so many hundreds of years seed from the tallest plants was selected in order to ensure long hemp fibers. Just as clandestine chemists have been turning out drugs in kitchen laboratories, however, so clandestine geneticists and horticulturists are already at work developing a shorter marijuana—less conspicuous to the police if grown outdoors and taking up less space indoors. Success should be fairly rapid; a marijuana strain growing only three to four feet tall has already been reported in London.[39]

Clandestine synthesis of THC is another potential development. A group of young underground chemists in London, indeed, has already succeeded in synthesizing a small quantity of an impure THC, which they proudly smoked in front of BBC television cameras.[40] It is almost certainly the relatively low price and relatively ready availability of natural marijuana and hashish that have to date discouraged further development of clandestine synthetic THC. If prices rise high enough, or marijuana and hashish become scarce enough, that curb on THC synthesis and distribution will no longer function.

The conclusion seems inescapable: as in the case of heroin, cocaine, the amphetamines, the barbiturates, LSD, and other illicit drugs, law enforcement can raise the price and thus the profits of the black market. Indeed, availability is *increased* when rising prices attract additional entrepreneurs. But no measures are currently visible, nor can any be foreseen, likely to curb availability for a longer time than it takes clandestine suppliers to adjust to the new measures.

60.

The Le Dain Commission Interim Report (1970)

It is often said that little is known about the psychological and physical effects of marijuana on the human user. This is a simple error of fact. In addition to many hundreds of significant papers reporting marijuana research through the past century, an impressive series of official investigating bodies have reviewed all of the available evidence and have presented their findings at length. The most important of these official marijuana investigation reports are listed here.

• *The Indian Hemp Drugs Commission Report* (1894). This 3,281-page, seven-volume report, published in Simla, India, in 1893–1894, has been justly called "the most complete and systematic study of marijuana undertaken to date." [1] The seven commissioners—four of them British and three of them Indian, including one rajah—secured testimony on every aspect of cannabis use from 1,193 witnesses. A digest of the findings of the Commission by Dr. Tod H. Mikuriya can be found in the Spring 1968 issue of the *International Journal of the Addictions*. A reprint of the final (Summary) volume, edited by Professor John Kaplan of the Stanford University Law School, was published by the Jefferson Press, Silver Springs, Maryland, in 1969.

• *The Panama Canal Zone Military Investigations* (1916–1929). A succession of military boards and commissions inquired into marijuana smoking by American military personnel stationed in the Canal Zone, beginning in 1916 and concluding with a full-scale investigation in 1929 under the chairmanship of Colonel J. F. Siler, M.D., of the Army Medical Corps. Sitting with him were two lieutenant colonels, a major, a naval commander, and the chief of the Canal Zone's Board of Health Laboratory. Colonel Siler and his associates reported the findings of their own and earlier Canal Zone investigations in the *Military Surgeon* in 1933 (volume 73, pages 269–280).

• *The LaGuardia Committee Report* (1939–1944). In 1939, at the request of Mayor Fiorello LaGuardia of New York City, the New York Academy of Medicine established a committee composed of eight physicians, a psychologist, and four New York City health officials. The committee studied marijuana smoking both under natural conditions in the city's "tea pads" and other marijuana centers, and in the laboratory. Its report was published in 1944, and reprinted in *The Marijuana Papers*

(Indianapolis: Bobbs-Merrill, 1966). This report is second only to the Indian Hemp Drugs Commission report in scope and thoroughness, and explores many areas of interest not considered by the Indian report. It is of particular contemporary importance because the pattern of marijuana smoking in New York City in the late 1930s that it describes was quite similar in many respects to the national pattern of marijuana smoking today.

• *The Baroness Wootton Report* (1968). In April 1967, the Advisory Committee on Drug Dependence of the United Kingdom Home Office appointed a subcommittee under Baroness Wootton of Abinger (formerly Barbara Wootton, a member of the House of Commons) to inquire into marijuana and hashish use in the United Kingdom. Her eleven fellow members included several of Britain's most eminent drug authorities. The report of the subcommittee, published in 1968, confirmed in all substantial respects the findings of the Indian Hemp Drugs Commission, the Panama Canal Zone investigations, and the LaGuardia Committee report.

• *The Interim Report of the Canadian Government's Le Dain Commission* (1970). In May 1969, on the recommendation of Minister of National Health and Welfare John Munro, the Government of Canada appointed a Commission of Inquiry into the Non-Medical Use of Drugs. The commission became known as the Le Dain Commission after its chairman, Dean Gerald Le Dain. The 320-page *Interim Report* of the commission, published in April 1970, marked a turning point in official North American thinking about psychoactive drugs in general—and about marijuana in particular. The commission's *Final Report* is scheduled for publication in 1972.

• In 1970 a sixth official body—the National Commission on Marijuana and Drug Abuse—was established by Congress and President Nixon, under the chairmanship of Raymond P. Schafer, former governor of Pennsylvania. Its initial findings, scheduled for 1972, were not yet available when this Consumers Union Report was completed.

In addition to these official investigations, four outstanding books on marijuana by individual authorities, and one important symposium, were published in 1970 and 1971. In alphabetical order by author, they are:

• *The Marijuana Smokers,* by Erich Goode, associate professor of sociology, State University of New York at Stony Brook (New York and London: Basic Books, 1970).

• *Marijuana Reconsidered,* by Lester Grinspoon, M.D., then associate clinical professor of psychiatry, Harvard Medical School, and director of psychiatry (research), Massachusetts Mental Health Center (Cambridge, Massachusetts: Harvard University Press, 1971).

• *Marijuana: The New Prohibition,* by Professor John Kaplan of the Stanford University Law School (New York: Crown, 1970).

• *The Strange Case of Pot,* by Michael Schofield, a member of the Baroness Wootton subcommittee and author of numerous works on psychology (Baltimore: Penguin Books, 1971).

• *The New Social Drug—Cultural, Medical, and Legal Perspective on Marijuana,* edited by David E. Smith, M.D., medical director of the Haight-Ashbury Medical Clinic, assistant clinical professor of toxicology at the University of California–San Francisco Medical Center, and editor of the *Journal of Psychedelic Drugs*—with contributions by Gilbert Geis, Frederick H. Meyers, Roger C. Smith, Andrew T. Weil, Norman E. Zinberg, and others (Englewood Cliffs, New Jersey: Prentice-Hall, 1970).

Remarkable as it may appear, all five of the reports of investigating bodies listed above, ranging in date from 1894 to 1970, and all of the books listed are in substantial agreement on substantially all major points of fact.

We have chosen, accordingly, to summarize and review in some detail only one of these major studies: the *Interim Report* of the Le Dain Commission. This decision was reached on several grounds:

(1) The Le Dain Commission's *Interim Report* is the most recent of the official investigations and therefore takes account of recent research not available for the earlier investigations.

(2) The findings and conclusions of the Le Dain Commission *Interim Report* are a fair sample of the findings and conclusions of the other studies.

(3) The drug scene in Canada on which the Le Dain Commission focuses is very similar in many respects to the comparable drug scene in the United States; and the problems Canada faces are very similar to United States problems.

(4) In our opinion, the methodology followed by the Le Dain Commission, in collecting data concerning other drugs as well as marijuana, is a model that future investigating bodies in the United States might well follow.

(5) Finally, the marijuana recommendations of the Le Dain Commission's *Interim Report* seem to us in many respects directly applicable to United States conditions.

Four of the five members of the Canadian Commission of Inquiry brought to their task a broad experience in public affairs and social problems, but relatively little knowledge of drug use: Gerald Le Dain, Q.C., Chairman, Dean of the Osgoode Hall Law School, York University, Toronto; Marie-Andrée Bertrand, Associate Professor of Criminology, University of Montreal; Ian L. Campbell, Dean of Arts, Sir George Williams University, Montreal; and J. Peter Stein, social worker, Vancouver.

The fifth member of the commission, Dr. Heinz E. Lehmann, Clinical Director of the Douglas Hospital in Montreal, is an internationally known authority on drugs, a Fellow of the American Psychiatric Association, a past president of the American College of Neuropsychopharmacology, and the author of more than 140 medical papers and publications.

Like the Indian Hemp Drugs Commission three-quarters of a century earlier, the Le Dain Commission adopted at the outset of its inquiry a "policy of the open ear." It held twenty-one days of formal hearings in twelve Canadian cities from coast to coast, traveling some 17,000 miles. Equally important, the commission listened to young people actually familiar with the drug scene, including many drug users. For this purpose it held numerous informal hearings on college and university campuses and in coffeehouses located near the heart of the drug scene of various cities (much as an 1884 Royal Commission had held hearings in a British Columbia opium den). To protect witnesses, an understanding was reached with the Royal Canadian Mounted Police, Canada's federal police agency, that appearances and statements "would not be exploited for law enforcement purposes." [2] In addition, witnesses were permitted to testify anonymously, some of them in private, and to submit anonymous statements; the press cooperated by refraining from publishing photographs. In all, the commission estimated, nearly 12,000 Canadians had attended these formal and informal hearings up to February 1, 1970.

Opinions and feelings have poured forth in the hearings with great spontaneity, particularly in the more informal settings [the *Interim Report* notes]. The Commission has been deeply impressed, and on several occasions, moved by the testimony which it has heard. It has been struck by the depth of feeling which [drug use] and the social response to it have aroused. As a result of the initial phase of its inquiry, the Commission is more than ever convinced that the proper response to the non-medical use of psychotropic drugs is a question which must be worked out by the people of Canada, examining it and talking it over together. It goes to the roots of our society and touches the values underlying our whole approach to life. It is not a matter which can be confined to the discrete consultation of experts, although experts obviously have their role, and a very important one, to play. [3]

Experts did play an important role in the Le Dain Commission deliberations. Scores of eminent Canadian scientists concerned with all aspects of drug use—the biochemical and pharmacological as well as the sociological and psychological—either testified personally or participated in the preparation of written submissions on behalf of the Royal Canadian Mounted Police, the Addiction Research Foundation of Ontario, the Narcotic Addiction Foundation of British Columbia, l'Office de la Prévention et du Traitement de l'Alcoolisme et des Autres Toxicomanies, numerous religious groups, and other respected Canadian organizations. Experts and organizations from the United States also submitted data and opinions; and members of the commission visited western European countries, consulting with drug authorities there and examining the European drug scene for themselves. Thus the inquiry was truly international.

The strictly psychopharmacological data were coordinated by a staff member specially trained in drug research, Dr. Ralph D. Miller. Chapter 2 of the *Interim Report*, entitled "Drugs and Their Effects," [4] prepared by Dr. Miller with the assistance of Dr. Charles Farmilo, is one of the most authoritative short statements of drug effects (beneficial and damaging) available, and is central to the conclusions that the commission reached.

Despite intensive American and Canadian law-enforcement efforts, the Le Dain Commission learned, marijuana smoking has become endemic in Canada—and here it cites high-school, college, and general population surveys showing levels of use quite comparable to those in the United States, reviewed above. Also as in the United States, use has spread from the "youth culture" to older age groups:

> The Commission has . . . been made aware of what appears to be an extensive and growing marijuana use by adults. The evidence of such use has come to us largely from the statements of individuals, many of whom have given private testimony, and from a large volume of correspondence received at the Commission's office. . . . Most were married and on the whole claimed to have reached an average or above average level of education. The Commissioners have spoken to physicians, lawyers, bankers, politicians, teachers, scientists, pilots, business executives and journalists, to mention only a few, who have smoked marijuana or hashish. Many of these reported using the drug with colleagues and many expressed the opinion that the use of these drugs would increase among their friends and associates.[5]

Why do so many *young* people smoke marijuana?
In the United States, a variety of reasons have been suggested:

• The general revolt of youth in the 1960s against their parents and parental taboos.
• The sense of "alienation" or of "anomie" among youth in the 1960s.
• The sense of impending nuclear doom, the draft, the war in Vietnam, and other factors leading youth to look to the immediate present rather than the future for satisfactions.
• The widespread advertising of mind-affecting drugs on radio and television.
• The widespread use of stimulants, depressants, and tranquilizers by parents.

- Parental and educational "permissiveness"; progressive education.
- The alleged breakdown of moral fiber among youth today.

The Le Dain Commission's *Interim Report* cites a quite different set of factors. In this as in other respects, the commission goes far beyond previous official reports and, largely as a result of its willingness to listen directly to young people, pioneers new ground. While many of its findings will come as a surprise and shock to nonsmokers of marijuana, these findings deserve careful consideration if the contemporary marijuana explosion is to be understood. "A major factor appears to be the simple pleasure of the experience," the Le Dain Commission explains. "Time after time, witnesses have said to us in effect: 'We do it for fun. Do not try to find a complicated explanation for it. We do it for pleasure.' " [6]

This pleasure explanation, the report adds, is offered not only by college students but also by adults in the working world.

A mother of four and a teacher said: "When I smoke grass I do it in the same social way that I take a glass of wine at dinner or have a drink at a party. I do not feel that it is one of the great and beautiful experiences of my life; I simply feel that it is pleasant and I think it ought to be legalized." [7]

A witness directly involved in work with drug users is quoted in much the same vein:

I think maybe it is time we stopped all the sociological nonsense about social milieus, and how your daddy fell off a horse, and how your mommy burnt the pablum or whatever it is—or what kind of sociological trip you want to blast off on, and just say . . . what you mean which is "I get loaded because I love to do it." [8]

The commission partially accepts this "we do it for fun" explanation.

We feel it would be a serious error, at least as far as cannabis use is concerned [the *Interim Report* declares] to think of use as symbolic of or manifesting a pathological, psychological or even sociological state. Simple pleasure, similar to that claimed for the moderate use of alcohol, or food, or sex, is frequently offered as the general explanation for most current drug use. This is particularly true of the growing number of adult users (who share perhaps little else but their taste for cannabis with the members of the "hip" culture). It is no doubt true that for some the use of drugs is a reflection of personal and social problems. But the desire for certain kinds of psychological gratification or release is not peculiar to the drug user or to our generations. It is an old and universal theme of human history. Man has always sought gratifications of the kind afforded by the psychotropic drugs. [9]

This use of marijuana for pleasure, the *Interim Report* continues, must not be interpreted as meaning that the motivation is trivial. On the contrary, it is one among many indications that the younger generation has profoundly reevaluated the proper role of pleasure in human life:

Young people speak often of a desire to overcome the division of life into work and play, to achieve a way of life that is less divided, less seemingly schizophrenic, and more unified. They seem to be talking about the increasingly rare privilege of work that one can fully enjoy—of work that is like one's play. They claim to be prepared to make considerable renunciation or sacrifice of traditional satisfactions like status and material success for work in which they can take pleasure. Indeed, one of their frequent commentaries on the older generation is that it does not seem to enjoy its work, that it does not seem to be happy. This is said sadly, even sympathetically. It is not said contemptuously. The young say, in effect, "Why should we repeat this pattern?" The use of drugs for many is part of a largely hedonistic life style in which happiness and pleasure are taken as self-evidently valid goals of human life.[10]

In addition to this happiness-and-pleasure motive, however, the Le Dain Commission notes that a number of young people also cite self-improvement as a reason for drug use:

In the case of *cannabis,* the positive points which are claimed for it include the following: it is a relaxant; it is disinhibiting; it increases self-confidence and the feeling of creativity (whether justified by objective results or not); it increases sensual awareness and appreciation; it facilitates concentration and gives one a greater sense of control over time; it facilitates self-acceptance and in this way makes it easier to accept others; it serves a sacramental function in promoting a sense of spiritual community among users; it is a shared pleasure; because it is illicit and the object of strong disapproval from those who are, by and large opposed to social change, it is a symbol of protest and a means of strengthening the sense of identity among those who are strongly critical of certain aspects of our society and value structure today.[11]

In these respects, the *Interim Report* adds, marijuana is seen as quite different from alcohol:

In our conversation with [students and young people], they have frequently contrasted marijuana and alcohol effects to describe the former as a drug of peace, a drug that reduces tendencies to aggression while suggesting that the latter drug produces hostile, aggressive behavior. Thus marijuana is seen as particularly appropriate to a generation that emphasizes peace and is, in many ways, anti-competitive.[12]

Feeling this way about his drug, the report continues, the cannabis user naturally "seeks to convert others to what he sincerely believes to be a superior outlook and life style. The smoking of cannabis becomes a rite of initiation to a new society and value system. These are aspects of cannabis use, particularly among the younger, more idealistic members of our society, which merit serious consideration in any attempt to measure its potential for growth." [13] LSD users, of course, voice these self-improvement and other idealistic themes with even more fervor than marijuana users.

On the whole, the *Interim Report* views these idealistic claims with some sympathy:

While pleasure, curiosity, the desire to experiment, and even the sense of adventure, are dominant motivations in drug use, there is no doubt that a search for self-knowledge and self-integration and for spiritual meanings are strong motivations with many.[14]

The *Interim Report* notes that drug use is not indispensable for achieving these new insights, and that it may in some cases be only a temporary stage in reaching fresh insight:

Some people are fortunate enough to be what users call a natural "turn on". It is conceded that you can be "turned on" without drugs—vital, human, and aware of all your senses, enjoying authentic, non-exploitative human relations, and alive to beauty and the possibilities of the moment. Indeed, there is an active doctrine of transcendence which sees drug use as a catalytic or transitional thing to be abandoned as soon as it has enabled you to glimpse another way of looking at things and of relating to life and people. The doctrine of transcendence carries much hope for the future. One witness said: "I don't do too many drugs anymore because I have gone beyond them. They have taught me the lesson and there isn't so much need for them anymore. I mean it's still fun to get stoned but there's a lot more to it. There is more to it than just fun. After you have learned the lesson, you have fun in virtually anything." [15]

Many former drug users, the Le Dain Commission continues,

have stated that the insights gained through drug use have carried over and remained with them. . . . In listening to these statements one cannot help feeling that this discovery was often made in other ways in the past—through traditional religious experiences, for instance.

Modern drug use would definitely seem to be related in some measure to the collapse of religious values—the ability to find a religious meaning of life. The positive values that young people claim to find in the drug experience bear a striking similarity to traditional religious values, including the concern with the soul, or inner self. The spirit of renunciation, the emphasis on openness and the closely knit community, are part of it, but there is definitely the sense of identification with something larger, something to which one belongs as part of the human race.[16]

Against this background, it is hardly surprising that the Le Dain Commission opposes the imprisonment of young people for the possession or use of marijuana. It is in exploring a wide range of alternatives to suppression and imprisonment that the commission makes its second major contribution to a reasonable consideration of marijuana.

We see non-medical drug use generally [the commission states] as presenting a complex social challenge for which we must find a wise and effective range of social responses. We believe that we must explore the full range of possible responses, including research, information and education; legislation and administrative regulation; treatment and supportive services; personal and corporate responsibility and self-restraint; and generally individual and social efforts to correct the deficiencies in our personal relations and social conditions which encourage the non-medical use of drugs. We attach importance to the general emphasis in this range of social responses. We believe that this emphasis must shift, as we develop and strengthen the non-coercive aspects of our social response, from a reliance on suppression to a reliance on the wise exercise of freedom of choice.[17]

As a first step toward improving the social response to the nonmedical use of drugs, the *Interim Report* suggests, society must abandon the transparent pretense that it considers all such use of drugs as *ipso facto* and *per se* evil and in need of suppression. This pretense is no longer tenable:

Alcohol is a sedative which is widely used for the relief of tension. Have we taken a strong moral position against its use? Some have done so and still do, but they are obviously in a minority, and the vast majority of the society pays little attention to them. As for the stimulants, we take in enormous quantities of caffeine and nicotine. We stimulate our systems and modify our mood by cup after cup of coffee through the day. The nicotine in tobacco is clearly a psychotropic drug used to modify one's mood. Have we adopted a moral position against the use of caffeine and nicotine? Hardly. We are beginning to react against tobacco because of its clear danger to health, but the effect on sales is so far unimpressive.[18]

In place of the pretense that the alcohol, caffeine, and nicotine one generation uses are nondrugs while the marijuana its children use is evil, the *Interim Report* recommends that each drug be judged on its merits: *"The extent to which any particular drug use is to be deemed to be undesirable will depend upon its relative potential for harm, both personal and social."* [19]

Against this background, the Le Dain Commission reviews the allegations traditionally made against marijuana, and reaches conclusions generally similar to those reached by the Indian Hemp Drugs Commission, the Panama investigating committees, the LaGuardia Committee, the Wootton Subcommittee, and other responsible bodies which have critically reviewed the evidence. It concludes, for example, that marijuana is not an addicting drug. Users do not develop tolerance in the classical sense—the kind of tolerance that leads to increasing the dosage. The Commission takes note, however, of the statements of some users "that if they stay 'high' for several days in a row the drug experience loses much of its freshness and clarity and, consequently, they prefer intermittent use." [20] Whether or not this is a tolerance effect, it is clearly a beneficent one.

Physical dependence on marijuana, the report adds, has not been demonstrated; "it would appear that there are normally no adverse physiological effects or withdrawal symptoms occurring with abstinence from the drug, even in regular users." [21] Reports to the contrary from the East are suspect. "Since hashish is smoked with large quantities of tobacco and other drugs in many Eastern countries, these mixtures could be responsible for the minor symptoms reported." [22] Marijuana, it is true, may in some cases produce *psychological* dependence—but "psychological dependence may be said to exist with respect to anything which is part of one's preferred way of life. In our society, this kind of dependency occurs regularly with respect to such things as television, music, books, religion, sex, money, favourite foods, certain drugs, hobbies, sports or games and, often, other persons. Some degree of psychological dependence is, in this sense, a general and normal psychological condition." [23]

The short-term physiological effects of marijuana use, the report continues, "are usually slight and apparently have little clinical significance." [24] Even overdose produces little acute physiological toxicity; "sleep is the usual somatic consequence of overdose. No deaths due directly to smoking or eating cannabis have been documented. . . ." [25]

The stepping-stone theory that marijuana use leads to heroin use is stated but given little credence. "In Canada . . . it appears that heavy use of sedatives (alcohol and barbiturates) rather than cannabis has most frequently preceded heroin use." [26] And again: "Persons dependent on opiate narcotics generally have a history of heavy alcohol consumption." [27] The same, as noted in Part I of this Consumers Union Report, is true in the United States.

The commission takes notice of the fear that marijuana smoking, like cigarette smoking, might lead to lung cancer and other lung pathology. No evidence currently exists, it points out, to support this view. Moreover, "the quantity of leaf consumed by the average cigarette smoker in North America is many times the amount of cannabis smoked by even heavy users. The present pattern of use by regular cannabis smokers in North

America is more analogous to intermittent alcohol use (e.g., once or twice a week), than to the picture of chronic daily use presented by ordinary tobacco dependence." [28] The commission adds, however, that "the deep inhalation technique usually used with cannabis might add respiratory complications." [29]

With respect to psychoses and other adverse psychological effects associated with marijuana, the Le Dain Commission report is on the whole quite reassuring. "Although there are some well documented examples of very intense and nightmarish short-term reactions (usually among inexperienced users in unpleasant situations and with high doses), these cases seem to be relatively rare and generally show a rapid recovery. Although many regular users have had an experience with cannabis which was in some way unpleasant, 'freak-outs' are apparently rare." [30] A Montreal psychiatrist of broad experience with adverse reactions to other drugs, Dr. J. R. Unwin, is quoted as reporting in the *Canadian Medical Association Journal* in 1969: "I have seen only three adverse reactions in the past two years; all following the smoking of large amounts of hashish and all occurring in individuals with a previous history of psychiatric treatment for psychiatric or borderline conditions." [31]

The United States experience, the commission notes, has in general been similar. Thus Dr. David E. Smith of the Haight-Ashbury Clinic in San Francisco is cited as reporting that he had not observed any cases of "cannabis psychosis" among the 35,000 marijuana users attending that clinic.[32]

True, the commission adds, there are some reports pointing in the other direction. But reports from the Eastern countries are of dubious value, since no control groups were studied; the question is not whether some marijuana smokers (like some nonsmokers) develop psychoses, but whether the use of marijuana *increases the incidence* of psychoses. Dr. J. T. Ungerleider (later appointed a member of President Nixon's National Commission on Marijuana and Drug Abuse) reported observing 1,887 "adverse reactions" to marijuana in Los Angeles—but "'these data are difficult to interpret since no clear definition of adverse reaction is provided and no follow-ups were made." * [34] A few psychoses reported

---

* Other Los Angeles observers have failed to confirm the Ungerleider findings. Thus Dr. George D. Lundberg, associate professor of pathology at the University of Southern California School of Medicine, and two colleagues, with the aid of a computer, searched the records of 701,057 consecutive admissions to the Los Angeles County–University of Southern California Medical Center from July 1, 1961, to January 1, 1969. Nine admissions involved marijuana. "Total marijuana users in the region served by this hospital during this time period are estimated to be in the hundreds of thousands, with tens of thousands of frequent or chronic users." Of the nine admissions, three were marijuana smokers, who experienced "mild illnesses . . . transient euphoria, a dream state, dizziness, confusion, and hallucinations." Two patients recovered rapidly. "The third later was diagnosed as a chronic paranoid schizophrenic, a state

among United States forces in Vietnam may or may not have been traceable to cannabis use; they involved "individuals who have consumed large doses of potent material under conditions of increased physical and psychological stress." [35] It is hardly necessary to invoke marijuana as an explanation for a few psychoses among soldiers billeted in a distant land and fighting on foreign fields. To the extent that psychoses do occur on rare occasions following cannabis use, they appear to be "a reflection of very special personality difficulties in the subjects involved or exceptional dose levels." [36]

The Canadian report also notes two public-health considerations that have generally been lost from sight in the American antimarijuana literature. The first concerns the somewhat greater hazard of eating marijuana and hashish as compared with smoking them. " 'Grass' and 'hash' are generally used interchangeably and great variations in potency of different samples are accommodated by the experienced user through a 'titration' of dose—i.e., intake is stopped when the smoker reaches a personally comfortable level of intoxication. Such precision is generally not possible with oral use, however, due to the long delay in action, and a 'non-optimal' effect is much more likely to occur with this practice." [37] In the United States this message rarely gets through to young people— primarily because the channels of public-health communication are overloaded with generalized antimarijuana propaganda, much of it unreliable and counterproductive.

The second public-health consideration noted in the Canadian report concerns the relative hazards of marijuana and hashish. As has already been noted, the two are related much as beer or wine is related to whisky or gin; the effects of equivalent doses are rather similar, but it is somewhat easier to overdose with whisky, gin, or hashish than with beer, wine, or marijuana. While a prudent and experienced cannabis smoker can limit his hashish "high" to the level of his customary marijuana "high," the *Interim Report* cautiously suggests the possibility that a nationwide conversion from marijuana to hashish might significantly increase the incidence of deleterious effects. "Moderate use of the milder forms is one thing; excessive use of the stronger forms may be quite another." [38]

---

which preceded his marijuana-induced hospitalization." Another patient ingested "a 'handful of marijuana leaves,' which produced drowsiness and headache with recovery following intravenously given fluid and cathartic therapy." Five patients had "mainlined" marijuana—four a seed extract and the fifth a leaf "juice"; they became acutely ill with "nausea, vomiting, fever, chills, shock, tachycardia [rapid heartbeat], weakness, headache," and an increase in white blood cells; all recovered following the "intravenous administration of fluids, antibiotics, and steroids. . . . a variety of comparative studies indicated that hospital admissions due to alcohol, tobacco, barbiturates, amphetamines, tranquilizers, and certain nonprescription drugs (all legal) were much more frequent and the cases much more serious medically. . . ." [33]

In this context, the American and Canadian trend from marijuana toward hashish, beginning in 1969, was naturally a cause of concern for the Le Dain Commission. It attributes this trend in considerable part to American law-enforcement policies:

The [Royal Canadian Mounted] Police representatives of the Department of Justice, and a number of witnesses have reported that marijuana, long the staple of the drug-using subculture, is now being replaced by hashish as the widely used illegal drug in some parts of the country. This shift in popularity can probably be attributed to a growing difficulty in obtaining marijuana (American and Mexican authorities lately have been intensifying their efforts to control its cultivation and prevent smuggling activities), the greater ease with which hashish, a concentrated form of cannabis, can be hidden and thus transported, and the greater profits in hashish trafficking. Hashish can be purchased at its source for around $50 a kilo and resold in Canada at $1,400 a kilo, while marijuana costs from $20 a kilo in Mexico to $100 a kilo in Southern California and can be resold in Canada for about $300 a kilo; an ounce of hashish sells for between $75 and $100 in contrast to about $20 an ounce for marijuana.[39]

As marijuana repression becomes more efficient, of course, the cost of marijuana rises and the relative competitive advantages of smuggling hashish instead become even greater.

The Le Dain Commission does *not* conclude that marijuana is harmless. The available evidence, it indicates, warrants a cautious approach. Additional problems may arise as marijuana research proceeds and as experience accumulates. Even so, the commission points out, reliance on the "hazards" theme to curb marijuana smoking has proved fruitless or worse in the past and is unlikely to prove more effective in the future.

"Many of the young people who have appeared before us have been critical of the drug education to which they have been exposed," the *Interim Report* notes. "In particular, they have said that the attempts to use 'scare tactics' have 'backfired' and destroyed the credibility of sound information." [40] The commission itself fully endorses these complaints from its young witnesses:

The conclusion we draw from the testimony we have heard is that it is a grave error to indulge in deliberate distortion or exaggeration concerning the alleged dangers of a particular drug, or to base a program of drug education upon a strategy of fear. It is no use playing "chicken" with young people; in nine cases out of ten they will accept the challenge.[41]

In place of the traditional deterrents to drug use—imprisonment and scare campaigns—the Le Dain Commission's *Interim Report* then proceeds to outline in the broadest terms, yet with many detailed recommendations, a major reorientation of attitudes toward the nonmedical use of psychoactive drugs, and major changes in laws and public policies. Many of these recommendations apply to the opiates, the amphetamines, the barbiturates, LSD, and other psychoactive drugs as well as to marijuana, and they closely parallel suggestions to be made in Part X, Conclusions and Recommendations, of this Consumers Union Report; they will therefore be noted there. The Le Dain Commission's comments on some of the special problems of marijuana legislation and marijuana law enforcement closely parallel comments in the Wootton subcommittee report and other recent publications, and are considered here.

The victim of a crime against person or property [the Commission points out] usually complains to the police, gives them information, and assists them to commence an investigation. The police react to what they have been told about a specific offense. If, on the other hand, someone has a drug in his possession, and has bought it from someone else, it is rare that anyone will feel affected enough to lay a complaint. Hence, instead of reacting to a specific request, the police must go out themselves and look for offenses. Moreover, it is difficult to discover these offenses. Because the parties to the offense or transaction are all willing participants, they can agree to carry out the prohibited conduct in a place of privacy where it is not likely to be seen either by witnesses or the police.[42]

Legislators, the report continues, have responded to these special drug-law enforcement difficulties by widening police powers of search and seizure in extraordinary ways. "Under the ordinary law, a person can be searched only after an arrest has been made, and in order to discover any evidence of the crime for which the arrest is made. Where there is not an arrest, there is no power to search premises without a search warrant. Again, such warrants assume specific evidence that the particular premises contain something incriminating. The point of these rules is to prevent indiscriminate interference with privacy in an attempt to turn up evidence of a crime and to prevent such interference by requiring cogent evidence that the person or premises affected are peculiarly worthy of search, before such search is authorized by an independent judicial officer who reviews the evidence." [43]

Under the Canadian *drug* laws, in contrast, "there is no longer a real requirement that the police obtain external review and confirmation of their judgment. . . . Any police officer can enter and search any place other than a dwelling house without a warrant. . . ." [44]

Even with respect to dwelling houses, moreover, Canadian drug law since 1929 has made available a legal device called a "writ of assistance." Such writs, as most United States schoolchildren learn in an early grade, were one of the causes of the American Revolution. An enforcement officer must apply to a judge for such a writ in the first instance, as in the case of a search warrant or warrant for arrest; but the writ of assistance does not specify any particular premises. "It remains valid so long as the officer retains his authority and it empowers him to enter any dwelling in Canada at any time, with such assistance as he may require, and search for narcotics and other proscribed drugs." [45]

Canadian drug law has also had a "no-knock" clause like the one enacted by the United States Congress in 1970; this clause provides that a peace officer armed with either a warrant or a writ of assistance may, "with such assistance as he deems necessary, break open any door, window, lock, fastener, floor, wall, ceiling, compartment, plumbing, box, container or any other thing," [46] may search any person found in such a place; and may seize and take away any narcotic or other proscribed drug in such place, as well as anything that may be evidence of the commission of a drug offense. (The possession of such extraordinary powers has not made the Canadian police forces noticeably more effective than American police forces in stamping out illicit drug trafficking.)

The difficulties of drug-law enforcement, the Le Dain Commission adds, have led to yet another "unusual practice—what is known in other jurisdictions as 'entrapment' but which may be described as 'police encouragement.' A person is encouraged by a police agent to commit an offense [and is then prosecuted for that offense]. It is impossible to say how extensive this practice is, but it is reflected in a number of cases." [47]

Many people approve such laws and practices, of course, on the ground that the "drug evil" must be stamped out at any cost. The Le Dain Commission points out that the cost is very high:

During the initial phase of our inquiry, we have heard bitter complaints and criticisms of the use of entrapment and physical violence to obtain evidence. We have not verified the particular circumstances of these complaints and criticisms, so that we make no charge of any kind at this time but we deplore the use of such methods to the extent that they may be resorted to on occasion. We believe that such methods are not only a serious violation of respect for the human person, but they are counter-productive in that they create contempt for law and law enforcement. The price that is paid for them is far too great for any good that they may do.

We recommend that instructions be given to police officers to abstain from such methods of enforcement, and that the RCMP use its influence with other police forces involved in the enforcement of the drug laws to try to assure that there is a uniform policy in this regard.[48] [The emphasis here and in the quotations below is in the original.]

The commission reviews the arguments in favor of legalizing marijuana, and indicates that serious consideration should be given to them. They are summarized in the *Interim Report* as follows:

1. The use of marijuana is increasing in popularity among all age groups of the population, and particularly among the young;

2. This increase indicates that the attempt to suppress, or even to control its use, is failing and will continue to fail—that people are not deterred by the criminal law prohibtion against its use;

3. The present legislative policy has not been justified by clear and unequivocal evidence of short term or long term harm caused by cannabis;

4. The individual and social harm (including the destruction of young lives and growing disrespect for law) caused by the present use of the criminal law to attempt to suppress cannabis far outweighs any potential for harm which cannabis could conceivably possess, having regard to the long history of its use and the present lack of evidence;

5. The illicit status of cannabis invites exploitation by criminal elements, and other abuses such as adulteration; it also brings cannabis users into contact with such criminal elements and with other drugs, such as heroin, which they might not otherwise be induced to consider.

For all of these reasons, it is said, cannabis should be made available under government-controlled conditions of quality and availability.[49]

The commission concludes, however, that legalization is not warranted *at this time* (spring of 1970). One reason for postponing the decision is that the scientific evidence concerning marijuana is not yet all in—but the *Interim Report* adds a cogent warning:

"How long can society wait for the necessary information? It is very serious that the scientific information concerning cannabis lags so far behind the rapidly developing social problem caused by its illegal status." [50]

One reason for this lag in scientific information, the commission notes, is government restraints on research. "Many scientists interested in such research have expressed feelings of dissatisfaction and frustration with governmental research policy. They have stated to the commission that they have been unable to carry out such work under their own authority as scientists in the present atmosphere of restraint. They say that they have been frustrated by the administration of the formal and unwritten governmental policies which surround the right to undertake research in this field." [51]

Many American scientists, of course, have expressed similar dissatisfaction and frustration.* One reason for this governmental repression of

* An example of the perils of marijuana research in the United States was reported in *Medical World News* in 1969:

"At ten minutes before midnight last June 27, [a psychiatrist] was rousted out of bed`. . . by callers from the narcotics division of the Texas Department of Public Safety and the local police, callers armed with a warrant for the psychiatrist's arrest on a charge of marijuana possession and for a search of his home.

"[The psychiatrist] informed them that he did, indeed, have marijuana in his possession, not in his residence but in his adjoining office, where he used it in fully research, the Le Dain Commission suggests (though it does not actually state) is the fear that sound research may fail to support the traditional allegations against marijuana and may thus lead to a change in public policy. "The public, including interested scientists, are justly dissatisfied and impatient with the present state of research. The public does not know whom to blame, *but it will not lightly tolerate an indefinite reliance on inadequate knowledge to justify a social policy which is coming under increasingly severe criticism.*" [53] (Emphasis added.)

A second reason given by the Le Dain Commission for not recommending the immediate legalization of marijuana was a purely practical one: public opinion was not yet ready (in the spring of 1970) for so drastic a change, and the recommendation would no doubt be rejected. " . . . It is our impression that there has not yet been enough informed public debate. Certainly there has been much debate, but all too often it has been based on hearsay, myth and ill-informed opinion about the effects of the drug. We hope that this report will assist in providing a basis for informed debate. . . ." [54]

A third reason for delaying the legalization decision, the *Interim Report* adds, is that "further consideration should be given to what may be necessarily implied by legalization. Would a decision by the government to assume responsibility for the quality control and distribution of cannabis imply, or be taken to imply, approval of its use* and an assurance as to the absence of significant potential harm?" [55] Finally, the commission

---

authorized research. He removed it from his office safe and turned it over to the officers, who confiscated it and arrested him. They also seized 208 *Cannabis sativa* plants the doctor showed them growing in his backyard.

"But he also showed them his permit to import marijuana, his Class 4 and Class 5 federal tax stamps covering marijuana used in research, and the paragraph in a booklet issued by the federal bureau of narcotics stating that Class 5 researchers 'may produce such quantities of marijuana and compound or manufactured marijuana preparations as are necessary for their research, instruction, or analysis.' [The psychiatrist] was nevertheless arrested, spent the night in the [county] jail and was released the next morning on $1,000 bond.

"Although it appeared unlikely that he would be prosecuted, [the psychiatrist] considers his research to have been effectively stopped, and himself to have been all but run out of town. 'My patients have been scared away,' he says, 'and my experimental subjects are afraid to come in because it was reported in the local papers that I was under surveillance for a month and that the police are watching me with binoculars.'" [52]

* In other situations, it should be noted, the repeal of a punitive law does *not* imply official approval of the behavior that is legalized. Thus the New York state legislature years ago repealed that state's law punishing suicide attempts, a number of state legislatures have in the past few years repealed state laws against homosexual acts between consenting adults, and the Oregon legislature in 1971 repealed that state's law restricting cigarette smoking by minors—not because the legislatures approved or wanted to encourage suicide attempts, homosexual acts, and cigarette smoking by minors, or because they thought such acts harmless, but because they recognized that criminal penalties are an unwise and ineffective response to such acts.

cites "jurisdictional and technical questions involved in the control of quality and availability." [56]

Both in the United States and Canada, the argument is sometimes made that international treaty obligations under the United Nations *Single Convention on Narcotics Drugs,* 1961, prevent the legalization of marijuana. The Le Dain Commission gives short shrift to this argument. Any country can withdraw from the Single Convention on January 1 of any year by giving six full months' notice; withdrawal "would not, of course, be in violation of international obligations since it is a right expressly provided for in the Convention." [57]

One step short of legalizing marijuana would be the abolition of all penalties for the *possession* of marijuana—leaving trafficking a criminal offense. The *Interim Report* concludes that this policy merits conscientious study, with respect not only to marijuana but to the psychoactive drugs in general, including heroin.

One Le Dain Commission argument in favor of abolishing the offense of simple possession is the high cost of enforcing the possession law: "Its enforcement would appear to cost far too much, in individual and social terms, for any utility which it may be shown to have. . . . The present cost of its enforcement, and the individual and social harm caused by it, are in our opinion, one of the major problems involved in the non-medical use of drugs." [58]

Unenforceability, the commission continues, is another argument in favor of abolishing all penalties against possession. "Insofar as cannabis, and possibly the stronger hallucinogens like LSD, are concerned, the present law against simple possession would appear to be unenforceable, except in a very selective and discriminatory kind of way. This results necessarily from the extent of use and the kinds of individual involved. It is obvious that the police can not make a serious attempt at full enforcement of the law against simple possession. . . ." [59]

It is often argued that, just as the continued commission of murder is not a sound reason for repealing the murder laws, so the smoking of marijuana is not a good reason for repealing the marijuana laws. The Le Dain Commission distinguishes the two cases:

> The law which appears to stand on the statute book as a mere convenience to be applied from time to time, on a very selective and discriminatory basis, to "make an example" of someone, is bound to create a strong sense of injustice and a corresponding disrespect for law and law enforcement. It is also bound to have an adverse effect upon the morale of law enforcement authorities.
>
> Moreover, it is doubtful if its deterrent effect justifies the injury inflicted upon the individuals who have the misfortune to be prosecuted under it. It is, of course, impossible to determine the extent to which the law against simple possession has deterrent effect, but certainly the increase in use, as well as the statements of users, would suggest that it has relatively little. The relative risk

of detection and prosecution may be presumed to have a bearing upon deterrent effect.[60]

The likelihood that a marijuana user will be brought to court for possession, the commission adds, "may be under one percent" [61]—hardly an effective deterrent.*

On the question of deterrence the *Interim Report* also cites a 1967 opinion of the Ontario Court of Appeal: "Those, of whom the accused is one, who have accepted the use of psychedelic drugs as socially desirable as well as personally desirable course of conduct are not as likely to be discouraged by the type of punishment ordinarily meted out to other traffickers. Such treatment will likely serve to confirm them in their belief in the drug cult. . . ." [62]

Yet another reason for repealing the possession laws is briefly stated in the *Interim Report*: "The extreme methods which appear to be necessary in the enforcement of a prohibition against simple possession—informers, entrapment, Writs of Assistance, and occasionally force to recover the prohibited substance—add considerably to the burden of justifying the necessity or even the utility of such a provision." [63]

But the Le Dain Commission waxes most eloquent in attacking the possession laws on the ground of the direct harm they do, not only to their victims but to respect for law and order:

The harm caused by a conviction for simple possession appears to be out of all proportion to any good it is likely to achieve in relation to the phenomenon of non-medical drug use. Because of the nature of the phenomenon involved, it is bound to impinge more heavily on the young than on other segments of the population. Moreover, it is bound to blight the life of some of the most promising of the country's youth. Once again there is the accumulating social cost of a profound sense of injustice, not only at being the unlucky one whom the authorities have decided to prosecute, but at having to pay such an enormous price for conduct which does not seem to concern anyone but oneself. This sense of injustice is aggravated by the disparity in sentences made possible by the large discretion presently left to the courts.[64]

Despite these impressive reasons for repealing the laws against mere possession of marijuana and other psychoactive drugs, a majority of the commission resolved not to recommend *immediate* repeal. More time was needed, the majority concluded, to study arguments *against* repeal made by the police. The commission indicated, however, that it would announce a decision in 1972.

* In the United States, where an estimated five million marijuana cigarettes were smoked daily in 1971, the likelihood of being arrested on any particular occasion of use was far less than one chance in five thousand—and for many users the risk approached zero.

This was the only point on which the *Interim Report* was not unanimous. The one woman member of the Le Dain Commission, Professor Bertrand, did not want to postpone the repeal recommendation even for one year. She wrote:

I find myself in disagreement with my colleagues on the Commission in respect of the offence of simple possession of cannabis. In my opinion the prohibition against such possession should be removed altogether. I believe that this course is dictated at the present time by the following considerations: the extent of use and the age groups involved; the relative impossibility of enforcing the law; the social consequences of its enforcement; and the uncertainty as to the relative potential for harm of cannabis.[65]

In lieu of recommending immediate repeal of the laws against simple possession, the Le Dain Commission majority recommended the immediate abolition of *imprisonment* as a penalty for simple possession:

. . . The Commission is of the opinion that no one should be liable for imprisonment for simple possession of a psychotropic drug for non-medical purposes.[*][66]

To replace imprisonment the commission recommended *"as an interim measure, pending its final report, that the Narcotic Control Act and the Food and Drugs Act be amended to make the offense of simple possession under these acts punishable upon summary conviction by a fine not exceeding a reasonable amount. The Commission suggests a maximum fine of $100."* [67]

A prisoner who cannot pay his fine or who refuses to pay it is ordinarily liable to imprisonment. To prevent imprisonment in such cases, the commission *"also recommends that the power . . . to impose imprisonment in default of payment of a fine should not be exercisable in respect of offenses of simple possession of psychotropic drugs. In such cases, the Crown should reply on civil proceedings to recover payment."* [68]

The proposal that offenders found guilty of possessing marijuana should not be imprisoned may seem radical indeed to some readers of this Consumers Union Report. But, as the Le Dain Commission points out, the courts of Canada had reached much the same conclusion on their own initiative in 1969, without waiting for the *Interim Report*. Canadian court statistics for the period from August through December 1969, this report declares, "reveal that imprisonment is now being rarely, if at all, resorted to in cases of simple possession of marijuana and hashish and, it would

---

[*] This recommendation, the commission made clear, applies to simple possession of heroin and other illicit drugs as well as to marijuana.

appear, LSD, and that such cases are now generally disposed of by suspended sentence, probation or fine." [69] Thus the key Le Dain Commission marijuana recommendation, far from representing a radical departure from current Canadian policy, does little more than recommend that the current practice of most Canadian courts be made uniform and mandatory.

Much the same trend appears to be under way in the United States courts, though at a slower pace. As the Select Committee on Crime of the United States House of Representatives commented in its *First Report on Marijuana,* dated April 6, 1970: "We have observed that the penalties for marijuana possession or even for selling are generally not imposed and that jail sentences are the rare exception rather than the rule."* [72]

To reduce without delay the damaging effects of law enforcement on drug users, the Le Dain Commission went on to recommend *"that the police, prosecutors and courts exercise the discretion entrusted to them at various stages of the criminal law process so as to minimize the impact of the criminal law upon the simple possessor of psychotropic drugs, pending decision as to the whole future of possessional offenses in this field."* [73]

The commission also recommended a substantial reduction in the penalties for trafficking and for possession for the purpose of trafficking—and a major restriction of the definition of "trafficking." Canadian penalties at the time of the *Interim Report* included a maximum of life imprisonment for either trafficking in marijuana or possession for the purpose of trafficking. This maximum could be meted out to a young person sharing a marijuana cigarette with a friend or giving marijuana

---

* Judge Charles W. Halleck of the District of Columbia Court of General Sessions, in testimony before the House of Representatives Special Subcommittee on Alcoholism and Narcotics on September 18, 1969, explained why he no longer gives jail sentences to youthful marijuana smokers:

"If I send [a long-haired marijuana offender] to the jail even for 30 days, Senator, he is going to be the victim of the most brutal type of homosexual, unnatural, perverted assaults and attacks that you can imagine, and anybody who tells you it doesn't happen in that jail day in and day out, is simply not telling you the truth. . . .

"How in God's name, Senator, can I send anybody to that jail knowing that? How can I send some poor young kid who gets caught by some zealous policeman who wants to make his record on a narcotics arrest? How can I send that kid to that jail?

"I can't do it. So I put him on probation or I suspend the sentence and everybody says the judge doesn't care. The judge doesn't care about drugs, lets them all go. You just simply can't treat these kinds of people like that." [70]

Dr. David E. Smith of the Haight-Ashbury Medical Clinic reported in June 1971 that among the psychiatric patients served by his clinic were 25 young men with serious psychoses—all of whom were imprisoned for possession of marijuana and all of whom suffered psychiatric breakdowns following homosexual rape while they were incarcerated. [71]

to a friend—a gift defined as "trafficking" in Canadian law and as a "sale" in United States law.

In Canada, importers and exporters of cannabis were also subject to a maximum of life imprisonment—and to a minimum mandatory sentence, which the judge could not reduce, of seven years' imprisonment. In lieu of these penalties, the Le Dain Commission recommended that minimum mandatory sentences be abolished altogether and that the *maximum* sentence be eighteen months for all cannabis offenses including importing, exporting, and trafficking. "*We further recommend that the definition of trafficking be amended so as to exclude the giving, without exchange of value, by one user to another of a quantity of cannabis which could reasonably be consumed on a single occasion. Such an act should be subject at most to the penalty for simple possession*" [74]—that is, a reasonable fine not to exceed $100.

In yet another respect the Le Dain Commission sought to minimize the impact of the criminal law on young marijuana offenders—indeed, on offenders generally:

> Great concern has been expressed during the initial phase of our inquiry concerning the serious effects of a criminal conviction and record upon the lives of drug users, particularly the young. These effects are cited, in the case of cannabis, as indicating that the harm caused by the law exceeds the harm which it is supposed to prevent. A criminal record may mar a young life, forever being an impediment to professional or other vocational opportunity and interfering with free movement and the full enjoyment of public rights. We believe this reasoning applies to all criminal convictions, and we do not believe that there should be a special rule in favour of drug offenders. *For this reason, we recommend the enactment of general legislation to provide for the destruction of all records of a criminal conviction after a reasonable period of time.*[75]

The *Final Report* of the Le Dain Commission was not available when this Consumers Union Report was completed. The guidelines laid down by the commission's *Interim Report*, however, are sound guidelines for the formation of policy in the United States. Consumers Union's own detailed recommendations, which go considerably further, appear below in Part X.

Part IX
The Drug Scene

61.

Scope of drug use

We have now completed our drug-by-drug review of the psychoactive drugs in common use, especially those frequently used for recreational, nonmedicinal purposes. In this and the next two chapters, we shall present some data on the relative popularity of the drugs we have been describing; and we shall offer some comments on the vague and shifting line which separates "good" from "bad" drugs, prescription from nonprescription drugs, medicinal from nonmedicinal use. In subsequent chapters, we shall concentrate on the relatively small portion of the overall drug scene that is of the greatest current concern to most Americans—the *youth* drug scene.

By far the most popular mind-affecting drugs in the United States today are caffeine, nicotine, and alcohol. This is true on every significant measure: number of people who have ever used, number of regular users, number of daily users, number of man-hours spent under the influence of the drug, and money spent for the drug.* The amount of harm done to the human body by nicotine and alcohol, moreover, vastly exceeds the physical harm done by all of the other psychoactive drugs put together (see Parts III and IV). Further, the amount of damage done to the human mind by alcohol alone, as measured by mental hospital admissions, vastly exceeds the mental harm done by all of the other psychoactive drugs put together. Nor is caffeine necessarily a "harmless" drug (see Part II).

These facts are commonly masked by the categorization of caffeine, nicotine, and alcohol as nondrugs. Society might equally well seek to solve its amphetamine, barbiturate, and marijuana problems by treating those substances as nondrugs; indeed, as discussed below, there is substantial reason to believe that the United States is moving in that direction. Whether or not such substances are legally defined as drugs however, they are all closely related components of our national drug problem.

Americans have long known that the current drug scene is vast; but its truly gargantuan dimensions came into clearer perspective as data began to emerge, late in 1971, from the computers of a long-term "Psychotropic

* In 1970, for example, Americans spent $15.7 billion for alcoholic beverages, $9 billion for tobacco, and $3.2 billion for the caffeine beverages, coffee, tea, and cocoa—a total of almost $28 billion.[1]

Drug Study" funded by the National Institute of Mental Health in cooperation with two academic research organizations—the Social Research Group of George Washington University in Washington, D.C., and the Institute for Research in Social Behavior in Berkeley, California. In charge of the study are Dr. Mitchell B. Balter for the NIMH, Drs. Hugh J. Parry and Ira H. Cisin for the Social Research Group, and Drs. Dean I. Manheimer and Glenn D. Mellinger for the Institute for Research in Social Behavior.

A part of the project, under the direction of Drs. Parry and Cisin, is seeking to determine the facts about psychoactive drug use in the population aged eighteen through seventy-four, excluding those hospitalized or in the armed forces—based on a probability sample of 2,552 respondents interviewed during the fall of 1970 and spring of 1972. Some of the findings follow (some columns total more or less than 100 percent because of rounding).

Caffeine (coffee and tea). Some 82 percent of respondents in the Parry-Cisin study reported that they drank coffee and 52 percent that they drank tea during the previous year.[2]

Amount	Users of Coffee (percentage)	Users of Tea (percentage)
None	18	48
Less than 1 cup daily	6	22
1 or 2 cups daily	30	21
3 or 4 cups daily	24	6
5 or 6 cups daily	12	2
7 or more cups daily	9	1

When use of the two caffeine beverages is considered in combination, it appears that very few Americans aged eighteen and over drink neither coffee nor tea, and that 25 percent drink six or more cups daily.[3]

Amount	Users of Coffee and/or Tea (percentage)
None	9
One cup or less a day	7
Two cups	24
Three cups	21
Four cups	7
Five cups	8
Six cups	11
Seven cups or more	14

These figures are consistent with sales figures showing that enough coffee (excluding decaffeinated coffee) was sold in the United States in 1970 to provide every man, woman, and child over the age of ten with 2.4 cups per day—or about 180 *billion* doses of caffeine a year.

The above figures, moreover, exclude hot chocolate and cocoa, caffeine-containing soft drinks (mostly cola drinks), and over-the-counter preparations containing caffeine (such as *NoDoz*).

Nicotine. Some of the Social Research Group findings for cigarette smoking have already been cited in Part III; they appear below in greater detail.[4]

Status	Men (percentage)	Women (percentage)
Current smokers	43	34
Never smoked	25	51
Ex-smokers	32	15

The paucity of women ex-smokers in the table above is worthy of particular comment. Women smokers, however, smoke fewer cigarettes than men.[5]

Amount	Men (percentage)	Women (percentage)
½ pack per day or less	12	16
About 1 pack per day	19	15
About 1½ packs or more	12	4

The number of cigarettes smoked in the United States in 1970, as noted earlier, totaled 542 *billion.* Thus, while there are far more coffee and tea drinkers in the United States than cigarette smokers, the number of *doses* of nicotine consumed is almost certainly greater than the number of doses of caffeine.

Alcohol. The Parry-Cisin study asked respondents whether they drank alcohol last year, whether their usual drink was wine, beer, or liquor, how often they drank during the year, and how much they drank. The replies were then grouped under six headings.[6]

Consumption	Men (percentage)	Women (percentage)
Did not drink alcohol last year	22	37
Drank very infrequently	8	14
Light drinkers	13	17
Moderate drinkers	21	18
Heavy drinkers	24	11
Very heavy drinkers	10	3

[477]

Sales figures add some details.[7] Almost 18 gallons of beer were consumed during 1969 for every man, woman, and child in the United States. More than a gallon of wine was consumed. And distilled spirits consumption totaled 1.8 gallons per capita.

Beer, as might be expected, is the most popular drink among men; surprisingly, hard liquor is the most popular among women. When asked what alcoholic beverage they *usually* consumed during the past year, respondents answered as follows.[8]

Choice of beverage	Men (percentage)	Women (percentage)
Didn't drink last year	22	37
Mostly beer	41	14
Mostly wine	14	17
Mostly hard liquor	23	31

Psychoactive prescription drugs. Though these drugs show substantial use, the Parry-Cisin data suggest that they hardly compare in popularity with caffeine, nicotine, or alcohol.[9]

First, respondents were asked whether they had used *any* psychoactive prescription drug even once during the past year.

Answer	Men (percentage)	Women (percentage)
Yes	13	29
No	87	71

The greater number of females using these drugs will be commented on below.

Among the users, a substantial proportion of the respondents used psychoactive prescription drugs only occasionally rather than daily.[10]

Frequency of use	Men (percentage)	Women (percentage)
Occasionally	5	12
Daily	7	17

Among the occasional users, moreover, a substantial proportion used psychoactive prescription drugs ten times or less during the year.[11]

Frequency of use	Men (percentage)	Women (percentage)
10 times or less	2	5
11 to 30 times	1	4
31 or more times	2	3

Similarly among the daily users, quite a few used psychoactive prescription drugs daily for less than six months in the year.[12]

Duration of use	Men (percentage)	Women (percentage)
Less than 1 month	1	4
1 month	1	2
2 to 5 months	1	3
6 months or more	4	7

When asked what *kinds* of psychoactive prescription drugs they used during the past year, the user-respondents answered as follows.[13]

Type of drug	Men (percentage)	Women (percentage)
Sedatives and minor tranquilizers	8	20
Stimulants	2	8
Sleeping drugs (hypnotics)	3	4
Antidepressants	2	2

Thus it appears that the use of sedatives and minor tranquilizers by women (20 percent) is the dominant form of psychoactive prescription drug use in the United States.

Finally, the age distribution of users of psychoactive prescription drugs proved of considerable interest. Respondents who had used any psychoactive prescription drug at any time during the previous year were distributed as follows.[14]

Age group	Users (percentage)
18 through 29	15
30 through 44	24
45 through 59	23
60 through 74	27

Frequency of use was also somewhat greater in the older age brackets. Thus 8 percent of those aged sixty through seventy-four reported taking a psychoactive prescription drug daily for six months or more during the previous year as compared with only 2 percent of those aged eighteen through twenty-nine.[15]

The figures above, it must be stressed, apply only to psychoactive drugs *secured on prescription.* When over-the-counter and black-market stimulants, depressants, and tranquilizers are added in (see below) a quite different picture emerges. Further, the figures above should be corrected to allow for underreporting by respondents.[16] This is a point to which we shall return.

Marijuana. This drug, as noted above, has been used at least once by an estimated 12,000,000 to 20,000,000 Americans; annual consumption was estimated in 1970 at five million marijuana cigarettes a day, or 1.8 billion a year. The Parry-Cisin study, together with a study by Dr. Jack Ellinson of the Columbia–Presbyterian Medical Center in New York City, covering young people under the age of eighteen, indicates that age is a major determining factor in marijuana use.[17]

Age group	Ever used marijuana (percentage)
12 through 17	15
18 through 20	19
21 through 24	20
25 through 29	10
30 through 34	4
35 through 74	less than 1

Among respondents aged eighteen to twenty-nine the frequency of use was reported as follows.[18]

Frequency	Percentage
Smoked marijuana 1 to 4 times	7
Smoked marijuana 5 to 49 times	4
Smoked marijuana 50 or more times	5

Other illicit drugs. While the Parry-Cisin study did not cover other illicit drugs such as LSD, heroin, illicit barbiturates, illicit amphetamines, and so on, it is clear from data in earlier chapters (and in the following chapter) that the amounts of those drugs used is trivial compared with the amounts of caffeine, nicotine, alcohol, and marijuana used. One conclusion is thus inescapable: the United States has been focusing an overwhelming proportion of its anxiety and concern on a very small corner of the drug scene.

Another obvious inference to be drawn from the above estimates is that we Americans—like almost all other human cultures, ancient and modern, primitive and civilized—are a drug-using people. Indeed, *Homo sapiens* is a drug-using species, and has been for thousands of years.

A third obvious inference is the relative rarity of non-drug-users in our culture. No estimate has been made of the number of American adults who have *never* used a mind-affecting drug, including caffeine, nicotine, and alcohol—but the number must be very small, a few percent of the population at most. The nonuse of mind-affecting drugs, indeed, can be described as aberrant behavior, deviating from the norms of American society.

Caffeine, nicotine, and alcohol were universally recognized as drugs during the nineteenth century, and were denounced as such. Their treatment as nondrugs today protects them from prohibitionist proposals and other repressive measures; it also enables coffee, tea, and alcohol drinkers, along with cigarette smokers, to decry the widespread use of "drugs."

62.

Prescription, over-the-counter, and black-market drugs

Americans tend to distinguish drugs by the channels through which they are distributed as well as by their chemistry and their pharmacological effects. Three major channels are recognized:

(1) The legal over-the-counter market. This is by far the biggest channel of drug distribution, delivering caffeine, nicotine, and alcohol plus vast quantities of psychoactive drugs sold over the counter in drugstores, supermarkets, and service stations.

(2) The prescription market. This market delivers barbiturates and other sedatives and hypnotics, minor tranquilizers (antianxiety drugs), amphetamines and other stimulants, and antidepression drugs—plus some narcotics. In 1964, 149 million prescriptions (including refills) for psychotherapeutic drugs were filled in American drugstores. During the next six years, such prescriptions increased by about 7 percent a year, to a total of 214 million in 1970.[1] The great bulk of the increase, however, was accounted for by antianxiety drugs, as shown in Figure 13 below. In 1970, minor tranquilizers accounted for 38.8 percent of all psychotherapeutic drug prescriptions and refills, hypnotics ("sleeping pills") 17.5 percent, stimulants 13.2 percent, sedatives 11.1 percent, and antidepressants 9.2 percent. The remaining 10.2 percent were for antipsychotic drugs (major tranquilizers), not covered in this Report.

(3) The black market. This route of distribution handles marijuana chiefly, plus relatively small amounts of LSD and LSD-like drugs, amphetamines and other stimulants, barbiturates and other depressants, heroin and other opiates, and bootleg alcohol.

How many people secure their stimulants, depressants, and tranquilizers by prescription? Over the counter? From the black market? Fresh light is thrown on these questions by the data assembled in another portion of the NIMH "Psychotropic Drug Study"—that under the direction of Drs. Manheimer, Mellinger, and Balter.

"In 1967-68 several polling studies of the Gallup type—including two that we were involved in—indicated that during the previous year 25 percent of adult Americans had used some psychotropic drug, either a prescription or over-the-counter preparation," Dr. Balter of the NIMH reports. "We now have good reason to believe that this figure of 25 percent is low. Through fortunate circumstances we have been able to

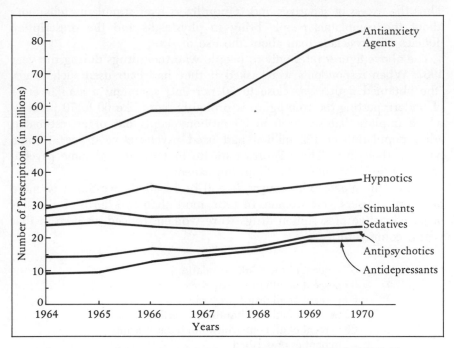

FIGURE 13. Psychotherapeutic Drugs: Prescriptions Filled in U.S. Drug Stores (1964–1970)[2]

do some validity studies on the polling type of approach and find it to be quite a bit in error in the direction of underreporting. If one adjusts for probable error of underreporting, the figures for 1967 would range between 33 and 35 percent, which translates into 35–40 million people."[3]

The most popular psychoactive drugs, the same surveys show, are the antianxiety drugs (minor tranquilizers). Next came the sedatives and hypnotics, and then the stimulants and antidepression drugs. (Some people of course, take drugs of more than one type.)

Some 75 to 80 percent of the psychoactive drugs prescribed by physicians in private practice, Dr. Balter notes, "were prescribed for the purposes of sedation, tranquility and sleep. Americans, in the main, at least those [who] visit physicians, come with problems that require calming down; it's peace that is desired, it's tranquility or sleep that is being sought. Only 20 to 25 percent of the prescriptions involved called for drugs that produce an increase in energy or elevation of mood. From these data it appears that the major American malady is tension or agitation rather than depression."[4] As will be shown below, however, stimulants from nonprescription sources substantially alter these proportions.

Thus the excess of sedatives and tranquilizers over stimulants tells more about the complaints people bring to physicians and the prescription policies of physicians than about the use of drugs.

The above figures refer only to people who took drugs during the year 1967. When respondents were asked if they had *ever* used such drugs, "the obtained figure was close to 50 percent; assuming a similar error of underreporting the true figure is probably more like 60 to 70 percent, which implies that some 80 to 90 million people out of an estimated adult population of 122 million had used psychoactive drugs at some point in their lives. These figures indicate that the use of some psychoactive drug is the rule rather than the exception." [5]

During the nineteenth century, it will be recalled, two-thirds or more of all opiate users were women. In 1967, more than two-thirds of all users of psychoactive prescription drugs were women. Indeed, women in that year accounted for: [6]

> 53 percent of the adult population
> 59 percent of all visits to doctors
> 60 percent of all drugs prescribed
> 63 percent of all barbiturates prescribed
> 66 percent of all nonbarbiturate sedatives and
>   hypnotics prescribed
> 68 percent of all antianxiety drugs (minor
>   tranquilizers) prescribed
> 68 percent of all psychoactive drugs prescribed
> 71 percent of all antidepressants prescribed
> 80 percent of all amphetamines prescribed

"As you move toward drugs used to treat the more frankly psychological or functional disorders," Dr. Balter notes, "you get an increasingly higher proportion of the drug prescriptions going to females." [7] If *nonprescription* stimulants, depressants, and tranquilizers are added in, however, the male-female ratios change, as we shall show below.

There are also clear-cut differences in psychoactive drug prescriptions between the young and the middle-aged. "Amphetamines are typically used by the younger age groups," Dr. Balter points out, "with the peak between 20 and 49.

Some 65% of all the amphetamine prescriptions go to people in this age range. However, there are marked male and female differences. Interestingly enough, prescribing of amphetamines for females reaches a relatively high level at age 20, stays relatively constant until age 49, and then drops off rather sharply. Prescribing of amphetamines for males shows a progressive increase until about age 40, stays constant between 40 and 49, and then drops off rapidly. With respect to male-female age differences on the amphetamines there's a real question whether we're dealing with esthetics, obesity, incidence of other medical problems, or a differential disposition to come to the physician with certain problems at various ages. The tranquilizers are mid-life drugs, that are frequently prescribed for ages 30 to 59. They have a relatively flat distribution, with a major peak in use between 40 and 60. Sedatives are popular in late middle age and show a steady increase into the 60's. Sleeping pills, which have a similar pattern, are infrequently prescribed to people under 30. At age 40, we begin to see a sharp increase in their use.

In a [1967] polling study in California, which covered the entire state, we found that men had a particularly clear-cut pattern of drug use: stimulants in the 30's; tranquilizers in the 40's and 50's; sedatives and hypnotics in the 60's. If these data reflect stresses in life and the distribution of problems and needs in the population at large, ours is a highly patterned, if not morbidly predictable existence.[8]

For the use of psychoactive prescription drugs among men and women aged sixty-five or older, we must turn to a study made by the United States Department of Health, Education, and Welfare's Task Force on Prescription Drugs. That study indicates that during the year 1966, the average American aged sixty-five or older secured 3.6 prescriptions for psychoactive drugs during the year—a higher rate than the rate for adults under sixty-five.[9] And a substantial proportion of the psychoactive drugs they use are the very same drugs that young people purchase on the black market—narcotics, barbiturates, and amphetamines. The study makes it clear that Americans aged sixty-five and older rarely have to patronize the black market for drugs; they can and do secure substantial supplies of psychoactive drugs on prescription at pharmacies.

Much more detailed information concerning the people who use various types of psychoactive drugs, and where they get them, was obtained as part of the NIMH project by interviewing 1,026 Californians aged twenty-one and over—a carefully selected cross-section of the state's noninstitutionalized residents. This survey was concerned with stimulants, sedatives, and tranquilizers taken on prescription, purchased over the counter, or secured from friends or in other ways—for example, on the black market.

A respondent will answer in one way if asked to name the stimulants, sedatives, or tranquilizers he has ever used. He may answer quite differently if asked to name the drugs he has used *within the past twelve months*—and give yet another answer if asked which drugs he uses *frequently*. Californians were asked all three questions. The percentages are given below.[10]

Category	Ever	Past 12 months	Frequently
Stimulants	19	9	6
Sedatives	29	16	7
Tranquilizers	29	19	10
Any of the above	51	29	17

As in the national studies, women mentioned almost twice as many drugs as men in the California study. "The greater use of drugs by women contrasts sharply with the available evidence regarding drinking," [11] the survey group noted. Just as in the nineteenth century, when women took opiates at home while their husbands drank liquor in saloons, so in California in 1967, women took prescribed stimulants, sedatives, and especially tranquilizers at home.

Marital status, it turned out, had a marked effect on drug use: "Eighteen percent of those who are divorced or separated say they have used tranquilizers frequently, as compared with 10 percent of married persons and only 3 percent of those who are single. These findings are consistent with studies showing that divorced members of our society have a disproportionate share of physical and mental health problems. Although they seldom use tranquilizers, single persons are close to the overall average in their use of stimulants and sedatives. Persons who are widowed tend to use sedatives somewhat more often than others—a reflection, perhaps, of their older age." [12]

Yet another feature of the NIMH-funded "Psychotropic Drug Study" was a survey conducted late in 1967 and early in 1968 of a cross-section of San Francisco residents aged eighteen or over—1,104 of them. One finding concerned the very widespread use of over-the-counter psychoactive drugs. About 12 percent of all drugs mentioned by respondents, for example, were over-the-counter stimulants such as *NoDoz* (caffeine), 11 percent were over-the-counter sleeping pills such as *Sominex* or *Sleep-Eze*, and 5 percent were over-the-counter tranquilizers such as *Compoz*. Of all the mentions of psychoactive drugs by respondents in the sample, 28 percent were over-the-counter proprietary remedies.[13]

A substantial proportion of respondents used *both* prescription and over-the-counter drugs. The preponderance of women using psychoactive drugs was more evident for prescription drugs than for over-the-counter drugs.

By far the most remarkable finding of the San Francisco study, however, concerned the existence of a substantial "gray market" as well as a black market in psychoactive drugs.

Most people think of a prescription drug as one that is prescribed for an individual patient by a physician and is taken solely by that patient. But in the San Francisco study 27 per cent of the prescription psychoactive drugs most recently used were obtained through informal ("gray-market") channels. In 17 percent of the cases the informal channel was a friend. The user's spouse was mentioned much less frequently (3 percent), and in most of these cases it was the wife, not the husband, who was the informal supplier. The remaining informal sources were divided about equally between relatives and other miscellaneous persons.[14]

The non-medical source mentioned most often [Dr. Mellinger reports] is someone described by the respondent as "a friend." In most cases, this designation can probably be taken at face value. Respondents often described the friend as a roommate, a boy friend or girl friend, and so on. In other cases, the relationship of the friend to the respondent was not quite so clear. We were curious, naturally, about the possibility that the friend might be "the friendly neighborhood pusher." However, other parts of the interview were really more important for our purposes, so we resisted the temptation to ask respondents to be more explicit. In short, I cannot tell you how many of these drugs were obtained through truly illegal channels. Suffice it to say that a good many of the prescription drugs are being obtained through channels that we can at least describe as "informal." [15]

Who are the people who secure their psychoactive drugs through these "informal" or "gray-market" channels? Though women use more psychoactive drugs than men do, men are much more inclined to rely on informal channels for obtaining their prescription drugs. Thus 41 percent of the prescription psychoactive drugs used by men were obtained through such channels, as compared with 20 percent of the prescription psychoactive drugs used by women.

Young people, the San Francisco survey also indicates, are much more likely to secure their psychoactive prescription drugs through "informal" channels, without a prescription. Here are the figures: [16] under thirty, 51 percent; thirty to forty-four years old, 24 percent; forty-five and older, 10 percent.

If both age and sex are considered together, the figures are even more startling. For example, 69 percent of all psychoactive prescription drugs secured by males under thirty were secured without a prescription!

These figures clearly suggest the progressive breakdown of the distinction society has tried to draw between psychoactive drugs secured on prescription (good) and psychoactive drugs secured in other ways (bad). The generation under thirty (at least those polled in San Francisco) simply refuses to abide by this distinction; a majority of them secure their psychoactive prescription drugs without bothering about a prescription.

The Parry-Cisin studies indicate a much lower use of prescription drugs without a prescription in their *national* sample. In many respects, however, San Francisco drug use in one year tends to foreshadow patterns that become visible elsewhere a few years later.

What will the picture be a decade or two hence? Will the generation now under thirty, as it matures, change its ways? Or is the securing of psychoactive drugs on prescription a fading custom, likely to decline further as prescription-users die off and nonprescription cohorts take their place? Indeed, are we only one generation away from defining the amphetamines, the barbiturates, the tranquilizers (and perhaps also marijuana) as nondrugs, like caffeine, nicotine, and alcohol?

A closely related question also arises: will the present generation of young people, who use most of the stimulants, continue to use stimulants as they age—or will they shift first to tranquilizers and then to sedatives like their elders today? Only time will tell—and only time will tell whether a new generation of physicians, who have themselves been using stimulant drugs, will be more willing to prescribe these drugs to their patients than today's physicians are. (No study has been found of the relative proportion of sedatives, tranquilizers, and stimulants prescribed by young, middle-aged, and elderly physicians.) In any event, the relative unwillingness of today's physicians to prescribe stimulants may be one of the reasons why young people, especially young males, are securing these drugs primarily over the counter, or from the "gray market," or from the black market.

Another reason why so high a proportion of prescription drugs are secured without a prescription may be simple consumer economics. Many prescription drugs—especially the barbiturates and the amphetamines—are quite inexpensive at wholesale. Here are some typical 1970 wholesale prices, as presented by Dr. Richard Burack in his *New Handbook of Prescription Drugs*: [17]

Drug	Strength	Price
Dextroamphetamine sulfate, U.S.P.	5-milligram tablets	$0.70 to $3.36 per thousand tablets
Sodium pentobarbital, U.S.P.	100-milligram capsules	$3.20 to $8.88 per thousand capsules
Sodium secobarbital, U.S.P.	100-milligram capsules	$4.00 to $12.36 per thousand capsules

Those wholesale prices, it should be noted, already include a considerable markup above the manufacturers' prices. When a patient secures such drugs on prescription, however, several factors combine to increase the cost.

In the first place, many physicians prescribe a heavily promoted drug by brand name rather than by generic name. The price ranges above are for generic-name drugs. If a physician specifies the Dexedrine brand of dextroamphetamine sulfate in a prescription, its cost reflects a wholesale price of $22.60 per thousand tablets.[18] Sodium pentobarbital under the brand name Nembutal carries a wholesale price of $16.20 per thousand capsules;[19] the Pulvule brand of the same drug commands a wholesale price of $22.50 per thousand capsules.[20] The wholesale price for a thousand capsules of the Seconal brand of sodium secobarbital is $18.30.[21]

Next, most pharmacies have a minimum charge for a prescription—often two or three dollars, sometimes more. On drugs such as the U.S.P. amphetamines and barbiturates, this minimum may multiply the wholesale cost per thousand many times over. A $3.00 charge for 50 dextro-amphetamine tablets on prescription is not unusual; the wholesale price of those 50 tablets, in lots of 1,000, is somewhere between 3½ and 17 cents.

Also, the purchaser who buys on prescription must often pay the physician a fee. Sometimes the prescription is refillable; sometimes it is not. Even if it is refillable, the total cost of the prescription plus the physician's fee is likely to be as high as, or higher than, the price of the same drug on the black market. And there is no long wait in the physician's reception room followed by a trip to the drugstore when you buy on the black market.

Another reason why some young people secure psychoactive prescription drugs without first securing a prescription is that they just don't like doctors. They may either know from experience or suspect on general principles that if *they* were to ask for the psychoactive drugs their parents are taking, they would be turned down—perhaps gently, perhaps brusquely, perhaps angrily.

These lines of thought suggest that American medicine may be facing a crisis, or rather, failing to face it. Many members of the generation now entering maturity in San Francisco have formed the habit of securing their psychoactive drugs—a substantial proportion of all drugs—without bothering to obtain a prescription. If the habit continues as these young people mature, and if it spreads across the country, the psychoactive prescription drugs will inevitably become "nondrugs," rather than continuing to be considered medicines for which one turns to a physician.

The fact that American physicians are currently writing some 260,000,-000 psychoactive-drug prescriptions a year raises the question: are they overprescribing these drugs? Perhaps they are. But the figures cited above, and the existence of booming black and gray markets in psychoactive prescription drugs, suggests that they may simultaneously be *underprescribing* certain drugs to certain patients—particularly the stimulants, and particularly for the needs of the young. The result is *not* to curtail the use of psychoactive drugs by young people. Rather, the clear effect is to increase the use of such drugs by young people *without medical supervision.*

It is possible to argue that the use of prescription drugs, even under medical supervision, constitutes a national peril and should be discouraged.* It is equally possible to argue that tens of millions of patients would not continue to take these drugs, and pay vast sums for them, if they did not serve a useful purpose; and that physicians would not continue to prescribe them, despite the many hazards, if they did not perceive substantial benefits to their patients. The issue need not here be decided. The important point from the perspective of this Report is that the use of "good drugs"—prescribed sedatives, hypnotics, and antianxiety drugs (minor tranquilizers), and prescribed stimulants and antidepression drugs—constitutes an essential feature of the American drug scene, along with the "nondrugs" (caffeine, nicotine, alcohol) and the "bad drugs" (marijuana, LSD, the black-market barbiturates, the black-market amphetamines, and the black-market narcotics). The goal of a sound national policy must be to maximize the benefits and minimize the hazards of *all* psychoactive drugs rather than to single out for condemnation a handful of drugs that happen at the moment to be illicit and to be attracting the wavering spotlight of public hostility.

This, in brief, is how the drug scene of the 1970s looks through a panoramic lens. In the chapters that follow, we shall focus more closely on a small segment of the panorama—the *youth* drug scene.

---

* Even where the prescribed drugs are clearly doing harm, however, the question must be asked whether, without the drugs, even more devastating consequences might not follow—alcoholism, disruption of family relationships, child abuse, loss of job, mental hospitalization, suicide, etc.

63.

The Haight-Ashbury, its predecessors and its satellites

During the 1960s, young people in substantial numbers—most of them middle-class and white—migrated to the Haight-Ashbury district in San Francisco. Adopting strange hair and clothing styles, they rejected the platitudes of their parents and of the "square" communities from which they came, coining unconventional platitudes of their own. The mass media called them *hippies*. A major feature of the hippie life-style was the use of illicit drugs—many different illicit drugs.

Nothing quite like this, it was commonly believed, had ever happened before—but that belief was mistaken. The "youth drug scene" of the 1960s was a continuation, under a new name and with minor changes in external style, of a continuing social process. Even in external appearance, the hippies of the 1960s—and the Beatniks of a decade earlier—markedly resembled the "Bohemians" who made their first appearance in Paris in the 1840s, founding a movement that spread to the United States. Male Bohemians, like male hippies, let their hair grow long; they and their female counterparts dressed in a manner deemed uncouth by the *bourgeoisie*. Bohemians lived in poverty in attics resembling today's hippie "pads." They held unconventional philosophies and flaunted unorthodox sexual mores.

The Timothy Leary of the Bohemian movement was Henri Murger (1822-1861), a Parisian whose *Scènes de la vie de Bohème* (1848) established and popularized the Bohemian life-style; but Murger's greatest influence, and the peak popularity of Bohemianism, came after 1898—when Puccini's opera *La Bohème*, based on Murger's *Scènes*, achieved worldwide renown.

Like today's hippies, the turn-of-the-century Bohemians were conspicuously drug-oriented. One of the drugs that the Bohemians (like their elders) used was alcohol. Murger himself became an alcoholic at an early age, and died in a sanitarium at the age of thirty-nine. In addition to alcohol, the Bohemians used coffee. They drank vast quantities of this stimulant, were preoccupied with coffee, and suffered coffee as well as alcohol hangovers. Respectable citizens of that era were as horrified by the Bohemian coffee cult as today's respectable citizens are horrified by marijuana smoking. Eminent scientists, it will be recalled, echoed this horror; for it was at the height of the Bohemian coffee cult that the public was being warned: "The sufferer [from coffee addiction] is tremulous and loses his self-command; he is subject to fits of agitation and depression. He loses color and has a haggard appearance. . . . As with other such agents, a renewed dose of the poison gives temporary relief, but at the cost of future misery." [1]

The Haight-Ashbury of the 1960s also resembled New York City's Greenwich Village of the 1920s, another center to which rebellious young people migrated. In the Greenwich Village era, it was the short, "boyish-bobbed" hair of the girls (rather than the long hair of the boys) along with their miniskirts, lipstick, and breastless "John Held, Jr." silhouettes, that shocked society. Necking, petting, and nonmarital sexual adventures were widely publicized features of the Greenwich Village scene and lifestyle.

The Greenwich Village subculture of the 1920s featured two drugs. One of them was alcohol. During the Prohibition years, socially rebellious young people from all over the United States thronged Greenwich Village's illicit "speakeasies" to drink "bootleg" liquor. The fact that young *women* were getting drunk in public, and could be seen staggering out of speakeasies at all hours (for a part of the cost of Prohibition was an end to the enforcement of legal closing hours) added to the popular revulsion.

The other Greenwich Village drug habit that deeply outraged the respectable was cigarette smoking. In 1921, it will be recalled, cigarettes were illegal in fourteen states and 92 anticigarette bills were pending in twenty-eight states. Smoking cigarettes in speakeasies and other public places was almost as alarming to some respectable members of society as engaging in nonmarital sexual encounters. Young women (Edna St. Vincent Millay among them) were expelled from college for smoking cigarettes much as in the 1960s young women were expelled for smoking marijuana.

In each generation, moreover, the drug-subculture phenomenon was not limited to the Bohemian Quarter of Paris, to Greenwich Village in New York, or to Haight-Ashbury in San Francisco. "Little Bohemias," patterned on Murger's Parisian original, could be found all over the Western world—including American cities from New York to California. Similarly, bush-league Greenwich Villages sprang up throughout the country during the 1920s, and bush-league Haight-Ashburys followed in the 1960s. These deviant youth cultures, characterized by bizarre clothing, unconventional hair styles, sexual nonconformity, and illicit or "bad" drug use, were not only national but international. London, Stockholm, Copenhagen, Amsterdam, Rotterdam, Montreal, Vancouver—all have hippie neighborhoods.

Finally, each of these life-styles also attracted "internal migrants," who patterned themselves on the deviant youth-drug-cult style of life without actually leaving home. Retired schoolteachers now in their seventies can no doubt remember the early 1920s, when almost every high school, even in Iowa and Kansas, had its "Greenwich Village crowd"—drinking bootleg alcohol, smoking cigarettes, "necking," "petting," reading the *American Mercury,* and writing poetry, to the distress of respectable citizens. Today, many (perhaps most) high schools have their pot-smoking, acid-dropping deviant youth subcultures composed of "internal migrants" who stay at home. In what follows, references to "youth-drug-scene migrants" will include these internal migrants.

What happened to rebellious young people in between these luridly publicized waves of youth-culture migration and internal migration? While the available evidence is sparse, it suggests that essentially the same process continued, on a smaller scale, with less flamboyance and less popular alarm. Every large city in the nineteenth and early twentieth century had its crowded, rundown "roominghouse district," sheltering not only its alcoholics, brothels, and streetwalkers but also youthful migrants in large numbers. Young artists, young writers, and young musicians— along with even larger numbers of would-be artists, writers, and musicians —flocked to these "Skid Roads," "Tenderloins," and "red-light districts." While prostitution was generally limited to such neighborhoods, only rarely were the red-light districts limited to prostitution. Low rents and the sense of freedom and adventure attracted countless youthful migrants to the same areas. Many eminent Americans, such as Stephen Crane, Theodore Dreiser, and Ben Hecht, participated in this scene. The drugs in most common use were usually alcohol and nicotine—though youthful deviants at times (as noted above) also turned to opium smoking and to cocaine, morphine, heroin, or a combination of such drugs.

The use here of the term *deviant* should not be deemed a value judgment; it is a purely descriptive term. In any generation, a majority of young people tend to follow the path marked out for them by the society in which they find themselves. A minority deviate from this path. One group, for example, drops out of junior high school; another group continues through graduate school. Both groups, in this context, are *deviants* from the usual path.

During the nineteenth and early twentieth century, sermons, newspapers, and sensational popular fiction were the chief media informing young people of the perils of Bohemias and of roominghouse and red-light districts—and incidentally publicizing their precise locations. The movies added their influence during the Greenwich Village era. The TV screen, the popular musicians and singers, and the mass media *en masse* played a generally similar role in publicizing the youth drug scene during the 1960s—and with similar results. It is hard to say whether romantic glorifications of such scenes or moralistic warnings against their perils contribute more to attracting rebellious young people to them.

In all eras, law enforcement has also played a crucial role in publicizing Greenwich Villages and Haight-Ashburys. The periodic nineteenth-century "vice squad" crackdowns on roominghouse and red-light districts, the Prohibition agents' raids on speakeasies during the 1920s, and the multitudinous drug raids by narcotics agents during the 1960s—each wave of raids accompanied by a wave of sensational publicity, and by pictures of young people defiantly confronting the police—added to the glamor of the youth cult centers, and made it certain that even the naïvest teenager in the remotest country village knew (and currently knows) precisely where to go and approximately how to behave, including what drugs to try, when he or she reaches the scene.

Against this briefly sketched historical background (let us hope future social historians will fill in the details), the current youth drug scene can perhaps be more objectively understood and evaluated.

One potentially fruitful way to view the youth drug scene today, like the Bohemias, roominghouse districts, and Greenwich Villages of earlier generations, is as a *competing* way of life. Such scenes compete with conventional institutions and life-styles for the allegiance of each youthful generation. The more young people find unattractive the way of life mandated by their elders at any moment in time, the more they are likely to run off, or wander off, or embark on an internal migration toward what appear to be greener pastures.

A curious fact about deviant youth subcultures must next be noted. *In each generation, respectable society itself dictates the direction that much of the deviance will take.* During alcohol Prohibition, for example, hostility was focused on alcohol—and it was alcohol that rebellious young people drank. Through the 1960s, society dictated *drug* deviance to young people, and that was the path youthful deviants followed.

This concept of *dictated deviance* can best be understood through a prototype example. Consider the anxious parents who keep watch over their unmarried teen-age daughter for fear the daughter will become pregnant out of wedlock. The parents harp on dire warnings of the perils of illicit intercourse, accompanied by emotion-laden accusations and predictions: "Where were you all evening? Whom were you out with? Why weren't you home on time? You're going to get yourself pregnant and ruin your life and ours—we can see it all coming."

The daughter gets the message loud and clear: "If you want to get even with your parents (or with society in general) for grievances real or imagined, the best way is to get yourself pregnant." The peril becomes a lure, and the prophecy proves self-fulfilling. In almost precisely this way, society as a whole dictated drug use as the dominant mode of deviance for disaffected young people during the 1960s. "Watch your step. Be careful. We can see it all coming. You're going to start smoking marijuana and progress to heroin. You're going to end up a hippie!"

No doubt a few years in a nineteenth-century Bohemia or in Greenwich Village in the 1920s contributed positively to the maturing of many young people of those generations. Certainly a number of distinguished writers, artists, musicians, even philosophers, came through such deviant youth scenes. Whether the same will prove true of contemporary Haight-Ashburys remains to be seen.

There can be little doubt, however, that future histories of music will cite the youth drug scene of the 1960s as one of the transforming influences on musical development. Whether psychedelic art will similarly survive seems less certain. Future histories of religious mysticism may well hail the current Haight-Ashburys as the sites of a major religious resurgence comparable to New England Transcendentalism in the days of Emerson and Thoreau. Canada's Le Dain Commission in particular has stressed this possibility:

We have been profoundly impressed by the natural and unaffected manner in which drug users have responded to the question of religious significance. They are not embarrassed by the mention of God. Indeed, as Paul Goodman has observed, their reactions are in interesting contrast to those of the "God is dead" theologian. It may be an exaggeration to say that we are witnessing the manifestations of a genuine religious revival, but there does appear to be a definite revival of interest in the religious or spiritual attitude towards life. As one drug user put it: "The whole culture is saying, 'Where is God?' I don't believe in your institutions, but now I know it's there someplace." Another witness said, "I just find that a lot of people are becoming a lot more aware of what's happening and joining in on a universal cause, a cosmic sort of joyousness and people are getting interested in spiritual things as well, because this is what our generation and the previous generations have lacked. . . ." [2]

Society's evaluation of today's Haight-Ashburys may ultimately be raised, as the accepted evaluation of the Greenwich Villages of the 1920s has already been raised. For now, many view the youth drug scene as an unmitigated evil and want to know what can be done about it. Three suggestions arise out of the above analysis.

First, a good way to lessen the likelihood that young people will migrate to the youth dug scene, or to any other form of social deviance, is to make the conventional pattern of life back home more attractive and challenging to young people—better able to compete with the deviant alternatives.

Second, a good way to decrease the likelihood that young people will select the youth drug scene rather than some other mode of deviance is to turn off the propaganda and the warnings that center so much attention on drugs—and thereby in effect dictate *drug* deviance.

Third, the number of participants in the youth drug scene at any moment depends only in part on how many young people enter it; the other determining factor is how many graduate from it and how soon they graduate. Thus one way to curb the Haight-Ashburys, large and small, is to keep the door wide open so that drug users can emerge from the scene. Indeed, affirmative steps can be taken to encourage and facilitate emergence. We shall review these possibilities in more detail in Chapter 67.

64.

Why a youth <u>drug</u> scene?

If the view is accepted, at least tentatively, that each generation spawns a larger or smaller proportion of deviant young people, and that these young people through the decades have sought for and found a deviant scene and life-style, complete with their own costume, hair styles, drugs, and sexual mores, a further question arises: why do *drugs* play so central a role in the currently dominant pattern of deviance?

The data are not yet available for a definitive answer. But a few factors are already clearly visible. The first concerns, not the deviant scene itself, but one's perception of it. Throughout the past century, society has tended to focus its dismay on two areas of youthful behavior—drugs and sex—and to condemn deviance from generally accepted standards in either area. In recent years, while still on occasion deploring sexual non-conformity, society appears to be much more concerned with illicit drug use among deviant subcultures.

Again, young people discovered during the 1960s that the conventional drug sequence prescribed by society—from caffeine and nicotine to alcohol—is not an inexorable law of nature. As discussed earlier, many young people had excellent reasons for seeking alternatives to alcohol. The use of other drugs by some young people in the 1960s can thus be viewed as a well-intentioned effort to escape the evils of alcohol.

LSD and marijuana were the first alternatives to alcohol to be widely publicized. Once freedom of choice and black markets were established, however, the spectrum broadened enormously. Young people, white and middle-class, began to experiment with a wide variety of different drugs—including, after about 1969, heroin. Unfortunately, that concept of choice and that experimentation arose at precisely the time when this country's antidrug propaganda was furthest out of touch with reality and therefore least credible.

To sum up, national drug policy throughout the 1960s contributed to the rise of the current youth drug scene in at least four major ways. First, by emphasizing "drug abuse," it virtually dictated youthful *drug* deviance rather than other forms of deviance. Second, by publicizing marijuana, LSD and LSD-like drugs, the amphetamines and other stimulants, the barbiturates and other depressants, and the opiates as well, these pronouncements informed an entire generation of the broad range of mind-affecting drugs from which a choice could be made. Third, for many the warnings actually served as lures. And finally, the supposed facts provided to inform and guide young people turned loose in the contemporary illicit-drug supermarket were almost invariably incredible, in conflict with everyday experience. Hence young people were left to flounder along without guidance they could trust—to learn by their own trials and errors and those of their peers.

The errors young drug users made, of course, were numerous—and some of them were tragic. This we all now know. But the extent to which well-meant, sincere, but disastrous antidrug policies contributed to the tragedies is still only vaguely perceived, or not perceived at all.

65.

First steps toward a solution: innovative approaches by indigenous institutions

Young people have many problems, whether or not they use drugs. They get sick and need medical care. They get toothaches and need a dentist. They get in trouble and need a lawyer. They get lonesome and need friends, plus a place to meet with their friends. They need food and a place to sleep. They get confused and need wise counseling. In addition, if they use drugs imprudently, their problems may become more complex.

The first waves of youthful migrants to Haight-Ashbury in San Francisco, to the East Village of New York City, and to the other youth drug scenes during the 1960s brought with them their full share of such problems, and acquired new ones in the drug scene. To help them with these problems, indigenous institutions arose—centers that were themselves a part of the drug scene, and that were established to meet the needs of drug-scene participants rather than the needs of the "square" society outside. Some of the institutions were staffed by ex-drug users (some of whom might still smoke marijuana on occasion); others were founded by sensitive adults who recognized hippies as human beings with many human needs.

The indigenous service agencies set up to help drug users are so numerous and so varied as almost to defy description. We shall here describe, accordingly, only a few significant prototypes. We shall consider them at some length and with great seriousness, however; for out of these youth-oriented service centers there are currently emerging both the first reliable insights into the nature of the deviant youth drug subculture and the most hopeful approaches toward solving the manifold problems of illicit drug use. In contrast to high-sounding policy formulations at the national level, the drug scene's indigenous institutions are evolving policies out of their day-by-day confrontation with the practical problems of today's young people, including but not limited to their problems with drugs. When effective approaches to this country's "drug crisis" are ultimately adopted, they will almost certainly include solutions currently being pioneered by these informal, loosely organized, and apparently haphazard local institutions within the drug scene itself.

"Switchboards" and "hot lines." During San Francisco's 1967 "Summer of Love," when adolescent "flower people" descended upon the city from

all over the United States, a young resident of the Haight-Ashbury named Al Rinker realized that there was an urgent need for a primitive communication system—a place where young migrants could get answers to pressing questions:

"I'm sick; how do I get to a doctor?"

"I'm broke. Where can I get a pad for tonight? A hot meal? A bath?"

"I'm pregnant; now what do I do?"

"My girl friend has just slashed her wrists. Help!"

Parents, too, needed a communications center:

"Where can I find my daughter? She's fifteen, has red hair, and wears lavender-tinted glasses."

"Can you find my son and tell him his mother died last night?"

In an effort to meet such needs, young Rinker publicized his personal telephone number in the underground press and elsewhere; calls promptly came pouring in. Volunteers, some of them drug users, helped him man the phone around the clock. Friends contributed small sums of money. Additional phone lines were installed. The service moved to larger quarters in the Haight-Ashbury. Thus arose one of the first and most urgently needed of the indigenous drug-scene institutions, the San Francisco Switchboard. Similar "hot lines" were soon in operation in other drug centers. Today there are several hundred hot lines, at a rough estimate, operating in towns as small as 20,000 as well as in most large cities. The best of them are concerned not only with drug problems but with the countless other problems young people today confront.

"Rap centers" and "crash pads." Alcohol drinkers have countless places to meet, talk, and drink—saloons, taverns, cocktail lounges, roadhouses, and night clubs, to mention only a few. The first migrants to the youth drug scenes had only their overcrowded pads and the streets. Help soon came, however, from a limited number of broad-minded churches, neighborhood centers, libraries, and other helping agencies, which set up "rap centers" where young people could meet, talk, rest, listen to music, escape from the streets. Some rap centers took the form of coffeehouses, others adopted other patterns. Many, not all, have rules against using illicit drugs on the premises; * all or nearly all have rules against dealing in illicit drugs on the premises.

---

* A number of cities in the United States and other countries have also tolerated places—sometimes called "coffeehouses"—where young drug users can congregate and smoke marijuana; but these are not subsidized public agencies. "Turning on" has been similarly tolerated at some rock-music festivals and other large-scale youth gatherings. The city of Amsterdam in the Netherlands has gone considerably further; it has made available public buildings and subsidies from tax funds for "rap centers" and music centers (such as the widely publicized Paradiso) where marijuana and hashish are publicly smoked. Many visitors to Amsterdam are amazed by this tolerance. One explanation is that city officials want to keep young people off the streets; another possible

"Crash pads"—that is, rooms with cots or at least mattresses where young migrants can spend a night or two—have similarly sprung up within the drug scene, in association with hot lines and rap centers or independently, sponsored by churches and other helping institutions or founded by drug users themselves. The rap centers and crash pads may be staffed by concerned volunteers, or they may boast a paid (minimally paid) staff of "indigenous nonprofessionals."

The useful functions of these centers are numerous. For one thing, they serve as news centers where young people can find out what is going on. (The scene is rarely the same from one season to another; new drugs, new ways of using and misusing them, and new nondrug problems are constantly turning up.) The centers also disseminate important information—such as warnings against a fresh shipment of worthless drugs, or of especially damaging drugs. Again, these centers are the places where peer standards are generated and peer pressures applied. The pot smoker who stays stoned all day, for example, or the "head" who drops acid too often, or the "speed freak" who shoots too much amphetamine over too long a period, or who engages in other forms of self-defeating, group-endangering behavior, can here be called to account by his fellow drug users.

Such peer pressures within the drug scene are far more effective than official or educational warnings. They do not, it is true, work miracles. They do not convert a compulsive drug user into a total abstainer. But neither does the conventional warning: "If you take LSD, you'll end up in a mental hospital." The goal of the rap centers, crash pads, and other indigenous drug-scene institutions is to *minimize the damage* done to young people by drugs and by other adverse influences. This goal, however modest, has at least the merit of being achievable.

The need for meeting places for young people was set forth in a speech by Canada's Minister of Health John Munro before the British Columbia Medical Association on October 5, 1970:

Most of all, drop-in centers—drug-free, harassment-free spots where young people can come around to mix and talk with people whom they consider their brothers and sisters—are an absolute must. Many people feel that their development should go hand in hand with the erection of the proposed national hostelling network.[1]

---

motive may be a desire to strengthen the marijuana-hashish culture at the expense of the opiate culture, the amphetamine culture, perhaps even the alcohol culture. Perhaps, too, Amsterdam's city fathers genuinely want to help meet the needs of young people as they try to meet the needs of other segments of the population. The fact that Amsterdam's young people have their own political party and elect their own representatives to the city council is probably also relevant. It is possible that the recent lowering of the voting age to eighteen here in the United States may have similar results.

This Munro speech, quoted further below, is particularly important because it demonstrates how a wholly new approach to the problem of illicit drugs, replacing traditional methods of repression, can be made *politically* palatable to voters. The *Canadian Medical Association Journal,* which called it "one of the most forceful and understanding speeches of [Munro's] political career," reprinted it at length in its November 7, 1970, issue.

"Crisis intervention centers." Young drug users, like other human beings, young and old, face crises from time to time. A crisis may be drug-related —an LSD "bad trip," for example, or a "crash" following a prolonged "speed run." Or a crisis may be simple exhaustion due to sleeplessness and malnutrition rather than drugs. Again, the presenting symptom may be mental depression, drug-associated or not; such depressions can reach suicidal intensity among young people as well as older people, among abstainers as well as drug users.

Such crises outside the drug scene are ordinarily handled by the emergency rooms of local hospitals; and before the rise of the indigenous drug-scene institutions we are describing, participants in the youth drug scene also tried the hospital emergency rooms. They also sought help at first from established clinics, welfare agencies, social work organizations, and other helping institutions. With some notable exceptions, however, these agencies proved poorly adapted to the needs of youth-drug-scene participants.

Many established agencies tended to view the crisis as essentially a *drug* problem, and sought to solve it by persuading the young patient or client to abstain from drugs altogether. Young drug users responded by walking out and staying away.

Many established agencies at first disapproved of the hippies' hair style, costume, sex mores, and style of life generally—and did not hesitate to make their disapproval known. Young long-hairs responded by staying away.

Many hospital emergency rooms and other established agencies asked questions and adhered to rules and regulations. Many refused to serve minors, for example, without written parental consent. Proof of local residence was also often required. Many participants in the youth drug scene were both minors and migrants; they responded to the questions and regulations by simply staying away.

Many established agencies felt called upon (as required by some state laws) to report drug users to the police. Once such police reports were made, the grapevine spread the news—and young drug users stayed away.

The youthful drug user who went to an indigenous "crisis intervention center" instead of to a hospital emergency room met with very different treatment. This was *his* place, set up to serve *his* interests. No questions were asked. The staffs of the indigenous centers, moreover, gradually learned from day-to-day experience improved methods of handling crises. In hospitals, for example, LSD "bad trips" or "freakouts" and other LSD emergencies were generally treated in the early days by administering tranquilizers and other medication. The staffs of the crisis intervention centers learned instead to "talk a man down," using reassurance, friendliness, diversion of attention, and other simple psychological methods to calm the panic. Only the most serious cases required a physician, or hospitalization. Unlike the hospitals, the crisis intervention centers did not simply turn patients loose after the crisis was over, or call the police. Post-crisis counseling was available—at the moment when it was most likely to be effective.

"Free clinics." Just as Al Rinker founded the original San Francisco Switchboard on his own initiative, so Dr. Joel Fort founded the first "free clinic" in San Francisco in 1966; and Dr. David E. Smith and a few physician associates, acting as volunteers, founded the Haight-Ashbury Medical Clinic during San Francisco's 1967 "Summer of Love," to meet the medical needs of the youth drug scene migrants. Currently an estimated 50 to 80 other "free clinics," modeled more or less closely on the Fort and Haight-Ashbury patterns, are functioning in major drug centers from coast to coast. Some are subsidized by voluntary contributions, others also receive funds from local health departments. These clinics are "free" in the sense that no charge, or only a nominal charge, is made for services. The term "free" also indicates, however, a clinic free of the traditional rules, regulations, and attitudes.

The following 1970 prospectus for a Montreal "youth clinic" illustrates the principles common to most free clinics:

As you may be aware, there exists today a large population of youth who are not seeking the advice and help of established medical facilities for their problems. These problems include . . . normal difficulties found in that population, as well as specific disorders related to the non-medical use of drugs and to sexual activity, e.g. drug-induced mental disturbances, unwanted pregnancies, venereal diseases, etc.

One approach to the problems mentioned above has been the establishment of "Youth Clinics," organized and directed by the youth population, and located in a community centre setting, which patients do not regard as foreign or hostile. 4424 Youth Clinic is such an establishment and is now in operation. It is permanently staffed by a physician and a psychiatric social worker. Clinics are held in general medicine, gynecology and psychiatry. Additional staff work on a voluntary basis and include residents from the Queen Elizabeth and Montreal Children's Hospital as well as volunteers from the youth centre. A full range of medical services is provided; referrals to specialists in the out-patients' departments are made when necessary. There is no fee for service and medications are provided free of charge if the patient is unable to pay.

One of the major factors in the success of this type of clinic is that complete confidence between patient and doctor is maintained: parents are not informed without the knowledge of the patient.

The aim of the clinic is threefold:

1. Treatment
2. Prevention
3. Crisis Intervention

Typical illnesses treated include mouth and chest infections, skin diseases, allergies, venereal infections, etc. as well as psychiatric problems of adolescence and disturbances related to drug use.

Prevention Includes the Following:

1. Information on drug hazards given in a factual and non-dogmatic manner, i.e. the most recent scientific data concerning drug hazards.
   a) dangerous drugs currently being sold in the street.
   b) procedure in case of bad drug reaction.
2. Information on venereal disease and birth control.
3. Drug information to parents and the community at large, thus narrowing the "generation gap" aspect which motivates many youths to risk taking dangerous drugs to defy their "straight" parents.

Crisis Intervention will include a 24 hour telephone service where a doctor can be reached to treat a bad drug reaction, as treatment in hospital emergency wards are not only often inadequate but may even be detrimental.[2]

By common consent, anyone coming to a free clinic for help is deemed to be eighteen years of age—or whatever age is locally required for treatment without parental consent. There are no local residency requirements. No unnecessary questions are asked. The police are not informed. If requested, only the patient's nickname is recorded. Even the shabby psychedelic décor of the clinic is designed to make participants in the youth drug scene feel welcome and at home. The physicians staffing the free clinics are mostly young volunteers who give their spare time or else are minimally paid; few have short haircuts or other stigmata of respectability.

Canada's Health Minister John Munro vividly described these free clinics, known in Canada as *street clinics,* in his 1970 address:

Perhaps the best answer is one which blends in emergency drug care with the rest of the spectrum of medical practice. I refer to the street clinic. After all, many illnesses crop up among drug users which are only indirectly related to the drugs they take. They come more from the dropout life-style of the heavy user, which is itinerant and mendicant. They include malnutrition from a diet rendered insufficient either by personal poverty or by the type of drug used. They also include the full gamut of respiratory ailments, from coughs and flu to chronic bronchitis and pneumonia, stemming from over-exposure to inclement weather in inadequate clothing, and compounded by nutritional deficiencies. They also include VD. They include hepatitis and other varieties of vascular infection resulting from dirty needles.

To deal with this constant demand for basic health care, the street clinic locates itself in the neighbourhood of its primary clientele. As a matter of fact, its staff members may more closely resemble the clientele than they do regular health personnel. As in one case we ran into recently, the central doctor may have shoulder-length hair, and wear a headband and serape. So located and staffed, the clinic takes care of medical problems of all varieties, not just crises. And it doesn't require documentary proof of Medicare coverage* before extending treatment. Thus it is more than a clinic; it is a refuge for those who are not welcome at numerous regular sources of care, or mistrust them, or want at all costs to avoid the identification procedures which are followed there.

Thus, these centres are vital, and I hope that they will spread. I also hope that their development is plotted hand-in-hand with municipal and regional health planning agencies, so that the clinics have the necessary back-up for major cases, which may lie beyond the scope of their own capacity.[3]

The quality of the medical care delivered by these free clinics is not always high; *but it gets delivered.* In the process, it subtly affects the attitudes and behavior of youth drug scene participants. A warning against a new drug shipment which has just hit town, for example, achieves an altogether different credibility rating if it comes from a free clinic rather than from a traditional agency—for several reasons: First, the free clinic does not destroy its own credibility by issuing unrealistic warnings. Second, the free clinic has earned respect as a truly helping agency; its warnings are therefore perceived as designed to serve the best interests of drug users themselves rather than repressive goals. Third, the free clinic's advice is based on its own experience. It can therefore be readily confirmed by a drug user's personal observations within the scene. Much the same is true of warnings circulated by other institutions indigenous to the drug scene; but because of its medical orientation, the free clinic is the most authentic source of reliable drug information, and is perceived as such by its patients.

Most medical problems handled by the free clinics are not drug-related at all. Indeed, when asked what service drug users need most urgently, clinic physicians often cite dental care.

As the free clinics and other indigenous institutions have established their usefulness and earned respect from both the "square" and the "hip" communities, they have been increasingly successful in bridging the chasm between drug users and established institutions. The clinics have accomplished this in part by interpreting the drug users to the established hospitals, clinics, welfare and other agencies, and in part by interpreting the established institutions to the drug users. As a result, patients and clients requiring medical or other services beyond the scope of the free clinics are now being referred to established institutions with much less

* Medicare in Canada covers all ages.

of a "hassle," and with greater likelihood of a favorable outcome. Where drug users feel they are being treated unfairly, the free clinic can sometimes intervene effectively in their behalf.

Comprehensive drug scene centers. The newest, rarest, and most hopeful development among the drug scene's indigenous institutions is the appearance of a few *comprehensive* centers combining all of the functions described above, from hot line and rap center to free clinic—and offering in addition a wide range of other services including education and prevention. In particular, these comprehensive centers are concerned with two as yet unanswered questions:

How can emergence from the youth drug scene be encouraged and facilitated?

How can the recruitment of additional participants be discouraged?

Some comprehensive center approaches to these questions will be described in the following chapters.

Are these indigenous institutions, from hot lines to comprehensive youth centers, worthy of public support—even though their primary goal is to help drug users rather than to repress drug use? Canada's Minister of Health John Munro eloquently stated the case for generous support in his 1970 speech:

After all, it is our children we are talking about. And some of the drug users of today will be the leaders of tomorrow. Will they come to power with a fierce dedication to destroy everything we now represent—the good along with the bad—because of the way we now treat the drug problem? Or is there still time to show them that the "system" is flexible enough to understand them, help them, and accommodate their valid opinions about the necessity of social change?[4]

66.

Alternatives to the drug experience

Staff members of the indigenous institutions just described are concerned with the roles that drugs play in the lives of youth drug scene participants, and the human needs that drugs satisfy. Two roles and needs are of particular significance. Drugs are used, on-the-scene observers quite generally report, for *mood-altering* and for *achieving altered states of consciousness*. As several chapters in this Report have demonstrated, *Homo sapiens* over the centuries has employed drugs to attain those effects. Recently, some observers—and some drug users—have considered a provocative question: can other methods be found to alter moods and to achieve altered states of consciousness—methods not dependent upon drugs?

Dr. Vincent Nowlis, psychologist at the University of Rochester, provides one thoughtful answer. A change in mood, he points out, is a "change in the way in which the individual is *disposed* to feel, to think, to evaluate, and to behave. . . . A drug which alters mood alters the self. . . . Man is frequently dissatisfied with his present self, with the current status of his mood, and seeks to change this mood—at least temporarily." [1]

This normal, natural, human desire to alter mood from time to time, Dr. Nowlis continues, is not limited to drug users. "A search through the literature shows that throughout history man has found many ways to change mood—through physical exercise, spiritual exercise, prayer, sex, diet, health nostrums, rest, recreation, bathing, massage, travel, rehabilitation, active and passive participation in all art forms, commercial entertainment, rituals, games, and drugs." [2] Television is perhaps the mood-changing nostrum in most common use today.

Much the same, Dr. Nowlis adds, is true of the common human desire —among abstainers as well as drug users—to achieve altered states of consciousness:

There are gradations of the intensity of such states and in the amount of behavior and experience which is affected. Some trance states are defined negatively, as in highway hypnosis, when you suddenly realize even though you are driving the car you seem to have paid no attention to the highway or thruway for the preceding 50 miles and you don't know whether you are now between Rochester and Syracuse or Rochester and Buffalo. Or as in playing the piano, you suddenly realize that you have been aware neither of the printed notes nor of the sounds you have been producing for the preceding 5 or 10 minutes, but no one listening to you has been aware that you were in a trance. Most trance states are more positively defined, in terms of the *presence* of some phenomena. In the hypnogogic state, for example, just before falling asleep, strange, symbolic images may appear, like amoebae, or towering figures; or in the break-off phenomenon, you suddenly find yourself above your bed or outside your airplane looking at yourself there in the bed or there in the plane. Recent studies by Shor, Ås, Lee, and others find that these and other trance-like phenomena occur normally and spontaneously in a majority of adolescent and adult Americans, sometimes to the level of intensity which Maslow calls a peak experience or even to the very intense level called ecstasy. Here the person reports that he found himself "completely immersed in nature or art and had a feeling of awe, inspiration and grandeur sweep over" him and felt that his whole state of consciousness was somehow altered. Some of the more common circumstances in which these intense experiences occur spontaneously involve love, religion, the contemplation of art, landscape, music, moving colored lights, deep involvement in cooperating with others, and other conditions leading to strong motivation or a high level of concentration.

In other words, spontaneous trances or trips *(without drugs)* are not rare and are psychologically normal in many Americans.[3]

The falling-in-love experience, the ecstasy of sexual fulfillment, and the mystical religious experience are familiar examples of such "altered states of consciousness." Dr. Andrew T. Weil adds that in his opinion this

desire to alter consciousness is an innate psychological drive arising out of the neurological structure of the human brain. Strong evidence for this idea comes from observations of very young children, who regularly use techniques of consciousness alteration on themselves and each other when they think no adults are watching them. These methods include whirling until vertigo and collapse ensue, hyperventilating and . . . fainting. Such practices appear to be universal, irrespective of culture, and present at ages when social conditioning is unlikely to be an important influence (in two and three years olds, for example). Psychiatrists have paid little attention to these activities of all children. Freud noted them and called them "sexual equivalents," which they may be, although that formulation is not very useful.[4]

Adults offer children many mood-altering and consciousness-altering "trips," of course—ranging from the cradle, the merry-go-round, the swing, and the teeter-totter to the roller coaster and the ski slope. Anyone who has watched a four-year-old on a swing can see for himself the delight produced by consciousness alteration. The child is experiencing a "high."

"Until a few years ago," Dr. Weil adds, "most children in our society who wanted to continue [in adolescence] to indulge in these states were content to use alcohol, the one intoxicant we make available legally. Now, large numbers of young people are seeking chemical alterations of consciousness by means of a variety of illegal and medically disapproved drugs." To understand this change, society must "listen to what many drug users, themselves, say: they say they choose illegal drugs over alcohol in order to get better highs." [5] And, we might add, fewer fights, fewer accidents, less devastating hangovers.

However, Dr. Weil continues:

Most societies, like our own, are uncomfortable about having people go off into trances, mystic raptures, and hallucinatory intoxications. Indeed, the reason we have laws against possession of drugs in the first place is to discourage people from getting high. But innate, neuropsychological drives cannot be banned by legislation. They will be satisfied at any cost. And the cost in our country is very great: by trying to deny young people these important experiences, we maximize the probability that they will obtain them in negative ways—that is, in ways harmful to themselves and to society.[6]

At youth drug centers throughout Western civilization, the obvious moral of all this is being put to practical use. From San Francisco and Vancouver to London and Amsterdam, innovative institutions serving youthful drug users have begun to introduce nonchemical ways of "turning on" or "getting high"—nonchemical routes to altered states of consciousness. Here are a few:

Sensitivity training
Encounter therapy
Zen Buddhism
Yoga
Transcendental meditation
Massage
Hypnosis and self-hypnosis

One youth drug center is even contemplating the introduction of a program of parachute-jumping.

Ordinary religious services appear to have little appeal in this connection. But special services stressing ritual, mystical insight, and the emotional aspects of religion—"religious highs"—attract large audiences in the youth drug centers. The Eastern religions at first appeared to have the greatest appeal; but recent reports suggest that esoteric and fundamentalist forms of Christianity such as Jehovah's Witnesses are also attracting some youthful drug users. In the Jewish tradition, a return to the Chassidic mode of "singing and dancing God's ecstasy" is enjoying a revival; and the Catholic Mass has on occasion been similarly adapted to the ecstatic goal. Long-haired denizens of the youth drug scene who have turned from drugs to Christianity became numerous enough by the early 1970s to earn a distinctive title—"Jesus freaks." These nonchemical routes to mood-altering and to altered states of consciousness, of course, may bring their own problems.

These and other "alternatives to the drug experience" are gaining favor among young people primarily because they are superior to drugs, not because they are safer than drugs. An experienced drug user, Dr. Weil points out, "often finds that some form of meditation more effectively satisfies his desire to get high. *One sees a great many drug takers give up drugs for meditation, but one does not see any meditators give up meditation for drugs."* [7] (Italics supplied.) "Once you have learned from a drug what being high really is, you can begin to reproduce it without the drug; all persons who accomplish this feat testify that the non-drug high is superior." [8]

Canada's Le Dain Commission places similar emphasis on alternatives to the drug experience as a superior form of high: "One student [witness] said that he did not feel any desire for drugs for two weeks when he was on a canoe trip in the Canadian north." [9]

Dr. Allan Y. Cohen reported in 1969:

Perhaps the most understressed objective in any public health [drug] campaign is the *provision of alternatives.* In a sense, we have been hampered by taking a defensive posture, trying to eradicate drug abuse without providing for those opportunities which could reduce the desire for drugs. . . . It might be extremely wise to reorient our public health approach in home, school, and community so that we put special priority on developing and implementing nonchemical alternatives to the search for meaningful interpersonal relationships, enduring values, and inner experience. . . . Whenever attention is redirected to this kind of orientation, viable prospects begin to pop into view. Whether it involves broad curriculum changes, opportunities for political and social involvement, study in practical mysticism, growth-oriented individual and group counseling or whatever, the fact is that young people *will* cease using drugs if they are provided with some better nonchemical technique.[10]

At a board meeting of one crisis intervention center visited in the course of research for this Report, the evening's discussion was focused primarily on a drive to improve the local ecology and to curb pollution. Just why an institution set up to face "the drug menace" should wander off on an ecological tangent gradually became apparent: participation in this hot local political issue, which was raising tempers all over town, was itself a mood-altering and consciousness-altering "alternative to the drug experience." It was giving these young people a sense of *commitment* to something other than drugs.

A detailed review of the many possible alternatives to the drug experience falls outside the scope of this Report. But a word about their success is in order.

Several years ago, Dr. Herbert Benson of the Harvard Medical School and Thorndike Memorial Laboratory, Boston City Hospital, trained monkeys to control their own blood pressure, and wondered whether a technique known as transcendental meditation might not similarly lower the blood pressure of humans. To find out, he brought into the laboratory twenty young male volunteers aged twenty-one to thirty-eight, all of whom practiced this technique—a simple routine of sitting quietly and pondering in a prescribed manner for fifteen or twenty minutes twice a day. In talking with these men about their drug use, Dr. Benson turned up facts so astounding that he reported them in a 1969 letter to the editor of the *New England Journal of Medicine*.

Nineteen of the twenty volunteers told Dr. Benson that they had used drugs—marijuana, barbiturates, LSD, amphetamines, and in several cases heroin—*before* taking up transcendental meditation. Since they had begun meditating, however, "all [nineteen] reported that they no longer took these drugs because drug-induced feelings had become exceedingly distasteful as compared to those experiences during the practice of transcendental meditation." Perhaps, he added, "transcendental meditation should be explored prospectively by others . . . primarily interested in the alleviation of drug abuse." [11]

In the same year a graduate student in psychology at the University of California at Los Angeles, Thomas Winquist, prepared a report entitled *The Effect of the Regular Practice of Transcendental Meditation on Students Involved in the Regular Use of Hallucinogenic and "Hard" Drugs*. Winquist questioned 484 students who had been practicing transcendental meditation regularly for a minimum of three consecutive months. Out of the 484, he identified 143 (30 percent) who had been regular drug users and who reported the following changes in their drug use following their adoption of transcendental meditation: [12]

• *Marijuana:* Of the 143 subjects who used marijuana, 84 percent stopped, 14.5 percent decreased, and 1.5 percent increased.
• *LSD and LSD-like drugs* (DMT, STP, hashish, peyote, psilocybin, morning glory seeds, and wood rose seeds): Of the 111 subjects who regularly used one or more of these drugs, 85 percent stopped and 14 percent decreased.
• *Heroin, opium,** *Methedrine ("speed"), barbiturates*: Of the 42 subjects who used one or more of these drugs, 86 percent stopped and 14 percent decreased.

When asked *why* they gave up drugs or decreased their use, 115 of the subjects gave the following answers: [13]

• 49 percent stated that their use of drugs changed after transcendental meditation because life became more fulfilling.

---

* None of the subjects was addicted to heroin or opium.

• 24 percent stated that their use of drugs changed after transcendental meditation because the drug experience became less pleasurable.

• 8 percent stated that their use of drugs changed after transcendental meditation because the desire for drugs disappeared.

Participants were quoted as making remarks such as these: [14]

"Drugs have naturally fallen by. I didn't try to stop—after awhile I just found myself not taking them anymore."

"Life after meditation finally became satisfying. I no longer needed drugs."

"Because all aspects of my life have become better; in school, at work, my inner personal life—everything."

Back at Harvard, meanwhile, Dr. Benson launched a study on an even larger scale. He began with 1,862 practitioners of transcendental meditation, all of whom had meditated daily for three months or longer; the average length of time they had been practicing daily meditation was about twenty months. In this population, marijuana smoking declined from 78.3 percent before entering meditation to 26.9 percent after meditating from four to nine months, and to 12.2 percent after twenty-two or more months of meditation. Moreover, only one subject who had meditated for twenty-two or more months reported that he was still smoking marijuana daily, as compared with 417 (22.4 percent) who reported smoking marijuana daily *before* entering transcendental meditation.[15]

The LSD results were similar. In the sample as a whole, 48.3 percent reported having used LSD; among those who had meditated for twenty-two or more months only 3 percent were still using LSD. For the sample as a whole, 132 subjects (7.1 percent) reported having used LSD once a week or oftener before entering transcendental meditation; none of those who had meditated for more than twenty-two months was using LSD that frequently.[16] Dr. Benson reported his findings in November 1970 at a University of Michigan International Symposium on Drug Abuse.

These studies are subject to a number of qualifications.

First, the participants in both the Winquist and Benson studies were mostly college students or ex-students; the effects on other groups have not been similarly studied.

Second, the participants in both studies were *self-selected.* They were the students attracted to transcendental meditation. The remarkable results cannot be generalized to apply to drug users who are *not* voluntarily attracted to transcendental meditation.

Third, applicants were expected to refrain from drug use for fifteen days *before* entering a transcendental meditation program; many confirmed drug users (and all or almost all addicts) are no doubt screened out of the program by this condition.

Fourth, both studies were limited to participants who *continued* to practice transcendental meditation. How many dropped out of transcendental meditation instead of dropping out of drugs is not reported.

Fifth, both studies lacked controls. As the Benson study itself points out, the number of similar college students who formerly used drugs and who dropped out of the drug scene during the same period *without* embracing transcendental meditation is not known.

Finally, neither the Winquist nor the Benson study establishes the superiority of transcendental meditation as compared with *other* alternatives to drug use. Transcendental meditation happens to be the only alternative for which such statistics are available. Perhaps sensitivity training, or Yoga, or Zen, or other alternatives are even more effective; no one knows.

It should further be noted that young people use drugs—just as their elders use drugs—in order to achieve such specific effects as relief from anxiety, or from boredom, or from depression, or, in many cases, just for fun or for "kicks." An alternative to the drug experience is most likely to be effective if it fulfills the same need for which the drug was previously used.

Despite their limitations, the Winquist and Benson studies are still landmarks in consideration of the youth drug scene. They indicate how fragile is the tie that binds many marijuana smokers to their joints and many LSD users to their acid.

At youth drug centers across the country, and especially in comprehensive centers, these and other alternatives to the chemical high and to the chemical induction of altered states of consciousness are currently being offered, and accepted. In the course of research for this Report, young people were encountered in drug centers from Vancouver's Fourth Avenue to Amsterdam's Paradiso who sat "stoned on life" while those around them sat stoned on marijuana or LSD. They looked and dressed like drug users and spent their time in drug centers with drug users—but their highs came neither from a pharmacy nor from a "pusher."

Meanwhile, in a few high schools and other agencies, especially in California, educators and others who have seen the results achieved by alternatives to the drug experience have begun to ask what is obviously the next question:

Why should illicit drug use be required as a ticket of admission to the achievement of nondrug "highs" and to nondrug approaches to altered states of consciousness? Why should not schools and other agencies make sensitivity training, encounter therapy, nature study, transcendental meditation, skiing, enjoyment of music, enjoyment of art, and other nonchemical highs available *before* students migrate, physically or internally, to the country's Haight-Ashburys?

In a growing number of schools, churches, and other agencies, such programs have been instituted. It is too early to evaluate them. But they are surely more promising than traditional approaches to prevention—the imprisonment of drug users, dire (and incredible) warnings against the hazards of drug use, and the other futile and counterproductive measures described at length throughout the earlier chapters of this Report.

Many thoughtful observers within the youth drug scene, however, view alternatives to the drug experience, like the drug experience itself, as at best mere palliatives. The alternatives can no doubt prove enormously helpful in particular cases. They may be necessary in many communities. But the ultimate goal, perhaps, should be a way of life free of dependence on alternatives to the drug experience as well as free of dependence on drugs.

A satisfying way of life is thus the ultimate prescription, and the immediate goal should be improvements in the *quality of life*—a topic that falls outside the scope of this Consumers Union Report.

67.

Emergence from the drug scene

Even many young drug users who become abstainers—and there is a growing number of them—remain in the scene, according to staff members of indigenous institutions. "The community imprisons them here as if in a corral," [1] the director of one free clinic remarks.

The price of readmission to conventional society has been set very high. Young people feel that to reenter they must betray everything they have learned and stand for—their ideals, their concerns with peace and love and sharing, their life-style, even the way they like to dress and wear their hair. It is hardly surprising that, even among those who have given up drugs, some do not return to the fold.

Even if society were to open the doors of its schools and employment offices to ex-drug users without setting unacceptable conditions, there is little likelihood that they would flock back. Canada's Le Dain Commission has explored the reasons for this, at some depth and with much subtlety, in the course of its year-long dialogue with countless drug users and ex-users. The commission's 1970 *Interim Report* merits quotation on this point at some length.

Many former drug users, the commission first notes, "have stated that the insights gained through drug use have carried over and remained with them, continuing to shape their attitudes and outlook and style of relating when they were not using drugs. In other words, the drug has been a means of discovering a new way to be—more relaxed and self-accepting, more accepting and indeed loving, more appreciative of the intensity and value of being human in the moment, less anxious about time and specific goals. . . . [2]

"The drug-taking minority of this generation," the *Interim Report* continues, "cannot be inspired by the goals of their fathers. They do not feel the same urgency to achieve material success and do not seek self-fulfillment that way." [3] Nor do they see the need to achieve success in order to survive. "They envisage a society which will be obliged to assure a sufficient amount of material security to everyone in order to maintain itself politically and economically." [4] And further:

There is . . . a strong impression that young people are, as it were, unconsciously adapting or preparing themselves for a time when there will be much less work to go around. The rapid rate of technological change and the pervading threat of work obsolescence makes them very uncertain about their own occupational future. They seem to suspect that a high proportion of them may have to learn to live happily with relatively little work.[5]

To many readers, this may sound like laziness; the Le Dain Commission sees it instead as realism. "Those of us who are well-established in work," the *Interim Report* points out, "tend to talk glibly of a future in which there will be increasing leisure. Little thought or practical effort has been devoted to the problem of how to fill that leisure in constructive and satisfying ways. The exploration of the inner self, the expansion of consciousness, the development of spiritual potential, may well be purposes to which young people are turning—in anticipation of a life in which they will have to find sustaining interest in the absence of external demands and challenges." [6]

In addition to preparing to live with relatively little work, moreover, the young drug users and ex-users with whom the Le Dain Commission talked at length seemed (as noted earlier) to be highly selective about the *kind* of work they wanted:

Young people speak often of a desire to overcome the division of life into work and play, to achieve a way of life that is less divided, less seemingly schizophrenic, and more unified. They seem to be talking about the increasingly rare privilege of work that one can fully enjoy—of work that is like one's play. They claim to be prepared to make considerable renunciation or sacrifice of traditional satisfactions like status and material success for work in which they can take pleasure. Indeed, one of their frequent commentaries on the older generation is that it does not seem to enjoy its work, that it does not seem to be happy. This is said sadly, even sympathetically. It is not said contemptuously. The young say, in effect, "Why should we repeat this pattern?" [7]

Thus the boundaries of the drug-scene corral are doubly fenced. On the one side, society demands surrender before it will permit emergence. On the other side, would-be emigrants from the corral are seeking a kind of work and a life-style that are exceedingly rare.

The route of emergence most eagerly discussed among young drug users and ex-users themselves in 1970 and 1971 was to move out into the country, establish a rural commune, and support the commune through farming and through handicrafts. Countless young denizens of the country's Haight-Ashburys, like their predecessors in the nineteenth century, dreamed of such a "back-to-the-land" migration. Many rural areas, of course, saw such proposals as an invasion threat. Canada's Minister of Health John Munro, in contrast, saw them as a national opportunity.

"Young people talk of the meaninglessness of most of the work done by people in our society," he told the British Columbia Medical Association in October 1970. "Why not then offer them the opportunity to pursue work that is socially meaningful?" [8] After discussing arts and handicrafts as possibilities, Mr. Munro continued:

Another positive means of reconstituting drug-fractured lives lies in a recent development of youth themselves—the "return-to-the-soil" movement. Such movements are, of course, historically classic developments among those who either felt themselves persecuted, or believed in the necessity of isolation from the corrupting influences around them. From the Oneida and Amana communities in 19th century America, through the Nouveau Québec colonization movement of the early 20th century, to the establishment of the kibbutzim in Israel, people have sought to revitalize and radically improve society by example, through pioneer collectivist farming.

The commune movement among today's so-called hippies offers the same opportunity. I personally felt this point brought home to me the other day, while flying by helicopter from Cornwall to Ottawa. Passing over the Eastern Ontario farm landscape, I was struck by the advantages that an out-door life of solid work, in an unpolluted rural setting, could mean to drug rehabilitation. Many young people drift into the drug world through the depersonalizing atmosphere of our cities, combined with easy life-style and plentiful drug access within them. Rural group living could offer them a chance at true closeness to nature, with their own kind of people.

Accordingly I feel that we should consider support for rural farm communes, where through work that is truly their own, young people can find both peace from that in our society which they reject, as well as a worthwhile alternative to a state of constant intoxication. We should also be thinking of support for cooperative markets to handle the produce of all these enterprises, so that they can eventually become financially independent and truly self-run.[9]

This "Munro plan" may or may not make sense in the current Canadian economy. Certainly grave difficulties would have to be overcome to graft such youth communes onto the United States farm economy. But the *spirit* of the Munro plan—the honest effort to seek ways of facilitating emergence from Canada's dismal youth slums—is highly relevant to the dismal United States youth slums as well. Perhaps the time has come for the United States, like Canada, to devote to such practical measures some of the energy that has been devoted to arresting, prosecuting, and imprisoning young people for drug offenses.

Part X

Conclusions and Recommendations

68.

Learning from mistakes: six caveats

This nation's drug laws and policies have not been working well; on that simple statement almost all Americans seem agreed. During the fifty-seven years since passage of the Harrison Narcotic Act, heroin has become a national menace; its use has even spread to the middle class and the suburbs. After a third of a century of escalating penalties against marijuana and of antimarijuana propaganda, marijuana has reached an unprecedented peak of popularity. After a decade of agitation and legislation, LSD—a drug few people had even heard of before 1962—is now known universally and used by hundreds of thousands, even high-school students. The barbiturates, which a generation ago were thought of as sedatives, useful for calming and for sleep, have become "thrill drugs." So have the amphetamines, once used mainly to enable people to work longer hours at hard jobs.

These changes, clearly, are not the result of changes in the chemical composition of the drugs. They are the result of mistaken laws and policies, of mistaken attitudes toward drugs, and of futile, however well-intentioned, efforts to "stamp out the drug menace." This Consumers Union Report, accordingly, has been only partly concerned with the "drug problem." Large portions of our work have focused instead on what Dr. Helen Nowlis has aptly called "the *drug problem* problem"—the damage that results from the ways in which society has approached the drug problem.

To summarize here the entire contents of this Report would be an impossible undertaking. We therefore present instead a series of brief reminders of some of the central themes developed earlier, plus drug-by-drug recommendations growing out of those themes.

Our recommendations are not intended as a blueprint for solving overnight either "the drug problem" or "the *drug problem* problem." Rather, each proposal is put forward as an approach worthy of consideration and trial. As the drug scene changes, new recommendations will no doubt be called for. Consumers Union expects to report such changes and to make additional recommendations in the pages of *Consumer Reports*.

Mistakes in drug laws, policies, and attitudes are discussed and documented throughout this Report. Among the steps which might correct them, we suggest the following.

(1) Stop emphasizing measures designed to keep drugs away from people.

Prohibition—trying to keep drugs away from people—began with the enforcement of the 1914 Harrison Narcotic Act, and it has remained the dominant theme of both antidrug legislation and antidrug propaganda ever since.

Prohibition does not work. As the United States learned from 1920 to 1933, it didn't work with alcohol. As the country has been learning since 1914, it doesn't work with heroin. It isn't working today with marijuana, LSD, or any of the other illicit drugs. Nor is prohibition likely to prove more effective in the future.

What prohibition does accomplish is to raise prices and thus to attract more entrepreneurs to the black market. If the drug is addicting and the price escalation is carried to outrageous extremes (as in the case of heroin), addicts resort to crime to finance their purchases—at a tragic cost, not only in dollars but in community disruption.

What prohibition also achieves is to convert the market from relatively bland, bulky substances to more hazardous concentrates which are more readily smugglable and marketable—from opium smoking to heroin mainlining, from coca leaves to cocaine, from marijuana to hashish.

Again, prohibition opens the door to adulterated and contaminated drugs—methyl alcohol, "ginger jake," pseudo-LSD, adulterated heroin.

Worst of all, excessive reliance on prohibition, on laws and law enforcement, lulls the country decade after decade into a false confidence that nothing more need be done—except to pass yet another law, or to hire a few hundred more narcotics agents, or to license the agents to break down doors without knocking first, and so on.

This is not, obviously, a justification for repealing *all* drug laws tomorrow. A nation that has not learned to keep away from some drugs and to use others wisely cannot be taught those essential lessons merely by repealing drug laws. What is needed in the legal arena are two fresh insights:

• Physicians have a maxim: *Nihil nocere.* It means that a physician must guard against doing more harm than good. A *nihil nocere* guideline is needed for drug laws and law enforcement. A law-enforcement policy that converts marijuana smokers into LSD or heroin users (see chart on Page 442), to cite an obvious example, should be abandoned. The same is true of a law that turns marijuana smokers into convicts and ex-convicts, with all that the prison experience and the prison record implies. Nor can much be said in favor of a law-enforcement policy that results in raising the price of a nickel's worth of heroin to five dollars—with the further result that addicts must steal vast amounts in order to buy their heroin.

A complete revision of laws and enforcement policies in the spirit of the *nihil nocere* principle is called for. Laws and law enforcement cannot solve the drug problem; they should not be allowed to exacerbate it.

• A realistic understanding of what laws can and cannot do is needed. Laws cannot work miracles. They cannot, for example, keep heroin away from heroin addicts, nor marijuana away from marijuana smokers. The most laws can do in these cases is to punish and to alienate. Accordingly, laws and enforcement policies should be revised to concentrate on *achievable* goals. For example, in countries where heroin addicts do not have to patronize and support a black market, law-enforcement efforts can be directed solely toward curbing the flow of heroin to *nonaddicts*. Surely this is the essential goal.

In sum, valuable resources and energies should no longer be wasted chasing prohibition will-o'-the-wisps. Those goals that cannot be achieved by law enforcement should be assigned to other instrumentalities such as education and social reform.

(2) Stop publicizing the horrors of the "drug menace." Scare publicity has been the second cornerstone of national policy, along with law enforcement, since 1914. The effort to frighten people away from illicit drugs has publicized and thus popularized the drugs attacked. The impact on young eyes and ears of the constant drumming of drug news stories and antidrug messages is clearly discernible—just look around.*

* Ken Sobol wrote in the New York *Village Voice,* October 21, 1971: "In the past week we were entertained [on television] by seven dope discussion/documentaries, a dope agony ballet, two dope poetry readings, innumerable anti-dope commercials, and three dramatic series shows centering around junkies. Not to mention Rona Barrett revealing Hollywood's latest hophead horror, a variety show host wittily confusing grass and grass, Jim Jensen crackling gravely as he narrated the [New York Police Department's] 'biggest raid of the week' bit, LeRoi Jones accusing the Pope of dealing, and countless other pieces of programs. Reds, greens, ups, downs, agony, ecstasy, sniff, smoke, mainline, degradation, or rehabilitation—you name it, we had it, as usual.

"All of these items began with the assumption that since dope is an evil, its horrors must be portrayed as graphically as possible in order to educate the viewer. But the question which nobody seems to ask is just what is being taught by all this electronic moralizing—that drugs are bad, or that *Dope Is Exciting!* Like everything else on tv, dope 'education' is show biz. And like all show biz, it is glamorous form first, content second. One National Football League anti-drug spot begins with exciting field action, while up tempo, big band jazz blares over. Then, as the music recedes, the camera picks out one player smashing an opposing ballcarrier and we hear his voice over: 'This is Mike Reid . . . That's the way I like to crack down. I'd like to rack up the drug traffic, too.' Up jazz, building to crash climax. It's all groovy sounds and fast action, only slightly interrupted by some rich jock's [anti-drug comments]. Wham, bam, dope, man! Dope is so exciting that even the anti-dope swings.

"That impression is enhanced by the fact that only beautiful, vibrant people turn to drugs on entertainment tv. Last Friday, for one example, among many, the 'D.A.,' a new NBC law and order hour, had a show about a junkie witness. She was, of course, young, beautiful, intelligent, and paying for her mistakes. Decadence sells

As shown throughout this Report, sensationalist publicity is not only in-effective but counterproductive. Both the peril and the warning function as lures. At the same time, the antidrug campaigns have inflamed the hostile emotions of many non-drug users, making it harder to win support for calm, rational, nonpunitive, *effective* drug policies.

(3) Stop increasing the damage done by drugs. Current drug laws and policies make drugs more rather than less damaging in many ways. The alleged justification for this is, of course, to *deter* people from using drugs. Thus, the sale or possession of hypodermic needles without prescription is a criminal offense—a policy which leads to the use of nonsterile needles, to the sharing of needles, and to epidemics of hepatitis and other crippling, sometimes fatal, needle-borne diseases. Contaminated and adulterated illicit drugs circulate as freely as pure illicit drugs, with no greater penalty for selling them and no effective system for warning users against them. Only trifling efforts are made to find and eliminate the cause of the hundreds of deaths each year among heroin mainliners—deaths falsely attributed to "overdose." The establishment of methadone maintenance programs for heroin addicts is resisted and delayed in part because some people *want* heroin addiction to lead to disaster—as a deterrent to others. Loss of employment, expulsion from school, and exclusion from respectable society similarly serve to increase the damage done by drugs—and over all of the other penalties hovers society's ultimate sanction, imprisonment, the most damaging of all consequences of illicit drug use.

These and other drug laws and policies have succeeded in making drug use more damaging in the United States than in other countries, and vastly more damaging today than in the United States of a century ago (see Chapter 1). But as deterrents against drug use, these policies clearly have failed.

---

better than ever these days. It makes people romantically exciting, cool, tragic and *plugged in*—beautiful people, that is.

"Even documentary dope can be a gas. In Frederick Wiseman's 'Hospital,' shown last week on NET, a long sequence (which I am pulling out of context) shows a bad-tripping teenaged boy in the emergency room. He screams, moans, shakes, crawls in his own puke, begs the doctors not to let him die. All genuine, all riveting. Yet at the same time completely unreal, because the tv screen automatically distances us and makes it a performance—a show about a kid connecting with life in the rawest, most primal way. And again, I think that what may remain in the mind from it is the generalized excitement of that elemental connection, rather than its individual real-life horror. Because tv is not real life, and while it is surprisingly easy to ignore someone else's horror on film, it is no trick at all to get excited by it.

"So there you are. A small piece of last week's junk action. Next week there will be more of the same, and more the week after, and so on, until we have theoretically been 'educated' or frightened off dope—or on to it. Because if McLuhan is at all right, then some people are going about this all wrong. Maybe there is no right way to treat dope on television as it is presently constituted, but I wish to hell someone in a foundation or school somewhere would at least sit down and worry about it."

Accordingly, future efforts should be directed toward *minimizing* the damage done by drugs. A substantial part of that damage stems not from the chemistry of the drugs but from the ignorant and imprudent ways in which they are used, the settings in which they are used, the laws punishing their use, society's attitudes toward users, and so on. Once a policy of minimizing damage is adopted and conscientiously pursued, a substantial part of the "drug menace" will be eliminated—even though many people may continue to use drugs.

The choice is clear: to continue trying, ineffectively, to stamp out illicit drug use by making it as damaging as possible, or to seek to minimize the damage done by drugs, licit and illicit alike.*

(4) Stop misclassifying drugs. Misclassification lies close to the heart of the drug problem, for what teachers tell students about a drug, and how judges sentence drug-law violators, both depend on how the drug is classified. Most official and unofficial classifications of drugs are illogical and capricious; they therefore make a mockery of drug-law enforcement and bring drug education into disrepute.

A major error of the current drug classification system is that it treats alcohol and nicotine—two of the most harmful drugs—essentially as nondrugs.† Equating marijuana with heroin is a second shocking example—for it helps to encourage the switch from marijuana to heroin.

The entire jerry-built structure of official drug classification rests on a series of Congressional enactments beginning in 1914 and reaching a climax in the Comprehensive Drug Abuse Prevention and Control Act of 1970. The misclassifications built into this Act were not the results of scientific study but represented compromises between Senate and House committees, between Republican and Democratic legislators, between Congress and the Nixon administration. Worse yet, the Act authorizes the *Attorney General* of the United States to alter the classifications from time

---

* The first faint harbingers of a trend toward lessening drug damage are beginning to appear. Some people who thought a few years ago that imprisonment or death was good enough for "drug fiends" whose skin color was different or who lived in another part of town have begun to change their minds as they realize that the users of illicit drugs include their own children. Actions by both Congress and a number of state legislatures to reduce marijuana possession penalties in 1970 and 1971 were straws in this breeze of change. The concern expressed in 1971 for veterans returning from Vietnam addicted to heroin was another straw. The problem of minimizing the damage done by *licit* drugs, such as nicotine and alcohol, also attracted Congressional attention in 1970 and 1971; cigarette advertising was banned from television and new alcoholism treatment and research programs were authorized. Several states repealed their laws making public drunkenness a crime punishable by imprisonment.

† Some young people, baffled by the illogic, have concluded that corrupt legislators must have adopted the classifications to protect the tobacco and alcohol industries. Such distrust is perhaps understandable, though ignorance rather than venality seems the more likely explanation. The fact remains, however, that a significant part of American agriculture and industry is engaged, with government support, in the production and marketing of nicotine and alcohol products.

to time. Yet judges are bound by this political rather than scientific system of classification in assessing penalties; and educational programs generally take their cue from the official classification.

Propaganda programs contribute to the classification chaos in another way; they accent the distinction between licit and illicit drugs, while failing to draw distinctions between more hazardous and less hazardous illicit drugs. The result is to facilitate the use of the more hazardous illicit drugs.

A sound classification program should concern itself with *modes* of drug use as well as drugs themselves; it should recognize, for example, the vast difference between sniffing, smoking, or swallowing a drug and mainlining it. Society, laws, and law-enforcement policies already differentiate the occasional drinker of a glass of wine or beer, the social drinker, the problem drinker, the spree drinker, the chronic drunk, and the alcoholic. Similar distinctions should be made with respect to various modes of use of marijuana, LSD, the barbiturates, and the amphetamines. It is one thing to get stoned on marijuana on Saturday night; it is quite another to stay stoned all day every day. A sensible drug classification program would not only recognize but stress the difference.

Once a reasonable approach is adopted to the classification of drugs and modes of drug use, educators can begin to plan a *believable* program of drug education, based on truth—on what is known and not known. Such a program will be confirmed by what young people see around them, and by what they experience if and when they try drugs themselves. It will therefore no longer bring down ridicule and disrepute upon the whole concept of drug education. Until drugs are sensibly reclassified, no amount of public-relations expertise will restore credibility to governmental, medical, and educational drug pronouncements.

(5) Stop viewing the drug problem as primarily a national problem, to be solved on a national scale. In fact, as workers in the drug scene confirm, the "drug problem" is a collection of local problems. The predominant drugs differ from place to place and from time to time. Effective solutions to problems also vary; a plan that works now for New York City may not be applicable to upstate New York and vice versa. With respect to education and propaganda, the need for local wisdom and local control is particularly pressing. Warning children against drugs readily available to them is a risky business at best, requiring careful, truthful, unsensational approaches. Warning children against drugs used elsewhere, of which they may never have heard, can be like warning them against putting beans in their ears. The role of anti-glue-sniffing warnings in popularizing glue-sniffing (see Chapter 44) is the most striking of many examples.

The errors in drug policy under review here are also generalizations that may or may not be relevant in a particular community. An essential preliminary step in any local drug education program should be to identify the errors in policy currently being committed *locally*—and, if possible, to correct them locally.

(6) Stop pursuing the goal of stamping out illicit drug use. If, in 1937, efforts had been undertaken to *reduce* marijuana smoking over a period of years rather than to try to eradicate it immediately, such a program might well have succeeded. Instead, one of the greatest drug explosions in history—the marijuana eruption of the 1960s—was triggered (see Part VIII).

Attempts to stamp out illicit drug use tend to increase both drug use and drug damage. Here LSD is the prime example (see Part VII).

Finally, as we have shown, efforts to stamp out one drug shift users to another—from marijuana to LSD and heroin, from heroin to alcohol.

These, then, are the major mistakes in drug policy as we see them. This Consumers Union Report contains no panaceas for resolving them. But getting to work at correcting these six errors, promptly and ungrudgingly, would surely be a major step in the right direction.

69.

Policy issues and recommendations

Narcotics. The one overwhelming objection to opium, morphine, heroin, and the other narcotics is the fact that they are addicting. The other disastrous effects of narcotics addiction on mind, body, and society are primarily the results of laws and policies (see Part I).

Many American morphine and heroin addicts prior to 1914 led long, healthy, respectable, productive lives despite addiction—and so do a few addicts today. The sorry plight of most heroin addicts in the United States today results primarily from the high price of heroin, the contamination and adulteration of the heroin available on the black market, the mainlining of the drug instead of safer modes of use, the laws against heroin and the ways in which they are enforced, the imprisonment of addicts, society's attitudes toward addicts, and other nonpharmacological factors. It was the enforcement of the Harrison Act of 1914 that converted opiate addiction from what it had long been—a misfortune and a disgrace—into a disaster.

The time has come to recognize what should have been obvious since 1914—that heroin is a drug most users go right on using despite the threat of imprisonment, despite actual imprisonment for years, despite repeated "cures" and long-term residence in rehabilitation centers, and despite the risks of disease and even death. Heroin is a drug for which addicts will prostitute themselves. It is also a drug to which most addicts return despite a sincere desire to "stay clean," a firm resolve to stay clean, an overwhelming effort to stay clean—and even a success (sometimes enforced by confinement) in staying clean for weeks, months, or years. This is what is meant by the statement that heroin is an addicting drug.

The first and most important step in solving the heroin problem, accordingly, is to recognize at long last what addiction to heroin means. Society must stop expecting that any significant proportion of addicts will become ex-addicts by an act of will, or by spending five years in prison, or a year or two in a prison-like California, New York State, or federal "drug treatment center," or even in a "therapeutic community" like Synanon, Daytop, Phoenix House, Odyssey House, or any of the others (see Chapter 10).

Almost all heroin addicts, it is true, do stop taking heroin from time to time. But almost all subsequently relapse. Among those who do not relapse, roughly half become skid-row alcoholics. For the details, see Chapter 10. By publicizing the few conspicuous exceptions—the handful of successful ex-heroin addicts—and by assuming that others need only follow in their footsteps, harm is done in at least three tragic ways.

(1) Another generation of young people is persuaded that heroin addiction is temporary. They are falsely assured that the worst that can happen to them if they get hooked on heroin is that they may have to spend a year or two in a drug treatment center, or, better yet, in a therapeutic community like Synanon or Daytop—after which they will emerge, heads high, as certified ex-addicts.

(2) Hundreds of millions of dollars are wasted on vast "treatment programs" that almost totally fail to curb subsequent heroin use by addicts, while more pressing measures are skimped on.

(3) Law-enforcement resources are wasted on futile efforts to keep heroin away from heroin addicts instead of concentrating on the essential task: keeping heroin away from nonaddicts.

The ideal solution to the heroin problem, of course, would be a *cure* for opiate addiction—some means of erasing altogether both the physiological and the psychological traces of past drug use. But no such cure exists, nor is there one on the horizon—and there exist no clues to where such a miracle cure might be found. Accordingly, while scientists who want to search for a cure should certainly be encouraged to do so, it is folly to base national policy on the hope that they may succeed.

There is one major exception to the rule that most heroin addicts go right on using heroin or returning to heroin. A heroin addict can comfortably do without his drug if supplied with a related drug. Methadone is one such drug. Unlike heroin, it can be effectively taken orally rather than by injection; it need be taken only once a day instead of several times; it is legal; it is cheap; and it has other advantages. Like heroin, it has very little effect on either mind or body if taken regularly. An estimated 25,000 ex-heroin addicts were taking legal methadone instead of black-market heroin in 1971, and the number was rapidly growing.

Methadone maintenance is not a panacea. But it frees addicts from the heroin incubus, which is ruining their lives, and it is therefore capable of turning a majority of heroin addicts into law-abiding citizens (like pre-1914 addicts). One of the reasons it succeeds, of course, is that it is itself an addicting drug—that is, a drug that must be taken daily. For further details, see Chapters 14–19.

The conversion of heroin addicts into methadone maintenance patients is proceeding too slowly. Some communities have no methadone maintenance program; most programs have long waiting lists. Putting an addict on a waiting list for methadone has been likened to putting a drowning man on a waiting list for artificial respiration.

Ideally, addicts should be given a choice of treatment modalities, a choice between methadone maintenance and other programs offering a similar likelihood of rehabilitation. But first those effective alternatives must be found. Consumers Union enthusiastically endorses laboratory and clinical research into effective alternatives to methadone maintenance, including both drug-free approaches and rehabilitation programs using drugs other than methadone. But large sums should not again be spent on alternatives which—since the early "opiate cures" of the nineteenth century—have already repeatedly demonstrated their worthlessness. A program should be considered experimental until it has proved its effectiveness; there should be no further mass failures, such as the California and New York State programs, into which vast sums have been sunk with barely a trace of benefits.

To date, no program other than methadone maintenance has demonstrated its ability to rehabilitate more than a minute proportion of addicts. Failure rates in nonmethadone programs range from 90 to 100 percent, even when entrance is limited to select groups of highly motivated addicts. The failures return to the American black-market system of heroin distribution, paying exorbitant prices for dangerously adulterated and contaminated heroin. Surely methadone maintenance is better than that.

It is shocking, of course, to think of tens of thousands of newly addicted young people and of addicted Vietnam veterans taking a narcotic such as methadone daily, for months, years, perhaps for the rest of their lives (see Chapter 20). No one can look forward to such a prospect with satisfaction. But no better solution is in sight. And the alternative for those who are not rehabilitated by existing methods is a return to black-market heroin.

The heroin black market must be abolished in the only way it can be abolished: by eliminating the demand for black-market heroin.

On the central issue of narcotics addiction, accordingly, Consumers Union recommends (1) that United States drug policies and practices be promptly revised to insure that no narcotics addict need get his drug from the black market; (2) that methadone maintenance be promptly made available under medical auspices to every narcotics addict who applies for it; (3) that other forms of narcotics maintenance, including opium, morphine, and heroin maintenance, be made available along with methadone maintenance under medical auspices on a carefully planned, experimental basis.

The third of these recommendations—that opium, morphine, and heroin as well as methadone be made available to addicts under well-planned experimental conditions—is based in part on the unassailable fact that an addict is personally far better off on legal, low-cost, medicinally pure opium, morphine, or heroin than he is on exorbitantly priced, dangerously adulterated, and contaminated black-market heroin.

[530]

Similarly, society is better off when addicts receive their drugs legally and at low cost or free of charge.

Finally, reliable scientific data on the relative advantages and disadvantages of various maintenance drugs under actual conditions of use in the United States can be secured only by comparative-use studies. The experimental programs should be designed to determine, if possible on a blind or double-blind basis, (a) whether any other drug has any advantages over methadone for general use in narcotics maintenance programs, and (b) whether any particular subcategories of patients may do better on opium, morphine, heroin, or some other maintenance drug rather than on methadone. The tests should be designed to determine whether it is the heroin molecule itself or the mystique surrounding it that makes the difference.

The comparative trials should also be designed to determine whether, as in Britain, there is a proper role for *injectable* methadone in maintenance programs, or for other routes of administration (such as smoking) for the various opiates. Oral morphine and oral heroin should be among the drugs submitted to double-blind trials in competition with oral methadone.

Consumers Union's recommendation for experimental opium, morphine, and heroin maintenance programs is not based on any confidence that they will prove superior to maintenance on methadone or on newer, longer-acting versions of methadone (such as acetyl-alpha-methadol). All of the data so far indicate that methadone is very nearly the ideal maintenance drug—fully effective by mouth, effective for a full twenty-four hours, effective in stable doses, with minimal side effects, and with its safety, effectiveness, and acceptability to addicts already proved under actual field conditions in some 25,000 patients. But the ready availability of an excellent maintenance drug is *not* a sound reason for abandoning the search for an even better maintenance drug. And even if, in the end, the trials of opium, morphine, and heroin maintenance merely buttress the conclusion that methadone is the maintenance drug of choice, the research will have served a useful purpose, for oral methadone has so far only proved its worth in competition with black-market heroin. The next challenge oral methadone should be required to meet is a carefully controlled comparison with legal opium, morphine, and heroin, with injectable methadone, and perhaps with other drugs.*

Further, Consumers Union calls for three immediate steps to be taken in connection with the tragic deaths of many hundreds of heroin users each year from so-called "overdose" (see Chapter 12).

First, the dangerously wrong "heroin overdose" myth must be promptly

---

* Including dipipanone, pethidine [meperidine, Demerol], dextromoramide, levorphanol—all of which are narcotics and all of which are being tried as maintenance drugs in Britain.

exploded once and for all. Addicts and the public alike must be warned that sudden death can follow the intravenous injection of mixtures containing very little heroin—or possibly none at all.

Second, heroin addicts throughout the country should be warned by all means available, including the fullest possible use of the mass media, that deaths falsely attributed to heroin overdose *may* be due to injecting heroin while drunk on alcohol or barbiturates. Although the evidence linking the many hundreds of so-called "heroin overdose" deaths to alcohol and the barbiturates is not conclusive, the evidence *is* conclusive that an addict who injects heroin while drunk on alcohol or barbiturates is running a far greater risk than one who shoots up while sober. *This* should be the public health message.

Third, a full-scale research program must be promptly launched, under capable scientific leadership, to determine what is in fact causing these hundreds of deaths annually, and what measures can be taken to lower the addict death rate. These deaths must be viewed not merely as arguments against injecting heroin, but as the tragic events they are. Society must seek ways to avert them, just as ways are sought to prevent the untimely deaths of nonaddicts.

Some readers who turn to these conclusions without first having read Part I may have indignant objections to our recommendations on narcotics—objections that cannot be answered here. Readers are referred to Part I for the answers.

Cocaine and the amphetamines. These twin drugs must be considered together. In general, the less said about them, the better. Antiamphetamine laws and campaigns have been among the major factors popularizing the amphetamines (see Chapter 38); and recent law-enforcement efforts to suppress the amphetamines have opened wide the door to cocaine (see Chapter 41).

Among drug users and potential drug users, two facts about the amphetamines are worth stressing. First, they are much less likely to prove damaging if taken in modest doses; hence the dosage should be kept down. Second, they should be taken orally if at all; the *injection* of amphetamines or cocaine in large doses constitutes one of the most damaging forms of drug use known to man. The failure to draw these distinctions between small and large doses, between oral and intravenous use, discredits drug propaganda programs and encourages the "speed-freak" phenomenon. For details, see Chapter 37.

The latest data from the youth drug scene suggest that the speed-freak phenomenon—that is, the injection of amphetamines in large doses—has passed its peak. Many speed freaks are turning to heroin instead, and the recruitment of new speed freaks is falling off. If a fresh antiamphetamine campaign is not launched, there is every reason to hope that the next wave of youthful drug users will engage in less damaging forms of drug use. But a revival of the antiamphetamine campaign could well sabotage this hopeful outlook.

The barbiturates and alcohol. These are pharmacologically a single problem. Both make you drunk in the same way; both can be addicting in the same way; both can produce hangovers, and delirium tremens can occur after withdrawal from excessive and persistent use. The barbiturates have the effect, in most respects, of solid alcohol—and alcohol is from the pharmacological point of view a kind of liquid barbiturate (see Part IV). The persistent, excessive use of alcohol and barbiturates ranks with the speed-freak phenomenon in damage wrought, and affects vastly more people.

The great majority of users of alcoholic beverages are able to do so occasionally, in moderation, and with minimal adverse effects. But roughly 10 percent of the users become alcoholics (alcohol addicts) or "problem drinkers," with disastrous results to themselves and to society. As with the use of other addicting drugs, no one using alcohol can foretell if or when he will be among the addicted.

Alcohol Prohibition failed woefully from 1920 to 1933. Barbiturate repression is no more successful today. For these as for most other drugs, the ideal solution is to raise a generation of young people whose *needs* for such drugs are minimal. At moments when life is rich and challenging, who wants a mood-altering drug?

As an interim measure, Consumers Union recommends that the advertising and promotion of alcoholic beverages be prohibited. An appropriate hazard notice should be required on all alcoholic beverage labels; like the warning on cigarette packages, it might not deter use of alcohol, but such a notice would at least indicate society's recognition of the potentially harmful nature of alcoholic beverages.

Other interim measures that might palliate this country's alcohol problem—a far larger problem, no matter how measured, than all other drug problems added together—are beyond the scope of this Report.

In particular, the problem of driving automobiles and using machinery while drunk on alcohol is a major menace. A solution to the drunken-driving problem is urgently needed, along with a solution to the problem of driving while under the influence of other drugs. Prohibition of drugs, like prohibition of alcohol, is *not* the answer.

Nicotine. This, too, is an addicting drug. "The confirmed smoker acts under a compulsion which is quite comparable to that of the heroin user." [1] For the evidence, see Part III. Just as some heroin addicts can and do stop, so some cigarette smokers can and do stop. But the disastrous effect of basing public policy on these exceptional cases is evident from that fact that cigarette consumption, after seven years of anticigarette drives urging voluntary abstinence, is close to its all-time high.

The other evil effect of failure to recognize that nicotine is an addicting

[533]

drug is that it encourages young people to start smoking. A majority of teen-age smokers have been persuaded, at least in part by anticigarette campaigns, that they will be able to smoke for a few years and then "kick the habit" when they are ready to quit (see Chapter 26). It is hard to imagine a nastier trap than this one that society has set for its own children.

The anticigarette campaigns have succeeded in persuading both adults and teen-agers that cigarette smoking causes lung cancer and is damaging to health in numerous other ways. But this conviction is not deterring tens of millions of adults and teen-agers from smoking cigarettes. Despite the highly impressive anticigarette ads on television and other well-planned campaigns, the proportion of smokers among seventeen- and eighteen-year-olds is almost as high as among adults.

It is uncertain whether a ban on cigarette advertising by itself would significantly reduce the numbers of new recruits to cigarette smoking. But, while it may not by itself be sufficient, such a ban is a necessary precondition if other anticigarette measures are to be effective (see Chapter 26). This is the practical ground that leads Consumers Union to recommend that all cigarette advertising and promotion—including point-of-sale displays and cigarette vending machines—be banned altogether.

There is also an ethical ground for our recommendation: it is immoral to permit the advertising of an addicting product that causes lung cancer and other diseases.

In the absence of effective ways to curb cigarette smoking, a safer substitute for nicotine is needed. So far, scientists have hardly even begun to look for one. When they do start to look, the odds are excellent that they will find a safer nicotine substitute, as well as safer ways of using nicotine itself.

Prescription drugs. Adults are securing mind-affecting drugs on prescription in vast quantities—stimulants, sedatives, hypnotics, tranquilizers, and others. Whether they are getting too many, or not enough, or the wrong ones, deserves objective research.

Many members of the generation under thirty are using, among others, the same drugs their elders get on prescription—but without bothering to get a prescription first. If young adults continue this practice as they mature, many prescription drugs may gradually become "nondrugs" like caffeine, nicotine, and alcohol. This, indeed, may already be happening. For details, see Chapter 62.

LSD. Until 1962, this drug was a promising adjunct to psychotherapy, tried out on thousands of patients with few adverse effects (see Chapter 48). Then came the anti-LSD campaign and the anti-LSD laws, which helped convert LSD from a psychotherapeutic novelty to an illicit drug popular even among high-school students.

The anti-LSD publicity, the scare campaigns, and the laws also helped convert what had been until 1962 a relatively unknown and innocuous drug into a quite damaging one. As in the case of heroin, legal and social rather than pharmacological factors account for most of the LSD tragedies of the 1960s (see Chapter 51).

Now that the furor has died down, LSD appears to be becoming less damaging again. The latest data indicate that it is not (as was supposed) a way of life, but a stage through which some drug users pass. Most users either discontinue LSD altogether after a few months or years or else reduce their consumption to a few "trips" a year.

The scattered data available so far indicate that LSD use has not benefited users as much as they suppose—nor has it damaged them as much as has been alleged. The LSD "chromosome scare" is treated in Chapters 50 and 52.

It is still too early to map out a sensible program for making the LSD experience legally available to those who want it for self-betterment and self-exploration ("mind expansion"). That time, however, may come. Meanwhile, experimental use of LSD in therapy for alcoholism, for the palliation of terminal cancer, and perhaps for other indications, should be revived and objectively evaluated.

As matters stand, with only "street LSD" of unknown strength and purity available, and in the absence of skilled supervision, no prudent person will take LSD—just as no prudent person will get dead drunk on alcohol. And it is the height of imprudence to take LSD more than a few times a year—just as it is the height of imprudence to get drunk frequently. For schizophrenics, for borderline schizoid personalities, and perhaps for some others, LSD may prove particularly damaging.

Laws, policies, and attitudes should accordingly be shaped to minimize the damage done by LSD and LSD-like drugs to those imprudent enough to take them. Repressive and punitive laws that add the damage done by imprisonment and criminalization to whatever damage may be done by LSD are irrational and counterproductive.

Marijuana. It is now much too late to debate the issue: marijuana *versus* no marijuana. Marijuana is here to stay. No conceivable law-enforcement program can curb its availability. Accordingly, we offer these seven recommendations.

(1) Consumers Union recommends the immediate repeal of all federal laws governing the growing, processing, transportation, sale, possession, and use of marijuana.

(2) Consumers Union recommends that each of the fifty states similarly repeal its existing marijuana laws and pass new laws legalizing the cultivation, processing, and orderly marketing of marijuana—subject to appropriate regulations.

The term "legalization of marijuana" means many things to many people. As used here, it means that marijuana should be classed as a licit rather than an illicit drug.

We do *not* recommend legalization because we believe that marijuana is "safe" or "harmless." No drug is safe or harmless to all people at all dosage levels or under all conditions of use. Our recommendation arises out of the conviction that an orderly system of legal distribution and licit use will have notable advantages for both users and nonusers over the present marijuana black market. In particular it will separate the channels of marijuana distribution from heroin channels and from the channels of distribution of other illicit drugs—and will thereby limit the exposure of marijuana smokers to other illicit drugs. Even more important, it will end the criminalization and alienation of young people and the damage done to them by arrest, conviction, and imprisonment for marijuana offenses.

Three major questions are not answered by the above recommendation:

• What *kind* of distribution system should be substituted for the present black-market system?
• What specific regulations should govern the new system?
• What should be the respective roles of the state and federal governments?

Most discussions of legalizing marijuana anticipate that distribution will be turned over to the tobacco companies, or the alcoholic beverage companies, or to similar large commercial enterprises. We urge instead that individual states experiment with a wide range of distribution patterns.

Marijuana grows readily in fields, along highways, in backyards, in window boxes, and even in suitably illuminated closets and cellars. An informal distribution system has grown up that is, in considerable part, a sharing among friends, and that is patterned after native arts-and-crafts enterprise rather than large-scale commercial enterprise. If legalizing marijuana should mean turning over production and distribution exclusively to the tobacco companies or to other corporate giants, it is questionable whether all marijuana smokers would readily patronize such a system. Some would no doubt continue to harvest and distribute their own, illegally, just as mountaineers and others continue to make and sell their own whiskey. Bootlegging does not encourage respect for law.

Unfortunately, no body of experience exists in any Western country which might serve as a guide or model for an acceptable system of marijuana distribution. In the absence of experience, neither the states nor the federal government can foretell how a system will work. We therefore

[536]

believe that the fifty states—at least in the beginning—should be left free to devise their own systems and that a wide range of alternative systems should be tried out. Among the possibilities are distribution through a statewide marijuana monopoly (private or public), through small-scale enterprises resembling arts-and-crafts centers, through alcohol channels, and through tobacco channels.

The fifty states should similarly consider alternative answers to other pressing questions. At what age should young people be allowed to buy marijuana legally? Should only one grade and strength be permitted, or should varying strengths be legally marketable? Should marijuana smoking be permitted in public or only in private? If in public, should it be permitted in cocktail lounges, taverns, bars, and roadhouses or only in places where alcoholic beverages are *not* sold? How can the problem of operating an automobile or other machinery while under the influence of marijuana best be handled? Only a wide range of experience can provide the answers needed for wise long-term decisions on these and related issues.

This does not mean, however, that the federal government should play no role. Experience in other fields has shown federal regulation to have great advantages; and this is almost certain to prove true with marijuana regulation as experience with various regulatory approaches accumulates.

(3) **Consumers Union therefore recommends that a national marijuana commission be established to help provide the states with needed research information, to monitor the various plans evolved by the states, and to build, eventually, the best features of those plans into federal marijuana legislation.**

Adequately staffed and funded, the commission should coordinate federal and state research programs, including ongoing controlled studies into long-term effects of marijuana use.

If some aspect of one state's plan proves disastrous, the commission should recommend a federal law prohibiting the practice nationally. If some other aspect of a state's law proves to be an outstanding success, the successful feature can in due course be accepted as national policy and embodied in federal laws or regulations. Four possibilities in particular should concern the national marijuana commission from the beginning:

- A law making it a federal offense to transport marijuana into a state in violation of that state's own laws. (A similar provision concerning the transportation of intoxicating liquors is contained in Section 2 of the Twenty-first Amendment to the United States Constitution, which repealed the Eighteenth [Alcohol Prohibition] Amendment.)
- A law setting national standards of marijuana strength and purity.
- A law banning the advertising or promotion of marijuana anywhere in the United States.

• A law requiring a detailed warning notice on all marijuana package labels. Such a warning, like the warning on cigarette packages, is unlikely to deter use; but it will serve to remind users that the legalization of marijuana does not constitute official approval of marijuana or assurance of the drug's harmlessness.

Such a hybrid of state experimentation plus federal intervention is hardly a tidy arrangement, but our system of government has never been noted for its tidiness. In fact, as a welcome result of this untidiness, it is possible for a state to experiment with a new policy without the entire country being subjected to that experimentation.* Our marijuana proposals are designed to take the greatest possible advantage of this freedom to experiment—while also making it possible to terminate experiments that go sour and to adopt nationally those that succeed.

During the period of transition, the marijuana debate will no doubt wax even hotter than it has in the past. Even more attention will be focused on marijuana—even more people will be attracted to the drug. Perhaps it will prove unfortunate, but it is equally possible that one effect of the greater concern with marijuana will be a lessening of use of other drugs, licit as well as illicit. This may prove a major gain.

(4) **Consumers Union recommends that state and federal taxes on marijuana be kept moderate, and that tax proceeds be devoted primarily to drug research, drug education, and other measures specifically designed to minimize the damage done by alcohol, nicotine, marijuana, heroin, and other drugs.**

Both Congress and state legislatures over the years have tended to tax alcoholic beverages and cigarettes for all that the traffic will bear—in part on the theory that high prices may deter use. As we have shown, however, high drug prices do *not* deter use. High taxes similarly would be unlikely to deter marijuana use. Rather, their effect very probably would be to encourage the bootlegging and smuggling of marijuana to avoid the tax, as whiskey is bootlegged and cigarettes are smuggled today.

It is hardly likely, of course, that Congress will repeal federal marijuana laws tomorrow, or that state legislatures will legalize marijuana without lengthy debate. Some delay may be tolerable—provided that interim measures are taken to end the cruelty and irrationality of current laws. We accordingly propose these interim measures, which we urge Congress and the states to adopt *without* delay:

---

* United States Supreme Court Justice Louis D. Brandeis wrote (1931): "It is one of the happy incidents of the federal system that a single courageous State may, if its citizens choose, serve as a laboratory; and try novel social and economic experiments without risk to the rest of the country."[2]

(5) **Consumers Union recommends an immediate end to imprisonment as a punishment for marijuana possession and for furnishing marijuana to friends.** *

This recommendation rests on the *nihil nocere* principle set forth above. The imprisonment of youthful marijuana users has not curbed marijuana smoking. It does more harm than good (see Part VIII). When a physician finds that his prescription is doing more harm than good, he withdraws the prescription.

The usual argument for continuing to imprison marijuana offenders—that the results of further scientific research should be awaited—is sophistical and brings both the law and scientific research into disrepute. What it tells young marijuana smokers, in effect, is something like this: "We will continue to imprison you for marijuana offenses because scientists are searching feverishly for some justification for imprisoning marijuana smokers, and they will no doubt find one some day." Even if marijuana ultimately proves as damaging as alcohol, which seems very unlikely, imprisonment is hardly the treatment of choice for users.

(6) **Consumers Union recommends, pending legalization of marijuana, that marijuana possession and sharing be immediately made civil violations rather than criminal acts.** Including marijuana offenses under the criminal law has two major adverse effects on marijuana smokers, even if there is no imprisonment. First, a criminal record bars an individual from government employment and from a wide variety of other jobs and activities. Second, engaging in criminal behavior has a subtle but significant effect on the self-image of individuals. Because they are criminals under the law, they begin to think of themselves as criminals. Lacking respect for the marijuana laws, they may lose respect for other laws as well. Taking marijuana possession and sharing offenses out of the criminal law altogether will contribute to respect for law.

(7) **Consumers Union recommends that those now serving prison terms for possession of or sharing marijuana be set free, and that such marijuana offenses be expunged from all legal records.** It is hard to think of a more dramatic way to demonstrate this country's earnest desire to bridge the generation gap and to right grievous miscarriages of justice. Respect for law will surely increase.

---

* From the 1970 *Interim Report* of Canada's Le Dain Commission: "There is obviously a big difference between selling the drug for monetary consideration and giving it to a friend. Selling it at cost to an acquaintance is different from selling it to a variety of people to make a profit. Selling it on a small scale to make a marginal profit—perhaps to support one's own usage—is not the same as organizing and controlling a large entrepreneurial organization. As can be seen, trafficking activities range along a spectrum from a kind of act not far removed in seriousness from simple possession to the extensive activities of the stereotyped exploiter and profiteer whose image led to the kinds of penalties associated with trafficking." [3]

70.

A last word

Before long, the generation now in its teens and twenties will be in its thirties and forties. Judges, prosecutors, and even narcotics agents, along with legislators and teachers, will be drawn from the pot-smoking, acid-dropping generation. When that time comes, they will find themselves confronting the same basic drug issues their elders confront today. How can the damage done by alcohol, nicotine, and other drugs be minimized? How can young children be protected from drug excesses? How can adolescents be helped to exercise prudence? How can nonchemical alternatives to the drug experience be developed and popularized? How can human life be enriched?

We hope that when the next generation takes over, this Consumers Union Report will still remain useful—as a guide to how mankind has used and misused drugs in the past, and as a warning against repeating the errors society is making today.

Notes

A number of works are cited in this Report with great frequency. Rather than repeat the full reference each time, we have listed them in full immediately below and again when first footnoted. Thereafter they are cited in the abbreviated style indicated below.

Drug Addiction: Crime or Disease? Interim and Final Reports of the Joint Committee of the American Bar Association and the American Medical Association on Narcotic Drugs (Bloomington, Ind.: Indiana University Press, 1961). Hereinafter cited as *ABA-AMA Report*.

George H. Stevenson et al., "Drug Addiction in British Columbia: A Research Survey" (University of British Columbia, 1956); unpublished. Hereinafter cited as *British Columbia Study*.

Louis S. Goodman and Alfred Gilman, eds., *The Pharmacological Basis of Therapeutics* (New York: Macmillan Co.). Hereinafter cited as *Goodman and Gilman*, preceded by contributor's name and followed by edition number and year (3rd ed., 1965, or 4th ed., 1970).

Interim Report of the Commission of Inquiry Into the Non-Medical Use of Drugs (Ottawa: Queen's Printer for Canada, 1970). Hereinafter cited as *Le Dain Commission Interim Report*.

Proceedings of the First National Conference on Methadone Treatment, New York, June 1968, supported by Health Research Council, New York City; New York State Narcotic Addiction Control Commission; and National Association for the Prevention of Addiction (NAPAN); mimeographed; unpublished. Hereinafter cited as *Proceedings, First Methadone Conference*.

Proceedings, Second National Conference on Methadone Treatment, New York, October 1969, sponsored by National Association for the Prevention of Addiction to Narcotics (NAPAN) and co-sponsored by National Institute of Mental Health; mimeographed; unpublished. Hereinafter cited as *Proceedings, Second Methadone Conference*.

Proceedings, Third National Conference on Methadone Treatment, New York, November 1970, sponsored by National Association for the Prevention of Addiction to Narcotics (NAPAN) and co-sponsored by National Institute of Mental Health; U. S. Public Health Service Publication No. 2172 (Washington, D.C.: U.S. Government Printing Office, 1971). Hereinafter cited as *Proceedings, Third Methadone Conference*.

Charles E. Terry and Mildred Pellens, *The Opium Problem* (New York: Committee on Drug Addictions, Bureau of Social Hygiene, Inc., 1928). Hereinafter cited as *Terry and Pellens*. [A reprint edition of *The Opium Problem* was published in 1970 by Patterson Smith Publishing Corporation, Montclair, N.J.]

In addition, for the sake of brevity, the *Journal of the American Medical Association* is cited as *JAMA* throughout the Notes.

Chapter 1

1. Hubert S. Howe, "A Physician's Blueprint for the Management and Prevention of Narcotic Addiction," *New York State Journal of Medicine*, 55 (February 1, 1955): 341–348.
2. Charles E. Terry and Mildred Pellens, *The Opium Problem* (New York: Committee on Drug Addictions, Bureau of Social Hygiene, Inc., 1928), p. 18. Hereinafter cited as *Terry and Pellens*.

3. Ibid., pp. 61, 96.
4. Ibid., pp. 75, 123.
5. Charles B. Towns, "The Peril of the Drug Habit," *Century Magazine*, 84 (1912): 580–587.
6. *Terry and Pellens*, p. 670.
7. *Proceedings, American Pharmaceutical Association*, 13 (1865): 51.
8. Perry M. Lichtenstein, "Thirteen Years' Observation on Drug Addiction at the Tombs Prison," *Narcotic Education*, ed. H. S. Middlemiss, *Proceedings of the First World Conference on Narcotic Education, July 5–9, 1926, Philadelphia* (Washington, D.C., 1926), p. 123.
9. S. Dana Hays, quoted in *Annual Report of the State Board of Health, Massachusetts* (1871), cited in *Terry and Pellens*, p. 7.
10. D. M. R. Culbrith, *Materia Medica and Pharmacology*, 3rd ed. (1903), cited in *Terry and Pellens*, p. 7.
11. Opium Poppy Control Act of 1942, Public Law No. 400, 78th Cong.
12. Quoted by Alonzo Calkins, *Opium and the Opium Appetite* (Philadelphia, 1871), cited in *Terry and Pellens*, p. 6.
13. Quoted by Calkins, *Opium and the Opium Appetite*.
14. Virgil G. Eaton, "How the Opium Habit Is Acquired," *Popular Science Monthly*, 33 (1888): 666, cited in Alfred R. Lindesmith, *Opiate Addiction* (Evanston, Ill.: Principia Press, 1947), p. 105.
15. Quoted by F. E. Oliver, *Annual Report of the State Board of Health, Massachusetts* (1871), cited in *Terry and Pellens*, p. 9.
16. *Annual Report, Michigan State Board of Health* (1878), Table 1, cited in *Terry and Pellens*, p. 12.
17. W. Dodd, *The Factory System Illustrated* (1842), p. 149, cited in E. P. Thompson, *The Making of the English Working Class*, 1966 ed. (New York: Vintage Books, 1963), p. 328.
18. "Report by Dr. Henry Julian Hunter on the Excessive Mortality of Infants in Some Rural Districts of England," in *Public Health. Reports of the Medical Officer of the Privy Council*, 6th Report (1864), p. 459, cited in Karl Marx, *Capital*, ed. Friedrich Engels, trans. Samuel Moore and Edward Aveling (Moscow: Progress Publishers, 1965), I, 399.
19. Ibid., p. 460.
20. Karl Marx, *Capital*, I, 399.
21. *Medical Times and Gazette*, 2 (London: July 19, 1873): 73.
22. C. Fraser Brockington, *Public Health in the Nineteenth Century* (London: E. & S. Livingstone, Ltd., 1965), pp. 225, 226.
23. Anon., "The Opium Habit," in *Catholic World*, 33 (September, 1881): 828.
24. Ibid., p. 829.
25. Ibid., p. 834.

Chapter 2

1. H. H. Kane, *The Hypodermic Injection of Morphia. Its History, Advantages, and Dangers. Based on Experience of 360 Physicians* (New York, 1880).
2. J. R. Black, "Advantages of Substituting the Morphia Habit for the Incurably Alcoholic," *Cincinnati Lancet-Clinic* (1889), cited in Alfred R. Lindesmith, *Opiate Addiction* (Evanston, Ill.: Principia Press, 1947), p. 183.
3. *Heroin and Heroin Paraphernalia*, Second Report by the Select Committee on Crime, House Report No. 91–1808, 91st Cong., 2nd Sess., January 2, 1971.
4. J. R. Black, cited in Lindesmith, *Opiate Addiction*, p. 184.
5. *Medical Times and Gazette*, 2 (London: July 19, 1873): 73.
6. John A. O'Donnell, *Narcotics Addicts in Kentucky*, U.S. Public Health Service Publication No. 1881 (Chevy Chase, Md.: National Institute of Mental Health, 1969), p. 77.
7. Ibid., p. 88.

8. Ibid., p. 138.
9. Ibid., p. 140.
10. Ibid.
11. Lawrence Kolb, *Drug Addiction, A Medical Problem* (Springfield, Ill.: Charles C Thomas, 1962), pp. 55–59.
12. Richard Brotman and Alfred M. Freedman, *A Community Mental Health Approach to Drug Addiction*, U.S. Department of Health, Education, and Welfare, Social and Rehabilitation Service, Office of Juvenile Delinquency and Youth Development (Washington, D.C.: U.S. Government Printing Office, 1968), p. 36.
13. Horatio Day, *The Opium Habit* (1868), cited in *Terry and Pellens*, p. 5.
14. William Pepper, *System of Practical Medicine* (1886), cited in *Terry and Pellens*, p. 100.
15. J. C. Wilson and A. A. Eshner, *American Textbook of Applied Therapeutics* (1896), cited in *Terry and Pellens*, p. 104.
16. Thomas C. Allbutt, *A System of Medicine* (1905), cited in *Terry and Pellens*, p. 186.
17. L. L. Stanley, "Morphinism," *Journal of the American Institute of Criminal Law and Criminology*, 6 (November 4, 1915): 586.
18. U.S. Department of Health, Education, and Welfare, Public Health Service, *Narcotic Drug Addiction*, U. S. Public Health Service Mental Health Monograph No. 2, Publication No. 1021 (Washington, D.C.: U. S. Government Printing Office, 1963), p. 8.
19. George H. Stevenson et al., "Drug Addiction in British Columbia: A Research Survey" (University of British Columbia, 1956); unpublished. Hereinafter cited as *British Columbia Study*.
20. Ibid., p. 391.
21. James D. Hardy, Harold G. Wolff, and Helen Goodell, *Pain Sensations and Reactions* (Baltimore: Williams & Wilkins, 1952), p. 264.
22. Louis Lasagna, John M. von Felsinger, and Henry K. Beecher, "Drug-Induced Mood Changes in Man," in *JAMA*, 157 (March 19, 1955): 1006–1020; Henry K. Beecher, "Analgesics and the Reaction Component of Pain," in *Drugs and the Brain*, ed. Perry Black (Baltimore: Johns Hopkins Press, 1969), p. 169.
23. J. Yerbury Dent, in *British Journal of Addiction*, 49 (1952): 17.
24. Jerome H. Jaffe, in Louis S. Goodman and Alfred Gilman, eds., *The Pharmacological Basis of Therapeutics* (New York: Macmillan), 4th ed. (1970), pp. 285–286. Hereinafter cited as *Goodman and Gilman* preceded by contributor's name and followed by edition number and year (3rd ed., 1965, or 4th ed., 1970).

Chapter 3

1. *Annual Report, Michigan State Board of Health* (1878), cited in *Terry and Pellens*, p. 13.
2. C. W. Earle, "The Opium Habit," *Chicago Medical Review* (1880), cited in *Terry and Pellens*, p. 470.
3. J. M. Hull, *The Opium Habit, Report of the State Board of Health, Iowa* (1885), cited in *Terry and Pellens*, p. 470.
4. C. W. Earle in *Terry and Pellens*, p. 470.
5. L. P. Brown, "Enforcement of the Tennessee Anti-Narcotic Law," *American Journal of Public Health*, 5 (1914), cited in *Terry and Pellens*, p. 471.
6. Ibid., p. 476.
7. *Traffic in Narcotic Drugs*, Report of Special Committee of Investigation Appointed by the Secretary of the Treasury (1918), cited in *Terry and Pellens*, p. 472.
8. *Traffic in Opium and Other Dangerous Drugs*, U.S. Treasury Department, Bureau of Narcotics, for year ending Dec. 31, 1967 (Washington, D.C.: U.S. Government Printing Office, 1968), Table 12, p. 55.
9. C. W. Earle in *Terry and Pellens*, p. 475.
10. J. M. Hull in *Terry and Pellens*, p. 476.

11. L. P. Brown in *Terry and Pellens,* p. 476.
12. *Traffic in Opium and Other Dangerous Drugs,* Table 12, p. 55.
13. B. H. Hartwell, "The Sale and Use of Opium in Massachusetts," *Annual Report of the State Board of Health, Massachusetts,* 20 (1889): 137–156, cited in *Terry and Pellens,* p. 488.
14. Anon., "The Opium Habit," in *Catholic World,* 33 (September, 1881): 827.
15. J. M. Hull, quoted in *Terry and Pellens,* p. 17.
16. C. E. Terry, *Annual Report, Board of Health* (Jacksonville, Fla., 1913); and Lucius P. Brown, *American Journal of Public Health* (1915), cited in *Terry and Pellens,* pp. 25, 28.
17. Data supplied by Bureau of Narcotics and Dangerous Drugs, U. S. Department of Justice.

Chapter 4

1. *Robinson v. California,* 370 U.S. 660, 1962.
2. *British Columbia Study,* pp. 509–510.
3. Ibid., p. 510.
4. Ibid., pp. 510–511.
5. National Heroin Symposium, San Francisco, June 1971.
6. Arthur B. Light and Edward G. Torrance, *Opium Addiction* (Chicago: American Medical Association, n. d. [1929 or 1930?]).
7. Arthur B. Light and Edward G. Torrance, in *A.M.A. Archives of Internal Medicine,* 44 (1929): 876.
8. Light and Torrance, in *A.M.A. Archives of Internal Medicine,* 43 (1929): 331.
9. Ibid., p. 327.
10. Ibid., p. 690.
11. Ibid., p. 329.
12. *British Columbia Study,* p. 516.
13. Light and Torrance, in *A.M.A. Archives of Internal Medicine,* 43 (1929): 332.
14. George B. Wallace, "The Rehabilitation of the Drug Addict," *Journal of Educational Sociology,* 4 (1931): 347, quoted in Daniel M. Wilner and Gene G. Kassebaum, eds., *Narcotics* (New York: Blakiston Div., McGraw-Hill, 1965), pp. xix–xx.
15. Harris Isbell, in *Narcotic Drug Addiction Problems* (Bethesda, Md.: National Institute of Mental Health, 1958), U.S. Public Health Service Publication No. 1050.
16. Walter G. Karr, cited in *Drug Addiction: Crime or Disease? Interim and Final Reports of the Joint Committee of the American Bar Association and the American Medical Association on Narcotic Drugs* (Bloomington, Ind.: Indiana University Press, 1961), p. 47. Hereinafter cited as *ABA-AMA Report.*
17. Nathan B. Eddy, cited in Alfred R. Lindesmith, *Opiate Addiction* (Evanston, Ill.: Principia Press, 1947), p. 729.
18. Richard Brotman, Alan S. Meyer, and Alfred M. Freedman, "An Approach to Treating Narcotic Addicts Based on a Community Mental Health Diagnosis," *Comprehensive Psychiatry,* 6 (April, 1965): 108.
19. Vincent P. Dole, personal communication.
20. Ibid.
21. Lawrence Kolb and W. F. Ossenfort, "The Treatment of Drug Addicts at the Lexington Hospital," *Southern Medical Journal,* 31 (August, 1938): 916.
22. A. Z. Pfeffer and D. C. Ruble, "Chronic Psychosis and Addiction to Morphine," *Archives of Neurology and Psychiatry,* 56 (December, 1946): 665–672.
23. Marie Nyswander, *The Drug Addict as a Patient* (New York and London: Grune & Stratton, 1956).
24. *British Columbia Study,* pp. 514–515.
25. Ibid., p. 518.
26. Harris Isbell and H. F. Fraser, in *Pharmacological Reviews,* 2 (1950): 373.
27. *British Columbia Study,* p. 513.
28. Ibid.

29. Lawrence Kolb, *Drug Addiction, A Medical Problem* (Springfield, Ill.: Charles C Thomas, 1962), p. 120.
30. Henry Brill, "Misapprehensions About Drug Addiction: Some Origins and Repercussions," *Comprehensive Psychiatry*, 4 (June, 1963): 155.
31. Lawrence Kolb, "Pleasure and Deterioration from Narcotic Addiction," *Mental Hygiene*, 9 (1925): 711–713.
32. Ibid., p. 723.
33. *British Columbia Study*, p. 319.
34. Ibid., p. 99.
35. Ibid.
36. William F. Wieland and Michael Yunger, in *Proceedings, Third National Conference on Methadone Treatment*, New York, November 1970, sponsored by National Association for the Prevention of Addiction to Narcotics (NAPAN) and co-sponsored by National Institute of Mental Health; U.S. Public Health Service Publication No. 2172 (Washington, D.C.: U.S. Government Printing Office, 1971), pp. 50–53. Hereinafter cited as *Proceedings, Third Methadone Conference*.
37. Paul Cushman, Jr., in *Proceedings, Third Methadone Conference*, pp. 144–149.
38. Robert C. Wallach, Eulogio Jerez, and George Blinick, "Pregnancy and Menstrual Function in Narcotics Addicts Treated with Methadone," *American Journal of Obstetrics and Gynecology*, 105 (December 15, 1969): 1228.
39. George Blinick, Robert C. Wallach, and Eulogio Jerez, "Pregnancy in Narcotics Addicts Treated by Medical Withdrawal," *American Journal of Obstetrics and Gynecology*, 105 (December 1, 1969): 998.
40. Ibid., p. 1000.
41. Ibid., pp. 999–1001.
42. Saul Blatman, in *Proceedings, Third Methadone Conference*, p. 83.
43. Blinick, Wallach, and Jerez, "Pregnancy in Narcotics Addicts Treated by Medical Withdrawal," p. 1001.
44. George Blinick, in *Proceedings, Third Methadone Conference*, p. 82.
45. Saul Blatman, in *Proceedings, Third Methadone Conference*, pp. 82–85.
46. Avram Goldstein, in *Proceedings, Third Methadone Conference*, pp. 35–36.

Chapter 5

1. Wilder Penfield, "Halsted of Johns Hopkins, The Man and His Problem as Described in the Secret Records of William Osler," *JAMA*, 210 (December 22, 1969): 2215.
2. Ibid., p. 2214.
3. William Osler, quoted in Penfield, "Halsted of Johns Hopkins," p. 2216.
4. Cited by Sally Hammond, "The Famous Addicts," New York *Post*, July 22, 1970.
5. William Osler, quoted in Penfield, "Halsted of Johns Hopkins," p. 2217.
6. Windsor C. Cutting, "Morphine Addiction for 62 Years," *Stanford Medical Bulletin*, 1 (August, 1942): 39–41.
7. Harry J. Anslinger and Will Oursler, *The Murderers* (New York: Farrar, Straus and Cudahy, 1961), pp. 181–182.
8. Ibid., p. 169.
9. Eugene J. Morhous, "Drug Addiction in Upper Economic Levels: A Study of 142 Cases," *West Virginia Medical Journal*, 49 (July, 1953): 189.
10. *Proceedings, White House Conference on Narcotic and Drug Abuse*, September 27–28, 1962 (Washington, D.C.: U.S. Government Printing Office, 1962), p. 305.
11. Quoted in Nat Hentoff, *A Doctor Among the Addicts* (Chicago: Rand McNally, 1968), pp. 43–44.
12. Jerome H. Jaffe, in *Goodman and Gilman*, 4th ed. (1970), p. 286.
13. Eugene J. Morhous, "Drug Addiction in Upper Economic Levels," p. 189.
14. Report No. 72, Senate Committee on Government Operations, 89 Cong., 1st Sess., p. 78.

15. *Hearings Before the Select Committee on Crime,* House of Representatives, 91st Cong., 1st Sess., 1969, p. 291.
16. National Heroin Symposium, San Francisco, June 1971.
17. Cited in Edward A. Preble and John J. Casey, Jr., "Taking Care of Business—The Heroin User's Life on the Street," *International Journal of the Addictions,* 4 (March, 1969): 2.
18. Isador Chein et al., *The Road to H* (New York: Basic Books, 1964), cited in Preble and Casey, "Taking Care of Business," p. 2.
19. Richard A. Cloward and Lloyd E. Ohlin, *Delinquency and Opportunity* (Glencoe, Ill.: Free Press, 1960), cited in Preble and Casey, "Taking Care of Business," p. 2.
20. *British Columbia Study,* pp. 396–397.
21. Preble and Casey, "Taking Care of Business," pp. 2–3.
22. Ibid., pp. 21–22.

Chapter 6

1. H. H. Kane, *Opium Smoking in America and China* (New York, 1882), cited in *Terry and Pellens,* p. 73.
2. Jonathan Spence, "Opium Smoking in Ch'ing China," presented at the Conference on Local Control and Social Protest During the Ch'ing Period, Honolulu, 1971 (under the auspices of the American Council of Learned Societies and the University of California); unpublished.
3. *British Columbia Study,* pp. 498–500.
4. Kane, in *Terry and Pellens,* p. 73.
5. Ibid.
6. Ibid.
7. Cited in Alfred R. Lindesmith, *Opiate Addiction* (Evanston, Ill.: Principia Press, 1947), p. 186.
8. Kane, in *Terry and Pellens,* p. 808.
9. Ibid.
10. *Terry and Pellens,* p. 747.
11. Ibid., p. 748.
12. *Exec. Doc. No. 79,* House of Representatives, 50th Cong., 1st Sess., C. S. Fairchild to Mr. Carlisle, Jan. 12, 1888, cited in *Terry and Pellens,* p. 747.
13. *Terry and Pellens,* pp. 747–748.
14. Lawrence Kolb and A. G. Du Mez, *The Prevalence and Trend of Drug Addiction in the United States and Factors Influencing It,* Treasury Department, U.S. Public Health Service, Reprint No. 924 (Washington, D.C.: U.S. Government Printing Office, 1924), p. 14.
15. *Outlook,* 91 (February 6, 1909): 275; Public Law No. 221, 60th Cong., approved February 9, 1909.
16. Public Law No. 46, 63rd Cong., approved January 17, 1914.
17. Public Law No. 47, 63rd Cong., approved January 17, 1914.
18. Public Law No. 233, 63rd Cong., approved December 17, 1914.
19. Harry J. Anslinger and William F. Tompkins, *The Traffic in Narcotics* (New York: Funk and Wagnalls, 1953), p. 54.
20. Baruch Spinoza, quoted by Joel Fort in Richard Blum and Associates, *Utopiates* (New York: Atherton Press, 1968), p. 205.
21. Charles B. Towns, "The Peril of the Drug Habit," *Century Magazine,* 84 (1912): 583.
22. Jerome H. Jaffe, in *Goodman and Gilman,* 3rd ed. (1965), p. 285.
23. Charles B. Towns, "The Peril of the Drug Habit," p. 583.
24. Lawrence Kolb, "Pleasure and Deterioration from Narcotic Addiction," *Mental Hygiene,* 9 (1925): 719–720.

Chapter 7

1. Samuel Hopkins Adams, *The Great American Fraud: Articles on the Nostrum Evil and Quackery,* reprinted from *Collier's* (1905, 1906, 1907, 1912) by American Medical Association, 1913.
2. *Terry and Pellens,* p. 75.
3. See, for example, Lawrence Kolb and A. G. Du Mez, *The Prevalence and Trend of Drug Addiction in the United States and Factors Influencing It,* Treasury Department, U.S. Public Health Service, Reprint No. 924 (Washington, D.C.: U.S. Government Printing Office, 1924), p. 14, Table 2.

Chapter 8

1. *Terry and Pellens,* pp. 629–631.
2. Harry J. Anslinger and William F. Tompkins, *The Traffic in Narcotics* (New York: Funk and Wagnalls, 1953), p. 8.
3. *Congressional Record,* U.S. House of Representatives, June 26, 1913, p. 2205.
4. Public Law No. 223, 63rd Cong., approved December 17, 1914.
5. Ibid.
6. Ibid.
7. Ibid.
8. "Mental Sequelae of the Harrison Law," *New York Medical Journal,* 102 (May 15, 1915): 1014.
9. Editorial Comment, *American Medicine,* 21 (O.S.), 10 (N.S.) (November 1915): 799–800.
10. Quoted by Anon., in *Outlook,* 112 (June 25, 1919): 122.
11. Ibid.
12. Lawrence Kolb, "Pleasure and Deterioration from Narcotic Addiction," *Mental Hygiene,* 9 (1925): 724.
13. *Task Force Report: Narcotics and Drug Abuse* (Washington, D.C.: U.S. Government Printing Office, 1967), p. 3.
14. "Stripping the Medical Profession of Its Powers and Giving Them to a Body of Lawmakers. The Proposed Amendment to the Harrison Narcotic Act—Everybody Seems to Know All About Doctoring Except the Doctors," *Illinois Medical Journal,* 49 (June 1926): 447.
15. August Vollmer, *The Police and Modern Society,* (Berkeley, 1936), pp. 117–118.
16. Alfred R. Lindesmith, "Dope Fiend Mythology," *Journal of the American Institute of Criminal Law and Criminology,* 31 (July-August, 1940): 207–208.
17. Rufus King in *Yale Law Journal,* 62 (1953): 748–749.
18. Karl M. Bowman, "Some Problems of Addiction," in *Problems of Addiction and Habituation,* ed. Paul H. Hoch and Joseph Zubin (New York: Grune & Stratton, 1958), p. 171.
19. Robert S. de Ropp, *Drugs and the Mind* (New York: St. Martin's Press, Macmillan, 1957), pp. 157–158.
20. *ABA-AMA Report,* pp. 19–21.
21. Jerome H. Jaffe, in *Goodman and Gilman,* 3rd ed. (1965), pp. 292–293.

Chapter 9

1. *Opium and Narcotic Laws,* compiled by Gilman G. Udell (Washington, D.C.: U.S. Government Printing Office, 1968), pp. ii–iv.
2. Ingeborg Paulus, "History of Drug Addiction and Legislation in Canada," The Narcotic Addiction Foundation of British Columbia, Vancouver, November 1966, unpublished.
3. Ibid., p. 6.

4. Sec. 2103d, Connecticut General Statutes, effective May 1, 1955.
5. *British Columbia Study,* p. 569.
6. Quoted by Gertrude Samuels, "Pot, Hard Drugs, and the Law," New York *Times Magazine,* February 15, 1970, p. 14.
7. Quoted by Gertrude Samuels, "Pot, Hard Drugs, and the Law," New York *Times Magazine,* February 15, 1970, p. 16.
8. Ibid.
9. Clemency application, Gilbert Mora Zargoza to Attorney General Robert F. Kennedy, January 18, 1962.
10. Harry J. Anslinger and William F. Tompkins, *The Traffic in Narcotics* (New York: Funk and Wagnalls, 1953), pp. 165, 281.
11. New York *Times,* September 25, 1969.
12. *People* v. *Glass,* 16 Ill. (2d) 595; 158 N.E. (2d) 639, 640 (1959).
13. *People* v. *Robinson,* 14 Ill. (2d), 325; 153 N.E. (2d) 65, 69 (1958).
14. *British Columbia Study,* Appendix G, p. 14.
15. Federal Jones-Miller Act (1922), cited by Udell, *Opium and Narcotic Laws,* p. 17.
16. New York *Times,* December 5, 1969.
17. *Robinson* v. *California,* 370 U.S. 660, 1962.
18. *British Columbia Study,* p. 415.
19. Ibid., pp. 415–416.
20. Ibid., p. 551.
21. David Burnham, reporting in New York *Times,* January 2, 1970.
22. New York *Times,* September 28, 1971.
23. Lawrence Kolb and A. G. Du Mez, *The Prevalence and Trend of Drug Addiction in the United States and Factors Influencing It,* Treasury Department, U.S. Public Health Service, Reprint No. 924 (Washington, D.C.: U.S. Government Printing Office, 1924).
24. Data supplied by Bureau of Narcotics and Dangerous Drugs, U.S. Department of Justice.
25. Robert van Hoek, Associate Administrator for Operations, Health Services and Mental Health Administration, U.S. Department of Health, Education, and Welfare, Statement in *Narcotics Research, Rehabilitation, and Treatment,* Hearings before the Select Committee on Crime, June 3, 1971, House of Representatives, 92nd Cong., 1st Sess., p. 431.

Chapter 10

1. Jerome H. Jaffe, in *Goodman and Gilman,* 4th ed. (1970), pp. 287–288.
2. George B. Wood, *Treatise on Therapeutics and Pharmacology* (1856), cited in *Terry and Pellens,* p. 518.
3. *British Medical Journal* (1867), cited in *Terry and Pellens,* p. 519.
4. Hugh C. Weir, "The American Opium Peril," *Putnam's Magazine,* 7 (1909): 330–331.
5. Harry J. Anslinger and William F. Tompkins, *The Traffic in Narcotics* (New York: Funk and Wagnalls, 1953), p. 24.
6. G. H. Hunt and M. E. Odoroff, "Follow-up Study of Narcotic Drug Addicts after Hospitalization," *Public Health Reports,* 77 (January, 1962): 41–54.
7. Henrietta Duvall, Ben Locke, and Leon Brill, "Follow-up Study of Narcotic Drug Addicts Five Years after Hospitalization," *Public Health Reports,* 78 (March, 1963): 185–193.
8. George E. Vaillant, "A Twelve-Year Follow-Up of New York Narcotic Addicts: I. The Relation of Treatment to Outcome," *American Journal of Psychiatry,* 122 (1965): 729–730.
9. Ibid., p. 730.
10. Ibid., p. 734.
11. John C. Kramer and Richard A. Bass, "Institutionalization Patterns Among Civilly Committed Addicts," *JAMA,* 208 (June 23, 1969): 2297–2301.

12. Ibid., p. 2298.
13. John C. Kramer, in *New Physician*, 18 (March, 1969): 208.
14. Ray E. Trussell, *Proceedings, White House Conference on Narcotic and Drug Abuse*, Panel 2, September 27–28, (Washington, D.C.: U.S. Government Printing Office, 1962), p. 68.
15. Ray E. Trussell, *Proceedings, Second National Conference on Methadone Treatment*, New York, October 1969, sponsored by National Association for the Prevention of Addiction to Narcotics (NAPAN) and co-sponsored by National Institute of Mental Health; mimeographed; unpublished, p. 12. Hereinafter cited as *Proceedings, Second Methadone Conference*.
16. Ibid., p. 13.
17. Ibid.
18. Trussell, *Proceedings, White House Conference on Narcotic and Drug Abuse*, pp. 70–71.
19. Trussell, *Proceedings, Second Methadone Conference*, p. 15.
20. Ibid.
21. Ibid.
22. Ibid., p. 16.
23. Meyer H. Diskind, "New Horizons in the Treatment of Narcotic Addiction," *Federal Probation*, 24 (December, 1960): 56–63.
24. Meyer H. Diskind and George Klonsky, "A Second Look at the New York State Parole Drug Experiment," *Federal Probation*, 28 (December, 1964): 34.
25. Ibid., p. 38.
26. Ibid.
27. Meyer H. Diskind, Robert F. Hallinan, and George Klonsky, "Narcotic Addiction and Post-Parole Adjustment," unpublished Master's dissertation, Fordham University, 1963, cited by Diskind and Klonsky, "A Second Look," p. 38.
28. New York *Times*, May 30, 1966.
29. ·Peter Kihss, reporting in New York *Times*, February 22, 1971.
30. Ibid.
31. Ibid.
32. Ibid.
33. Quoted by Owen Moritz, "Drug Program at $250 Million, Deemed a Failure," *National Observer*, June 8, 1970.
34. Bernard J. Langenauer and Charles L. Bowden, "Success and Failure in the NARA Addiction Program" and "A Follow-up Study of Narcotic Addicts in the NARA Program," papers delivered at the Annual Meeting of the American Psychiatric Association, Washington, D.C., May 1971.
35. Quoted in *Addiction and Drug Abuse Report*, ed. Samuel Grafton, 2 (June, 1971): 2.
36. Personal communication.
37. George Nash, Dan Waldorf, Kay Foster, and Ann Kyllingstad, "The Phoenix House Program: The Results of a Two Year Follow-up," New York, February 1971, unpublished.
38. Vincent P. Dole, in *New York Law Journal*, 166 (December 6, 1971): 35.
39. Raymond M. Glasscote et al., *The Treatment of Drug Abuse* (Washington, D.C.: Joint Information Service of the American Psychiatric Association and the National Association for Mental Health, 1971; in press for 1972 publication), Chapter 15.
40. William R. Martin, in *New York Law Journal*, 166 (December 6, 1971): 34.
41. M. A. Hamilton Russell, "Cigarette Smoking: Natural History of a Dependence Disorder," *British Journal of Medical Psychology*, 44 (1971): 2.
42. *British Columbia Study*, p. 369.
43. J. B. Mattison, *The Mattison Method in Morphinism* (New York: E. B. Treat, 1902), p. 29.
44. *British Columbia Study*, pp. 372–376.
45. Ibid., p. 368.

46. Lawrence Kolb, *Drug Addiction, A Medical Problem* (Springfield, Ill.: Charles C Thomas, 1962), p. 55.
47. John A. O'Donnell, *Narcotics Addicts in Kentucky,* U.S. Public Health Service Publication No. 1881 (Chevy Chase, Md.: National Institute of Mental Health, 1969), pp. 31–32.
48. Ibid., p. 33.
49. Ibid., p. 205.
50. Ibid.
51. Ibid., p. 56.
52. Ibid., p. 60.
53. Ibid., p. 217.
54. Ibid., p. 205.
55. Charles W. Sheppard, George R. Gay, and David E. Smith, "The Changing Patterns of Heroin Addiction in the Haight-Ashbury Subculture," *Journal of Psychedelic Drugs,* 3 (1971): 22–30.

Chapter 11

1. *Heroin and Heroin Paraphernalia,* Second Report by the House Select Committee on Crime, House Report No. 91–1808, 91st Cong., 2nd Sess., January 2, 1971, p. 17.
2. "The World Heroin Problem: Report of Special Study Mission," House Report No. 92-298, Union Calendar No. 124, June 22, 1971.
3. New York *Times,* July 1, 1971.
4. "The World Heroin Problem: Report of Special Study Mission," June 22, 1971.
5. *Heroin and Heroin Paraphernalia,* p. 16.
6. *LBI Facts Book 1970* (New York: Licensed Beverage Industries, Inc., 1971), pp. 23, 34.
7. *Heroin and Heroin Paraphernalia,* p. 16.
8. New York *Post,* October 27, 1969.
9. Ibid.
10. *Heroin and Heroin Paraphernalia,* p. 20.
11. Edward A. Preble and John J. Casey, Jr., "Taking Care of Business—The Heroin User's Life on the Street," *International Journal of the Addictions,* 4 (March 1969): 7.
12. Harry J. Anslinger and William F. Tompkins, *The Traffic in Narcotics* (New York: Funk and Wagnalls, 1953), pp. 137–138.
13. Preble and Casey, "Taking Care of Business," p. 7.
14. Arthur D. Little, Inc., *Drug Abuse and Law Enforcement,* A Report to the President's Commission on Law Enforcement and Administration of Justice, January 18, 1967.
15. Arthur Howard, cited in "Drugs and Delinquency," *Medico-Legal Journal,* 33 (February 11, 1965): 58.
16. J. H. Willis, "Some Problems of Opiate Addiction," *Practitioner,* London, 200 (February 1968): 220–225.
17. Arthur D. Little, Inc., *Drug Abuse and Law Enforcement,* p. F-2.
18. Ibid., Table I-I, p. I-1.
19. Preble and Casey, "Taking Care of Business," pp. 8–12.
20. Arthur D. Little, Inc., *Drug Abuse and Law Enforcement,* Table I-IV, p. I-4.
21. New York *Times,* September 23, 1969.
22. New York *Post,* October 27, 1969.
23. Preble and Casey, "Taking Care of Business," p. 12.

Chapter 12

1. Jerome H. Jaffe, in *Goodman and Gilman,* 4th ed. (1970), p. 286.
2. Ibid.

3. Milton Helpern and Yong-Myun Rho, "Deaths from Narcotism in New York City," *New York State Journal of Medicine,* 66 (1966): 2393.
4. Ibid., Table XI, p. 2402.
5. Richard Severo in "News of the Week in Review," New York *Times,* February 1, 1970.
6. New York *Times,* December 30, 1970.
7. Michael M. Baden, quoted by Barbara Campbell in the New York *Times,* December 16, 1969; New York *Times,* December 30, 1970.
8. New York *Times,* December 30, 1970.
9. A. K. Reynolds and Lowell O. Randall, *Morphine and Allied Drugs* (Toronto: University of Toronto Press, 1957), p. 119.
10. Jerome H. Jaffe, in *Goodman and Gilman,* 4th ed. (1970), pp. 252, 268.
11. New York *Times,* June 21, 1970.
12. Reynolds and Randall, *Morphine and Allied Drugs,* pp. 176–177.
13. Jerome H. Jaffe, in *Goodman and Gilman,* 4th ed. (1970), p. 252.
14. Robert H. Dreisbach, *Handbook of Poisoning: Diagnosis and Treatment,* 7th ed. (Los Altos, Cal.: Lange Medical Publications, 1971), p. 247.
15. Reynolds and Randall, *Morphine and Allied Drugs,* p. 119.
16. William T. Salter, *A Textbook of Pharmacology* (Philadelphia and London: W. B. Saunders Company, 1952), p. 77.
17. Reynolds and Randall, *Morphine and Allied Drugs,* p. 119.
18. Lawrence Kolb and A. G. Du Mez, *U.S. Public Health Reports,* 46 (1931): 698.
19. A. B. Light and E. B. Torrance, *Archives of Internal Medicine,* 44 (1929): 875.
20. Ibid., pp. 377–379.
21. Ibid., p. 394.
22. Ibid., p. 381.
23. Mary Jane Kreek in *Proceedings, Second Methadone Conference,* p. A-72.
24. Donald B. Louria, "The Major Medical Complications of Heroin Addiction," *Annals of Internal Medicine,* 67 (1967): 2; also, Helpern and Rho, "Deaths from Narcotism in New York City," pp. 2405–2407.
25. Helpern and Rho, pp. 2405–2407.
26. Ibid., p. 2402.
27. Ibid., p. 2403.
28. Ibid.; see also Michael M. Baden, "Medical Aspects of Drug Abuse," *New York Medicine,* 24 (1968): 464–466.
29. Milton Helpern in *Pharmacological and Epidemiological Aspects of Adolescent Drug Dependence,* Proceedings of the Society for the Study of Addiction, ed. C. W. M. Wilson (London: Pergamon Press, 1968), p. 228.
30. Helpern and Rho, "Deaths from Narcotism in New York City," pp. 2402–2403.
31. Michael M. Baden, "Pathological Aspects of Drug Addiction," *Proceedings of the Committee on Problems of Drug Dependence* (Washington, D.C.: Division of Medical Sciences, National Academy of Science–National Research Council, 1969), p. 5792.
32. Michael M. Baden, "Medical Aspects of Drug Abuse," p. 466.
33. Ibid., p. 464.
34. Michael M. Baden, in *Proceedings, Second Methadone Conference,* pp. A-58, A-59.
35. Mary Jane Kreek, in *Proceedings, Second Methadone Conference,* p. A-72.
36. Michael M. Baden, in *Proceedings, Second Methadone Conference,* p. A-74.
37. Barbara Campbell, reporting in New York *Times,* December 16, 1969.
38. Milton Helpern, testifying at Hearings, House Select Committee on Crime, 91st Cong., 2nd Sess., June 27, 1970, p. 188.
39. Ralph W. Richter, John Pearson and Michael M. Baden, paper presented at 51st annual session, American College of Physicians, Philadelphia, 1970.
40. Milton Helpern, "Epidemic of Fatal Malaria Among Heroin Addicts in New York City," *American Journal of Surgery,* 26 (1943): 111.

41. Quoted by Milton Helpern in *Pharmacological and Epidemiological Aspects of Adolescent Drug Dependence*, p. 248.
42. Rudolph F. Muelling in *Pharmacological and Epidemiological Aspects of Adolescent Drug Dependence*, p. 248.
43. Robert Silber and E. P. Clerkin, "Pulmonary Edema in Acute Heroin Poisoning," *American Journal of Medicine*, 27 (July, 1959): 190.
44. George R. Gay et al., "Short Term Heroin Detoxification on an Outpatient Basis," mimeographed, unpublished, p. 9.
45. Harold Alksne, Ray E. Trussell, and Jack Elinson, *A Follow-up Study of Treated Adolescent Narcotics Users* (New York: Columbia University School of Public Health and Administrative Medicine, 1959), unpublished, p. 101.
46. Ibid.
47. William B. Deichmann and Horace W. Gerarde, *Toxicology of Drugs and Chemicals* (New York and London: Academic Press, 1969), pp. 407–408.
48. Charles E. Cherubin, Jane McCusker, Michael M. Baden, Florence Kavaler, and Zilu Amsel, "The Epidemiology of Death in Narcotics Addicts," *American Journal of Epidemiology*, in press.
49. George R. Gay et al., "Short Term Heroin Detoxification on an Outpatient Basis," p. 18.
50. George R. Gay at National Heroin Symposium, San Francisco, June 1971.
51. *Time*, October 19, 1970, p. 54.
52. Ramon Gardner, "Deaths in United Kingdom Opioid Users, 1965–1969," *Lancet* (September 26, 1970): 650–651.
53. Ibid., p. 651.
54. Personal communication, October 11, 1971.

Chapter 13

1. Lawrence Kolb and A. G. Du Mez, *The Prevalence and Trend of Drug Addiction in the United States and Factors Influencing It*, Treasury Department, U.S. Public Health Service, Reprint No. 924 (Washington, D.C.: U.S. Government Printing Office, 1924), pp. 2–3.
2. Ibid., p. 3.
3. August Vollmer, *The Police and Modern Society* (Berkeley, 1936), pp. 117–118.
4. *British Columbia Study*, Appendix A, p. 2.
5. Ibid.
6. Report on Narcotic Addiction to the Attorney General by the California Citizens' Advisory Committee, March 26, 1954, cited in *ABA-AMA Report*, p. 97.
7. Cited in *ABA-AMA Report*, p. 93.
8. Ibid., p. 95.
9. Ibid., p. 94.
10. Ibid.
11. Ibid., p. 102.
12. Ibid., p. 11.
13. *Proceedings, White House Conference on Narcotic and Drug Abuse*, September 27–28, 1962 (Washington, D.C.: U. S. Government Printing Office, 1962), p. 296.
14. Cited in *ABA-AMA Report*, pp. 94–95.
15. *Final Report*, President's Advisory Commission on Narcotic and Drug Abuse, Judge E. Barrett Prettyman, Chairman (Washington, D.C.: U.S. Government Printing Office, 1963), p. 58.
16. *Wall Street Journal*, April 17, 1963.
17. Isador Chein et al., *The Road to H* (New York: Basic Books, 1964), pp. 371–372, 379.
18. New York *Times*, February 27, 1965.
19. Ibid.
20. *ABA-AMA Report*, p. 101.

21. Harry Campbell, "The Pathology and Treatment of Morphia Addiction," *British Journal of Inebriety,* 20 (1922–23): 147.
22. Cited in Edwin M. Schur, *Narcotic Addiction in Britain and America* (Bloomington, Ind.: Indiana University Press, 1968), p. 71.
23. Ibid., p. 118.
24. Ibid., Table 1, p. 119.
25. Frederick B. Glaser and John C. Ball, "The British Narcotic 'Register' in 1970: A Factual Review," *JAMA,* 216 (May 17, 1971): 1177–1182.
26. T. H. Bewley, in *British Medical Journal,* 2 (November, 1965): 1285.
27. Edwin M. Schur, *Narcotic Addiction in Britain and America,* pp. 162–164.
28. United Kingdom Home Office press notices, "1969 Statistics of Drug Addiction and Drug Offenses," September 18, 1970; and "1970 Statistics of Drug Addiction and Drug Offenses," August 5, 1971.
29. Ibid.
30. Ibid.
31. Frederick B. Glaser and John C. Ball, "The British Narcotic 'Register,'" pp. 1177–1182.
32. Editorial, *British Medical Journal,* 2 (August 7, 1971): 321–322.
33. John A. O'Donnell, *Narcotics Addicts in Kentucky,* U.S. Public Health Service Publication No. 1881 (Chevy Chase, Md.: National Institute of Mental Health, 1969), p. 80.
34. Ibid., p. 81.
35. Ibid., Table 6-3, p. 81.
36. Ibid., pp. 81–82.
37. Ibid., Table 12-3, p. 185.
38. Ibid., pp. 223–224.
39. Ibid., p. 233.
40. Ibid., p. 95.
41. Ibid., pp. 95–96.
42. Ibid., pp. 97–98.
43. Ibid., p. 193.
44. Ibid.
45. John A. O'Donnell, personal communication, August 4, 1970.
46. Quoted in Nat Hentoff, *A Doctor Among the Addicts* (Chicago: Rand McNally & Co., 1969), p. 44.
47. O'Donnell, *Narcotics Addicts in Kentucky,* p. 226.
48. Ibid., p. 132.
49. Harry J. Anslinger and William F. Tompkins, *The Traffic in Narcotics* (New York: Funk and Wagnalls, 1953), p. 194.
50. O'Donnell, *Narcotics Addicts in Kentucky,* p. 115.
51. Ibid., p. 119.

Chapter 14

1. Quoted in Nat Hentoff, *A Doctor Among the Addicts* (Chicago: Rand McNally & Co., 1969), p. 26.
2. Ibid., p. 112.
3. Ibid., p. 113.
4. Ibid., p. 114.
5. Ray E. Trussell, in *Proceedings, Second Methadone Conference,* pp. 17–18.
6. Ibid., p. 17.
7. Ibid., p. 19.
8. Vincent P. Dole, testimony in *Crime in America—Heroin Importation, Distribution, Packaging and Paraphernalia,* Hearings before the Select Committee on Crime, U.S. House of Representatives, 91st Cong., 2d Sess., June 29, 1970, p. 264.
9. Vincent P. Dole, personal communication, January 25, 1971.
10. Ibid.

11. Ibid.
12. Ibid.

Chapter 15

1. Frances R. Gearing, "Successes and Failures in Methadone Maintenance Treatment of Heroin Addicts in New York City," in *Proceedings, Third Methadone Conference,* Table 1, p. 3.
2. Ibid.
3. Ibid., Appendix B, p. 16.
4. Ibid., Table 1, p. 3.
5. Ibid.
6. Frances R. Gearing, "Progress Report of Evaluation of Methadone Maintenance Program, as of March 31, 1968," in *Proceedings of the First National Conference on Methadone Treatment,* New York, June 1968, supported by Health Research Council, New York City; New York State Narcotic Addiction Control Commission, and National Association for the Prevention of Addiction (NAPAN); mimeographed, unpublished, p. 5. Hereinafter cited as *Proceedings, First Methadone Conference.*
7. Ibid.
8. Frances R. Gearing, "Successes and Failures," p. 8.
9. Vincent P. Dole, in *Proceedings, First Methadone Conference,* pp. 16–17.
10. Ibid., p. 17.
11. Ibid.
12. Vincent P. Dole, Marie E. Nyswander, and Alan Warner, "Successful Treatment of 750 Criminal Addicts," *JAMA,* 206 (December 16, 1968): 2710–2711.
13. Frances R. Gearing, "Data to Accompany Presentation Evaluation of Methadone Maintenance Treatment Program," paper presented at Second National Conference on Methadone Treatment, New York, October 1969, Fig. 11.
14. *Proceedings, First Methadone Conference,* p. 10-B.
15. Frances R. Gearing, in *Proceedings, Third Methadone Conference,* Fig. 9, p. 12.
16. *Proceedings, First Methadone Conference,* Fig. 3, p. 22.
17. Ibid., Fig. 1, p. 20.
18. Frances R. Gearing, in *Proceedings, Third Methadone Conference,* Fig. 10, p. 13.
19. Ibid., Fig. 11, p. 14.
20. Vincent P. Dole, in *Proceedings, First Methadone Conference,* p. 17.
21. Ibid.
22. Ronald Bayer, Letter to the Editor, New York *Times,* July 20, 1971.
23. Frances R. Gearing, in testimony before House Select Committee on Crime, April 27, 1971, p. 116.
24. Frances R. Gearing, "Evaluation of Methadone Maintenance Treatment Program, Progress Report Through March 31, 1969," unpublished, p. 7.
25. Carl D. Chambers, Dean V. Babst, and Alan Warner, "Characteristics Predicting Long-Term Retention in a Methadone Maintenance Program," *Proceedings, Third Methadone Conference,* pp. 140–143.
26. Ibid.

Chapter 16

1. William A. Bloom, Jr., and Brian T. Butcher, in *Proceedings, Third Methadone Conference,* pp. 44–46.
2. Avram Goldstein, in *Proceedings, Third Methadone Conference,* p. 30.
3. Ibid., p. 33.
4. Robert C. Wallach, Eulogio Jerez, and George Blinick, "Pregnancy and Menstrual Function in Narcotics Addicts Treated with Methadone," *American Journal of Obstetrics and Gynecology,* 105 (December 15, 1969): 1227.

5. William F. Wieland and Michael Yunger, in *Proceedings, Third Methadone Conference,* p. 51.
6. Ibid.
7. Ibid., p. 52.
8. Bloom and Butcher, *Proceedings, Third Methadone Conference,* p. 46.
9. Saul Blatman, in *Proceedings, Third Methadone Conference,* pp. 84–85.
10. Ibid., p. 85.
11. Ibid., pp. 84–85.
12. Ibid., p. 84.
13. Paul Cushman, Jr., in *Proceedings, Third Methadone Conference,* p. 147.
14. Ibid.
15. Ibid., p. 148.
16. Morton I. Davidson, in *Proceedings, Third Methadone Conference,* p. 79.

Chapter 17

1. *Science,* 173 (August 6, 1971): 505.
2. William R. Martin in *New York Law Journal,* 166 (December 6, 1971): 34.
3. John N. Chappel, Edward C. Senay, and Jerome H. Jaffe, "Cyclazocine in a Multi-Modality Treatment Program: Comparative Results," *International Journal of the Addictions,* 6 (September, 1971): 509–523.
4. Marie E. Nyswander, personal communication.
5. Vincent P. Dole, "Thoughts on Narcotics Addiction," *Bulletin, New York Academy of Medicine,* 41 (February, 1965): 212.
6. Ibid.
7. Vincent P. Dole and Marie E. Nyswander, "Rehabilitation of Heroin Addicts after Blockade with Methadone," *New York State Journal of Medicine* (August 1, 1966), p. 2015.
8. Vincent P. Dole and Marie E. Nyswander, "Narcotic Blockade—A Medical Technique for Stopping Heroin Use by Addicts," *Transactions of Association of American Physicians,* 79 (1966): 132.
9. Personal communication.

Chapter 18

1. *Proceedings, First Methadone Conference.*
2. *Proceedings, Second Methadone Conference.*
3. *Proceedings, Third Methadone Conference.*
4. Emmett P. Davis, in *Proceedings, Second Methadone Conference,* pp. 135–146.
5. Robert A. Maslansky, in *Proceedings, Second Methadone Conference,* pp. 84–90.
6. Personal communication.
7. Gordon Stewart, in *Proceedings, Third Methadone Conference,* p. 27.
8. Personal communication.
9. Maslansky, *Proceedings, Second Methadone Conference,* p. 89.
10. Ibid.
11. Ibid., p. 95.
12. Ibid.
13. Ray E. Trussell, *Proceedings, Second Methadone Conference,* p. 28.
14. *The Dolly* (Man Alive, Inc., August 1969), p. 3; personal communications.
15. Jerome H. Jaffe, in *Proceedings, Second Methadone Conference,* pp. 130–131.
16. Herbert D. Kleber, in *Proceedings, Second Methadone Conference,* p. A-6.
17. William A. Bloom, Jr., in *Proceedings, Second Methadone Conference,* p. A-36.
18. Ibid., p. A-39.
19. Jaffe, *Proceedings, Second Methadone Conference,* p. 59.
20. Ibid., p. 93.
21. Ibid., pp. 77–78.
22. Ibid., p. 79.
23. Ibid.

24. Vincent P. Dole, in *Proceedings, Second Methadone Conference*, p. 54.
25. Ibid., p. 38.
26. Ibid.
27. Ibid.
28. Ibid., pp. 38–39.
29. *U. S. News and World Report*, September 27, 1971, p. 43.
30. Senator Harold Hughes in "Federal Drug Abuse and Drug Dependence Prevention, Treatment and Rehabilitation Act of 1970," *Hearings before Special Subcommittee on Alcoholism and Narcotics of the Committee on Labor and Public Welfare*, U. S. Senate, 91st Cong., 2nd Sess., 1970, Part 2, p. 575.
31. Richard G. Adams et al., "Heroin Addicts on Methadone Replacement: A Study of Dropouts," *International Journal of the Addictions*, 6 (June, 1971): 269–277.
32. Ibid., p. 275.

Chapter 19

1. United Kingdom Home Office press notice, August 5, 1971.
2. William S. Greenawalt, quoted by Edward C. Burks, New York *Times*, March 24, 1970.
3. Robert G. Newman, in *Proceedings, Third Methadone Conference*, p. 123.
4. Ibid., p. 124.
5. Ibid.
6. Richard Severo, reporting in New York *Times*, April 18, 1971.

Chapter 20

1. C. W. Sheppard, G. R. Gay, and D. E. Smith, "The Changing Patterns of Heroin Addiction in the Haight-Ashbury Subculture," *Journal of Psychedelic Drugs*, 3 (Spring, 1971): 22–31.
2. Ibid., Table, p. 28.
3. Ibid., Chart, p. 23.
4. New York *Times*, May 16, 1971.
5. Major Eric Nelson, Letterman General Hospital, San Francisco, quoted in *Medical World News*, September 3, 1971, p. 17.
6. Norman E. Zinberg, in New York *Times* Magazine, December 5, 1971, pp. 37, 112–124; and in *New York Law Journal*, December 6, 1971, p. 43.
7. Zinberg, New York *Times* Magazine, December 5, 1971, p. 120.
8. Ibid.
9. Zinberg, *New York Law Journal*, December 6, 1971, p. 43.
10. Gloria Emerson, reporting in New York *Times*, September 12, 1971.
11. Zinberg, New York *Times* Magazine, December 5, 1971, p. 123.
12. Ibid., p. 120.
13. Ibid.
14. Zinberg, *New York Law Journal*, December 6, 1971, p. 43.
15. Ibid.
16. House Report No. 92–298, Union Calendar No. 124, 92nd Cong., 1st Sess., 1971, p. 3.
17. Zinberg, New York *Times* Magazine, December 5, 1971, p. 122.
18. Ibid., p. 116.
19. Harry Campbell, "The Pathology and Treatment of Morphia Addiction," *British Journal of Inebriety*, 20 (1922–23): 147.

Chapter 21

1. Andrew T. Weil, "Altered States of Consciousness, Drugs, and Society," September 18, 1970; unpublished.
2. Quoted by Ralph Holt Cheney, *Coffee* (New York: New York University Press, 1925), p. 207.

3. Ibid., p. 209.
4. *Encyclopaedia Britannica,* 11th ed., s.v. "Coffee," VI, 646.
5. Quoted by Edward Forbes Robinson, *The Early History of Coffee Houses in England* (London: Regan Paul, Trench, Trubner & Co., Ltd., 1893), pp. 19, 20.
6. Ibid., p. 26.
7. Robert S. de Ropp, *Drugs and the Mind* (New York: St. Martin's Press, Macmillan, 1957), p. 248.
8. T. D. Crothers, *Morphinism and Narcomanias from Other Drugs* (Philadelphia: W. B. Saunders & Co., 1902), p. 303.
9. Ibid., pp. 303–304.
10. Ibid., p. 304.
11. Sir T. Clifford Allbutt and Humphrey Davy Rolleston, eds., *A System of Medicine,* Vol. II, Part I (London: Macmillan, 1909), pp. 986–987.
12. Ibid., pp. 987–988.
13. Ibid.

Chapter 22

1. J. Murdoch Ritchie, in *Goodman and Gilman,* 4th ed. (1970), p. 359.
2. Ibid., p. 363.
3. Ibid.
4. Hobart A. Reimann, "Caffeinism," *JAMA,* 202 (December 18, 1967): 1105.
5. Ibid., p. 1106.
6. Ibid.
7. Avram Goldstein and Sophia Kaizer, "Psychotropic Effects of Caffeine in Man. III. A Questionnaire Survey of Coffee Drinking and Its Effects in a Group of Housewives," *Clinical Pharmacology and Therapeutics,* 10 (July 8, 1969): 478–479.
8. Ibid., p. 482.
9. Ibid., p. 483.
10. Ibid.
11. Avram Goldstein, Sophia Kaizer, and Owen Whitby, "Psychotropic Effects of Caffeine in Man. IV. Quantitative and Qualitative Differences Associated with Habituation to Coffee," *Clinical Pharmacology and Therapeutics,* 10 (July 8, 1969): 489–497.
12. Ibid., p. 490.
13. Ibid., pp. 495–496.
14. Ibid., p. 497.
15. J. Murdoch Ritchie in *Goodman and Gilman,* 4th ed. (1970), p. 363.
16. Ibid., p. 360.
17. Ibid., p. 368.
18. Ibid., p. 365.
19. Ibid.
20. Margaret C. McManamy and Purcell G. Schube, "Caffeine Intoxication," *New England Journal of Medicine,* 215 (1936): 616–620.
21. Ibid.
22. J. M. Peters, "Caffeine-Induced Hemorrhagic Automutilation," *Archives of International Pharmacodynamics,* 169 (1967): 141.

Chapter 23

1. Count Egon Caesar Corti, *A History of Smoking,* trans. Paul England (London: George G. Harrap & Co., Ltd., 1931), p. 69.
2. Jerome E. Brooks, *The Mighty Leaf* (Boston: Little, Brown and Co., 1952), pp. 33–34.
3. Louis Lewin, *Phantastica: Narcotic and Stimulating Drugs, Their Use and Abuse* (1924), trans. 1931 (New York: E. P. Dutton & Co., 1964, reprint), p. 290.

4. Bartolomé de las Casas, *Historia,* cited by Brooks, p. 14; *Histoire des Indes* (1520–1559), cited by Corti, pp. 42–43.
5. Edmund Gardiner, *Triall of Tobacco* (1610), cited by Corti, *History,* p. 89.
6. Francis Bacon, *Historia vitae et mortis* (1623), cited by Corti, *History,* p. 94.
7. Berthold Laufer, *Introduction of Tobacco into Europe,* Anthropology Leaflet 19 (Chicago: Field Museum of Natural History, 1924), p. 16.
8. Ibid.
9. Corti, *History,* p. 107.
10. Ibid., p. 116.
11. Johann Lassenius, *Adeligen Tischreden* (1661), cited by Corti, *History,* p. 117.
12. Jakob Balde, *Die truckene Trunkenheit* (Nuremberg, 1658), cited by Corti, *History,* pp. 118–119.
13. Report of the Hofkammer (Exchequer), August 1677, cited by Corti, *History,* p. 157.
14. Brooks, *The Mighty Leaf,* p. 105.
15. *Briefe der Herzogin Elisabeth Charlotte von Orleans,* ed. Hans F. Helmolt (Leipzig: 1924), p. 335, cited by Corti, *History,* p. 182.
16. Corti, *History,* pp. 129, 130.
17. Louis Lewin, *Phantastica,* p. 302.
18. Corti, *History,* pp. 113, 114, 123.
19. Ibid., pp. 138–139.
20. Adam Alearius, *Beschreibung der moskowitischen und persienischen Reise* (1696), cited by Corti, *History,* p. 141.
21. J. Crull, *Ancient and Present State of Muscovy* (1698), p. 145, cited by Laufer, *Introduction of Tobacco into Europe,* p. 59.
22. Corti, *History,* p. 145.
23. Ibid., pp. 146–147.
24. Edward H. Pinto, *Wooden Bygones of Smoking and Snuff Taking* (London: Hutchinson of London, 1961), pp. 56–57.
25. Smokeless Tobacco Council, Inc., New York, "Nothing to Sneeze At" (press release), January 1971.

Chapter 24

1. Ernest Jones, *The Life and Work of Sigmund Freud,* 3 vols. (New York: Basic Books, 1953).
2. Jones, *Freud,* I, 309.
3. Ibid., pp. 309–310.
4. Ibid., p. 311.
5. Jones, *Freud,* II, 96.
6. Jones, *Freud,* III, 89.
7. Ibid., p. 150.
8. Ibid., p. 202.
9. Ibid., p. 238.
10. Vincent P. Dole, personal communication.
11. New York *Times,* May 23, 1971.
12. Ibid.
13. John S. Tamerin and Charles P. Neumann, "Casualties of the Anti-Smoking Campaign," presented at the Annual Meeting of the American Psychiatric Association, Washington, D.C., May 1971; unpublished.
14. Ibid.
15. Ibid.
16. Daniel Horn, "Epidemiology and Psychology of Cigarette Smoking," *Chest,* 59 (May, 1971, supplement): 227.
17. Tamerin and Neumann, "Casualties of the Anti-Smoking Campaign."

Chapter 25

1. M. A. Hamilton Russell, "Cigarette Smoking: Natural History of a Dependence Disorder," *British Journal of Medical Psychology*, 44 (1971): 9.
2. Lennox M. Johnston, "Tobacco Smoking and Nicotine," *Lancet*, 243 (December 19, 1942): 742.
3. J. K. Finnegan, P. S. Larson, and H. B. Haag, "The Role of Nicotine in the Cigarette Habit," *Science*, 102 (July 27, 1945): 94–96.
4. Ibid.
5. B. Ejrup and P. A. Wikander, "Försök med Nikotin, Lobelin och Placebo," *Svenska Läkartidningen*, 56 (July 17, 1959): 2025–2034.
6. B. R. Lucchesi, C. R. Schuster, and G. S. Emley, "The Role of Nicotine as a Determinant of Cigarette Smoking Frequency in Man with Observations of Certain Cardiovascular Effects Associated with the Tobacco Alkaloid," *Clinical Pharmacology and Therapeutics*, 8 (1967): Table I, p. 791.
7. Ibid., Table II, p. 792.
8. C. D. Firth, in *Psychopharmacologia*, 19 (1971): 188–192.
9. B. L. Levinson, D. Shapiro, G. E. Schwartz, and B. Tursky, "Smoking Elimination by Gradual Reduction," *Behavior Therapy*, 2 (October, 1971): 477–487.
10. M. A. Hamilton Russell, "Cigarette Smoking," p. 1.
11. *Use of Tobacco*, National Clearinghouse for Smoking and Health, U.S. Department of Health, Education, and Welfare (Washington, D.C.: U.S. Government Printing Office, 1969), p. 306.
12. M. A. Hamilton Russell, "Cigarette Smoking," p. 8.
13. Ibid., p. 3.
14. Ibid.
15. Ibid., pp. 12–13.
16. Ibid., pp. 8–9.
17. Joan S. Guilford et al., *Factors Related to Successful Abstinence from Smoking: Final Report* (Pittsburgh: American Institutes, 1966): Table XXIX, pp. 114–115.
18. Ibid., Table XXX, pp. 116–117.
19. Peter H. Knapp, C. M. Bliss, and H. Webb, "Addictive Aspects in Heavy Cigarette Smoking," *American Journal of Psychiatry*, 119 (1963): 966–972.
20. M. A. Hamilton Russell, "Cigarette Smoking," p. 2.
21. Ibid., p. 3.
22. Ibid., pp. 3–4.
23. F. I. Arntzen, "Some Psychological Aspects of Nicotinism," *American Journal of Psychology*, 61 (1948): 425.
24. William A. Hunt and Joseph D. Matarazzo, "Habit Mechanisms in Smoking," in *Learning Mechanisms in Smoking*, ed. W. A. Hunt (Chicago: Aldine, 1970), p. 76.
25. Ibid.

Chapter 26

1. James L. Hedrick, *Smoking, Tobacco and Health*, prepared for National Clearinghouse for Smoking and Health, U.S. Department of Health, Education, and Welfare, Public Health Service, March 1969 (revised), p. 4.
2. Jerome E. Brooks, *The Mighty Leaf* (Boston: Little, Brown and Co., 1952), p. 274.
3. Ibid., pp. 274–275.
4. Statistical Bulletin No. 467, "Annual Report on Tobacco Statistics 1970," U.S. Department of Agriculture, Consumer and Marketing Service, 1971, Table 16, p. 30.
5. James L. Hedrick, *Smoking, Tobacco and Health*, p. 3.
6. Ruth and Edward Brecher, *Smoking—The Great Dilemma*, Public Affairs Pamphlet No. 361 (New York: Public Affairs Pamphlets, 1964), pp. 2, 3.

7. Moses Barron, reported to Minnesota State Medical Society, August 25, 1921, cited in Ruth and Edward Brecher et al., *The Consumers Union Report on Smoking and the Public Interest* (Mount Vernon, N.Y.: Consumers Union, 1963), pp. 13–14.
8. F. E. Tylecote in *Lancet*, cited in Ruth and Edward Brecher et al., *The Consumers Union Report on Smoking and the Public Interest*, p. 25.
9. C. M. Fletcher and Daniel Horn in *WHO Chronicle*, Geneva, Switzerland, 24 (1970): 345–370.
10. Ruth and Edward Brecher, *Smoking—The Great Dilemma*, pp. 2, 3.
11. *Use of Tobacco*, National Clearinghouse for Smoking and Health, U.S. Department of Health, Education, and Welfare, Washington, D.C., 1969, pp. 137 ff.
12. Daniel Horn, "The Smoking Problem in 1971," statement prepared for the American Cancer Society's 13th Annual Science Writers' Seminar, Phoenix, Arizona, April 6, 1971.
13. Data supplied by National Clearinghouse for Smoking and Health.
14. Data supplied by Bureau of Labor Statistics, U.S. Department of Labor.
15. Statistical Bulletin No. 467, "Annual Report on Tobacco Statistics 1970," p. 32.
16. Lieberman Research, Inc., "The Teenager Looks at Cigarette Smoking," conducted for the American Cancer Society, September 1969, Table 108, p. 212.
17. Ibid., Table 92, p. 196.
18. Ibid., Table 44, p. 141.
19. Ibid., Table 47, p. 145.
20. Ibid., p. 2.
21. Ibid., Table 28, p. 125.
22. Data supplied by National Clearinghouse for Smoking and Health.
23. Lieberman Research, Inc., "The Teenager Looks at Cigarette Smoking," Table 22, p. 118.
24. Carlo Vetere, National Ministry of Health, Italy, in *Summary of Proceedings*, World Conference on Smoking and Health (New York: National Interagency Council on Smoking and Health and American Cancer Society, 1967), p. 232.
25. M. A. Hamilton Russell, "Cigarette Smoking: Natural History of a Dependence Disorder," *British Journal of Medical Psychology*, 44 (1971): 11.
26. Data supplied by National Center for Health Statistics.
27. Data supplied by National Clearinghouse for Smoking and Health.
28. Data supplied by Social Research Group, George Washington University.

Chapter 27

1. James L. Hedrick, *Smoking, Tobacco and Health*, prepared for National Clearinghouse for Smoking and Health, U.S. Department of Health, Education, and Welfare, Public Health Service, March 1969 (revised), Figure 13, p. 27.

Chapter 28

1. Seth K. Sharpless, in *Goodman and Gilman*, 4th ed. (1970), p. 98.
2. W. E. Hambourger, "A Study of the Promiscuous Use of the Barbiturates," *JAMA*, 108 (April 8, 1937): 1343.
3. Jerome H. Jaffe, in *Goodman and Gilman*, 4th ed. (1970), p. 290.
4. Harris Isbell, personal communication, February 26, 1971.

Chapter 29

1. Harris Isbell et al., "Chronic Barbiturate Intoxication," *AMA Archives of Neurology and Psychiatry*, 64 (July 1950): 8.
2. Ibid., p. 9.
3. Ibid., p. 10.
4. Ibid., pp. 10–11.

 5. Ibid., p. 11.
 6. Ibid.
 7. Ibid.
 8. Ibid., p. 14.
 9. Ibid., p. 15.
10. Ibid., p. 27.
11. Ibid., p. 23.
12. Jerome H. Jaffe in *Goodman and Gilman,* 4th ed. (1970), p. 289.

Chapter 30

1. Dr. Sidney Cohen, in *Hearings Before the Subcommittee to Investigate Juvenile Delinquency of the Committee on the Judiciary,* U.S. Senate, 91st Cong., 1st Sess., September 17, 1969 (Washington, D.C.: U.S. Government Printing Office, 1969), p. 293.
2. Ibid.

Chapter 31

1. Placidyl package insert, rev. June 1971, Abbott Laboratories, North Chicago, Ill.
2. Murray E. Jarvik, in *Goodman and Gilman,* 4th ed. (1970), p. 174.
3. Ibid., pp. 175, 179.
4. *The Medical Letter,* 11 (October 3, 1969): 84.
5. *The Medical Letter,* 13 (March 5, 1971): 19.
6. Valium package insert, September 1971, Roche Laboratories, Nutley, N.J.
7. Seth K. Sharpless, in *Goodman and Gilman,* 4th ed. (1970), pp. 125, 127.

Chapter 32

1. Data supplied by National Institute on Alcohol Abuse and Alcoholism, National Institute of Mental Health, November 1971.
2. Thomas F. A. Plaut, Appendix I, *Task Force Report: Drunkenness,* President's Commission on Law Enforcement and Administration of Justice (Washington, D.C.: U.S. Government Printing Office, 1967), pp. 120–131.
3. Ibid.
4. Judge John M. Murtagh, Appendix E, *Task Force Report: Drunkenness,* pp. 65–67.
5. Plaut, Appendix I, p. 122.
6. L. M. Shupe, cited by Richard H. Blum assisted by Lauraine Braunstein, Appendix B, *Task Force Report: Drunkenness,* p. 41.
7. H. A. Bullock, cited by Blum, Appendix B, p. 40.
8. R. S. Fisher, cited by Blum, Appendix B, p. 40.
9. M. E. Wolfgang, cited by Blum, Appendix B, pp. 40–41.
10. Richard H. Blum, Appendix B, p. 41.
11. FBI "Uniform Crime Reports," 1961, cited by Blum, Appendix B, p. 40.
12. E. G. Palola, T. L. Dorpat, and W. R. Larsen, cited by Blum, Appendix B, p. 35.
13. J. R. McCarroll and W. Haddon, Jr., cited by Blum, Appendix B, p. 38.
14. W. Haddon, Jr., and V. Bradess, cited by Blum, Appendix B, ibid.
15. W. Haddon, Jr., P. Valien, and J. R. McCarroll, cited by Blum, Appendix B, ibid.
16. Richard H. Blum, Appendix B, p. 38.
17. Jerome H. Jaffe, in *Goodman and Gilman,* 3rd ed. (1965), p. 291.

Chapter 33

1. F. R. Menue, "Acute Methyl Alcohol Poisoning," *Archives of Pathology,* 26 (1938): 79–92.
2. Louis Lewin, *Phantastica: Narcotic and Stimulating Drugs, Their Use and Abuse,* 1924, trans. 1931 (New York: E.P. Dutton & Co., 1964, reprint), p. 235.

Chapter 34

1. Hector P. Blejer, "Coca Leaf and Cocaine Addiction—Some Historical Notes," *Canadian Medical Association Journal,* 93 (September 25, 1965): 701.
2. Ibid.
3. Ibid.
4. W. G. Mortimer, *Peru History of Coca, "The Divine Plant" of the Incas, With an Introductory Account of the Incas and Andean Indians of Today* (New York: J. H. Vail and Co., 1901), pp. 28 and 119; cited by Blejer, p. 701.
5. Jerome H. Jaffe in *Goodman and Gilman,* 3rd ed. (1965), p. 299.
6. J. L. Corning, *Local Anesthesia in General Medicine and Surgery, Being the Practical Application of the Author's Recent Discoveries* (New York: D. Appleton and Co., 1886), p. 21; cited by Blejer, p. 702.
7. Mortimer, *Peru History of Coca,* p. 179, cited by Blejer, p. 702.
8. Personal communication.

Chapter 35

1. *Remington's Pharmaceutical Sciences,* 14th ed. (Easton, Pa.: Mack Publishing Co., 1970), p. 1067.
2. Theodor Aschenbrandt, "Die physiologische Wirkung und die Bedeutung des Cocains," *Deutsche medizinische Wochenschrift* (December 12, 1883); cited by Ernest Jones, *The Life and Work of Sigmund Freud, Volume I (1856–1900)* (New York: Basic Books, 1953), p. 80.
3. Ernest Jones, *Life and Work of Sigmund Freud,* I, 80.
4. Ibid.
5. Ibid., p. 81.
6. Ibid.
7. Ibid., p. 84.
8. Ibid., p. 82.
9. Ibid., pp. 82–83.
10. Ibid., p. 83.
11. Jerome H. Jaffe in *Goodman and Gilman,* 3rd ed. (1965), pp. 298–299.
12. Ernest Jones, *Life and Work of Sigmund Freud,* I, 94.
13. Ibid., p. 91.
14. Charles B. Towns, "The Peril of the Drug Habit," *Century Magazine,* 84 (1912): 586.
15. Ibid., p. 583.

Chapter 36

1. John C. Kramer, "Introduction to Amphetamine Abuse," *Journal of Psychedelic Drugs,* vol. II, no. 2 (1969): 1.
2. Roger C. Smith, "The Marketplace of Speed: Violence and Compulsive Methamphetamine Abuse"; unpublished (1969), p. 6.
3. *Physicians' Desk Reference to Pharmaceutical Specialties and Biologicals,* 26th ed., 1972 (Oradell, N.J.: Medical Economics, 1972), pp. 202, 302, 308, 317.
4. Ian P. Innes and Mark Nickerson, in *Goodman and Gilman,* 4th ed. (1970), p. 502.
5. Ibid.
6. Iago Galdston, "Pep Teasers," *Hygeia,* 18 (October 1940): 878–880, cited by Roger C. Smith, "Marketplace of Speed," p. 8.

Chapter 37

1. *JAMA,* 183 (1963): 363.
2. Roger C. Smith, "The Marketplace of Speed: Violence and Compulsive Methamphetamine Abuse"; unpublished (1969), p. 9.

3. Ibid., p. 11.
4. Ibid., p. 13.
5. Ibid., p. 17.
6. John C. Kramer, "Introduction to Amphetamine Abuse," *Journal of Psychedelic Drugs,* vol. II, no. 2 (1969): 2.
7. Ibid., pp. 2–3.
8. Ibid., p. 3.
9. Ibid., p. 4.
10. Roger C. Smith, "Marketplace of Speed," p. 46.
11. John C. Kramer, "Introduction to Amphetamine Abuse," p. 4.
12. Ibid., p. 5.
13. Ibid., p. 6.
14. Ibid.
15. Roger C. Smith, "The World of the Haight-Ashbury Speed Freak," *Journal of Psychedelic Drugs,* vol. II, no. 2 (1969): 178.
16. John C. Kramer, "Introduction to Amphetamine Abuse," pp. 6–7.
17. Ibid., p. 7.
18. Roger C. Smith, "Marketplace of Speed," p. 54.
19. Ibid., p. 109.
20. Ibid., pp. 110–111.
21. Ibid., p. 111.
22. Ibid.
23. Ibid., p. 113.
24. Ibid., pp. 113–114.
25. Ibid., p. 120.
26. Ian P. Innes and Mark Nickerson in *Goodman and Gilman,* 4th ed. (1970), p. 504.
27. John C. Kramer, "Introduction to Amphetamine Abuse," pp. 9–10.
28. Ibid., p. 12.
29. Ibid., p. 13.
30. Ibid.
31. Ibid.
32. Ibid.
33. Ibid.
34. Ibid.

Chapter 38

1. Roger C. Smith, "U. S. Marijuana Legislation and the Creation of a Social Problem," *Journal of Psychedelic Drugs,* vol. II, no. 1 (1968): 52.
2. Allen Ginsberg, interview with Art Kunkin, in Los Angeles *Free Press,* December 1965, reprinted in *Speed Hurts,* ed. Art Wiener, Amphetamine Research Project, sponsored by National Institute of Mental Health, March 31, 1969, p. 2.
3. *Le Dain Commission Interim Report,* p. 50.
4. *Speed Hurts,* p. 4.
5. James R. Allen, Louis Jolyon West, and Joshua Kaufman, in *American Journal of Psychiatry,* 126 (November 1969): 165.
6. *Le Dain Commission Interim Report,* p. 168.

Chapter 39

1. Gunnar Inghe, "The Present State of Abuse and Addiction to Stimulant Drugs in Sweden," in *Abuse of Central Stimulants,* ed. Folke Sjöqvist and Malcolm Tottie (Stockholm: Almqvist and Wiksell, 1969), p. 187.
2. Ibid.
3. L. Goldberg, "Drug Abuse in Sweden," United Nations *Bulletin on Narcotics,* 2 (1968): 9–36.
4. Gunnar Inghe, "The Present State of Abuse and Addiction," p. 187.

5. Ibid., p. 189.
6. Ibid.
7. Ibid.
8. Ibid., p. 190.
9. Personal communication.
10. Gunnar Inghe, "The Present State of Abuse and Addiction," p. 190.
11. For example, Henry Brill and T. Hirose, "The Rise and Fall of a Methampheta-mine Epidemic: Japan 1945–55," *Seminars in Psychiatry,* 1 (1969): 179–194.

Chapter 40

1. Roger C. Smith, "The Marketplace of Speed: Violence and Compulsive Metham-phetamine Abuse"; unpublished (1969), p. 81.
2. Ibid., p. 83.
3. Ibid., p. 84.
4. Ibid.
5. Ibid., p. 85.
6. Ibid.

Chapter 41

1. New York *Times,* February 1, 1970.
2. Ibid.
3. Ibid.
4. New York *Times,* January 25, 1971.
5. Jerry Mandel, "Myths and Realities of Marijuana Pushing," *Marijuana Myths and Realities,* ed. J. L. Simmons (North Hollywood, Calif.: Brandon House, 1967), p. 73.
6. New York *Times,* February 1, 1970.
7. New York *Times,* January 25, 1971.
8. Ibid.
9. New York *Times,* February 1, 1970.

Chapter 43

1. Edward Preble and Gabriel V. Laury, "Plastic Cement: The Ten Cent Hallucino-gen," *International Journal of the Addictions,* 2 (Fall 1967): 271–272.
2. David R. Nagle, "Anesthetic Addiction and Drunkenness," *International Journal of the Addictions,* 3 (Spring 1968): 33.
3. Thomas Mitchell, *Elements of Chemical Philosophy* (Cincinnati: Corey and Fairbank, 1832), cited by Nagle, "Anesthetic Addiction and Drunkenness," p. 27.
4. Peter J. Cohen and Robert D. Dripps in *Goodman and Gilman,* 4th ed. (1970), p. 43.
5. Ibid.
6. Henry L. Price and Robert D. Dripps in *Goodman and Gilman,* 4th ed. (1970), p. 72.
7. *Psychiatric News,* December 15, 1971.
8. Edward J. Lynn et al., "Nitrous Oxide: It's a Gas!" presented at the 124th Annual Meeting of the American Psychiatric Association, May 1971.
9. *Encyclopaedia Britannica,* 11th ed., s.v. "Ether."
10. David R. Nagle, "Anesthetic Addiction and Drunkenness," p. 26.
11. W. Lewis, *Materia Medica* (London, 1761), cited by Nagle, "Anesthetic Addiction and Drunkenness," p. 26.
12. Nagle, p. 26.
13. T. Lee, "The Sedative Effects of Vaporous Ether Recognized Some Forty Years Since," *Lancet,* 1 (1847): 164, cited by Nagle, p. 26.
14. Nagle, p. 28.

15. Ibid.
16. E. Hart, "Ether Drinking," *British Medical Journal,* 2 (1890): 885, cited in Nagle, p. 29.
17. Select Committee on British and Foreign Spirits, 1890–1891, cited in Nagle, p. 27.
18. Nagle, p. 27.
19. Oliver Wendell Holmes, *Mechanism in Thought and Morals,* Phi Beta Kappa address, Harvard University, June 29, 1870 (Boston: J. R. Osgood and Company, 1871).
20. Peter J. Cohen and Robert D. Dripps in *Goodman and Gilman,* p. 44.
21. N. Kerr, "Ether Inebriety," *JAMA,* 17 (1891): 791, cited by Nagle, p. 30.
22. Axel Munthe, *The Story of San Michele* (New York: Dutton, 1929), cited by Nagle, p. 27.
23. *Bulletin, National Clearinghouse for Poison Control Centers,* U.S. Department of Health, Education, and Welfare, Public Health Service (February-March 1962), p. 2.
24. Nagle, p. 36.
25. Samuel Guthrie, "New Mode of Preparing a Spiritous Solution of Chloric Ether," *American Journal of Science and Arts* (Silliman's), 24 (1831): 64.
26. Henry L. Price and Robert D. Dripps in *Goodman and Gilman,* p. 83.
27. Nagle, pp. 31–32.
28. Ewart A. Swinyard, "Noxious Gases and Vapors," in *Goodman and Gilman,* 4th ed. (1970), pp. 937–938.
29. A. E. Hamilton, *Psychology and the Great God Fun* (New York: Julian Press, 1955), pp. 106–109.
30. Henry L. Verhulst and John J. Crotty in *Bulletin, National Clearinghouse for Poison Control Centers,* U.S. Department of Health, Education, and Welfare, Public Health Service (February-March 1962).

Chapter 44

1. Lenore R. Kupperstein and Ralph M. Susman, "Bibliography on the Inhalation of Glue Fumes and Other Toxic Vapors," *International Journal of the Addictions,* 3 (1968): 177–197.
2. Betty J. Fluke and Lillian R. Donato, "Some Glues Are Dangerous," *Empire* Magazine, supplement to Denver *Post,* August 2, 1959, p. 24.
3. Denver *Post,* June 12, 1960.
4. Denver *Post,* October 23, 1961.
5. State Representative Ben Klein, quoted in Denver *Post,* December 8, 1961.
6. Denver *Post,* April 13, 1962.
7. Denver *Post,* October 23, 1961.
8. Denver *Post,* April 13, 1962.
9. Denver *Post,* October 23, 1961.
10. Ibid.
11. Denver *Post,* December 8, 1961.
12. Al Arnold, in Denver *Post,* April 29, 1962.
13. Helen H. Glaser and Oliver N. Massengale, "Glue-Sniffing in Children," *JAMA,* 181 (July 28, 1962): 301.
14. Ibid., pp. 302–303.
15. Ibid., p. 301.
16. Denver *Post,* January 18, 1965.
17. Denver *Post,* March 21, 1965.
18. Denver *Post,* April 22, 1965.
19. Denver *Post,* April 29, 1965.
20. Denver *Post,* June 25, 1965.
21. Denver *Post,* July 2, 1965.
22. Denver *Post,* January 11, 1966.

23. Denver *Post,* May 18, 1966.
24. Denver *Post,* June 10, 1966.
25. Denver *Post,* October 30, 1966.
26. New York *Times,* October 6, 1961.
27. New York *Times,* April 25, 1963.
28. *International Journal of the Addictions* (January, 1966), p. 147.
29. *Bulletin, National Clearinghouse for Poison Control Centers,* U.S. Department of Health, Education, and Welfare, Public Health Services (February–March, 1962), pp. 1–2.
30. Phillip E. Norton, in *Wall Street Journal,* December 7, 1962.
31. Ordinance No. 1722, City of Anaheim, California, June 6, 1962, cited in *Bulletin, National Clearinghouse for Poison Control Centers* (July–August, 1964), p. 1.
32. H. Jacobziner and H. W. Raybin, *New York State Journal of Medicine,* 16 (1963), cited in *Bulletin, National Clearinghouse for Poison Control Centers* (July–August, 1964), p. 1.
33. *Time,* February 16, 1962, p. 55.
34. Ibid.
35. *Newsweek,* August 13, 1962, p. 42.
36. Ibid.
37. "Glue Sniffing," *Consumer Reports,* 28 (January, 1963): 40.
38. Jacob Sokol, "A Sniff of Death," *FBI Law Enforcement Bulletin,* 34 (October, 1965): 8.
39. Ibid.
40. Ibid.
41. Massachusetts Department of Public Health, "Glue Sniffing by Youngsters Fought by Department," *New England Journal of Medicine,* 267 (November 8, 1962): 993.
42. Henry L. Verhulst and John J. Crotty, in *Bulletin, National Clearinghouse for Poison Control Centers* (July–August, 1964).
43. Dorothy F. Berg, "Illicit Use of Dangerous Drugs in the United States," Drug Sciences Division, Office of Science and Drug Abuse Prevention, Bureau of Narcotics and Dangerous Drugs, U.S. Department of Justice (September, 1970), Table 5, p. 33.
44. Ibid.
45. *Advisory Commission Report on Drug Abuse,* Governor's Citizen Advisory Committee on Drug Abuse, State of Utah, cited in Berg, Table 5, p. 34.
46. Richard A. Bogg et al., Michigan Department of Public Health, 1968, cited in Berg, Table 5, p. 35.
47. Ibid., Table 5, p. 37.
48. Grace Lichtenstein, reporting in New York *Times,* July 20, 1971.
49. *Psychiatric News,* December 15, 1971, p. 10.

Chapter 45

1. Richard Evans Schultes, "Hallucinogens of Plant Origin," *Science,* 163 (January 17, 1969): 250.
2. Ibid.
3. Ibid.
4. Frank Barron, Murray E. Jarvik, and Sterling Bunnell, Jr., "The Hallucinogenic Drugs," *Scientific American,* 210 (1964): 32.
5. J. S. Slotkin, *The Peyote Religion* (Glencoe, Ill.: The Free Press, 1956), Table 1, p. 36.
6. Weston La Barre, *The Peyote Cult* (New York: Schocken Books, 1969), pp. 109–123.
7. William H. McGlothlin and David O. Arnold, "LSD Revisited—A Ten-Year Follow-up of Medical LSD Use," *Archives of General Psychiatry,* 24 (January, 1971): 35.

8. Bernard Roseman, *The Peyote Story* (Hollywood, Calif.: Wilshire Book Co., 1963), pp. 55–60.
9. Ibid.
10. Ibid.
11. J. S. Slotkin, *The Peyote Religion*, p. 44.
12. Ibid., pp. 52–53. See also Ruth Ernestine Cook [Brecher], "Indian Dance Ceremonials in Modern America: A Study of Governmental Policies and Civilian Attitudes, 1921–1933," senior thesis, Swarthmore College, 1933; unpublished.
13. J. S. Slotkin, *The Peyote Religion*, p. 53.
14. Weston La Barre, *The Peyote Cult*, pp. 223–224.
15. Ibid., p. 230.
16. Cited by David Solomon, ed., in *LSD: The Consciousness-Expanding Drug* (New York: G. P. Putnam's Sons, 1966), p. 63.
17. Robert L. Bergman, "Navajo Peyote Use—Its Apparent Safety," presented at the American Psychiatric Association Convention, Washington, D.C., May 6, 1971; later published, *American Journal of Psychiatry*, 128 (December, 1971): 695–699.
18. Richard Evans Schultes in *Science*, pp. 245-247.
19. Frank Barron, Murray E. Jarvik, and Sterling Bunnell, Jr., "The Hallucinogenic Drugs," p. 30.
20. Ibid.
21. Daniel H. Efron, ed., *Psychotomimetic Drugs* (New York: Raven Press, 1970), p. 47.
22. Richard Evans Schultes in *Science*, pp. 248–249.
23. *Le Dain Commission Interim Report*, p. 141.
24. Richard Evans Schultes in *Science*, pp. 251–252.

Chapter 46

1. Albert Hofmann, cited by John Cashman, *The LSD Story* (Greenwich, Conn.: Fawcett Publications, 1966), p. 31.
2. Ibid., p. 32.
3. Albert Hofmann, "LSD Discoverer Disputes 'Chance' Factor in Finding," condensed excerpt from *Discoveries in Biological Psychiatry*, ed. Frank J. Ayd, Jr., and Barry Blackwell, *Psychiatric News*, 6 (April 21, 1971): 23.
4. Harold A. Abramson, ed., in *The Use of LSD in Psychotherapy and Alcoholism* (New York: Bobbs-Merrill, 1967), p. vii.
5. William H. McGlothlin and David O. Arnold, "LSD Revisited—A Ten-Year Follow-up of Medical LSD Use," *Archives of General Psychiatry*, 24 (January, 1971): Table 5, p. 39.
6. Jerome Levine, paper presented at National Association of Student Personnel Administrators Drug Education Conference, Washington, D.C., November 7–8, 1966; unpublished, p. 3.
7. Humphrey Osmond, "A Review of the Clinical Effects of Psychotomimetic Agents," in David Solomon, ed., *LSD: The Consciousness-Expanding Drug* (New York: G. P. Putnam's Sons, 1966), p. 148.
8. M. Rinkel and H. C. B. Denber, eds., *Chemical Concepts of Psychosis* (New York: McDowell, 1958), cited by Morris A. Lipton, "The Relevance of Chemically-Induced Psychoses to Schizophrenia," in Daniel H. Efron, ed., *Psychotomimetic Drugs* (New York: Raven Press, 1970), p. 235.

Chapter 47

1. J. H. Rothschild, *Tomorrow's Weapons* (New York: McGraw-Hill, 1964), quoted in Seymour M. Hersh, *Chemical and Biological Warfare: America's Hidden Arsenal* (New York: Doubleday Anchor, 1969), p. 50.
2. Victor W. Sidel and Robert M. Goldwyn, "Chemical Weapons, What They Are, What They Do," *Scientist and Citizen*, 9 (August–September, 1967): Table 1, p. 144.

3. Ibid., pp. 45–48.
4. Sidney Cohen, *The Beyond Within: The LSD Story* (New York: Atheneum, 1968), p. 237.
5. A. K. Busch and W. C. Johnson, "Lysergic Acid Diethylamide (LSD-25) as an Aid in Psychotherapy," *Diseases of the Nervous System,* 11 (1950): 204.
6. M. Rostafinski, "Experimental Hallucination in Epileptic Patients," *Rocznik Psychiatryczny* (Poland), 38 (1950): 109; summarized in *Bibliography on Psychotomimetics, 1943–1966* (U.S. Department of Health, Education and Welfare, Public Health Service, 1966), p. 5.
7. Charles Savage, "Lysergic Acid Diethylamide (LSD-25): A Clinical-Psychological Study," *American Journal of Psychiatry,* 108 (1952): 898.
8. D. W. Liddell and H. Weil-Malherbe, "The Effects of Methedrine and of Lysergic Acid Diethylamide on Mental Processes and on the Blood Adrenalin Level," *Journal of Neurology, Neurosurgery and Psychiatry* (British), 16 (1953): 7, summarized in *Bibliography on Psychotomimetics,* p. 10.
9. J. D. P. Graham and Alaa Iddeen Khalidi, "The Action of d-Lysergic Acid Diethylamide (LSD 25), Part 1, General Pharmacology," *Journal of the Faculty of Medicine* (Baghdad), 18 (1954): 1, summarized in *Bibliography on Psychotomimetics,* p. 20.
10. Ibid., p. 14.
11. John Buckman, "Theoretical Aspects of LSD Therapy," in Harold A. Abramson, ed., *The Use of LSD in Psychotherapy and Alcoholism* (New York: Bobbs-Merrill, 1967), p. 96.
12. Ibid.
13. Sidney Cohen, "Psychotherapy with LSD: Pro and Con," in *The Use of LSD,* pp. 581–582.
14. Ibid., p. 578.
15. Ibid.
16. Daniel X. Freedman, "On the Use and Abuse of LSD," *Archives of General Psychiatry,* 18 (March, 1968): 331.
17. Oliver Wendell Holmes, *Mechanism in Thought and Morals,* Phi Beta Kappa Society address, Harvard University, June 29, 1870 (Boston: J. R. Osgood and Company, 1871).
18. Wilson Van Dusen, Wayne Wilson, et al., "Treatment of Alcoholism with Lysergide[1]," *Quarterly Journal Studies on Alcohol,* 28 (1967): 299, 302.
19. Albert A. Kurland et al., "The Therapeutic Potential of LSD in Medicine," in *LSD, Man and Society,* ed. Richard C. DeBold and Russell C. Leaf (Middletown, Conn.: Wesleyan University Press, 1967), p. 23.
20. Ibid.
21. Ibid., p. 24.
22. Ibid.
23. Ibid.
24. Ibid.
25. E. Kast, "Pain and LSD-25: A Theory of Attenuation of Anticipation," in *LSD: The Consciousness-Expanding Drug,* pp. 239–254.
26. Sidney Cohen, "LSD and the Anguish of Dying," *Harper's,* 231 (September, 1965): 69–78.
27. Albert A. Kurland et al., p. 31.
28. Ibid., pp. 31–33.
29. Ibid., p. 33.
30. Sidney Cohen in *Harper's,* p. 71.

Chapter 48

1. Sidney Cohen, "Lysergic Acid Diethylamide: Side Effects and Complications," *Journal of Nervous and Mental Diseases,* 130 (January, 1960): 30–40.
2. Ibid., pp. 30–31.

3. Ibid., pp. 31–32.
4. Ibid., p. 32.
5. Ibid.
6. Ibid.
7. Ibid.
8. Ibid., p. 36.
9. Ibid.
10. E. F. W. Baker, "The Use of Lysergic Acid Diethylamide (LSD) in Psychotherapy," *Canadian Medical Association Journal,* 91 (December 5, 1964): 1202.
11. Sidney Cohen, "Lysergic Acid Diethylamide," p. 39.
12. Ibid.
13. Jerome Levine and Arnold M. Ludwig, "The LSD Controversy," *Comprehensive Psychiatry,* 5 (1964): 318.
14. Nicolas Malleson, "Acute Adverse Reactions to LSD in Clinical and Experimental Use in the United Kingdom"; unpublished, provisional report, June, 1969.

Chapter 49

1. Richard H. Blum and Associates, *Utopiates: The Use and Users of LSD–25* (New York: Atherton Press, 1964).
2. Ibid., pp. 22–23.
3. Ibid., p. 23.
4. Ibid.
5. Ibid., p. 29.
6. Ibid., p. 31.
7. Ibid., p. 32.
8. Ibid., p. 35.
9. Ibid., p. 33.
10. Ibid., p. 34.
11. Ibid., p. 35.
12. Ibid., p. 41.
13. Ibid., p. 36.
14. Ibid.
15. Ibid., p. 49.
16. Ibid.
17. Ibid.
18. Ibid., pp. 42–43.

Chapter 50

1. Data supplied by Bureau of Narcotics and Dangerous Drugs, U.S. Department of Justice.
2. *The Amphetamines and Lysergic Acid Diethylamide (LSD),* Report by the Advisory Committee on Drug Dependence, Home Office, Department of Health and Social Security (London: Her Majesty's Stationery Office, 1970), p. 38.
3. *Le Dain Commission Interim Report,* p. 141.
4. William H. McGlothlin and David O. Arnold, "LSD Revisited—A Ten-Year Follow-up of Medical LSD Use," *Archives of General Psychiatry,* 24 (January, 1971): 35.
5. Arnold M. Ludwig and Jerome Levine, "Patterns of Hallucinogenic Drug Abuse," *JAMA,* 191 (January 11, 1965): 93.
6. Timothy Leary, *High Priest* (New York: World, 1968), p. 34.
7. New York *Times,* May 20, 1969.
8. C. W. Sandman, Jr., quoted by William H. McGlothlin, "Toward a Rational View of Hallucinogenic Drugs," MR–83, Institute of Government and Public Affairs (University of California, 1966), p. 4.
9. *Le Dain Commission Interim Report,* p. 139.

10. United Press International, in New York *Times,* October 4, 1969.
11. New York *Times,* April 7, 1966.
12. New York *Times,* April 12, 1966.
13. James T. Barter and Martin Reite, "Crime and LSD: The Insanity Plea," *American Journal of Psychiatry,* vol. 26, no. 4 (October, 1969): 532.
14. Reported by William H. McGlothlin, "Toward a Rational View of Hallucinogenic Drugs," paper distributed at National Association of Student Personnel Administrators Drug Education Conference, Washington, D.C., November 7–8, 1966; unpublished.
15. Ibid.
16. Ibid.
17. Washington *Post,* February 12, 1969.
18. Harold A. Abramson, ed., in *The Use of LSD in Psychotherapy and Alcoholism* (New York: Bobbs-Merrill, 1967), p. 328.
19. Ibid.
20. *Home Office Report* (1970), p. 41.
21. Ibid., p. 36.
22. Ibid., pp. 41–42.
23. M. M. Cohen, M. Marinello, and N. Bach, "Chromosomal Damage in Human Leukocytes Induced by Lysergic Acid Diethylamide," *Science,* 155 (1967): 1417–1419; and M. M. Cohen, K. Hirschhorn, and W. A. Frosch, "In Vivo and In Vitro Chromosomal Damage Induced by LSD–25," *New England Journal of Medicine,* 277 (1967): 1043–1049.
24. *Home Office Report* (1970), p. 34.

Chapter 51

1. Sidney Cohen, "Lysergic Acid Diethylamide: Side Effects and Complications," *Journal of Nervous and Mental Disease,* 130 (January, 1960): 39.
2. David E. Smith and Alan J. Rose, "LSD: Its Use, Abuse and Suggested Treatment," *Journal of Psychedelic Drugs,* vol. I, no. 2 (1967–1968): 122.
3. Ibid., p. 120.
4. *Le Dain Commission Interim Report,* p. 209.
5. Frederick H. Meyers, Alan J. Rose, David E. Smith, et al., "Incidents Involving the Haight-Ashbury Population and Some Uncommonly Used Drugs," *Journal of Psychedelic Drugs,* vol. I, no. 2 (1967–1968): 143.
6. Ibid.
7. Sidney Cohen, "Lysergic Acid Diethylamide," p. 31.
8. Mardi J. Horowitz, "Flashbacks: Recurrent Intrusive Images After the Use of LSD," *American Journal of Psychiatry,* 126 (October, 1969): 565–569.
9. Leon J. Hekimian and Samuel Gershon, "Characteristics of Drug Abusers Admitted to a Psychiatric Hospital," *JAMA,* 205 (July 15, 1968): 125–130.
10. George S. Glass and Malcolm B. Bowers, Jr., "Chronic Psychosis Associated with Long-Term Psychotomimetic Drug Abuse," *Archives of General Psychiatry,* 23 (August, 1970): 97–103.

Chapter 52

1. William H. McGlothlin and David O. Arnold, "LSD Revisited—A Ten-Year Follow-up of Medical LSD Use," *Archives of General Psychiatry,* 24 (January, 1971): 35–49.
2. Ibid., p. 40.
3. Ibid., p. 49.
4. Ibid., Table 5, p. 39.
5. Ibid.
6. Ibid., p. 48.
7. New York *Times,* January 17, 1971.

8. William H. McGlothlin and David O. Arnold, "A Ten-Year Follow-Up," p. 41.
9. Ibid., Table 8, p. 42.
10. Ibid.
11. Ibid.
12. Ibid., p. 42.
13. Ibid., pp. 43–45.
14. Ibid., p. 49.
15. Ibid., p. 46.
16. Ibid.
17. Ibid., p. 47.
18. Ibid.
19. Ibid.
20. Ibid., p. 46.
21. Ibid.
22. Ibid., p. 49.
23. Ibid.
24. William H. McGlothlin, David O. Arnold, and Daniel X. Freedman, "Organicity Measures Following Repeated LSD Ingestion," *Archives of General Psychiatry,* 21 (December, 1969): 704–709.
25. Ibid., p. 705.
26. Ibid., p. 707.
27. Ibid., table, p. 707.
28. Sidney Cohen and A. E. Edwards, "LSD and Organic Brain Damage," *Drug Dependence,* cited in "Organicity Measures," p. 709.
29. William H. McGlothlin, David O. Arnold, and Daniel X. Freedman, "Organicity Measures," table, p. 707.
30. Sidney Cohen and A. E. Edwards, cited in "Organicity Measures," p. 708.
31. William H. McGlothlin, Robert S. Sparkes, and David O. Arnold, "Effect of LSD on Human Pregnancy," *JAMA,* 212 (June 1, 1970): 1483–1487.
32. Ibid., p. 1486.
33. Ibid., p. 1487.
34. "Drugs in Pregnancy: Are They Safe?" *Consumer Reports,* 32 (August, 1967): 435.
35. William H. McGlothlin, Robert S. Sparkes, and David O. Arnold, "Effect of LSD," p. 1487.
36. Detroit *News,* June 4, 1970, p. 4-C.
37. *Medical World News* press release, undated.
38. H. A. Lubs and F. H. Ruddle, "Chromosomal Abnormalities in the Human Population: Estimation of Rates Based on New Haven Newborn Study," *Science,* 169 (July 31, 1970): 495–498.

Chapter 53

1. Robert P. Walton, *Marijuana, America's New Drug Problem* (Philadelphia: J. B. Lippincott, 1938), p. 2.
2. Richard Brotman and Alfred M. Freedman, "Perspectives on Marijuana Research," prepared for Center for Studies in Substance Use; unpublished, p. 7.
3. Robert P. Walton, *Marijuana, America's New Drug Problem,* p. 6.
4. Ibid., pp. 2, 3, 5.
5. Ibid., p. 6.
6. Ibid., p. 7.
7. Ibid., p. 8.
8. Ibid., p. 23.
9. C. Creighton, "On Indications of the Hachish-Vice in the Old Testament," *Janus,* 8 (1902): 241–246, 297–303.
10. Melvin Clay, "The Song of Solomon," in *The Book of Grass: An Anthology of*

Indian Hemp, ed. George Andrews and Simon Vinkenoog (New York: Grove Press, 1967), p. 19.
11. Robert P. Walton, *Marijuana, America's New Drug Problem,* p. 17.
12. *Encyclopaedia Britannica,* 11th ed., s.v. "Hemp."
13. François Rabelais, "The Herb Pantagruelion," trans. by Samuel Putnam, in *The Marijuana Papers,* ed. David Solomon (New York: Bobbs-Merrill, 1966), p. 105.
14. "Queries and Minor Notes," *JAMA,* 94 (1930): 1165.
15. Frances Ames, "A Clinical and Metabolic Study of Acute Intoxication with *Cannabis Sativa* and its Role in the Model Psychoses," *Journal of Mental Science,* 104 (1958): 975–976.
16. C. J. G. Bourhill, "The Smoking of Dagga (Indian Hemp) Among the Native Races of South Africa and the Resultant Evils"; unpublished dissertation, Edinburgh University, 1916, cited by Ames, "A Clinical and Metabolic Study," p. 976.
17. Louis Lewin, *Phantastica: Narcotic and Stimulating Drugs: Their Use and Abuse* (1924), trans. 1931 (New York: Dutton 1964, reprint), p. 109.
18. I. C. Chopra and R. N. Chopra, "The Use of Cannabis Drugs in India," United Nations *Bulletin on Narcotics,* 9 (1957): 13.
19. Ibid., p. 8.
20. Ibid., p. 7.
21. Ibid.
22. Ibid., pp. 10–11.
23. Ibid., p. 13.
24. Ibid.
25. Ibid., pp. 13–14.
26. Louis Lewin, *Phantastica,* p. 107.
27. J. Bouquet, "Cannabis," United Nations *Bulletin on Narcotics,* 3 (1951): 31.
28. Stanley Yolles, Testimony in *Narcotics Legislation,* Hearings before the Subcommittee to Investigate Juvenile Delinquency of the Committee on the Judiciary, U.S. Senate, 91st Congress, 1st Session, September 17, 1969 (Washington, D.C.: U.S. Government Printing Office, 1969), p. 267.

Chapter 54

1. J. Bouquet, "Cannabis," United Nations *Bulletin on Narcotics,* 3 (1951): 36.
2. Ibid.
3. Richard Brotman and Alfred M. Freedman, "Perspectives on Marijuana Research," prepared for Center for Studies in Substance Use, unpublished, p. 19.
4. S. S. Boyce, *Hemp, A Practical Treatise on the Culture of Hemp for Seed and Fiber with a Sketch of the History and Nature of the Hemp Plant* (New York: Orange Judd, 1900), p. 35.
5. Ibid.
6. Cited by George Andrews and Simon Vinkenoog, eds., *The Book of Grass: An Anthology of Indian Hemp* (New York: Grove Press, 1967), p. 34.
7. Ibid.
8. Ibid., pp. 35–36, 41.
9. James L. Allen, *The Reign of Law* (1900), cited by Robert P. Walton, *Marijuana, America's New Drug Problem* (Philadelphia: J. B. Lippincott, 1938), p. 45.
10. W. W. Robbins and F. Ramalay (1933), cited by Walton, *Marijuana,* p. 45.
11. *Crime in America—A Mid-America View,* Hearings before the Select Committee on Crime, House of Representatives, 91st Cong., 1st Sess., pursuant to H. R. 17, October 11, 1969, Lincoln, Nebraska (Washington, D.C.: U.S. Government Printing Office, 1969), p. 168.
12. Walton, *Marijuana,* p. 44.
13. Richard Colestock Pillard, "Medical Progress: Marijuana," *New England Journal of Medicine,* 283 (August 6, 1970): 294–295.

14. Ibid., p. 295.
15. Ibid.
16. Leo E. Hollister, "Marijuana in Man: Three Years Later," *Science,* 172 (April 2, 1971): 22.
17. *The Pharmacopoeia of the United States of America* (Easton, Pa.: Mack Printing, 1851), pp. 332–334.
18. *The Pharmacopeia of the United States of America,* 11th ed. (Easton, Pa.: Mack Printing, 1936), p. lxviii.
19. George B. Wood and Franklin Bache, eds., *The Dispensatory of the United States of America,* 9th ed. (Philadelphia: Lippincott, Grambo, 1851), pp. 310–311.
20. J. Russell Reynolds, "On the Therapeutic Uses and Toxic Effects of Cannabis Indica," *Lancet* (March 22, 1970): 637.
21. R. R. McMeens, "Report of the Committee on Cannabis Indica," from *Transactions of the 50th Annual Meeting of the Ohio State Medical Society* (Columbus, Ohio: Follett, Foster, 1860), pp. 75–100.
22. G. S. D. Anderson, "Remarks on the Remedial Virtues of Cannabis Indica, or Indian Hemp," *Boston Medical and Surgical Journal,* 67 (1863): 427–430.
23. Edward J. Waring, *Practical Therapeutics* (Philadelphia: Lindsay and Blakiston, 1874), pp. 157–161.
24. C. W. Suckling, "On the Therapeutic Value of Indian Hemp," *British Medical Journal,* 2 (1881): 12.
25. J. B. Mattison, "Cannabis Indica as an Anodyne and Hypnotic," *St. Louis Medical and Surgical Journal,* 61 (1891): 265–271.
26. A. A. Stevens, *Modern Materia Medica and Therapeutics* (Philadelphia: W. B. Saunders, 1903), pp. 77–78.
27. Tod H. Mikuriya, "Marijuana in Medicine, Past, Present and Future," *California Medicine,* 110 (January, 1969): 34–40.
28. W. Osler and T. MacCrae, *Principles and Practice of Medicine,* 8th ed. (New York: D. Appleton, 1916), p. 1089.
29. Marty Sasman, "Cannabis Indica in Pharmaceuticals," *Journal of the Medical Society of New Jersey,* 35 (1938): 51–52.
30. P. H. Blachly, "Use of Amphetamines, Marijuana and LSD by Students," *New Physician,* 15 (April, 1966): 90.
31. David Solomon, ed., *The Marijuana Papers* (New York: Bobbs-Merrill, 1966), p. 121.
32. Fitz Hugh Ludlow, "The Hasheesh Eater," quoted in Solomon, *The Marijuana Papers,* pp. 148–149.
33. Ibid., p. 149.
34. Ibid.
35. Ibid., p. 150.
36. *Scientific American,* 21 (September 18, 1869): 183.
37. Reprinted in the New York *Times* Magazine, December 13, 1970, p. 26.
38. H. H. Kane (according to *Oxford English Dictionary*), "A Hashish-House in New York," *Harper's New Monthly Magazine* (November, 1883), pp. 944–949.
39. Ibid., p. 945.
40. Ibid., p. 948.
41. Quoted by Michael R. Aldrich, *Heads Hidden in the Hemp Fields* (Mill Valley, Calif.: Marijuana Research Association, 1970), p. 7.
42. George Wheelock Grover, *Shadows Lifted or Sunshine Restored in the Horizon of Human Lives: A Treatise on the Morphine, Opium, Cocaine, Chloral and Hashish Habit* (Chicago, 1894, quoted in Tuli Kupferberg's *Birth* Magazine, no. 3, book 1 (Autumn, 1960), p. 48.
43. Victor Robinson, "Experiments With Hashish," cited in Solomon, *The Marijuana Papers,* pp. 201–215.
44. Walton, *Marijuana,* p. 25.
45. J. D. Reichard, "The Marijuana Problem," *JAMA,* 125 (June 24, 1944): 594–595.

Chapter 55

1. Mayor's Committee on Marijuana, "The Marijuana Problem in the City of New York," (1944), in *The Marijuana Papers,* ed. David Solomon (New York: Bobbs-Merrill, 1966), p. 246.
2. See New Orleans *Morning Tribune,* October 17, 19–23, 28, 1926; and New Orleans *Item,* October 22, 1926; February 4, 1927.
3. Robert F. Walton, *Marijuana, America's New Drug Problem* (Philadelphia: J. B. Lippincott, 1938), p. 29.
4. Ibid.
5. Ibid., p. 30.
6. Ibid., pp. 30–31.
7. Ibid., Table I, p. 37.
8. Ibid., p. 31.
9. Ibid.
10. Ibid., p. 32.
11. Ibid.
12. Ibid., p. 33.
13. Ibid., Table I, p. 37.
14. U.S. Treasury Department, *Traffic in Opium and Other Dangerous Drugs for the Year Ended December 31, 1931* (Washington, D.C.: U.S. Government Printing Office, 1932), p. 51.

Chapter 56

1. Bureau of Narcotics, U.S. Treasury Department, *Traffic in Opium and Other Dangerous Drugs for the Year Ended December 31, 1932* (Washington, D.C.: U.S. Government Printing Office, 1933), p. 13.
2. U.S. Treasury Department, *Traffic in Opium and Other Dangerous Drugs for the Year Ended December 31, 1931* (Washington, D.C.: U.S. Government Printing Office, 1932), p. 51.
3. Bureau of Narcotics, U.S. Treasury Department, *Traffic in Opium and Other Dangerous Drugs for the Year Ended December 31, 1935* (Washington, D.C.: U.S. Government Printing Office, 1936), p. 30.
4. David Solomon, in *The Marijuana Papers,* ed. David Solomon (New York: Bobbs-Merrill, 1966), p. xv.
5. Robert P. Walton, *Marijuana, America's New Drug Problem* (Philadelphia: J. B. Lippincott, 1938), Table I, p. 37.
6. Howard S. Becker, "Marijuana: A Sociological Overview," in Solomon, *The Marijuana Papers,* p. 62.
7. Ibid.
8. Harry J. Anslinger, with Courtney Ryley Cooper, "Marijuana: Assassin of Youth," *American Magazine,* 124 (July, 1937): 19, 150.
9. Cited by Walter Bromberg, "Marihuana: A Psychiatric Study," *JAMA,* 113 (1939): 9, reprinted in Solomon, *The Marijuana Papers,* p. 251.
10. Ibid.
11. Ibid., pp. 251–252.
12. James C. Munch, United Nations *Bulletin on Narcotics,* 18 (1966): 20.
13. Lawrence Kolb, *Drug Addiction, A Medical Problem* (Springfield, Ill.: Charles C Thomas, 1962), p. 55.
14. Public Law No. 238, 75th Cong., August 2, 1937, reprinted in Solomon, *The Marijuana Papers,* pp. 426–438.
15. *Taxation of Marijuana,* Hearings before the Committee on Ways and Means, U.S. House of Representatives, 75th Cong., 1st Sess., on H.R. 6385, April 27–30 and May 4, 1937 (Washington, D.C.: U.S. Government Printing Office, 1937), p. 7.
16. Cited by Alfred R. Lindesmith, in Solomon, *The Marijuana Papers,* p. xxiv.

17. Ibid.
18. Ibid.
19. Richard Brotman and Alfred M. Freedman, "Perspectives on Marijuana Research," prepared for Center for Studies in Substance Use; unpublished, p. 29.
20. "Federal Regulation of the Medicinal Use of Cannabis," *JAMA*, 108 (May 1, 1937): 1543.
21. Ibid., pp. 1543–1544.
22. Medical Center Hospital of Vermont, Burlington, *Progress and Care*, 20 (August, 1970): 1, 3.
23. *Cannabis,* Report by the Advisory Committee on Drug Dependence (London: Her Majesty's Stationery Office, 1968), p. 32.
24. "Report of Committee on Legislative Activities," *JAMA*, 108 (June 26, 1937): 2214.
25. *Taxation of Marijuana,* p. 88.
26. Ibid., pp. 27–30.
27. Ibid., p. 68.
28. Personal communication.
29. Data supplied by the Bureau of Narcotics and Dangerous Drugs, U.S. Department of Justice.
30. "Analysis of State Laws Governing Marijuana," *Congressional Record,* January 20, 1970, pp. S240–245.
31. Public Law No. 78-728, 84th Cong., 2nd Sess., July 18, 1956.
32. Personal communication.
33. New York *Times,* October 26, 1969.
34. New York *Times,* October 23, 1969.

Chapter 57

1. Stanley Yolles, testimony in *Narcotics Legislation,* Hearings before the Subcommittee to Investigate Juvenile Delinquency of the Committee on the Judiciary, U.S. Senate, 91st Cong., 1st Sess., September 17, 1969 (Washington, D.C.: U.S. Government Printing Office, 1969), p. 267.
2. Ibid., p. 277.
3. David Solomon, ed., *The Marijuana Papers* (New York: Bobbs-Merrill, 1966), Table 5, p. 30.
4. State of California, Department of Justice, Bureau of Criminal Statistics, Drug Arrests and Dispositions in California, 1967, Table a, p. 4; Table b, p. 5; and 1968, Table III-1, p. 61; Table I-4, p. 45.
5. Stanley Yolles, "Statement for the National Institute of Mental Health," presented to Subcommittee on Public Health and Welfare of the Interstate and Foreign Commerce Committee, U.S. House of Representatives, 91st Cong., 2nd Sess., February 4, 1970 (Washington, D.C.: U.S. Government Printing Office, 1970), p. 181.
6. New York *Times,* May 26, 1969.
7. New York *Times,* January 17, 1971.
8. Ibid.
9. New York *Times,* October 26, 1969.
10. James D. McKenzie, cited by B. J. Phillips in Washington *Post,* January 14, 1970.
11. Ibid.
12. Jack D. Blaine, Carl M. Lieberman, and Joseph Hirsh, "Preliminary Observations on Patterns of Drug Consumption Among Medical Students," *International Journal of the Addictions,* 3 (Fall, 1968): Table 4, p. 394.
13. Ibid.
14. Samuel G. Benson, "Marijuana Use by Medical Students," presented at the Annual Meeting of the American Psychiatric Association, Washington, D.C., May, 1971; unpublished.
15. Ibid.

16. Ibid.
17. Barry L. Morris, in *Columbia Law School News,* 24 (November 11, 1969): 1–2.
18. Dean I. Manheimer, Glen D. Mellinger, and Mitchell B. Balter, "Marijuana Use Among Urban Adults," *Science,* 166 (December 19, 1969): 1544–1545.
19. New York *Times,* April 4, 1970.
20. Ibid.
21. The Associated Press, in New York *Times,* June 22, 1971.
22. New York *Times,* March 29, 1970.
23. Richard A. Bogg, Roy G. Smith, and Susan D. Russell, "Some Sociological and Social-Psychological Correlates of Marihuana and Alcohol Use by Michigan High School Students," presented at the Ohio Valley Sociological Society and the Midwest Sociological Society Joint Meeting, Indianapolis, Ind., May 2, 1969; unpublished.
24. Ibid.
25. Ibid.
26. Sam Blum, "Marijuana Clouds the Generation Gap," New York *Times* Magazine, August 23, 1970, pp. 28–30, 45, 48, 55–58.
27. Ibid.

Chapter 58

1. Sam Blum, "Marijuana Clouds the Generation Gap," New York *Times* Magazine, August 23, 1970, pp. 28–30, 45, 48, 55–58.
2. Ibid.
3. Alfred R. Lindesmith, "Student Drug Use Viewed by a Sociologist," Loyola Conference on Student Use and Abuse of Drugs, Montreal, October 31–November 3, 1968; unpublished, p. 43.
4. John Kaplan, *Marijuana—The New Prohibition* (New York and Cleveland: World, 1970), pp. 293–294.
5. New York *Times,* August 9, 1970.
6. Seymour Halleck, quoted by John Kaplan, *Marijuana,* p. 294.
7. Hugh J. Parry, personal communication.

Chapter 59

1. New York *Times,* September 9, 1969.
2. Peggy J. Murrell, *Wall Street Journal,* September 11, 1969.
3. Ibid.
4. Ibid.
5. New York *Times,* September 22, 1969.
6. Ibid.
7. Ibid.
8. New York *Daily News,* September 29, 1969.
9. New York *Times,* September 25, 1969.
10. New York *Times,* September 28, 1969.
11. New York *Times,* October 10, 1969.
12. New York *Times,* October 8, 1969.
13. New York *Daily News,* September 29, 1969.
14. New York *Times,* October 2, 1969.
15. Robert Lindsey in the New York *Times,* November 30, 1971.
16. New York *Times,* October 2, 1969.
17. New York *Times,* October 10, 1969.
18. New York *Times,* October 11, 1969.
19. Robert Berrellez, Associated Press, in the *Reporter Dispatch,* White Plains, N.Y., October 1, 1969.

20. New York *Times*, October 24, 1969.
21. Charles R. Beye, Letter to the Editor, New York *Times*, October 30, 1969.
22. W. McGlothlin, K. Jamison, and S. Rosenblatt, "Marijuana and the Use of Other Drugs," *Nature* (London), 228 (December 19, 1970): 1227–1229.
23. Ibid.
24. Ibid.
25. Ibid.
26. Ibid.
27. New York *Times*, August 18, 1969.
28. New York *Times*, October 6, 1969.
29. New York *Times*, October 10, 1969.
30. Burlington, Vt., *Free Press*, March 17, 1970.
31. Edward B. Zuckerman in the *Wall Street Journal*, August 20, 1969.
32. New York *Times*, November 7, 1969.
33. Nicholas von Hoffman in the Washington *Post Star*, August 12, 1970.
34. *Crime in America—A Mid-America View*, Hearings before the Select Committee on Crime, U.S. House of Representatives, 91st Cong., 1st Sess., pursuant to H.R. 17, October 11, 1969, Lincoln, Nebraska (Washington, D.C.: U.S. Government Printing Office, 1969), pp. 165–168.
35. New York *Times*, October 6, 1970.
36. Nicholas von Hoffman, Washington *Post Star*, August 12, 1970.
37. Edward B. Zuckerman, *Wall Street Journal*, August 20, 1969.
38. Personal communication.
39. Personal communication.
40. Personal communication.

Chapter 60

1. Tod H. Mikuriya, "Physical, Mental and Moral Effects of Marijuana," *International Journal of the Addictions*, 3 (Fall, 1968): 253.
2. *Le Dain Commission Interim Report*, p. 8.
3. Ibid., p. 7.
4. Ibid., pp. 13–126.
5. Ibid., p. 145.
6. Ibid., p. 154.
7. Ibid., p. 155.
8. Ibid.
9. Ibid., pp. 155–156.
10. Ibid., p. 160.
11. Ibid., p. 156.
12. Ibid., p. 144.
13. Ibid., pp. 156–157.
14. Ibid., p. 157.
15. Ibid., p. 158.
16. Ibid.
17. Ibid., p. 195.
18. Ibid., p. 196.
19. Ibid., p. 197.
20. Ibid., p. 83.
21. Ibid.
22. Ibid.
23. Ibid., p. 26.
24. Ibid., p. 76.
25. Ibid.
26. Ibid., p. 85.
27. Ibid., p. 45.

28. Ibid., p. 77.
29. Ibid.
30. Ibid., p. 79.
31. Ibid.
32. Ibid., p. 80.
33. George D. Lundberg, Janeth Adelson, and Eric H. Prosnitz, "Marijuana-Induced Hospitalization," *JAMA*, 215 (January 4, 1971): 121.
34. *Le Dain Commission Interim Report,* p. 79.
35. Ibid., p. 80.
36. Ibid., p. 203.
37. Ibid., pp. 77–78.
38. Ibid., p. 200.
39. Ibid., p. 146.
40. Ibid., p. 230.
41. Ibid., p. 231.
42. Ibid., p. 183.
43. Ibid.
44. Ibid.
45. Ibid., p. 184.
46. Ibid.
47. Ibid.
48. Ibid., p. 250.
49. Ibid., p. 245.
50. Ibid., p. 247.
51. Ibid., p. 225.
52. *Medical World News,* September 19, 1969, pp. 15–16.
53. *Le Dain Commission Interim Report,* p. 225.
54. Ibid., p. 247.
55. Ibid.
56. Ibid.
57. Ibid., p. 248.
58. Ibid., p. 241.
59. Ibid.
60. Ibid., pp. 241–242.
61. Ibid., p. 241.
62. Ibid., p. 188.
63. Ibid., p. 242.
64. Ibid.
65. Ibid., p. 258.
66. Ibid., p. 242.
67. Ibid.
68. Ibid., p. 243.
69. Ibid., p. 187.
70. Charles W. Halleck, testimony in *Comprehensive Narcotic Addiction and Drug Abuse Care and Control Act of 1969,* Hearings before the Special Subcommittee on Alcoholism and Narcotics of the Select Committee on Labor and Public Welfare, U.S. Senate, 91st Cong., 1st Sess., September 18, 1969 (Washington, D.C.: U.S. Government Printing Office, 1969), pp. 105–106.
71. David E. Smith, "Testimony to National Commission on Marijuana and Drug Abuse," presented to National Commission on Marijuana and Drug Abuse, San Francisco, June 14, 1971; unpublished.
72. *First Report on Marijuana,* Select Committee on Crime, U.S. House of Representatives, April 6, 1970 (Washington, D.C.: U.S. Government Printing Office, 1970), p. 114.
73. *Le Dain Commission Interim Report,* p. 243.
74. Ibid., p. 250.
75. Ibid., p. 251.

Chapter 61

1. "Summary of 1970 Consumer Expenditures," *Supermarketing*, 26 (September, 1971): 39.
2. Data supplied by Social Research Group, George Washington University, Washington, D.C.; unpublished.
3. Ibid.
4. Ibid.
5. Ibid.
6. Ibid.
7. *The Liquor Handbook* (New York: Gavin-Jobson Associates, 1970), p. 18.
8. Data supplied by Social Research Group, George Washington University.
9. Ibid.
10. Ibid.
11. Ibid.
12. Ibid.
13. Ibid.
14. Ibid.
15. Ibid.
16. Hugh J. Parry, Mitchell B. Balter, and Ira H. Cisin, "Primary Levels of Underreporting Psychotropic Drug Use," *The Public Opinion Quarterly*, 34 (Winter, 1970–71): 582–592.
17. Data supplied by Social Research Group, George Washington University.
18. Ibid.

Chapter 62

1. Mitchell B. Balter and Jerome Levine, "Character and Extent of Psychotherapeutic Drug Usage in the United States," presented at the Fifth World Congress on Psychiatry, Mexico City, November 30, 1971; proceedings to be published in *Excerpta Medica*.
2. Ibid.
3. Mitchell B. Balter, "The Use of Drugs in Contemporary Society," 14th Annual Conference, Veterans Administration Cooperative Studies in Psychiatry, Houston, Texas, April 1, 1969, in *Highlights of the Conference* (Washington, D.C.: Veterans Administration, 1969), pp. 58–59.
4. Ibid., p. 59.
5. Ibid.
6. Ibid.
7. Ibid.
8. Ibid.
9. *The Drug Users*, Task Force on Prescription Drugs, U.S. Department of Health, Education, and Welfare (December, 1969), p. 33.
10. Dean Manheimer, Glenn D. Mellinger, and Mitchell B. Balter, "Psychotherapeutic Drug Use Among Adults in California," *California Medicine*, 109 (December, 1968): Table 1, p. 447.
11. Ibid., p. 449.
12. Ibid.
13. Glenn D. Mellinger, "The Psychotherapeutic Drug Scene in San Francisco," presented at the Western Institute of Drug Problems, Portland, Oregon, August 13, 1969; unpublished, Table 1.
14. Ibid., Table 2.
15. Ibid., p. 17.
16. Ibid., Table 3.
17. Richard Burack, *The New Handbook of Prescription Drugs* (New York: Pantheon Books, Random House, 1967, 1970), pp. 294–295, 309–310, 315.

18. Ibid., p. 295.
19. Ibid., p. 309.
20. Ibid., p. 310.
21. Ibid., p. 315.

Chapter 63

1. Sir T. Clifford Allbutt and Humphrey Davy Rolleston, eds., *A System of Medicine,* vol. II, part I (London: Macmillan, 1909), pp. 286–287.
2. *Le Dain Commission Interim Report,* pp. 157–158.

Chapter 65

1. John Munro, in *Canadian Medical Association Journal,* 103 (November 7, 1970): 1100.
2. *Interim Report for 4424, Inc.,* Youth Centre/Clinic, Montreal (1970); unpublished.
3. John Munro, in *Canadian Medical Association Journal,* 103: 1097.
4. Ibid., p. 1102.

Chapter 66

1. Vincent Nowlis, "Drugs, The Self and Society," paper presented at National Association of Student Personnel Administration Drug Education Conference, Region II, Philadelphia, March 13, 1967; unpublished.
2. Ibid.
3. Ibid.
4. Andrew T. Weil, "Altered States of Consciousness, Drugs, and Society," September 18, 1970; unpublished.
5. Ibid.
6. Ibid.
7. Ibid.
8. Ibid.
9. *Le Dain Commission Interim Report,* p. 163.
10. Allan Y. Cohen, "Inside What's Happening: Sociological, Psychological, and Spiritual Perspectives on the Contemporary Drug Scene," *American Journal of Public Health,* 59 (November, 1969): 2094.
11. Herbert Benson, "Yoga for Drug Abuse," Letter to the Editor, in *New England Journal of Medicine,* 281 (November 13, 1969).
12. W. Thomas Winquist, "The Effects of the Regular Practice of Transcendental Meditation on Students Involved in the Regular Use of Hallucinogenic and 'Hard' Drugs," Students' International Meditation Society, Los Angeles 90024; unpublished (1969).
13. Ibid.
14. Ibid.
15. Herbert Benson and R. Keith Wallace, "Decreased Drug Abuse with Transcendental Meditation," *Proceedings of the International Symposium on Drug Abuse* (Philadelphia: Lea and Febiger, in press).
16. Ibid.

Chapter 67

1. Personal communication.
2. *Le Dain Commission Interim Report,* p. 158.
3. Ibid., p. 159.
4. Ibid.
5. Ibid.

6. Ibid., pp. 159–160.
7. Ibid., p. 160.
8. John Munro, in *Canadian Medical Association Journal*, 103 (November 7, 1970): 1100–1102.
9. Ibid.

Chapter 69

1. Vincent P. Dole, personal communication.
2. U. S. Supreme Court Justice Louis D. Brandeis, dissenting opinion, *New State Ice Company* v. *Ernest A. Liebmann,* 1931 (285 U.S. 311).
3. *Le Dain Commission Interim Report,* p. 182.

Permission to quote

The authors wish to acknowledge their appreciation to the following authors, publishers, individuals, publications and institutions for permission to use selected materials from their works.

Harold A. Abramson, John Buckman, Sidney Cohen, and The Bobbs-Merrill Company, Inc. for "Theoretical Aspects of LSD Therapy," by John Buckman, and for "Psychotherapy with LSD Pro and Con," by Sidney Cohen (reprinted from *The Beyond Within: The LSD Story*, Atheneum, New York; copyright © 1964, 1967 by Sidney Cohen). Both published in *The Use of LSD in Psychotherapy and Alcoholism*, edited by Harold A. Abramson. Copyright © 1967 by Harold A. Abramson. The Bobbs-Merrill Company Inc., publisher.

Academic Press for *Toxicology of Drugs and Chemicals*, by William B. Deichmann and Horace W. Gerarde. Copyright © 1969 by Academic Press, Inc.

Addiction and Drug Abuse Report for permission to reprint material from *Addiction and Drug Abuse Report*, June 1971. Copyright © 1971, by Grafton Publications, Inc.

Aldine-Atherton, Inc. for "Habit Mechanisms in Smoking," by William A. Hunt and Joseph D. Matarazzo, published in *Learning Mechanisms in Smoking*, edited by W. A. Hunt. Copyright © 1970 by Aldine-Atherton, Inc.

Aldine-Atherton, Inc., for *Utopiates: The Use and Users of LSD-25*, by Richard H. Blum and Associates. Copyright © 1964 by Atherton Press. Reprinted by permission of the author and Aldine-Atherton, Inc.

Michael R. Aldrich for "Heads Hidden in the Hemp Fields." Copyright © 1970 by Marijuana Research Association.

Harold Alksne, Ray E. Trussell, and Jack Elinson for "A Follow-Up Study of Treated Adolescent Narcotics Users," 1959; unpublished.

Almqvist and Wiksell for "The Present State of Abuse and Addiction to Stimulant Drugs in Sweden," by Gunnar Inghe, edited by Folke Sjöqvist and Malcolm Tottie. Copyright 1969 by Almqvist & Wiksell.

American Cancer Society for "The Teenager Looks at Cigarette Smoking," research study conducted by Lieberman Research, Inc., September 1969.

American College of Physicians for paper presented by Ralph W. Richter, John Pearson and Michael M. Baden at the 51st Annual Session of the American College of Physicians, 1970.

American Institutes for Research for "Factors Related to Successful Abstinence from Smoking: Final Report," by Joan S. Guilford, et al. Copyright © 1966 by American Institutes for Research.

American Journal of Medicine for "Pulmonary Edema in Acute Heroin Poisoning," by Robert Silber and E. P. Clerkin, July 1959. Copyright © 1959 by *American Journal of Medicine*.

American Journal of Obstetrics and Gynecology for "Pregnancy in Narcotics Addicts Treated by Medical Withdrawal," by George Blinick, Robert C. Wallach, and Eulogio Jerez, December 1, 1969, and "Pregnancy and Menstrual Function in Narcotics Addicts Treated with Methadone," by Robert C. Wallach, Eulogio Jerez, and George Blinick, December 15, 1969. Copyright © 1969 by C. V. Mosby Company.

The American Journal of Psychiatry for "Lysergic Acid Diethylamide (LSD-25): A Clinical Psychological Study," by Charles Savage, 1952; "Addictive Aspects in Heavy Cigarette Smoking," by Peter H. Knapp, C. M. Bliss and H. Webb, 1963; "A

Twelve-Year Follow-up of New York Narcotic Addicts: I. The Relation of Treatment to Outcome," by George Vaillant, 1965; "Flashbacks: Recurrent Intrusive Images After the Use of LSD," by Mardi J. Horowitz, October 1969; "Crime and LSD: The Insanity Plea," by James T. Barter and Martin Reite, October 1969; an article by James R. Allen, Louis Jolyon West, and Joshua Kaufman, November 1969; and "Navajo Peyote Use—Its Apparent Safety," by Robert L. Bergman, December 1971. Copyright © 1952, 1963, 1965, 1969, 1971 by American Psychiatric Association.

American Psychiatric Association for *The Treatment of Drug Abuse*, by Raymond M. Glasscote, et al., 1971; in press for 1972 publication by Joint Information Service of the American Psychiatric Association and the National Association for Mental Health.

American Journal of Public Health for "Inside What's Happening: Sociological, Psychological and Spiritual Perspectives on the Contemporary Drug Scene," by Allan Y. Cohen, November 1969. Copyright © 1969 by American Public Health Association, Inc.

American Journal of Psychology for "Some Psychological Aspects of Nicotinism," by F. I. Arntzen, 1948. Copyright 1948 by University of Illinois Press.

American Journal of Surgery for "Epidemic of Fatal Malaria Among Heroin Addicts in New York City," by Milton Helpern, 1943. Copyright 1943 by *American Journal of Surgery*.

American Social Health Association for *The Opium Problem*, by Charles E. Terry and Mildred Pellens. Copyright 1928 by Committee on Drug Addictions, Bureau of Social Hygiene, Inc.

Annals of Internal Medicine for "The Major Medical Complications of Heroin Addiction," by D. D. Louria, T. Hensle, and J. Rose, 1967. Copyright © 1967 by American College of Physicians.

Harry J. Anslinger for personal communication and "Marijuana: Assassin of Youth," by Harry J. Anslinger and C. R. Cooper, July 1937, *American Magazine*.

Appleton-Century-Crofts for *Principles and Practice of Medicine*, 8th ed., by W. Osler and T. MacCrae. Copyright 1916 by Appleton-Century-Crofts.

Archives of General Psychiatry for "On the Use and Abuse of LSD," by Daniel X. Freedman, March 18, 1968; "Organicity Measures Following Repeated LSD Ingestion," by William H. McGlothlin, David O. Arnold, and Daniel X. Freedman, December 1969, "Chronic Psychosis Associated with Long-Term Psychotomimetic Drug Abuse," by George S. Glass and Malcolm B. Bowers, August 1970, and "LSD Revisited—A Ten Year Follow-up of Medical LSD Use," by William H. McGlothlin and David O. Arnold, January 1971. Copyright © 1968, 1969, 1970, 1971 by the American Medical Association.

Archives of Internal Medicine for articles by Arthur B. Light and Edward G. Torrance, *A.M.A. Archives of Internal Medicine*, vols. 43 (1929) and 44 (1930). Copyright 1929, 1930 by American Medical Association.

Archives of International Pharmacodynamics for "Caffeine-Induced Hemorrhagic Automutilation," by J. M. Peters, 1967. Copyright © 1967 by Archives Internationales de Pharmacodynamie et de Thérapie.

Archives of Neurology and Psychiatry for "Chronic Psychosis and Addiction to Morphine," by A. Z. Pfeffer and D. C. Ruble, December 1946, and "Chronic Barbiturate Intoxication," by Harris Isbell, et al., July 1950. Copyright © 1946, 1950 by American Medical Association.

Archives of Pathology for "Acute Methyl Alcohol Poisoning," by F. R. Menue, 1938. Copyright 1938 by American Medical Association.

Associated Press Newsfeatures for an article by Robert Berrellez, 1969. Published in the *Reporter Dispatch*, White Plains, New York, October 1, 1969.

Astor-Honor for *Chemical Concepts of Psychosis*, edited by M. Rinkel and H. C. B. Denber, 1958. Cited by Morris A. Lipton in "The Relevance of Chemically-Induced Psychoses to Schizophrenia," published in *Psychotomimetic Drugs*, Daniel H. Efron, ed., 1970. Reprinted by permission of Astor-Honor, Inc.

Atheneum, and Laurence Pollinger Limited for *The Beyond Within: The LSD Story* by Sidney Cohen. Copyright © 1964, 1967 by Sidney Cohen. Atheneum, and Martin Secker & Warburg, Ltd., publishers.

Michael M. Baden for "Pathological Aspects of Drug Addiction," from Proceedings of the Committee on Problems of Drug Dependence, 1969.

Mitchell Balter for "The Use of Drugs in Contemporary Society," paper presented at the 14th Annual Conference, Veterans Administration Cooperative Studies in Psychiatry, April 1, 1969; unpublished.

Mitchell Balter and Jerome Levine for "Character and Extent of Psychotherapeutic Drug Usage in the United States," paper presented at Fifth World Congress on Psychiatry, Mexico City, November 30, 1971.

Basic Books, Inc. for *The Road to H: Narcotics, Delinquency and Social Policy*, by Isidor Chein, Donald L. Gerard, M.D., Robert S. Lee, and Eva Rosenfeld. Copyright © 1964 by Basic Books, Inc., Publishers.

Ronald Bayer for Letter to the Editor, published in the New York *Times*, July 20, 1971.

Herbert Benson for Letter to the Editor, "Yoga for Drug Abuse," published in the *New England Journal of Medicine*, November 13, 1969.

Herbert Benson and R. Keith Wallace for "Decreased Drug Abuse with Transcendental Meditation," from *Proceedings of the International Symposium on Drug Abuse*, November 1970.

Samuel Benson for "Marijuana Use by Medical Students," paper presented at the Annual Meeting of the American Psychiatric Association, May 1971; unpublished.

Charles R. Beye for Letter to the Editor, published in the New York *Times*, October 30, 1969.

Brandon House for "Myths and Realities of Marijuana Pushing," by Jerry Mandel. Published in *Marijuana Myths and Realities*, edited by J. L. Simmons. Copyright © 1967 by Brandon House, Chatsworth, California.

British Journal of Addiction for an article by J. Yerbury Dent, 1952. Copyright 1952 by *British Journal of Addiction*.

British Journal of Medical Psychology for "Cigarette Smoking: Natural History of a Dependence Disorder," by M. A. Hamilton Russell, 1971. Copyright © 1971 by *British Journal of Medical Psychology*. Published by Cambridge University Press.

British Medical Journal for October 1922 issue, cited in New York *Post*, "The Famous Addicts—Article III: Freud and Halsted," by Sally Hammond, July 22, 1970; article by T. H. Bewley, November 1965; and Editorial, August 7, 1971. Copyright 1922, © 1965, 1971 by *British Medical Journal*.

Richard Brotman and Alfred M. Freedman for "Perspectives on Marijuana Research," work prepared for Center for Studies in Substance Use; unpublished.

Andrew G. Bucaro for personal communication.

Bulletin of the New York Academy of Medicine for "Thoughts on Narcotics Addiction," by Vincent P. Dole, February 1965. Copyright © 1965 by *Bulletin of the New York Academy of Medicine*.

Bulletin on Narcotics for "Cannabis," by J. Bouquet, 1951, and "The Use of Cannabis Drugs in India," by I. C. Chopra and R. N. Chopra, 1957.

California Medicine for "Psychotherapeutic Drug Use Among Adults in California," by Dean Manheimer, Glen D. Mellinger and Mitchell B. Balter, December 1968; and "Marijuana in Medicine, Past, Present and Future," by Tod H. Mikuriya, January 1969. Copyright © 1968, 1969 by California Medical Association.

Canadian Medical Association Journal for "The Use of Lysergic Acid Diethylamide (LSD) in Psychotherapy," by E. F. W. Baker, December 5, 1964; "Coca Leaf and Cocaine Addiction—Some Historical Notes," by H. P. Blejer-Prieto, September 25, 1965; and "What Society Must Do to Solve Problem of Drug Use Among Young," by Honourable John Munro, November 7, 1970. Copyright © 1964, 1965, 1970 by Canadian Medical Association.

Charles E. Cherubin for "The Epidemiology of Death in Narcotics Addicts," by Charles E. Cherubin et al., 1971; unpublished; in press.

Permission to Quote

Chest for "Epidemiology and Psychology of Cigarette Smoking," by Daniel Horn, May 1971. Copyright © 1971 by American College of Chest Physicians.

Clinical Pharmacology and Therapeutics for "The Role of Nicotine as a Determinant of Cigarette Smoking Frequency in Man with Observations of Certain Cardiovascular Effects Associated with the Tobacco Alkaloid," by B. R. Lucchesi, C. R. Schuster and G. S. Emley, 1967; and "Psychotropic Effects of Caffeine in Man," by Avram Goldstein and Sophia Kaizer, July 8, 1969. Copyright © 1967, 1969 by C. V. Mosby Company.

Sidney Cohen for "LSD and the Anguish of Dying," copyright © 1965 by Minneapolis Star and Tribune Co., Inc. Reprinted from the September, 1965 issue of *Harper's Magazine* by permission of the author.

Columbia Law School News for an article by Barry L. Morris, November 11, 1969. Copyright © 1969 by *Columbia Law School News.*

Comprehensive Psychiatry for "Misapprehension About Drug Addiction: Origins and Repercussions," by Henry Brill, June 1963; "The LSD Controversy," by Jerome Levine and Arnold M. Ludwig, 1964; "An Approach to Treating Narcotic Addicts Based on a Community Mental Health Diagnosis," by Richard Brotman, Alan S. Meyer, and Alfred M. Freedman, April 1965. Copyright © 1963, 1964, 1965 by Grune & Stratton, Inc.

The Controller of Her Britannic Majesty's Stationery Office for *Cannabis*—Report by the Advisory Committee on Drug Dependence, 1968; *The Amphetamines and Lysergic Acid Diethylamide (LSD)*—Report by the Advisory Committee on Drug Dependence, Department of Health and Social Security, 1970. Reprinted by permission of the Controller of Her Britannic Majesty's Stationery Office.

Crown Publishers for "The Herb Pantagruelion," by François Rabelais, translated by Samuel Putnam. Published in *The Marihuana Papers,* edited by David Solomon. The Bobbs-Merrill Company, Inc., publisher.

Diseases of the Nervous System for "Lysergic Acid Diethylamide (LSD-25) as an Aid in Psychotherapy," by A. K. Busch and W. C. Johnson, 1950. Copyright 1950 by *Diseases of the Nervous System.*

Denver Post, August 2, 1959; June 12, 1960; October 23, December 8, 1961; April 13, 29, 1962; January 18, March 21, April 22, 29, June 25, July 2, 1965; January 11, May 18, June 10, October 30, 1966. Copyright © 1959, 1960, 1961, 1962, 1965, 1966 *Denver Post.*

Meyer H. Diskind for "New Horizons in the Treatment of Narcotic Addiction," by Meyer H. Diskind, *Federal Probation,* December 1960 and "Narcotic Addiction and Post-Parole Adjustment," by Meyer H. Diskind, Robert F. Hallinan and George Klonsky, 1963, unpublished, cited in "A Second Look at the New York State Parole Drug Experiment," by Meyer H. Diskind and George Klonsky, *Federal Probation,* December 1964.

Vincent P. Dole for personal communication.

E. P. Dutton & Co., Inc. for *Story of San Michele,* by Axel Munthe. Copyright 1929 by E. P. Dutton & Co., Inc. Renewal 1932 by Axel Munthe and 1951 by Major Malcolm Munthe. Published by E. P. Dutton & Co., Inc. and used with their permission.

Encyclopaedia Britannica for "Hemp," "Ether," and "Coffee," 11th edition. Copyright 1910, 1911 by *Encyclopaedia Britannica.*

Farrar, Straus & Giroux, Inc. for *The Murderers* by Harry J. Anslinger and Will Oursler. Copyright © 1961 by Farrar, Straus & Giroux, Inc.

Fawcett Publications, Inc., for *The LSD Story* by John Cashman, published by Gold Medal Books. Copyright © 1966 by Fawcett Publications, Inc.

4424 Youth Clinic, Montreal, for Interim Report for 4424, Inc., 1970; unpublished.

Free Press, March 17, 1970. Copyright © 1970 by *Free Press,* Burlington, Vermont.

W. H. Freeman and Company for "The Hallucinogenic Drugs," by Frank Barron, Murray E. Jarvik, and Sterling Bunnell, Jr. Copyright © 1964 by Scientific American, Inc. All rights reserved.

Funk & Wagnalls Co., Inc. for *The Traffic in Narcotics,* by Harry J. Anslinger and William F. Tompkins. Copyright 1953 by Funk & Wagnalls Co., Inc. Used with permission of the publisher, Funk & Wagnalls, Inc., Publishers.

[586]

Gavin-Jobson Associates for *The Liquor Handbook,* 1970. Copyright © 1970 by Gavin-Jobson Associates.

George R. Gay for paper presented at National Heroin Symposium, June 1971.

George R. Gay et al. for "Short Term Heroin Detoxification on an Outpatient Basis"; unpublished.

Allen Ginsberg for interview, Los Angeles *Free Press,* December 1965.

Grove Press and Peter Owen Ltd. for *The Book of Grass: An Anthology of Indian Hemp,* edited by George Andrews and Simon Vinkenoog. Copyright © 1967 by Peter Owen. Published by Peter Owen, London. Reprinted by permission of Grove Press, Inc.

Grune & Stratton, Inc. for *The Drug Addict as a Patient,* by Marie Nyswander. Copyright © 1956 by Grune & Stratton, Inc.

Grune & Stratton, Inc. for "Some Problems of Addiction," by Karl M. Bowman. Published in *Problems of Addiction and Habituation,* edited by Paul H. Hock and Joseph Zubin. Copyright © 1957 by Grune & Stratton, Inc.

Seymour Halleck, quoted in *Marijuana—The New Prohibition,* by John Kaplan.

George G. Harrap & Company Ltd. for *A History of Smoking,* by Count Egor Caesar Corti, trans. Paul England, 1931. Copyright 1931 by George G. Harrap & Co., Ltd.

Daniel Horn for "The Smoking Problem in 1971," presented at American Cancer Society's Thirteenth Annual Science Writers Seminar, 1971.

Hutchinson of London for *Wooden Bygones of Smoking and Snuff Taking,* by Edward H. Pinto. Copyright © 1961 by the Hutchinson Publishing Group.

Illinois Medical Journal for "Stripping the Medical Profession of Its Powers and Giving Them to a Body of Lawmakers. The Proposed Amendment to the Harrison Narcotic Act—Everybody Seems to Know All about Doctoring except the Doctors," June 1926. Copyright 1926 by *Illinois Medical Journal.*

Indiana University Press for *Drug Addiction: Crime or Disease? Interim and Final Reports of the Joint Committee of the American Bar Association and the American Medical Association on Narcotic Drugs.* Introduction Copyright © 1969 by Indiana University Press.

Indiana University Press for *Narcotic Addiction in Britain and America,* by Edwin M. Schur. Copyright © 1968 by Indiana University Press.

The International Journal of the Addictions, January 1966; "Plastic Cement: The Ten Cent Hallucinogen," by Edward Preble and Gabriel V. Laury, Fall 1967; "Anesthetic Addiction and Drunkenness," by David R. Nagle; and "A Bibliography on the Inhalation of Glue Fumes and Other Toxic Vapors," by Lenore R. Kupperstein and Ralph M. Susman, both Spring 1968; "Physical, Mental and Moral Effects of Marijuana," by Tod H. Mikuriya, Fall 1968; "Preliminary Observations on Patterns of Drug Consumption Among Medical Students," by Jack D. Blaine, Carl M. Lieberman, and Joseph Hirsh, Fall 1968; "Taking Care of Business—The Heroin User's Life on the Street," by Edward Preble and John J. Casey, Jr., March 1969; "Heroin Addicts on Methadone Replacement: A Study of Dropouts," by Richard G. Adams et al., June 1971; and "Cyclazocine in a Multi-Modality Treatment Program: Comparative Results," by John N. Chappel, Edward C. Senay, and Jerome H. Jaffe, September 1971. Copyright © 1967, 1968 by the Institute for the Study of Drug Addiction. Copyright © 1969, 1971 by Marcel Dekker, Inc. Reprinted by courtesy of Marcel Dekker, Inc.

The Johns Hopkins Press for "Analgesics and the Reaction Component of Pain," by Henry K. Beecher. Published in *Drugs and the Brain,* edited by Perry Black. Copyright © 1969 by The Johns Hopkins Press.

Harris Isbell for personal communication.

Mrs. Katharine Jones, The Hogarth Press, and Basic Books, Inc. for *The Life and Work of Sigmund Freud* by Ernest Jones. Copyright © 1953 by Ernest Jones, Basic Books, Inc., and The Hogarth Press Ltd., publishers.

Journal of Criminal Law and Criminology for "Morphinism," by L. L. Stanley, November 1915, and "Dope Fiend Mythology," by Alfred R. Lindesmith, July–August 1940, both in *Journal of the American Institute of Criminal Law and Criminology.*

Permission to Quote

Copyright 1915, 1940 by the *Journal of Criminal Law and Criminology* (including the *American Journal of Police Science*).

Journal of Nervous and Mental Diseases for "Lysergic Acid Diethylamide: Side Effects and Complications," by Sidney Cohen, January 1960. Copyright © 1960 by The Williams & Wilkins Co.

Journal of Psychedelic Drugs for "LSD: Its Use, Abuse and Suggested Treatment," by David E. Smith and Alan J. Rose, and "Incidents Involving the Haight-Ashbury Population and Some Uncommonly Used Drugs," by Frederick H. Myers, Alan J. Rose, and David E. Smith, both published in vol. 1, no. 2 (1967–68); "U.S. Marijuana Legislation and the Creation of a Social Problem," by Roger C. Smith, vol. 2, no. 1 (1968); "The World of the Haight-Ashbury Speed Freak," by Roger C. Smith, and "An Introduction to Amphetamine Abuse," by John C. Kramer, both vol. 2, no. 2 (1969); "The Changing Patterns of Heroin Addiction in the Haight-Ashbury Subculture," by Charles W. Sheppard, George R. Gay, and David E. Smith, vol. 3, Spring (1971); Proceedings of the National Heroin Symposium, June 19–20, 1971, vol. 4, issue 1 (1971). Copyright © 1967, 1968, 1969, 1971 by *Journal of Psychedelic Drugs*.

The Journal of the American Medical Association for "Queries and Minor Notes," 1930; "A Study of the Promiscuous Use of the Barbiturates," by W. E. Hambourger, April 1937; "Federal Regulation of the Medicinal Use of Cannabis," May 1, 1937; "Report of Committee on Legislative Activities," June 26, 1937; "Marijuana: A Psychiatric Study," by Walter Bromberg, July 1, 1939; "The Marijuana Problem," by J. D. Reichard, June 24, 1944; "Drug-Induced Mood Changes in Man," by Louis Lasagna, John M. von Felsinger, and Henry K. Beecher, March 19, 1955; "Glue-Sniffing in Children," by Helen H. Glaser and Oliver N. Massengale, July 28, 1962; "Patterns of Hallucinogenic Drug Abuse," by Arnold M. Ludwig and Jerome Levine, January 11, 1965; "Caffeinism," by Hobart A. Reimann, December 18, 1967; "Characteristics of Drug Abusers Admitted to a Psychiatric Hospital," by Leon J. Hekimian and Samuel Gershon, July 15, 1968; "Successful Treatment of 750 Criminal Addicts," by Vincent P. Dole, Marie E. Nyswander, and Alan Warner, December 16, 1968; "Institutionalization Patterns Among Civilly Committed Addicts," by John C. Kramer, June 23, 1969; "Halsted of Johns Hopkins, The Man and His Problem as Described in the Secret Records of William Osler," by Wilder Penfield, December 22, 1969; "Effects of LSD on Human Pregnancy," by William H. McGlothlin, Robert S. Sparkes, and David O. Arnold, June 1, 1970; "Marijuana-Induced Hospitalization," by George D. Lundberg, Janeth Adelson, and Eric H. Prosnitz, January 4, 1971; and "The British Narcotic 'Register' in 1970: A Factual Review," by Frederick B. Glaser and John C. Ball, May 17, 1971. Copyright 1930, 1937, 1939, 1944, © 1955, 1962, 1965, 1968, 1969, 1970, 1971 by the American Medical Association.

The Journal of the Medical Society of New Jersey for "Cannabis Indica in Pharmaceuticals," by Marty Sasman, 1938. Copyright 1938 by The Medical Society of New Jersey.

The Julian Press for *Psychology and the Great God Fun,* by A. E. Hamilton. Copyright © 1955 by The Julian Press, Inc.

The Lancet for article by F. E. Tylecote, 1927; "Tobacco Smoking and Nicotine," by Lennox M. Johnston, December 19, 1942; "On the Therapeutic Uses and Toxic Effects of Cannabis Indica," by J. Russell Reynolds, March 22, 1970; and "Deaths in United Kingdom Opioid Users," by Ramon Gardner, September 26, 1970. Copyright 1927, 1942, © 1970 by The Lancet Ltd.

Lange Medical Publications for *Handbook of Poisoning: Diagnosis and Treatment,* 7th ed., Robert H. Dreisbach. Copyright © 1971 by Lange Medical Publications.

Jerome Levine for paper presented at National Association of Student Personnel Administrators Drug Education Conference, November 7–8, 1966; unpublished.

Licensed Beverage Industries, Inc. for *LBI Facts Book 1970.*

Alfred R. Lindesmith for *Opiate Addiction.* Copyright 1947 by Alfred R. Lindesmith. Published by Principia Press.

Alfred R. Lindesmith for "Student Drug Use Viewed by a Sociologist," October 1968; unpublished.

J. B. Lippincott Company for *Marijuana, America's New Drug Problem,* by Robert P. Walton. Copyright 1938 by J. B. Lippincott.

Little, Brown and Company for *The Mighty Leaf,* by Jerome E. Brooks. Copyright 1952 by Little, Brown and Company.

E. & S. Livingstone, Ltd. for *Public Health in the Nineteenth Century,* by C. Fraser Brockington. Copyright © 1965 by E. & S. Livingstone, Ltd.

Los Angeles *Times-*Washington *Post* News Service for an article published in *Detroit News,* June 4, 1970.

Edward J. Lynn for "Nitrous Oxide: It's a Gas!" presented at 124th Annual Meeting of American Psychiatric Association, 1971; unpublished.

William H. McGlothlin for "Toward a Rational View of Hallucinogenic Drugs," by William H. McGlothlin. Paper distributed at National Association of Student Personnel Administrators Drug Education Conference, November 7–8, 1966; unpublished.

McGraw-Hill Book Company for "The Rehabilitation of the Drug Addict," by George B. Wallace, published in *Journal of Educational Sociology,* 1931. Quoted in *Narcotics,* edited by Daniel M. Wilner and Gene G. Kassebaum. Copyright © 1965 by Blakiston Division of McGraw-Hill Company.

Rand McNally & Company for *A Doctor Among the Addicts,* by Nat Hentoff. Copyright © 1968 by Nat Hentoff; published by Rand McNally & Company.

The Macmillan Company for "Marijuana: A Sociological Overview," from *Outsiders* by Howard S. Becker. Copyright © 1963 by The Free Press of Glencoe, a division of The Macmillan Company. Published in *The Marihuana Papers,* edited by David Solomon. Copyright © 1966 by David Solomon. The Bobbs-Merrill Company, Inc., publisher.

The Macmillan Company for *The Peyote Religion,* by J. S. Slotkin. Copyright © 1956 by The Free Press of Glencoe, a division of The Macmillan Company.

The Macmillan Company for *The Pharmacological Basis of Therapeutics,* by Louis S. Goodman and Alfred Gilman, editors, 3rd edition (1965) and 4th edition (1970). Copyright © 1965, 1970 by The Macmillan Company.

The Macmillan Company for *Delinquency and Opportunity* by Richard A. Cloward and Lloyd E. Ohlin, cited in Preble and Casey, "Taking Care of Business—The Heroin User's Life on the Street," *International Journal of the Addictions,* March 1969. Copyright © 1964 by The Free Press of Glencoe, a division of The Macmillan Company.

Nicolas Malleson for "Acute Adverse Reactions to LSD in Clinical and Experimental Use in the United Kingdom," provisional report, June 1969; unpublished. Later published in *The British Journal of Psychiatry,* February 1971. Copyright © 1971 by Royal Medico-Psychological Association.

Medical Center Hospital of Vermont for *Progress and Care,* August 1970.

Medical Economics for Physicians' Desk Reference to Pharmaceutical Specialties and Biologicals, 26th ed., 1972. Copyright © 1972 by Medical Economics Company.

The Medical Letter, October 3, 1969 and March 5, 1971. Copyright © 1969, 1971 by *The Medical Letter.*

Medical Tribune, January 12, 1969, July 7, 1969 and October 10, 1969. Copyright © 1969 by Medical Tribune, Inc. Reprinted by courtesy of *Medical Tribune.*

Medical World News, September 19, 1969, and September 3, 1971. Copyright © 1969, 1971 by *Medical World News.*

The Medico-Legal Journal for "Drugs and Delinquency," February 11, 1965. Copyright © 1965 Medico-Legal Society.

Glen D. Mellinger for "The Psychotherapeutic Drug Scene in San Francisco," August 13, 1969; unpublished.

Mental Hygiene for "Pleasure and Deterioration from Narcotic Addiction," by Lawrence Kolb, 1925. Copyright 1925 by National Association for Mental Hygiene.

Ministry of National Health and Welfare of Canada for *Interim Report of the Commission of Inquiry Into the Non-Medical Use of Drugs,* 1970. Copyright © 1970 Information Canada, Ottawa.

Minnesota State Medical Association and Moses Barron for report to the Minnesota State Medical Society, by Moses Barron, August 25, 1921.

Narcotic Addiction Foundation of British Columbia for *History of Drug Addiction and Legislation in Canada* by Ingeborg Paulus. Copyright © November 1966 by Narcotic Addiction Foundation of B.C.

George Nash for "The Phoenix House Program: The Results of a Two Year Follow-up," by George Nash, Dan Waldorf, Kay Foster, and Ann Kyllingstad, February 1971; unpublished.

National Observer for "Drug Program at $250 Million, Deemed a Failure," by Owen Moritz, June 8, 1970. Copyright © 1970 Dow Jones Company, Inc.

Nature and William McGlothlin for "Marijuana and the Use of Other Drugs," by William McGlothlin, K. Jamison, and S. Rosenblatt, December 19, 1970. Copyright © 1970, *Nature* (London).

New England Journal of Medicine for "Caffeine Intoxication," by Margaret C. McManamy and Purcell G. Schube, 1936; "Glue Sniffing by Youngsters Fought by Department," November 8, 1962; "In Vivo and In Vitro Chromosomal Damage Induced by LSD-25," by M. M. Cohen, K. Hirschhorn, and W. A. Frosch, October 1967; Letter to the Editor "Yoga for Drug Abuse," by Herbert Benson, November 13, 1969, and "Medical Progress: Marijuana," by Richard Colestock Pillard, August 6, 1970. Copyright 1936, © 1962, 1967, 1969, 1970 by *New England Journal of Medicine*.

New Orleans *Item* for New Orleans *Morning Tribune*, October 17, 19, 23, 28, 1926; and New Orleans *Item*, October 22, 1926 and February 4, 1927.

The New Physician for "Use of Amphetamines, Marijuana and LSD by Students," by P. H. Blachly, April 1966, and an article by John C. Kramer, March 1969. Copyright © 1966, 1969 by Student American Medical Association.

New Republic for "The Risks of Marijuana," by David Sanford. Copyright © 1967 by Harrison-Blaine of New Jersey, Inc.

New York Daily News, September 29, 1969 and March 11, 1966. Copyright © 1966, 1969 by the *New York Daily News*. Reprinted by courtesy of the *New York Daily News*.

New York Law Journal for articles by Vincent P. Dole, William R. Martin, and Norman E. Zinberg, December 6, 1971. Copyright © 1971 by *New York Law Journal*.

New York Medicine for "Medical Aspects of Drug Abuse," by Michael M. Baden, 1968. Copyright © 1968 by *New York Medicine*.

New York Post for "49 Agents Quit in Drug Probe," by Warren Hoge, October 27, 1969. Copyright © 1969 by New York Post Corporation. Reprinted by permission of *New York Post*.

New York State Journal of Medicine for "Mental Sequelae of the Harrison Law," May 15, 1915; "A Physician's Blueprint for the Management and Prevention of Narcotic Addiction," by Hubert S. Howe, February 1, 1955; "Rehabilitation of Heroin Addicts After Blockade with Methadone," by Vincent P. Dole and Marie E. Nyswander, August 1, 1966; and "Deaths from Narcotism in New York City," by Milton Helpern and Yong-Myun Rho, September 15, 1966. Copyright 1915, © 1955, 1966 by Medical Society of the State of New York. Reprinted by permission of the *New York State Journal of Medicine*.

The New York Times, October 6, 1961, April 25, 1963, February 27, 1965, April 7, 12, May 30, 1966, May 20, 26, August 18, September 5, 9, 22, 23, 25, 28, October 2, 4, 6, 8, 10, 11, 23, 24, 26, 30, November 7, December 5, 16, 1969, January 2, February 1, 15, March 24, 29, April 4, June 21, August 9, 23, October 6, December 13, 30, 1970, January 17, 25, February 22, April 18, May 16, 23, June 22, July 1, 20, September 12, 28, November 30 and December 5, 1971. Copyright © 1961, 1963, 1965, 1966, 1969, 1970, 1971 by The New York Times Company. Reprinted by permission.

New York University Press for *Coffee*, by Ralph Holt Cheney. Copyright 1925 by New York University Press.

Newsweek, August 13, 1962. Copyright © 1962 by Newsweek, Inc.

Vincent Nowlis for "Drugs, The Self and Society," presented at National Association of Student Personnel Administration Drug Education Conference, Philadelphia, March 13, 1967; unpublished.

Marie Nyswander for personal communication.

John A. O'Donnell for personal communication.

Hugh J. Parry for "Caffeine, Nicotine, Alcohol and Psychoactive Prescription Drugs," by Social Research Group, The George Washington University; unpublished.

Pharmacological Reviews for an article by Harris Isbell and H. F. Fraser, vol. 2 (1950). Copyright 1950 by The Williams & Wilkins Co.

The Practitioner for "Some Problems of Opiate Addiction," by J. H. Willis, February 1968. Copyright © 1968 by *The Practitioner.*

Psychiatric News for "LSD Discoverer Disputes 'Chance' Factor in Finding," April 21, 1971, and an article, December 15, 1971. Copyright © 1971 by *Psychiatric News.*

Psychopharmacologia for an article by C. D. Frith, 1971. Copyright © 1971 by Springer-Verlag, publishers.

Public Opinion Quarterly for "Primary Levels of Underreporting Psychotropic Drug Use," by Hugh J. Parry, Mitchell B. Balter, and Ira H. Cisin, Winter 1970–71. Copyright © 1970, 1971 by *Public Opinion Quarterly.*

G. P. Putnam's Sons for "A Review of the Clinical Effects of Psychotomimetic Agents," by Humphrey Osmond, and "Pain and LSD-25: A Theory of Attenuation of Anticipation," by E. Kast. Published in *LSD, The Consciousness-Expanding Drug* edited by David Solomon. Copyright © 1964, 1966 by David Solomon. G. P. Putnam's Sons, publishers.

Quarterly Journal of Studies on Alcohol for "Treatment of Alcoholism with Lysergide[1]," by Wilson Van Dusen, Wayne Wilson, et al., 1967. Copyright © 1967 by Journal of Alcohol Studies, Inc.

Random House, Inc. for *The Big Drink: The Story of Coca-Cola,* by E. J. Kahn, Jr. Copyright © 1960 by Random House, Inc.

Random House, Inc. for *The New Handbook of Prescription Drugs,* by Richard Burack, M.D. Copyright © 1967, 1970 by Richard Burack, M.D. Published by Pantheon Books, a division of Random House, Inc.

Random House, Inc. for *The Making of the English Working Class,* by E. P. Thompson. Copyright © 1963 by E. P. Thompson. Published by Pantheon Books, a division of Random House, Inc.

Raven Press for *Psychotomimetic Drugs,* edited by Daniel H. Efron. Copyright © 1970 by Raven Press.

Remington's Pharmaceutical Sciences, 14th ed., 1970. Copyright © 1970 by *Remington's Pharmaceutical Sciences,* published by Mack Publishing Company.

The Ronald Press Company for "The Marijuana Problem in the City of New York," by the Mayor's Committee on Marijuana. Copyright 1944 by The Ronald Press Company. Published in *The Marihuana Papers,* edited by David Solomon. Copyright © 1966 by David Solomon. The Bobbs-Merrill Company, Inc., publishers.

J. H. Rothschild, and McIntosh and Otis, Inc. for *Tomorrow's Weapons.* Copyright © 1964 by J. H. Rothschild. Cited in *Chemical and Biological Warfare: America's Hidden Arsenal* by Seymour M. Hersh. Copyright © 1968, by Seymour M. Hersh. The Bobbs-Merrill Company, Inc., publishers.

Routledge & Kegan Paul, Ltd. for *Phantastica: Narcotic and Stimulating Drugs, Their Use and Abuse,* by Louis Lewin, 1924, trans. 1931; reprint, 1964, E. P. Dutton & Co. Copyright © 1964 by Routledge & Kegan Paul, Ltd.

St. Martin's Press, Inc. for *Drugs and the Mind,* by Robert S. de Ropp. Copyright © 1957 by St. Martin's Press, Inc., Macmillan & Co., Ltd.

W. B. Saunders Company for *Textbook of Pharmacology,* by William T. Salter. Copyright 1952 by W. B. Saunders Company, publishers.

Richard Evans Schultes for personal communication.

Science for "The Role of Nicotine in the Cigarette Habit," by J. K. Finnegan, P. S. Larson, and H. B. Haag, July 27, 1945; "Chromosomal Damage in Human Leukocytes Induced by Lysergic Acid Diethylamide," by M. M. Cohen, M. Marinello, and N. Bach, March 17, 1967; "Hallucinogens of Plant Origin," by R. E. Schultes, January 17, 1969; "Marijuana Use Among Urban Adults," by Dean I. Manheimer, G. D. Mellinger, and M. B. Balter, December 19, 1969; "Chromosomal Abnormalities in the

Human Population: Estimation of Rates Based on New Haven Newborn Study," by H. A. Lubs and F. H. Ruddle, July 31, 1970; "Marijuana in Man: Three Years Later," by L. E. Hollister, April 2, 1971, and "Narcotic Antagonists: New Methods to Treat Heroin Addiction," by A. L. Hammond, August 6, 1971. Copyright 1945, © 1967, 1969, 1970, 1971 by American Association for the Advancement of Science.

Scientist and Citizen for "Chemical Weapons, What They Are, What They Do," by Victor W. Sidel and Robert M. Goldwyn, August–September, 1967. Copyright © 1967 by Committee for Environmental Information.

The Shoe String Press for *The Peyote Cult*, by Weston LaBarre. Copyright © 1959, 1964 by The Shoe String Press, Inc. Preface Copyright © 1969 by Weston LaBarre. Reprinted by permission of the publishers, The Shoe String Press, Inc., Hamden, Connecticut.

David E. Smith for "Testimony to National Commission on Marijuana and Drug Abuse," San Francisco, 1971; and for remarks at National Heroin Symposium, San Francisco, 1971.

Roger C. Smith for "The Marketplace of Speed: Violence and Compulsive Methamphetamine Abuse"; unpublished.

Society for the Study of Addiction to Alcohol and Other Drugs for *Pharmacological and Epidemiological Aspects of Adolescent Drug Dependence,* edited by C. W. M. Wilson, 1966. Copyright © 1968 by Pergamon Press, Inc.

Southern Medical Journal for "The Treatment of Drug Addicts at the Lexington Hospital," by Lawrence Kolb and W. F. Ossenfort, August 1938. Copyright 1938 by *Southern Medical Journal.*

Jonathan Spence for "Opium Smoking in Ch'ing China," 1971; unpublished.

Stanford Medical Bulletin for "Morphine Addiction for 62 Years," by Windsor C. Cutting, August 1942. Reprinted by permission *Stanford M.D.*

George H. Stevenson for "Drug Addiction in British Columbia: A Research Survey," 1956; unpublished. Reprinted by permission of the author.

Supermarketing for "Summary of 1970 Consumer Expenditures," September 1971. Copyright © 1971 by C. M. Business Publications, Inc.

Svenska Läkartidningen for "Försök med Nikotin, Lobelin och Placebo," by B. Ejrup and P. A. Wikander, July 17, 1959. Copyright © 1959 by Swedish Medical Association.

John S. Tamerin for paper presented by John S. Tamerin and Charles P. Neumann at the Annual Meeting of the American Psychiatric Association, May 1971; unpublished.

Charles C Thomas for *Drug Addiction, A Medical Problem,* by Lawrence Kolb. Copyright © 1962 by Charles C Thomas, Publishers. Courtesy of Charles C Thomas, Publisher, Springfield, Illinois.

Time for "The New Kick," February 16, 1962, and "Blues for Janis," October 19, 1970. Reprinted by permission of *Time, The Weekly Newsmagazine.* Copyright © 1962, 1970 by Time Inc.

Today's Health for "Pep Teasers," by Iago Galdston, published in *Hygeia,* October 1940, by The American Medical Association. Copyright 1940 by The American Medical Association.

Transactions of Association of American Physicians for "Narcotic Blockade—A Medical Technique for Stopping Heroin Use by Addicts," by Vincent P. Dole and Marie E. Nyswander, 1966. Copyright © 1966 by *Transactions of Association of American Physicians.*

University of Toronto Press for *Morphine and Allied Drugs,* by A. K. Reynolds and Lowell O. Randall. Copyright © 1957 by University of Toronto Press.

U.S. News and World Report and Gerald E. Davidson for article of September 27, 1971.

The Village Voice for article by Ken Sobol, October 21, 1971. Reprinted by permission of *The Village Voice.* Copyright 1971 by The Village Voice, Inc.

The Wall Street Journal, December 7, 1962, article by Phillip E. Norton; April 17, 1963, Editorial; August 20, 1969, article by Edward B. Zuckerman; September 11,

1969, article by Peggy J. Murrell. Copyright © 1962, 1963, 1969 by *The Wall Street Journal.*

Washington Post, February 12, 1969; January 14, 1970, article by B. J. Phillips; August 12, 1970, article by Nicholas von Hoffman. Copyright © 1969, 1970 by *The Washington Post.*

Andrew T. Weil for "Altered States of Consciousness, Drugs, and Society," September 18, 1970; unpublished.

Wesleyan University Press, and Faber and Faber, Ltd., for "The Therapeutic Potential of LSD in Medicine," by Albert A. Kurland et al. Published in *LSD, Man and Society,* edited by Richard C. DeBold and Russell C. Leaf. Copyright © 1967 by Wesleyan University.

West Virginia Medical Journal for "Drug Addiction in Upper Economic Levels: A Study of 142 Cases," by Eugene J. Morhous, July 1953. Copyright 1953 by *West Virginia Medical Journal.*

Grenville B. Whitman for *The Dolly,* August 1969. Published by Man Alive, Inc.

WHO Chronicle for "Smoking and Health," by C. M. Fletcher and Daniel Horn, 1970. Copyright © 1970 by World Health Organization.

The Williams & Wilkins Co. for *Pain Sensations and Reactions,* by James D. Hardy, Harold G. Wolff, and Helen Goodell. Copyright 1952 by The Williams & Wilkins Co.

Wilshire Book Company for *The Peyote Story,* by Bernard Roseman. Copyright © 1963 by Wilshire Book Company.

W. Thomas Winquist for "The Effects of the Regular Practice of Transcendental Meditation on Students Involved in the Regular Use of Hallucinogenic and 'Hard' Drugs," 1969; unpublished.

World Publishing Company, and Brandt & Brandt for *Marijuana—The New Prohibition,* by John Kaplan. Copyright © 1970 by John Kaplan. World Publishing Company, publishers.

World Publishing Company for *High Priest,* by Timothy Leary. Copyright © 1968 by World Publishing Company. The New American Library, publishers.

The Yale Law Journal for "The Narcotics Bureau and the Harrison Act: Jailing the Healers and the Sick," by Rufus King, 1953. Reprinted by permission of the Yale Law Journal Company and Fred B. Rothman & Company.

The authors are also grateful to the following persons for permission to quote from their papers, presented at the following conferences.

Vincent P. Dole and Frances R. Gearing for papers presented at First National Conference on Methadone Treatment, June 1968.

Michael M. Baden, William A. Bloom, Jr., Emmett P. Davis, Vincent P. Dole, Frances R. Gearing, Jerome H. Jaffe, Herbert Kleber, Mary Jane Kreek, Robert A. Maslansky, and Ray Trussell for papers presented at Second National Conference on Methadone Treatment, October 1969.

Saul Blatman, George Blinick, William A. Bloom, Jr., Dean V. Babst, Paul Cushman, Jr., Morton I. Davidson, Frances R. Gearing, Avram Goldstein, Robert G. Newman, Gordon T. Stewart, and William F. Wieland for papers presented at Third National Conference on Methadone Treatment, November 1970.

Index

Abbott Laboratories, 256–257, 282–283
Abraham, Dr. Karl 214
Abramson, Dr. Harold A., 372
abstinence, drug, 515–517; and methadone maintenance, 141–142, 170; speed, 289
Abu Mansur Muwaffaq, 398
acetic acid, 1, 95
acetyl-alpha-methadol, 161n, 531
Adams, Richard G., 172
Adams, Samuel Hopkins, 47
Adams, Tom, 323
addict, 39–41; new-style (white middle-class), 89, 100, 183–188, 491, 497; differences between opium, morphine, or heroin, 95; black inner-city, 100; and overdose death, 101–114; and legal narcotics maintenance, 115–134; British, 121–125, 127; in Kentucky, 129–134; as a patient, 135–136; and methadone maintenance, 135–152, 176; role of in methadone maintenance programs, 166; teen-age, 169; historical antecedents for new-style, 491–492
addicting drug, definitions of, 65, 84–85
addiction, alcohol, *see* alcoholism
addiction, narcotics, 15, 64–89, 528; effects of, 1–2, 21–32, 101; famous users, 5, 33–37; and 19th-century morality, 6–7; preceded by alcohol use, 9–10, 85; from medically administered narcotics, 16; sex ratio, 17; age, 18; socioeconomic status, 18, 38; among blacks, 18–19; characteristics of user, 19–20; and drug laws, 22; morphine, 23; health, 23–25, 36; and mental health, 25–28, 101; adequate supply and legitimate functioning of user, 38; and Vietnam, 39; and detection, 39; the street addict, 39–41; and opium, 42–46; and impurities in the drugs, 47; present-day attitudes toward, 52–55; a crime by "status laws," 59; statistical increase since 1914, 62–63; derivation of word-use, 64; medical theories of, 64–66; and withdrawal syndrome, 65; "cures," 66–67; psychological theories of, 67, 68, 83; sociological theories of, 67–68, 83; biochemical

theories of, 68, 83–84, 135; treatment, 69–71; federal and state rehabilitation programs, 69–78; and alcoholism, 85–89; and overdose, 101–114, 157–158; and methadone, 159, 161; and non-addicting antagonist, 160; caffeine, 197–198, 203, 492; barbiturate, 250; cocaine, 274–276; and LSD, 335, 348; and marijuana, 396, 416, 460
addiction, nicotine, 209, 210, 211, 213–244 *passim*; and Freud, 214–215; compared to heroin addiction, 216, 217; and "hidden smoker," 217–219; use pattern, 223; and tolerance, 224–226; and behavior, 226–227; relapse rate, 227–228; and teen-agers, 236–238, 241
Addiction Research Center, U.S. Public Health Service, Lexington, Kentucky, 83–84, 160n. See also Lexington, Kentucky
Addiction Research Foundation of Ontario, 454
Addiction Research Unit (ARU), London, 84, 126, 222–223, 225, 226, 238
Ad Hoc Panel on Narcotic and Drug Abuse (1962), 38, 119
Adler, Dr. Martin, 83n
administration, drug: route of, 1; and pleasure effect, 12–13; and likelihood of addiction, 15; equipment for, 59; preferred route (intravenous), 101; for cocaine and amphetamines, 267, 279; and sniffing, 311–334; and LSD, 335
adulteration, 524; heroin, 47, 96, 97, 101, 114, 115, 528; and quinine, 110; LSD, 376
Advisory Commission on Narcotics and Drug Abuse (1963 — Kennedy Administration), 119, 134
Advisory Committee on Drug Dependence, United Kingdom Home Office, 360, 418n; and U.S. black-market LSD, 366–367; and LSD research, 372–373; and Baroness Wootton Report on marijuana and hashish use, 452
aerosol-sniffing, 333–334
Africa, 91, 209, 211, 398
age, 37, 224; of 19th-century user, 18; and

methadone issue, 169; and new-style addict, 187; and LSD user, 363; of prescription drug user, 479, 484–485; and marijuana use, 480; and "gray market" psychoactive prescription drugs, 487. *See also* youth

Alabama, marijuana laws, 419

Albert Einstein College of Medicine, 424

alcohol, 8–11, 43n, 63, 64, 195, 203, 205, 206, 247–253, 260–266, 276, 402, 475, 480; 19th-century opiate use as substitute for, 8–10, 85n; use prior to opiate addiction, 9–10, 87, 263; and ex-heroin addicts, 16, 70, 85–89, 150; 19th-century attitudes toward female use of, 17; and brain damage, 26, 261, 475; and organic deterioration, 27, 261, 475; and babies of addicted mothers, 30; and Volstead Act, 45, 410; and physical dependence, 65; federal failure to prevent illegal distillation of, 92; inelasticity in demand, 94; in combination with heroin, 111–113, 532; and methadone maintenance, 150, 153, 154; and youth, 183; in European culture, 195; described, 245; risk of addiction, 245; history of use, 247; similarities to barbiturates, 249–253; cross-tolerance with barbiturates, 252–253; similarities to sedatives and tranquilizers, 256–259; arguments for prohibition, 260–264; and homicide, 262; and suicide, 262–263; and automobile accidents, 263; leading to narcotic addiction, 263; and marijuana user, 263, 264, 410–412, 427–428, 431–433; and pregnancy, 263–264; and college students, 264; unworkability of prohibition, 265–266; "bootleg," 265; and peyote, 341; and LSD, 385; in Le Dain Commission report, 459; categorization as nondrug, 475, 481, 525; in Parry-Cisin study, 477–478; in Greenwich Village of twenties, 491–492; alternatives to for the young, 497; CU recommendations concerning, 533

alcoholism, 8–10, 197, 260–262; public attitudes toward, 9, 10; and ex-heroin addicts, 16, 70; correlation with drug abstinence, 85–89; and barbiturate addiction, 87n; incidence and prevalence, 260; biochemical studies, 260n; physical and mental deterioration, 261; law-enforcement, 261–262; and the American Indians, 338, 339; and LSD treatment, 351–353, 385, 535; and marijuana use, 431–433

Aldrich, Dr. Michael, 408n

Alksne, Harold, 111

Allbutt, Dr. T. Clifford, his *System of Medicine* (1905), 11, 198, 200

Allen, Dr. James R., 292, 403–404

Alpert, Dr. Richard, 368, 369

A.M.A. Archives of Internal Medicine, 23

Ambrose, Myles J., 443

American Bar Association: committee on narcotics, 53; Joint Committee (with AMA) on Narcotic Drugs, 54, 118; and drug-maintenance programs, 118, 122, 134

American Cancer Society, 232, 233, 236, 242

American Institutes of Research, 224–225

American Journal of Psychiatry, 340

American Journal of Psychology, 226

American Magazine, 414, 416

American Medical Association, 23, 54; Joint Committee (with American Bar Association) on Narcotic Drugs, 54, 118; drug-dependency committees, 107–108; and narcotic-maintenance programs, 118, 122; Council on Mental Health, 118, 134; Committee on Narcotic Drugs, 140; Council on Drugs, 281; and marijuana, 416, 417, 418; Committee on Legislative Activities, 417

American Medicine, 50–51

American Psychiatric Association, 217, 314, 340, 343

American Textbook of Applied Therapeutics (1896), 11

Ames, Dr. Frances, 398

amitriptyline (Elavil), 267

"Amphetamine Abuse: Pattern and Effects of High Doses Taken Internally" (Kramer, Fischman and Littlefield), 283

amphetamines, 33, 63, 96, 204n, 277, 278–280, 521; and methadone patient, 154; and caffeine, 199, 203; experience with alcohol prior to, 263; described, 267; effects, 267, 274, 278–279, 281; and "catarrh cures," 276, 278; history, 278, 281–282; combined with barbiturate or tranquilizer, 279, 286–287; users, 280, 484–485; cost, 280; home-made, 280, 283, 297; intravenous injection of (speed), 281–290 (*see also* Speed); abuse, 281; as treatment for heroin addiction, 282; Swedish experience, 294–298; federal ban proposal, 294, 305; distribution, 302, 482; and cocaine revival, 304–305; in adulteration of LSD, 376; CU recommendations concerning, 532–533

brain damage, 22, 25–26; in overdose death, 109; nicotine concentration, 223; and LSD, 388–389
Brandeis, Louis D., 538n
Brazil, 195, 403
Brecher, Edward, 323n
Brecher, Ruth, 323n
Brent, Reverend Charles H., 48
Brent Commission, 48
Brill, Dr. Henry, 27, 140
Britain, 94–95, 137, 140, 192; 19th-century use of opiates, 5; and "opium wars," 48; legal prescribing of drugs to addicts, 95; and overdose deaths, 113–114; opiate maintenance program, 115, 117, 120–129, 162, 531; Dangerous Drugs Act (1920), 120; known addicts, (1935-1951) 121–122, (1967-1970) 127; and American maintenance program proponents, 122–123; and heroin subculture (1960s), 123–126, 128; study of American methods, 124–125; and methadone maintenance, 125, 127, 162, 176–177; changes in policy (1970), 126–127; compulsory-notification law (1968), 127; view of nicotine addiction, 222, 238–239; LSD research, 360–361, 372; and U.S. black-market LSD in 366–367; and LSD hazards, 373–374; reevaluation of cannabis as medicine, 418n
British Columbia, study of addiction in, 11, 117, 135; and effects of narcotic drugs, 21, 22, 24; and addict's mental health, 25–27; and effect of drugs on sexual potency, 28–29; characterization of street addict, 40; and drug laws, 56n–57n; on failure of deterrent effect of drug laws, 60; on relationship between alcoholism and abstinence from narcotics, 85–86
British Columbia Medical Association, 501, 516–517
British Medical Journal, 66, 128, 316
British Medico-Legal Society, 95n
British Pharmacopoeia, 418n
Brockington, Dr. C. Fraser, 6
Bromberg, Dr. Walter, 415
bromide salts, 247
bronchitis, 232
Brooks, Jerome E., 209n
Brotman, Dr. Richard, 10, 25
Brown, Pat, 370
Bryan, William Jennings, 49
Bucaro, Andrew, 163
Buerger's disease, 215–216
Buffalo Medical Journal, 409

Bulgaria, 90
Bulletin of the Menninger Clinic, 318
Burack, Dr. Richard, 488
Bureau of Customs, *see* United States Bureau of Customs
Bureau of Food and Drugs, 270
Bureau of Narcotics and Dangerous Drugs, *see* Federal Bureau of Narcotics (and Dangerous Drugs)
Burkett, B. J., 334
Burnham, David, 61
Burlington (Vermont) *Free Press*, 443
Burroughs, Wellcome, 283, 406
Busch, Dr. Anthony K., 349
Bushmen, Africa, 398
Butcher, Dr. Brian T., 153
BZ, hallucinogen, 349; described, 349n

caffeine, 193–206, 402, 475, 480; described, 193; early history, 195–198; dangers of, 199; hazards and desirable effects of, 199–200, 205; and metabolic rate, 200; withdrawal syndrome, 201–203; and children, 202–203; addictive qualities, 203; toxic effects, 203–205; fatal dose, 203; tablet, 204; citrate, 204; behavioral effects, 205; domestication of, 205; in cola drinks, 270, 271; in Le Dain Commission report, 459; categorization of as nondrug, 475, 481; in Parry-Cisin study, 476–477; distribution route, 482. *See also* coffee
caffeinism, 197–198, 200, 204
California, 4, 90, 126, 403; and civil commitment, 60, 71–72; and narcotics maintenance, 118; methadone program, 154, 530; and new-style addict, 187–188 (*see also* Haight-Ashbury); and speed freak, 284–293 *passim*, 306–307; LSD legislation, 370–371; study of "LSD babies," 373; marijuana laws, 421, 422; study of users of psychoactive drugs, 485–486; investigations into nonchemical alternatives to drug mood effects, 513
California Rehabilitation Center (CRC), 71–72, 76, 77, 281; and speed freak, 289
Campbell, Dr. Harry, 120–121
Campbell, Dr. Ian L., 453
Camps, Dr. F. E., 110
Canada, 51, 129, 369; antinarcotics laws, 56, 59n, 60; and establishment of narcotics clinics, 117–118; U.S. black market LSD in, 366; and Le Dain Commission *Interim Report*, 453; marijuana smoking, 455; "street clinics," 503–504

Index

adaptive mechanism, 84; for cigarettes (nicotine), 136n, 209, 214–215, 217, 220–228; and methadone maintenance, 138, 159, 162, 169–170; and caffeine, 193; and cocaine, 274
Creighton, Dr. C., 398
crime, 38, 522; "victimless," 45; and drug-price escalation, 58; and legal opiates, 133; and methadone programs, 142–143, 152; and marijuana, 411, 416
"crisis intervention centers," 502–503, 510
cross-tolerance, 2; and methadone blocking effect, 162; and xanthine beverages, 193, 203; between alcohol and barbiturates, 252–253
Crothers, Dr. T. D., 197, 204
Crotty, Dr. John J., 320, 331, 332
Cushman, Dr. Paul, Jr., 156–157
Cutting, Dr. Windsor, 35, 36
"cutting," heroin, *see* Adulteration, heroin
cyclamates, 64
cyclazocine, 159, 160n, 167
cyclopropane, 317
Czechoslovakia, 372

Dahoon, 196
Dangerous Drugs Act (1920), Britain, 120
David, Sister, 166
Davidson, Dr. Gerald E., 170–171
Davidson, Dr. Morton I., 157
Davis, Dr. Emmett P., 163
Day, Dr. Horatio, his *The Opium Habit*, 11
Dayle, Dennis, 302
Daytop, 67, 78, 79, 82, 167, 168, 528, 529
Davy, Sir Humphrey, 312
dealer in weight, 97
death, 2; overdose, 32; rate among heroin addicts, 101. *See also* overdose
Dederich, Charles E., 78, 81, 216
Deichmann, Dr. William B., 111
Delaware Indians, 338
delirium tremens, 246, 274, 348; from barbiturates, 249, 251–252; and alcohol-barbiturate cross-tolerance, 253; cocaine, 276
Delinquent and the Law, The (R. and E. Brecher), 323n
delta-9-tetrahydrocannabinol, *see* THC
de Maupassant, Guy, 316–317
Demerol, 157, 531n
Denmark, 120
Denny, Robert V., 447
Dent, Dr. J. Yerbury, 14n
Denver, Colorado, 321–327; Poison Control Center, 321; Juvenile Police Bureau,

322; Police Crime Laboratory, 322; Juvenile Court, 323
Denver *Post*, 321–322, 324
dependence, physical, 13, 65; on medically administered narcotics, 16; and caffeine, 193, 201, 203; nicotine, 220–228; barbiturate, 248, 256; and LSD, 384; marijuana, 460. *See also* addiction
depressant, 111, 114; nonbarbiturate, 256–257, 260
depression, 139; in postaddiction syndrome, 14, 15, 71, 82; and drug-seeking behavior, 89; and methadone, 159, 162; and caffeine, 203; and cigarettes, 217; and cocaine, 272–273, 276; and amphetamines, 278–279; and intravenous amphetamines (speed), 284–285
De Quincey, Thomas, his *Confessions of an English Opium-Eater*, 5, 406; and use of word "tranquilizer," 11
de Ropp, Dr. Robert S., 54, 197
Des Moines, Iowa, 171–172
Desoxyn, 267; ampules, 283
detoxification, 74–75, 143; approved technique, 137; and methadone programs, 167
Detroit *News*, 392n, 412
deviance, cultural, 491–496; dictated, 494–496; and national drug policy (1960s), 497–498
dexamphetamine, 296
Dexamyl, 279
Dexedrine, 267, 488–489
dextroamphetamine (Dexedrine), 267, 488–489
dextromoramide, 531n
diarrhea, narcotic relief of, 1, 8, 31; and caffeine, 203
diazepam (Valium), 245, 257, 258
Diaz Ordaz, Gustavo, 434, 438
diet drugs, 267, 285
diethylpropion (Tenuate, Tepanil), 267, 296
digestion, 31; and caffeine, 203–206 *passim*
Dingell, John, 416
Dioscorides, 398
dipipanone, 531n
disease, 22
Diskind, Meyer H., 75–76
distribution system, opium, 4–5; in 19th-century Britain, 5–6; heroin, 19, 92–93, 185–186; New York City, 97–98; marijuana, 185, 186, 448, 482, 536–537; of alcohol during Prohibition, 266; speed, 283; cocaine, 302–304; peyote, 339–340; LSD, 366–367, 371, 482; over-the-

counter data, 482; prescription data, 482. *See also* black market

diuretics, 193, 203

Division of Narcotic and Drug Abuse Control, New Jersey Department of Health, 80n

Dixon, Dr. Walter Ernest, 198, 200

dizziness, 2, 346

d-lysergic acid diethylamide, 346, 376. *See also* LSD

DMT (*Yurema*), 344, 357n, 370, 511

Dole, Dr. Vincent P., 25, 80, 83n, 158; research on addict's resistance to overdose, 104; his research on obesity, 135, 136; his methadone research (with Nyswander), 136–139, 140–151, 162, 163, 165, 167, 169, 171, 174, 180; on cost of methadone maintenance, 165; and maintenance for teen-age addict, 169; and "weaning" patients from methadone, 169–170; on nicotine addiction, 216, 217

Done, Dr. Alan K., 329

Doors of Perception, The (Huxley), 362

Doriden, 245, 256

dosage, 102, 104–105; maintenance, 104, 137; methadone, 153–154, 161–162, 174; barbiturate, 251; cocaine, 275; amphetamine, 279, 532; speed, 283–284, 288–289; nitrous oxide, 312; ether, 314; LSD, 346, 347–348, 375–376. *See also* overdose

Dreiser, Theodore, 493

drop-in centers, *see* indigenous institutions

Drug Abuse Control Amendments, *see* Federal Drug Abuse Control Amendments

Drug Abuse Council, 188

Drug Addict as a Patient, The (Nyswander), 135

"Drug Addiction in British Columbia — A Research Study," 11–12. *See also* British Columbia

Drug Hang-Up: America's Fifty-Year Folly (King), 53n

drug laws, *see* laws

drug policy, 521–527; policy issues and recommendations, 528–540

drug-seeking behavior, 71, 162, 170; and craving, 14, 68, 89

drugstores, as dispensers of opiates, 3

Dumas *père*, Alexandre, 406

Du Mez, Dr. A. G., 51; and number of opiate addicts prior to Harrison Act, 62; research on dosage necessary for overdose death, 104

Durkin, William, 435

dysentery, 8

dysphoria, 2

East Lansing (Michigan) Drug Information Center, 314

East Village, New York, 499

Ecuador, 269n

Eddy, Dr. Nathan B., 25

Edison, Thomas A., 230, 232

education, level of new-style addict, 89, 187

Edwards, Dr. A. E., 389

Effect of the Regular Practice of Transcendental Meditation on Students Involved in the Regular Use of Hallucinogenic and "Hard" Drugs (Winquist), 511

Eggston, Dr. Edward E., 118

Egypt, 197

Eighteenth (Prohibition) Amendment, U.S. Constitution, 265, 410

Elan, Boston drug-free therapeutic community, 170

Elavil, 267

Elizabeth Charlotte, princess of Orleans, 211

Ellinson, Dr. Jack, 480

Ellis, Havelock, 362

emaciation, 23–24

Emerson, Gloria, 189–190

Emley, Dr. G. S., 221

emphysema, 36, 207, 216, 232

"encounter therapy," 81, 509, 513

endocarditis, 101

England, 84, 315; investigation of opiate deaths in, 110; tobacco smoking, 210, 213n; ether inhalation, 316. *See also* Britain

Equanil, 8, 245, 257

ergot, 409

Ejrup, Dr. B., 221

Erlenmeyer, Emil, 274

Erythroxylon coca, 269

Eskimos, 195

ethchlorvynol (Placidyl), 245, 256

ether, 311, 314–317, 351n; recreational use, 310, 315–316; dosage, 314; sniffing, 315; hazards, 316; prohibition attempts in Britain, 316; inhalation, 316–317

Ethiopia, 196

ethnobotany, 337

ethyl alcohol, 265

ethyl chloride, 317

ethylene, 317

euphoria, 2, 95n; and methadone blockade effect, 142; and cocaine, 267, 269,

Index

273–274; and amphetamines, 278; and intravenous amphetamine (speed), 284–285; from Preludin, 296

Europe: introduction of mind-affecting drugs in, 195–196; introduction of coffee, 197; spread of tobacco use, 211; U.S. black market LSD to, 366; introduction of marijuana into, 398

Extract of Cannabis (*Extractum Cannabis*), 396, 405

eye, constriction of pupils, 2, 31

Eysenck neuroticism scale, 352

Factory System Illustrated, The (Dodd), 5

Fairfield Hills Hospital, Newtown, Connecticut, 81–82

Farmilo, Dr. Charles, 455

FBI Law Enforcement Bulletin, 330

FDA, *see* United States Food and Drug Administration

fear, 2

Federal Bureau of Investigation, 330

Federal Bureau of Narcotics (and Dangerous Drugs), 18, 38–39, 116, 413; and narcotics maintenance programs, 118, 120, 132n; new addicts reported to (1964), 124; regulations governing research, 137; and amphetamine smuggling, 302, 306; and cocaine smuggling, 302, 304; and marijuana, 413–415, 435

Federal Drug Abuse Control Amendments (1965), 299, 305

females, *see* women

fertility, *see* pregnancy

Finnegan, Dr. J. K., 220, 221

First Report on Marijuana (1970), House Select Committee on Crime, 471

Fischer, Dr. Emil, 247

Fischman, Dr. Vitezslav, 283

flashback, 378–379, 387–388

Fleischl-Marxow, Dr. Ernst von, 272, 274, 280, 282, 284, 285n

Fleiss, Dr. Wilhelm, 214

Fletcher, Dr. C. M., 232

Florida, 4, 196; narcotics-dispensing clinics (1912), 115; anticigarette laws, 231

fly agaric (*Amanita muscaria*), 343

Food and Drug Administration, *see* United States Food and Drug Administration

Food and Drugs Act, Canada, 470

Ford, Henry, 230

Fordham University School of Social Service, 76

Foreign Policy Association, 415

formication, 275, 280; in speed psychosis, 285n

Fort, Dr. Joel, 503

Fort Worth, Texas, U.S. Public Health Service Hospital at, 69

France, 91n, 94; morphine-to-heroin converters in, 92, 97; ether inhalation, 317

Fraser, Dr. H. F., 26

free clinics, *see* clinics

Freedman, Dr. Alfred M., 10, 25

Freedman, Dr. Daniel X., 351, 388

Freon Products Division, E. I. du Pont de Nemours & Co., 334

Freud, Dr. Sigmund: cancer of jaw, 214–215; "tobacco angina," 215; and cocaine, 272–275, 278–279, 282, 303

Frith, Dr. C. D., 222

Fry, Edith G., 23

Gallup poll, 384n, 421, 423. *See also* public opinion

gasoline, 310, 318–319, 332

gastric acids, 199

gastrointestinal system, 253, 279. *See also* digestion

Gautier, Théophile, 406

Gay, Dr. George R., 111–113

Gardner, Dr. Ramon, 113–114

Gearing, Dr. Frances Rowe, 140, 141, 143, 148; on securing jobs for methadone patients, 149; on drug abuse by methadone patients, 150

Geis, Gilbert, 453

George III, of England, 213

Georgia, 4, 90, 403; anticigarette laws, 231; antimarijuana legislation, 419; domestic marijuana crop, 445

Gerarde, Dr. Horace W., 111

Germany, 94, 211, 226–227; ether drinking, 316

ghettos, black inner-city, 100

Gildenberg, Dr. Philip, 83n

Gilliam, Philip, 324

Gilman, Dr. Alfred, 16, 38, 54, 65, 101, 199, 203, 252, 257–258, 263, 274, 278, 318

Ginsberg, Allen, 292, 368, 408n

Giordano, Henry, 38

Glaser, Dr. Frederick B., 123n, 128

Glaser, Dr. Helen, 324–325

Glass, Dr. George S., 379

glue-sniffing, 310–334; historical antecedents, 311–320; popularization of, 320–334, 368; laws against, 324, 326, 328–329; research studies, 324–326

glutethimide (Doriden), 245

Godfrey's Cordial, 6

Golden, Colorado, 323

[604]

Index

Jones, Dr. Ernest: his *Life and Work of Sigmund Freud,* 214–215, 272–273, 275
Jones, LeRoi, 523n
Joplin, Janis, 113
Journal of Inebriety, 197
Journal of Psychedelic Drugs, 281, 453
Journal of the American Institute of Criminal Law and Criminology, 11
Journal of the American Medical Association, 71, 128, 200, 283, 318, 325–326; on LSD, 367, 392; and marijuana, 415–417
juggler (pusher), 98–100

Kahn, E. J., his *The Big Drink: the Story of Coca-Cola,* 270n
Kaizer, Dr. Sophia, 200–203
Kane, Dr. H. H., his *The Hypodermic Injection of Morphia,* 8, 408n
Kansas, 231; domestic marijuana crops in, 444–446
Kaplan, John, 451; his *Marijuana — The New Prohibition,* 432–433, 453
Kariri Indians, Brazil, 344
Karlsruhe, 211
Karolinska Institute, Stockholm, 295
Karr, Dr. Walter G., 23, 24
Kast, Dr. Eric C., 353
Katz, Larry, 435
Kaufman, Joshua, 292
Kennedy, David M., 435
Kennedy, John F., 38, 58, 119
Kentucky, 9, 87; legal opiates in, 129–134, 137, 162; hemp cultivation, 403–404
Kerr, Dr. Frederick W. L., 83n
Khazan, Dr. Naim, 83n
Kifner, John, 444–445
kilo connection, 97
King, Rufus, Esq., 53
King's College Hospital, London, 95n
Kiowas, 338
Kleber, Dr. Herbert D., 166
Klein, Ben, 324
Kleindienst, Richard G., 440, 441
Klonsky, George, 75–76
Knapp, Dr. Peter, 225
kola nut, 196, 270
Kolb, Dr. Lawrence, 10, 25, 27, 415; and effect of opiates on sexual potency, 28n; on opium-to-heroin pattern, 46n, 51; and number of opiate addicts prior to Harrison Act, 62; on alcohol-opiate correlation, 87; research on dosage necessary in overdose death, 104
Korea, 281
Kornetsky, Dr. Conan, 83n

Kramer, Dr. John C., 71, 72, 281, 283–286; evaluation of California CRC program, 72n; and deaths attributable to speed, 288; and recovery from speed-induced paranoia, 289; on value of enforced abstinence for speed freak, 289–290
Kupperstein, Lenore R., 321, 329
Kurland, Dr. Albert A., 352, 353, 355

LaGuardia, Fiorello, 451
LaGuardia Committee Report (1939-1944), 451, 452, 460
Lamb, Charles, 235
Lancet, 220, 232, 405
Laos, 90
Lapps of Inari, 343
Larson, Dr. P. S., 220
Latin America, 91, 302–304; and Operation Intercept, 438, 440
laudanum (opium in alcohol), 4, 5, 66
Laury, Gabriel V., 311
law enforcement, 51, 56–58, 529; accomplishments of, 58–62; alternatives to, 63; and black-market heroin, 91–94; agents' honesty, 93n; and black-market profitability, 94; and addicts' conversion from opium or morphine to heroin, 95; and black-market manufacture of narcotic concentrates, 96; British, 122; and alcoholism, 261–262; during Prohibition, 266; and amphetamines, 280; and speed, 282; Sweden, 296; and perpetuation of syndicate operations, 304, 306; and cocaine revival, 304–305; and LSD, 370, 377, 382; and marijuana, 422, 450, 464–465, 468–472; and trend from marijuana to hashish, 463; and publicizing of youthful subculture, 494; and *nihil nocere* principle, 522–523
Lawrence, Kansas, 444–445
laws: antinarcotic, 7, 22, 42–63, 467n, 528; and shift in age and sex of user, 18; 19th-century anti-opium smoking, 42–44, 46; failures of, 45–46, 60–63, 417, 422–423, 521–527; Pure Food and Drug Act, 47; Harrison Narcotic Act, 48–56; state, 51, 59; critics of, 52–55, 57; penalty provisions, 56–58; parole provisions, 58; accomplishments of, 58; and conviction of offenders, 58–60, 59n–60n; concerning possession, 59, 73, 177, 468–471; and burden of proof, 59; "status laws," 59; "no-knock" law, 60, 465; and civil commitment, 60, 73; to facilitate arrest of suspects, 60; failure of deterrent effect, 60–63, 521, 524;

[608]

Torrance, Dr. Edward G., 23
Towns, Dr. Charles B., 46, 275n–276n, 276
  toxicity: of caffeine, 203–205; of nicotine, 226; LSD, 376; marijuana, 460
Toxicology of Drugs and Chemicals (Deichmann and Gerarde), 111
Traffic in Narcotics (Anslinger and Tompkins), 21, 69
tranquilizers, 245, 534; addiction hazards, 245; and delirium tremens, 253; minor, 257–258, 260, 479, 482–483; experience with alcohol prior to, 263; combined with amphetamines, 279; female users, 479; distribution route, 482–486; over-the-counter, 486
tranquilization, 1, 11, 24, 131; and morphine, 8; and heroin, 12; nicotine, 209
transcendental meditation, 509–512
Trasov, George E., 12
Travia, A. J., 370
Treanor, Major John J., 425
treatment, 53, 66, 69–83; and aftercare, 70; and relapse, 71; federal and state programs, 72–78; Synanon-type, 78–83
"trip," hallucinogenic, 312; bad, 352–353, 357–361, 375–380
Trussell, Dr. Ray E., 73, 74–75, 111; and Beth Israel Medical Center, 138n–139n; and methadone research, 138, 140; and methadone diversion, 165
Tulane Medical School, methadone maintenance program, 168–169
Turkey, 90, 97, 196; price of opium, 90–91; and American black-market suppliers, 91; ban on production of opium, 91
Twenty-first (Prohibition Repeal) Amendment, U.S. Constitution, 265, 266, 537
Tucson, Arizona, 321
Tylecote, Dr. F. E., 232

UCLA, 441–442
ulcer formation, 199–200
Underwood, Wilbur, 303
Unger, Dr. Sanford, 352
Ungerleider, Dr. J. T., 461
"Uniform Anti-Narcotics Act," 413
United Kingdom, *see* Britain
United Nations: Commission on Narcotic Drugs, 22; *Bulletin on Narcotics*, 399, 415; estimates of world marijuana users, 402; Single Convention on Narcotics Drugs, 468
United Press International, 369–370
United States Army, *see* Army, U.S.
United States Bureau of Customs, 61, 91n, 92, 93; seizure of heroin, 93–94,

96; and stimulant smuggling, 302, 306; cocaine seizures, 302–303
United States Defense Department, 188
United States Department of Agriculture, 196, 220, 404
United States Department of Health, Education, and Welfare, 321, 327; Task Force on Prescription Drugs, 485
United States *Dispensatory*, 405, 407
United States Food and Drug Administration, 64; suppression of nonprescribed barbiturates, 254; and amphetamine ampules, 283, 302; antispeed campaign, 291; IND (investigational new drug) regulations, 366; and LSD, 366, 367, 368–369
United States Justice Department, 440
United States–Mexican Border Cities Association, 437
United States Navy, 350
United States Pharmacopoeia, 115; and medicinal use of marijuana, 405; Committee on Revision of, 418–419
United States Public Health Service, 11, 62; treatment of addict, 69; anticigarette campaigns, 233, 234. *See also* Lexington, Kentucky
United States State Department, 48, 440
United States Supreme Court; characterization of the narcotic addict, 21, 33; and drug "status laws," 59
United States Treasury Department, 412, 440; Narcotics Unit, 69, 116
United States v. Forty Barrels and Twenty Kegs of Coca-Cola, 271
United States War Department Commission of Inquiry, *see* Brent Commission
University of Colorado Medical Center, Adolescent Clinic, 324–325
University of Illinois, 445
University of Kansas, 445
University of Michigan, International Symposium on Drug Abuse, 512
University of Mississippi, 404
University of Vermont College of Medicine, research on medicinal use of cannabis, 417n–418n
University of Zurich, 347
Unwin, Dr. J. R., 461
Urban VIII, Pope, 211
Utah, 333, 420
Utopiates (Blum), 362

Vaillant, Dr. George E., 70–71, 76
Valium, 245, 257, 258; hazards of, 258, 259
Vancouver, British Columbia, 11, 117,

NO'

HETERICK MEMORIAL LIBRARY
362.29 B829I c.2
Brecher, Edward M./Licit and illicit dru   onuu

3 5111 00028 2503